CYSTIC FIBROSIS IN ADULTS

CYSTIC FIBROSIS IN ADULTS

Editors

James R. Yankaskas, M.D.
Professor of Medicine
Director, Critical Care Medicine Program
Co-Director, Adult Cystic Fibrosis Program
University of North Carolina School of Medicine
Chapel Hill, North Carolina

Michael R. Knowles, M.D.
Professor of Medicine
Director, Adult Cystic Fibrosis Program
University of North Carolina School of Medicine
Chapel Hill, North Carolina

Foreword by

Thomas F. Boat, M.D.
Chairman, Department of Pediatrics
University of Cincinnati College of Medicine
Director, Research Foundation
Children's Hospital Medical Center
Cincinnati, Ohio

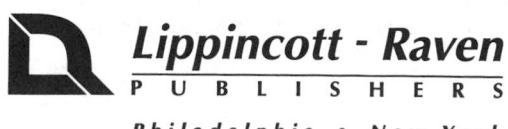

Lippincott - Raven
P U B L I S H E R S
Philadelphia • New York

Acquisitions Editor: Joyce-Rachel John
Developmental Editor: Lesa E. Ramsey
Manufacturing Manager: Kevin Watt
Supervising Editor: Carolyn Foley
Production Service: P.M. Gordon Associates
Indexer: Nancy Newman
Compositor: Compset Inc.
Printer: Maple Press

Library of Congress Cataloging-in-Publication Data
Cystic fibrosis in adults / editors, James R. Yankaskas, Michael R. Knowles; foreword by Thomas F. Boat.
    p.   cm.
  Includes bibliographical references and index.
  ISBN 0–7817–1011–1.
  1. Cystic fibrosis. I. Yankaskas, James R. II. Knowles, Michael R.
  [DNLM: 1. Cystic Fibrosis—in adulthood. WI
820C9984 1999]
RC858. C95C966 1999
616.3'7—dc21
DNLM/DLC
for Library of Congress   98–29116
                                                     CIP

Contents

Section I. Pathogenesis

Section II. Pulmonary

Section III. Gastrointestinal

Section IV. Other Systems

Contributors

Robert J. Beall, Ph.D.   *President and CEO, Cystic Fibrosis Foundation, 6931 Arlington Road, Bethesda, Maryland 20814*

Melvin Berger, M.D., Ph.D.   *Chief of Immunology and Allergy, Rainbow Babies and Children's Hospital, Case Western Reserve University School of Medicine, 11100 Euclid Avenue, Cleveland, Ohio 44106–2624*

Richard C. Boucher, M.D.   *Professor of Medicine, Director, Cystic Fibrosis/Pulmonary Research and Treatment Center, Division of Pulmonary and Critical Care Medicine, University of North Carolina School of Medicine, 7011 Thurston-Bowles Building, CB# 7248, Chapel Hill, North Carolina 27599–7248*

Barry Bresnihan, M.D.   *Professor of Medicine, Department of Rheumatology, St. Vincent's Hospital, Elm Park, Dublin 4, Ireland*

Allan L. Coates, M.D.   *Professor of Pediatrics, University of Toronto Faculty of Medicine, Director, Division of Pediatric Respiratory Medicine, The Hospital for Sick Children, 555 University Avenue, Toronto, Ontario M5G 1X8, Canada*

Morty Cohen, B.S.   *Coordinator, Investigational Drug Service, Children's Hospital and Regional Medical Center, 4800 Sand Point Way, N.E., Seattle, Washington 98105*

Carla Colombo, M.D.   *Associate Professor, Department of Pediatrics, University of Sassari, Viale San Pietro, 12, 01700 Sassari, Italy*

Stefania Comi, M.D.   *Clinical Fellow, Department of Pediatrics, University of Milan, Via Commenda, 9, 20122 Milan, Italy*

Andrea Crosignani, M.D.   *Clinical Fellow, Istituto di Scienze Biomediche, San Paolo Hospital, University of Milan, Via di Rudini', 8, 20142 Milan, Italy*

Pamela B. Davis, M.D., Ph.D.   *Professor of Medicine and Pediatrics, Department of Pediatrics, Case Western Reserve University School of Medicine, Chief, Pediatric Pulmonary Division, Rainbow Babies and Children's Hospital, 2109 Adelbert Road, Cleveland, Ohio 44106– 4223*

Peter R. Durie, M.D.   *Professor, Department of Pediatrics, University of Toronto Faculty of Medicine, Head, Division of Gastroenterology/Nutrition, Senior Scientist, The Research Institute, The Hospital for Sick Children, 555 University Avenue, Toronto, Ontario M5G 1X8, Canada*

Thomas M. Egan, M.D., M.Sc.   *Professor of Surgery, Director, Lung Transplant Program, Associate Division Chief, General Thoracic Surgery, Division of Cardiothoracic Surgery, University of North Carolina School of Medicine, 108 Burnett-Womack Building, CB# 7065, Chapel Hill, North Carolina 27599–7065*

Gerald W. Fernald, M.D.   *Professor of Pediatrics, Director, Cystic Fibrosis Center, Department of Pediatrics, University of North Carolina School of Medicine, 509 Burnett-Womack Building, CB# 7220, Chapel Hill, North Carolina 27599–7220*

Patrick A. Flume, M.D. *Assistant Professor of Medicine and Pediatrics, Director, Adult Cystic Fibrosis Program, Division of Pulmonary and Critical Care Medicine, Medical University of South Carolina, Room 812-CSB, 171 Ashley Avenue, Charleston, South Carolina 29425*

Gordon G. Forstner, M.D. *Professor, Department of Pediatrics, University of Toronto Faculty of Medicine, Senior Scientist, The Research Institute, The Hospital for Sick Children, 555 University Avenue, Toronto, Ontario M5G 1X8, Canada*

Kenneth J. Friedman, Ph.D. *Department of Pathology and Laboratory Medicine, 4027 Thurston-Bowles Building, CB# 7525, University of North Carolina School of Medicine, Chapel Hill, North Carolina 27599–7525*

Kevin John Gaskin, M.D. *Professor of Paediatrics, James Fairfax Institute of Paediatric Nutrition, Royal Alexandra Hospital for Children, Corner Hawkesbury Road & Hainsworth Street, Westmead, Sydney, New South Wales 2145, Australia*

Peter H. Gilligan, Ph.D. *Professor of Microbiology-Immunology and Pathology-Laboratory Medicine, University of North Carolina School of Medicine, Director, Clinical Microbiology-Immunology, University of North Carolina Hospitals, 1035 East Wing, CB# 7600, Chapel Hill, North Carolina 27514*

Annamaria Giunta, M.D. *Associate Professor, Department of Pediatrics, University of Milan, Via Commenda, 9, 20122 Milan, Italy*

Larry G. Johnson, M.D. *Associate Professor of Medicine, Cystic Fibrosis/Pulmonary Research and Treatment Center, Division of Pulmonary and Critical Care Medicine, University of North Carolina School of Medicine, 7123 Thurston-Bowles Building, CB# 7248, Chapel Hill, North Carolina 27599–7248*

Kim Jones, M.D., Ph.D. *Assistant Professor of Surgery, Division of Otolaryngology, University of North Carolina School of Medicine, 610 Burnett-Womack Building, CB# 7070, Chapel Hill, North Carolina 27599–7070*

Daina Kalnins, R.D., C.N.S.D. *Clinical Dietician, Division of Respiratory Medicine, Department of Pediatrics and The Research Institute, The Hospital for Sick Children, 555 University Avenue, Toronto, Ontario M5G 1X8, Canada*

Michael R. Knowles, M.D. *Professor of Medicine, Director, Adult Cystic Fibrosis Program, Cystic Fibrosis/Pulmonary Research and Treatment Center, Division of Pulmonary and Critical Care Medicine, 7019 Thurston-Bowles Building, CB# 7248, University of North Carolina School of Medicine, Chapel Hill, North Carolina 27599–7248*

Michael W. Konstan, M.D. *Assistant Professor of Pediatrics, Director, Cystic Fibrosis Center, Case Western Reserve University School of Medicine, 2101 Adelbert Road, Cleveland, Ohio 44106–2624*

Larry C. Lands, M.D., Ph.D. *Associate Professor, Department of Pediatrics, McGill University Health Centre, Montreal Children's Hospital, 2300 Tupper Street, Suite D380, Montreal, Quebec H3H 1P3, Canada*

Margaret W. Leigh, M.D. *Professor of Pediatrics, Chief, Division of Pulmonary Medicine and Allergy, Department of Pediatrics, 635 Burnett-Womack Building, CB# 7220, University of North Carolina School of Medicine, Chapel Hill, North Carolina 27599–7220*

Matthew A. Mauro, M.D.   *Professor of Radiology and Surgery, Vice Chairman, Clinical Affairs, University of North Carolina School of Medicine, 2006 Old Clinic Building, CB# 7510, Chapel Hill, North Carolina 27599–7510*

Maria Luisa Melzi, M.D.   *Clinical Fellow, Department of Pediatrics, University of Milan, Via Commenda, 9, 20122 Milan, Italy*

Peadar G. Noone, M.D.   *Assistant Professor of Medicine, Cystic Fibrosis/Pulmonary Research and Treatment Center, Division of Pulmonary and Critical Care Medicine, University of North Carolina School of Medicine, 7123 Thurston-Bowles Building, CB# 7248, Chapel Hill, North Carolina 27599–7248*

David A. Ontjes, M.D.   *Professor of Medicine and Pharmacology, Division of Endocrinology, University of North Carolina School of Medicine, 348A MacNider Building, CB# 7170, Chapel Hill, North Carolina 27599–7170*

Linda J. Paradowski, M.D.   *Assistant Professor of Medicine, Division of Pulmonary and Critical Care Medicine, 724 Burnett-Womack Building, CB# 7020, University of North Carolina School of Medicine, Chapel Hill, North Carolina 27599–7020*

Paul B. Pencharz, M.D., Ph.D.   *Professor of Pediatrics, Unversity of Toronto, and Division of Gastroenterology and Nutrition, The Hospital for Sick Children, 555 University Avenue, Toronto, Ontario M5G 1X8, Canada*

Giovanna Pizzamiglio, M.D.   *Clinical Fellow, Department of Internal Medicine, ICP, University of Milan, Via Commenda, 10–12, 20122 Milan, Italy*

Paul M. Quinton, Ph.D.   *Professor of Biomedical Sciences, University of California at Riverside School of Medicine, Professor, Department of Pediatrics, University of California at San Diego School of Medicine, 220 Dickinson Street, San Diego, California 92103*

Bonnie W. Ramsey, M.D.   *Director, Cystic Fibrosis Research Program, Professor of Pediatrics, Department of Pediatrics, University of Washington School of Medicine, 4800 Sand Point Way, Seattle, Washington 98105*

Mark K. Robbins, M.D.   *Assistant Professor of Medicine, Medical Director, Lung Transplant, Medical Director, Adult Cystic Fibrosis Program, Pulmonary/Critical Care Medicine, Private Clinic Building, 6th floor, Hospital Drive, University of Virginia Health System, Charlottesville, Virginia 22908*

Lawrence M. Silverman, Ph.D.   *Professor of Pathology and Laboratory Medicine, Department of Pathology and Laboratory Medicine, University of North Carolina Hospitals, 1045 East Wing, CB# 7525, Chapel Hill, North Carolina 27599–7525*

Arnold L. Smith, M.D.   *Professor and Chairman, Department of Molecular Microbiology and Immunology, University of Missouri–Columbia School of Medicine, M653 Medical Science Building, Columbia, Missouri 65212*

Robert C. Stern, M.D.   *Professor of Pediatrics, Rainbow Babies and Children's Hospital, Case Western Reserve University School of Medicine, 11100 Euclid Avenue, Cleveland, Ohio 44106*

Cynthia Stewart, R.D.   *Adult Cystic Fibrosis Program, St. Michael's Hospital, 294 Stelbrake Boulevard, Toronto, Ontario M4P QB6, Canada*

M. Jackson Stutts, Ph.D.   *Professor of Medicine, Cystic Fibrosis/Pulmonary Research and Treatment Center, Division of Pulmonary and Critical Care Medicine, University of North*

Carolina School of Medicine, 6023 Thurston-Bowles Building, CB# 7248, Chapel Hill, North Carolina 27599–7248

Elizabeth Tullis, M.D.   *Professor, Division of Respirology, Department of Medicine, University of Toronto; Director, Adult Cystic Fibrosis Program, University of Toronto Faculty of Medicine, St. Michael's Hospital, 160 Wellesley Street East, Toronto, Ontario M5G 1X8, Canada*

James R. Yankaskas, M.D.   *Professor of Medicine, Co-Director, Adult Cystic Fibrosis Program, Cystic Fibrosis/Pulmonary Research and Treatment Center, Division of Pulmonary and Critical Care Medicine, University of North Carolina School of Medicine, 7007 Thurston-Bowles Building, CB# 7248, Chapel Hill, North Carolina 27599–7248*

Foreword

Most of the medical care for patients with cystic fibrosis (CF), over the nearly 60 years since its description as a distinct medical disorder, has been provided by pediatricians. As in other areas of medicine, things have changed. CF is now the object of considerable interest and participation by adult caregivers. As outlined in this book, approximately one third of all patients with CF currently meet age criteria for adulthood. However, as with many other progressive disorders, the medical challenge intensifies as individuals with CF make the transition into adulthood.

This transition is a critical time in many ways. Most adults with CF need some level of support to accommodate the tasks of living. This support often comes from family, friends, and even the community. However, a knowledgeable and responsive medical care system for young adults with CF is a key element. The adult CF team can provide the reassurance and the stability that allows individuals with this disorder to move out and engage in the process of living.

From this perspective, it is essential that internists with pulmonary and other subspecialty training become increasingly involved in providing adult care options for patients with CF. Further, the next generation of internists must be better informed and, in some cases, highly trained to take on the challenging tasks of adult CF care.

It also is important that the research expertise of physicians trained in adult medicine be brought to bear on the basic science and clinical problems of individuals with CF. This disorder must be understood more thoroughly at both a molecular and a clinical level to more favorably affect diagnosis and therapy.

Cystic Fibrosis in Adults represents a benchmark in the 60-year medical history of CF. It is a statement that the care of adults is, in many ways, different from that of children. It is a statement that adult care now is not a by-product; it is in the mainstream of the struggle to conquer this disease. Cystic fibrosis truly has "grown up."

The editors of this textbook, for 15 years and more, have been leaders in the area of adult CF care. They have trained many of the current CF caregivers. They are to be complimented for recognizing an important healthcare niche and for steadfastly committing their efforts to develop this important area of medicine.

Thomas F. Boat

Preface

Once considered a childhood disease, cystic fibrosis (CF) now also is a disease of adults. Before 1950, gastrointestinal, nutritional, and pulmonary complications resulted in a median survival of 1 year. The recognition of abnormal sweat electrolytes provided an early diagnostic test that allowed clear identification of patients with CF. The foresight of the national Cystic Fibrosis Foundation to cluster care of patients with CF in defined centers of clinical excellence fostered the development and use of improved treatments for the major clinical problems. By 1996, the median survival had increased to 31 years, and 36% of patients registered with the Cystic Fibrosis Foundation were adults. Patients with CF clearly have benefited from clinical and basic science advances.

Research has been a hallmark of the comprehensive approach to CF. Definition of abnormal ion transport in sweat glands and airways in the early 1980s focused attention on deranged ion transport as a basis for the disease. The CF gene was identified in 1989 by positional cloning, and it provided an essential element in the quest to better understand disease pathogenesis. The normal cystic fibrosis transmembrane conductance regulator (CFTR) protein functions as an ion channel and as a regulator of other ion channels, explaining earlier observations. These and other functions of the CFTR are being evaluated as possible contributors to disease pathogenesis. This information has provided a foundation for further exploration of disease pathobiology and for the development of new therapeutic strategies.

Increased longevity has resulted in more age- and disease-related medical problems, and the growing number of adults with CF has increased medical care needs. These needs are being met by dedicated CF pediatricians and by a growing number of internists, adult pulmonologists, and other specialists. This book was written as a comprehensive text for the diagnosis and care of adults with CF. It is directed at physicians who are developing expertise in the myriad aspects of this disease. It also will be useful to the nurse specialists, respiratory and physical therapists, social workers, dietitians, and others who provide the care that has become a model of healthcare excellence.

Cystic Fibrosis in Adults is organized by the organ systems most affected by CF. The first section describes the molecular and cellular bases of disease pathogenesis. The second section deals with pulmonary disease, which is the major cause of morbidity and mortality. The third section deals with the gastrointestinal system, including nutrition. The final section deals with other organ systems that are affected by CF and includes chapters on social issues and the U.S. National Cystic Fibrosis Foundation. The chapters include descriptions of integrated molecular, cellular, tissue, and organ-level physiology and disease manifestations of cystic fibrosis. Differential diagnoses, diagnostic approaches, and treatment options are provided and are supplemented with practical suggestions. The authors are internationally recognized experts in the pathophysiology of disease and the clinical care of adults with cystic fibrosis. They have provided up-to-date summaries of the state of knowledge and guidelines for the evaluation and care of the adult with CF.

We hope that this book will expand the expertise of healthcare providers for adults with CF, encourage further insights into the mechanisms of disease, and foster the development of improved treatments. We anticipate that advances in these areas will further increase the quality of life and survival of adults with CF. As these goals are achieved, the hopes and hard work of our mentors, patients, and coworkers will be met and amply rewarded.

James R. Yankaskas
Michael R. Knowles

Acknowledgments

Our interest in cystic fibrosis (CF) arose from a research focus on pulmonary defense mechanisms associated with airway epithelial ion transport physiology and the clinical challenges of disease in patients with CF. These interests led to the development of major research and clinical programs for patients with CF at the University of North Carolina (UNC) at Chapel Hill. This book is a product of those ongoing efforts. It marks a way point in the decades-long effort to understand and effectively treat the complications of CF.

Many people have contributed to our education about CF. Our clinical and scientific mentors and colleagues Gerald W. Fernald, M.D., Thomas F. Boat, M.D., Al Spock, M.D., John Gatzy, Ph.D., and Richard C. Boucher, M.D., provided the support, the environment, and the intellectual rigor necessary to address these research and clinical challenges. Many individuals with CF and their families provided stimuli to advance this work. They made insightful observations about the clinical problems of CF and volunteered for numerous laboratory and clinical studies. We owe special thanks to the nurses and social workers who were key to the development of the UNC adult CF clinical program and to the smooth transition of patients from pediatric to adult care. Our professional colleagues on the CF team have provided continuing support in solving problems and in developing effective clinical care. Many pulmonary trainees participated in the care of adults with CF at UNC. Some have gone on to lead other adult CF programs and have contributed to chapters in this book. Colleagues at other CF centers provided patients and *ad hoc* research facilities for early and ongoing electrophysiology studies *in vivo* and in excised CF tissues. The Cystic Fibrosis Foundation contributed ideas and support in many tangible ways.

The professional staff at Little, Brown and Company recognized the need for this book and stimulated its production. They and their peers at Lippincott–Raven Publishers provided the expert guidance and reasonable patience required by new editors. We thank the authors for providing up-to-date chapters and for responding promptly to our requests, and we thank the colleagues who reviewed chapters. Beth Godwin and Lisa Brown provided excellent secretarial and artistic support throughout the preparation of this book. Finally, we thank our wives, Bonnie and Marilyn, for their unwavering support of our work.

SECTION I

Pathogenesis

Cystic Fibrosis in Adults,
edited by J. R. Yankaskas and M. R. Knowles,
Lippincott-Raven Publishers, Philadelphia, 1999.

1

Cystic Fibrosis Gene and Functions of CFTR

Implications of Dysfunctional Ion Transport for Pulmonary Pathogenesis

M. Jackson Stutts and Richard C. Boucher

Cystic Fibrosis/Pulmonary Research and Treatment Center, Division of Pulmonary and Critical Care Medicine, University of North Carolina School of Medicine, Chapel Hill, North Carolina

Cystic fibrosis (CF) is an inherited autosomal recessive disease that disrupts ion transport in epithelial-lined organs, including pulmonary airways, sweat ducts, pancreatic ducts, and intestine (1–3). Because obstruction of pulmonary airways is the cause of death of more than 90% of patients with CF, understanding the pathophysiology of CF lung disease is an urgent goal. Since the CF gene was identified in 1989 (4), there has been rapid progress in understanding the structure and functions of the CF gene product, the cystic fibrosis transmembrane conductance regulator (CFTR), and in understanding how mutations in the CF gene generate the array of organ-specific pathophysiologies that make up CF. This knowledge has generated ideas for novel therapeutic approaches, including pharmacologic maneuvers to normalize defective ion transport functions and efforts to transfer the normal CF gene into the airway cells of patients with CF (see Chapter 11).

The CFTR functions as a cyclic adenosine monophosphate (cAMP)-dependent chloride (Cl^-) channel in the apical membrane of the epithelia affected in CF (5,6). This discovery prompted expectation that CF pathogenesis could be understood in unified terms of defective or missing Cl^- conductance that is necessary for normal transepithelial Cl^- movement in each of the organs affected in CF. However,

each manifestation of CF cannot be attributed solely to defective Cl^- conductance. For some organs, this may mean that the basic physiology of the epithelium is not understood sufficiently for the role of a cAMP-dependent Cl^- channel to be appreciated. Alternatively, it may mean that a normal CFTR regulates the functions of other proteins; thus, a defective CFTR causes secondary abnormalities that contribute variably to organ-specific CF pathogenesis (7–9) (also see Chapter 2). Nowhere is this conundrum more evident than in the lung, where fundamental questions about the etiology of CF airways disease remain unresolved. These questions include the identification of the airway region(s) in the lung where CF disease is initiated, the relative contributions of airway surface and submucosal glandular epithelium to surface liquid metabolism, the link between abnormal ion transport and bacterial infection, and the significance of the effects of CFTR on other ion channels.

In this chapter, knowledge resulting from the discovery of the CF gene is summarized, including the structure of the CFTR and its functions as a Cl^- channel and as a regulator of other channels and transporters. The potential contributions of CFTR to the normal physiology of salt and water transport airway surface cells and submucosal gland epithelia will be assessed. Finally, we will review several hypotheses relating the loss of CFTR function to the etiology of CF airways disease, and identify remaining gaps in understanding the molecular, cellular, and organ-level physiology of CFTR.

THE CYSTIC FIBROSIS GENE

Identification

The CF gene locus was first located on the long arm of human chromosome 7 through linkage analysis (10) and then identified through linkage disequilibrium analysis and chromosome walking (8,11). This approach formed a paradigm called positional cloning, which allows disease genes of unknown function to be identified (12). The CF gene consists of 250 kB of genomic DNA containing 27 exons (13). Introns in the CF gene contain information that allows alternative splicing of CFTR mRNA. Alternative splicing is of clinical significance principally because it may decrease the quantity of mature CFTR protein expressed (14–18) (see Chapter 2, Genotype/phenotype). Although shortened versions of CFTR transcripts and protein have been detected in various tissues [kidney (19), heart (20)], there is little indication that alternative splicing results in CFTR proteins that function. An important observation is that the quantity of normally spliced full-length CFTR mRNA in some tissues can be as little as 10% of total CFTR mRNA (14). Because CFTR heterozygotes ("carriers") typically are asymptomatic with approximately 50% of the normal level of CFTR, this observation suggests that the quantity of normal length CFTR required for normal epithelial function is much less than 50% of the wild-type level.

Characteristics

Once the human CF gene was cloned, its species' homologues were detected across a wide range of vertebrates (13,21). Within a given species, the expression of CFTR is highly regulated in epithelial cells of the lung, pancreas, intestine, gallbladder, kidney, salivary and sweat glands, testis, and uterus. Exceptions to this rule exist; CFTR is expressed in cardiac tissue of some species, including humans (22), and in human lymphocytes (23), but the pathophysiology of CF appears to be limited to epithelial-lined organs. In certain epithelial tissues, such as airway submucosal glands, CFTR expression appears concentrated within specific cell types (24). Attempts have been made to identify transcriptional control elements in the CF gene that determine this limited pattern of expression. The candidate promoter region (3,700 bp immediately 5' to the presumed site for initiation of transcription) resembles promoters for "housekeeping" genes in several ways: a high content of guanine and cytosine, the lack of a TATA box, and the lack of a RNA polymerase recognition site (25). However, the expression of CFTR is downregulated by activators of protein kinase C (PKC) (26) and upregulated by activators of protein kinase A (PKA) (27,28). Examination of the gene structure of eight mammalian species revealed conserved cAMP- and phorbol myristate acetate (PMA)-responsive elements within the putative promoter region (21). Activation of cAMP-dependent protein kinase or PKC, *in vivo*, may regulate CFTR expression levels (29).

CYSTIC FIBROSIS TRANSMEMBRANE CONDUCTIVE REGULATOR: STRUCTURE/FUNCTION RELATIONSHIPS AND CELLULAR LOCALIZATION

Structure

Important predictions for structure were derived immediately from the sequence of the coding region of the CF gene (4). A protein of 1,480 amino acids was predicted, which bore 35% homology to P-glycoprotein, the product of the MDR1 gene located nearby on the long arm of human chromosome 7. Based on this homology and the predicted amino acid sequence, it appeared that the CF gene encoded a membrane protein with 12 membrane-spanning regions (Fig. 1–1). The highest degree of amino acid homology to P-glycoprotein was within two predicted intracellular domains that represented conserved adenine nucleotide binding cassette (ABC) sequences (4). These characteristics placed the CF gene in the ABC transport protein superfamily with the MDR1 gene (3,8). The members of this gene super-family use energy from hydrolysis of adenosine triphosphate (ATP) to move a wide variety of specific substrates against a concentration gradient. The CF gene product has an additional and unique intracellular domain, which is rich in consensus sites for phosphorylation by PKA and PKC. This region was presumed to be important for regulation of CFTR by phosphokinases and therefore was called the R domain.

Given these predicted features, the known ability of other ABC superfamily members to transport regulatory peptides, and reports that epithelia affected in CF were defective in several ion transport processes, the investigators who discovered the CF gene named its protein product the cystic fibrosis transmembrane conductance regulator, or CFTR (4). Remarkably, most of the structural predictions based on analysis of the predicted amino acid sequence of CFTR have been verified experimentally and support the topographic model originally proposed.

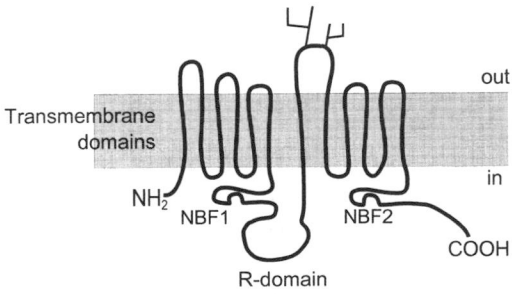

FIG. 1–1. CFTR structure. Twelve hydrophobic membrane-spanning domains, two nucleotide-binding folds (NBF1 and NBF2), and an intracellular regulatory region (the R domain) with many phosphorylation sites comprise a membrane-associated protein.

Hydropathy plots and careful comparison to P-glycoprotein predicted that CFTR would cross the plasma membrane 12 times, and this prediction has been verified in several ways. Mature CFTR protein runs as a broad band when subjected to polyacrylamide gel electrophoresis, consistent with glycosylation of its extracellular domains (30). When two consensus sites for N-glycosylation in putative extracellular loop 1 and 4 were eliminated by mutagenesis, CFTR no longer appeared glycosylated on polyacrylamide gel electrophoresis (31). A second method of assessing CFTR topography is an engineered cysteine mutation mapping strategy devised by Akabas et al. (32). Mutant CFTR molecules, in which single wild-type residues of putative transmembrane segments systematically were replaced by cysteine, were expressed heterologously and exposed to reactive sulfhydryl reactive reagents. These hydrophilic compounds permeate the pore of CFTR and inactivate its Cl⁻ conductance if they encounter the engineered cysteine. This procedure has allowed identification of specific residues of transmembrane segments that are accessible within the ion conductive pore of CFTR (32). Others have shown that certain natural disease-causing mutations of CFTR within putative membrane-spanning regions result in CFTR Cl⁻ channels with altered conduction properties (33,34).

The nucleotide-binding folds (NBFs) contained in CFTR are highly homologous to sequences within other ABC transport proteins that have been shown to bind and hydrolyze ATP (35). Although no substrate that is transported actively by CFTR has been identified, this remains a formal possibility (see pp. 9–10). However, CFTR has been shown to hydrolyze ATP (36), and the concentration of ATP and adenosine diphosphate at the cytosolic face of the plasma membrane can markedly affect CFTR-mediated Cl⁻ conductance (37). ATP binding and hydrolysis at first and second NBFs (NBF1 and NBF2) are proposed to cause conformational changes in CFTR that are associated with identifiable kinetic states of Cl⁻ channel opening and closing (38). Models of these kinetic states give predictions that are compatible with observed inhibitory effects of adenosine diphosphate (39) and induction of prolonged open times by nonhydrolyzable ATP analogues (40).

The 240 amino acids between the end of NBF1 and the beginning of transmembrane-spanning segment 7 correspond to exon 13 and make up the R domain. The location between the intracellular NBF1 and the transmembrane segment 7 projects this region to be intracellular. The overall hydrophobicity of this region of CFTR suggests that it may assume a globular conformation. Within this sequence are consensus sites for phosphorylation by PKA (41) and PKC (42), and phosphorylation of the R domain plays an essential role in regulation of Cl^- transport via PKA and, to a lesser extent, PKC. Deletion of a portion of the R domain produced a constitutively active Cl^- conductance (43), leading to the hypothesis that the R domain acted as a plug for the conducting pore of CFTR that was regulated by phosphorylation. The role of the R domain in CFTR Cl^- channel function has been tested by several approaches. Mutation of 11 consensus sites for PKA, for example, decreased CFTR Cl^- channel activity and nearly eliminated its activation by PKA (44). Moreover, the R domain has been generated as a separate protein and shown to block CFTR Cl^- channels, but only after it was phosphorylated by PKA (45).

Membrane Localization and Cellular Expression

The CFTR protein is likely a low abundance protein, based on the Cl^- conductance of individual CFTR molecules, the prevalent gradients for Cl^- movement, and the macroscopic Cl^- conductance of airway surface epithelia. Thus, CFTR function (Cl^- conductance) is easily demonstrable in epithelia that line the surface of airways, but native CFTR protein has been difficult to demonstrate by conventional immunocytochemical approaches using a variety of antibodies. Airway surface staining has been reported by Puchelle et al., using immunogold labeling (46). Interestingly, CFTR

appeared to be expressed at higher levels in certain specialized epithelial cells of airway submucosal glands. These observations are consistent with *in situ* hybridization of CFTR mRNA within the lung, which also detected hot spots of CFTR expression in isolated cells of airway submucosal glands but undetectable levels in surface epithelia (24).

In contrast to the difficulty of detecting CFTR expression in surface airway epithelia, the CFTR was visualized by immunocytochemistry in the apical cell membrane of normal pancreatic and sweat ducts (47). Immunocytochemical localization using the same probes in the same tissues from patients with CF revealed mostly perinuclear staining. This important observation has been confirmed and explained by the discovery that the most frequent mutation of the CF gene results in unstable CFTR protein that is not delivered to the plasma membrane (48,49). Rare CF mutations result in a dysfunctional CFTR that normally is trafficked to the luminal membrane (50). One conclusion from these studies is that most patients with CF lack a functional CFTR in the apical membrane of affected epithelia. These observations identified the processes that govern CFTR processing as a target for pharmacologic therapy of CF. Several groups are actively seeking compounds that increase the proportion of a mutant CFTR that is processed successfully to the apical cell membrane (51,52) (also see Chapter 11).

FUNCTIONS OF THE CYSTIC FIBROSIS TRANSMEMBRANE CONDUCTANCE REGULATOR

Although the CFTR functions as a cAMP-regulated Cl^- channel, the CFTR also affects the activity of several other ion transport processes. So far, there is no well-established link from defective Cl^- conductance, or any other missing function of the CFTR, to CF lung disease. Thus, each of the functions of the CFTR must be identified and characterized and their roles determined in normal lung defense mechanisms. If it could be determined that a single function of CFTR is crucial for maintaining the lung free of infection, researchers could focus on pharmacologic strategies to restore this function in the airways of patients with CF.

Chloride Channel

The CFTR definitively functions as a cAMP-regulated Cl^- channel in cells in which it is expressed endogenously or heterologously. Heterologous expression of the CFTR in several model cells that did not natively express the CF gene caused the appearance of small conductance nonrectifying cAMP-regulated Cl^- channels (53,54). Moreover, the genetic transfer of the wild-type CFTR into cells endogenously expressing the mutant ΔF508 CFTR "corrected" the cultured cell CF phenotype of reduced Cl^- conductance and absence of activation of Cl^- conductance by cAMP (55–57), and thus established the principle that CF can be treated by gene therapy. Expression of CFTR cDNA with introduced mutations produced cAMP-dependent Cl^- channels with characteristics different from the wild-type CFTR, strongly indicating that the CF gene product was a cAMP-dependent Cl^- channel (34,58). Ultimately, purified CFTR protein was reconstituted in artificial lipid bilayers and demonstrated to function as a Cl^- channel (6).

The CFTR Cl^- channel clearly is subject to regulation by kinases and phosphatases. There are up to 11 consensus sites for PKA phosphorylation, and mutagenesis of these sites severely reduces CFTR Cl^- channel open probability (44). Some of these sites also are phosphorylated by PKC (42), and PKC phosphorylation of membrane patches, possibly of CFTR, potentiates and/or enables activation of the CFTR by PKA activity (59). The CFTR can be phosphorylated and activated by cyclic guanine monophosphate (cGMP)-dependent kinase (60), and CFTR single channel gating is affected by exogenous src-kinase applied to excised patches (61). Not surprisingly, CFTR activity is sensitive to phosphatase activity (62,63). The NBFs of the CFTR bind and hy-

drolyze ATP, with distinct effects on channel gating (38). The details of these regulatory events are important because several classes of drugs appear to activate the CFTR, including phosphatase inhibitors (64), phosphodiesterase inhibitors (65), genistein-type compounds (66), and cyclopentyl xanthine (CPX) (67), and therefore may be able to maximize the performance of limited quantities of the mutant CFTR or genetically transferred CFTR (see Chapter 11).

Regulator of Other Ion Channels

Because the CFTR functions as a Cl^- channel, and because CF epithelia generally are characterized by a decreased Cl^- conductance, the initial inclination has been to construe organ-specific CF pathophysiology as the result of missing CFTR Cl^- channel function. This reasoning assumes a well-defined role of CFTR Cl^- channels in the normal physiologic functions of the epithelial targets of CF. However, it has been difficult to identify a requirement for transcellular Cl^- movement in the normal function of surface airway epithelia. Moreover, there currently are several well-documented examples in which the CFTR alters the activity of other ion channels or transporters, and some of these functions of the CFTR probably contribute to normal epithelial physiology. Thus, the possibility exists that abnormal activities of other epithelial ion channels or transporters, secondary to the absence of the CFTR, participate in organ-specific pathophysiology.

The presence of CFTR function alters the activity and/or regulation of at least 3 distinct ion channels: epithelial sodium (Na^+) channels (ENaC); outward-rectifying Cl^- channels (ORCC); and potassium (K^+) channels. Of these channels, ENaC has the best-understood role in normal physiology of airway epithelia, and its misregulation is potentially important in CF lung disease. These clearly demonstrable effects of the CFTR on other ion channels may provide clues as to the biochemical mechanism of the interactions of the CFTR with other proteins.

Epithelial Sodium Channels (ENCs)

In vitro studies of freshly excised proximal airways from many species revealed that ouabain- and amiloride-sensitive Na+ absorption was a consistent physiologic function of adult mammalian airways (1,68,69). Available evidence also supports the concept that bronchiolar surface cells exhibit Na+ absorption as the basal function (70–74). These observations are consistent with *in situ* hybridization for ENaC subunits, which are present throughout the conducting airways (75).

The earliest human studies *in vivo*, which established raised transepithelial electrical potential difference (PD) as a hallmark of abnormal ion transport in CF airways, also found the amiloride-sensitive PD to be greater in patients with CF than in healthy subjects (76). The interpretation of this observation, that amiloride-sensitive Na+ absorption is increased in CF, has been confirmed by measurement of ion fluxes in freshly excised tissues (77) and by microelectrode analyses performed in freshly excised (78) and cultured epithelia (79,80). Most recently, Na+ absorption was found to be increased across the nasal epithelia of CFTR knockout mice (81). Because Na+ conductance is increased in the absence of a functional CFTR, the simplest interpretation of these results is that the presence of a functional CFTR decreases Na+ conductance. This notion has been tested formally in several heterologous systems, in which coexpression of the CFTR with the ENaC decreased amiloride-sensitive Na+ conductance (82–84).

The interaction of the CFTR and the ENaC appears to involve the regulation of the ENaC by cAMP. In some epithelia, cAMP is the second messenger that results in increased apical membrane Na+ conductance in response to vasopressin (85,86). Repeated studies in normal airway epithelia revealed that amiloride-sensitive Na+ absorption was not increased by elevating cAMP or other signal transduction pathways (77). However, raising cAMP in CF airway epithelia increased the already abnormally high rate of Na+ absorption (77). Moreover, in recent studies, cAMP-induced activation of Cl− conductance was associated with downregulation of ENaC-mediated Na+ conductance in CFTR-expressing intestinal cells (87) and M1 kidney cells (88). The mechanism by which the CFTR influences regulation of the ENaC by cAMP-dependent protein kinase is not known. In fibroblasts expressing a heterologous ENaC, PKA increased the open probability of individual ENaCs in both cell-attached and excised membrane patches from cells lacking the CFTR but inhibited open probability of ENaCs in patches from CFTR-expressing cells (89).

The mechanism of this effect is not yet agreed on, but evidence already has been presented for direct interactions between the CFTR and the ENaC (90), as well as an indirect connection via CFTR-mediated ATP release (91). From published information, however, it seems clear that the CFTR does not downregulate ENaCs in each cell in which the two proteins are coexpressed. For example, CFTR Cl− conductance and ENaC-mediated conductance both appear to be activated coordinately by PKA activity in the sweat ductal epithelium (92). Tissue-variable occurrence of CFTR regulation of ENaCs suggests that the mechanism uses additional proteins that are not expressed in each tissue in which the two ion channels are found.

Outward-Rectifying Chloride Channels

ORCCs were shown to be misregulated in cells derived from patients with CF before the cloning of the CFTR (93,94). In fact, the ORCC was a candidate for the CF gene product because in epithelial cells from patients with CF, PKA did not activate ORCCs (93,94). The CFTR later was shown to be distinct from ORCCs, but the former was required for cAMP regulation of ORCCs (95,96). The physiologic role of this CFTR-mediated regulation of ORCCs in airway surface epithelia has been debated because of the extensive nonepithelial distribution of ORCCs (97). However, the concept that the CFTR mediates the coordinate regulation of a parallel Cl⁻ conductance in the apical cell membrane is important when considering therapeutic approaches to restoring normal epithelial functions in patients with CF (98).

Potassium Channels

Coexpression of the CFTR in heterologous cells induces the ROMK2 K⁺ channel to become sensitive to the K⁺ channel-blocking agent glibenclamide (99). Another ABC protein, the sulfonylurea receptor, similarly affects KIR K⁺ channels *in vivo* (100). In the latter case, the mechanism of interaction appears to involve tight and specific protein:protein association between the ABC transport ATPase and the regulated ion channel (101). Although the CFTR has similar effects on ROMK2 channels (i.e., conveyance of glibenclamide sensitivity), it is not known whether the CFTR physically associates with ROMK2 channels. CFTR expression in oocytes activates an endogenous K⁺ conductance (102). The physiologic significance of CFTR interactions with K⁺ conductances may involve the coordinated increases in Cl⁻ and K⁺ conductances observed with stimulation of Cl⁻-secreting epithelia.

Cystic Fibrosis Transmembrane Conductance Regulator Effects on Other Ion Transport Mechanisms

Evidence is accumulating that CFTR alters the function/regulation of Na⁺/hydrogen (H⁺) exchangers (NHEs) and Cl⁻/bicarbonate (HCO_3^-) exchangers [anion exchangers (AEs)] in epithelia, where these exchangers play an important role in normal physiology. In intestinal epithelium, Na⁺ absorption is mediated, in part, by electroneutral processes. NHE3 is on the luminal membrane and operates in parallel with Cl⁻/HCO_3^- exchange to account for an absorptive flow of salt and water. In normal epithelia (i.e., in the presence of CFTR), the activity of NHE3 is inhibited by stimuli that increase intracellular cAMP. This effect of PKA requires the presence of another protein, NHERF (103). Its molecular role in regulation

of NHE3 is not known. In mouse intestine, cAMP-dependent inhibition of NHE requires a CFTR (104).

In other CFTR-expressing cells, such as pancreas and intrahepatic biliary epithelial (IBE) cells, the addition of cell-derived bicarbonate to the luminal liquid is an important physiologic function. The CFTR long has been hypothesized to operate as a Cl⁻ channel in parallel with an anion exchanger in the apical membrane (105). In this model, the CFTR provides Cl⁻ to the lumen through electrogenic Cl⁻ secretion, which then is exchanged electroneutrally for cellular bicarbonate. As a result, the concentration of bicarbonate in pancreatic juice can approach 100 mmol/L, which is critical for the solubility and activity of secreted enzymes (106). Recently, Jefferson and colleagues (107) reported a more direct functional interaction between the CFTR and the anion exchanger in the apical membrane of IBE cells. In normal IBE cells, introduction of luminal Cl⁻-free solution imposed a gradient for Cl⁻ exit from the cells that ran the Cl⁻/HCO_3^- exchanger backward, resulting in alkalinization of the cell due to HCO_3^- uptake. This response was not seen in IBE cells derived from patients with CF, although the cells expressed the appropriate anion exchanger. However, this response was restored by transfection of the cells with the wild-type CFTR. These data strongly implicate the CFTR as a positive regulator of AE activity and suggest that the absence of this regulatory function of the CFTR contributes to hepatic pathophysiology in CF. This regulatory function of the CFTR could be important in other bicarbonate-secreting tissues affected in CF, such as the pancreas, and it could play a role in determining the composition of airway surface liquid.

The Cystic Fibrosis Transmembrane Conductance Receptor May Transport Regulatory Molecules

Because the CFTR belongs to the ABC transport ATPase family, there has been interest in the possibility that the CFTR can transport substances other than inorganic anions. The appeal of this idea rests in its potential to explain some of the effects of CFTR expression on the activity of other transport molecules or to explain how airway surface liquid is modified by the CFTR to prevent bacterial infection. One controversial possibility is the participation of the CFTR in the gated release of ATP from epithelial cells (108,109). Independent observations indicate that ATP released from epithelial cells into the airway lumen will occupy purinergic receptors linked to phospholipase C and thereby enhance fluid secretion by activating calcium (Ca^{2+})-activated Cl^- conductance (110) and inhibiting amiloride-sensitive Na^+ channels (91). Moreover, extracellular ATP also stimulates ciliary beat frequency and particulate clearance from the lung (111,112). Thus, CFTR-mediated ATP release could play a central role in coordinating the activities of multiple elements of lung defense against bacterial infection. Whereas some investigators have reported that the CFTR conducts negatively charged ATP (113), and thereby accounts for cAMP-stimulated release of ATP from CFTR-expressing cells, other investigators find no conduction of ATP through the CFTR (114) or no connection between expression of the CFTR in a cell and ATP release in response to any stimulus (115). Most recently, data linking the CFTR to regulated release of ATP suggest that the actual movement of ATP across the plasma membrane occurs not through the CFTR but through an unidentified protein that is itself regulated by the CFTR (116).

SALT AND WATER TRANSPORT BY NORMAL AIRWAY SURFACE EPITHELIA

Historic Context/Overview

Before the molecular identity of any of the ion transport elements in airway epithelia was known, functional assays were used to describe the pattern of ion transport across airway mucosa. These studies revealed pathways for active ion transport (i.e., Na^+ absorption and Cl^- secretion) in proximal conducting airways and upper respiratory (nasal) epithelia of adult mammalian species (1,69). Early reliance on studies of canine tracheal epithelium, which has an exaggerated capacity for Cl^- secretion, fostered the view that the predominant function of lower airway epithelia was Cl^- secretion (117–121) (see "Transepithelial Chloride Conductive Path," p.13). When the CFTR was identified as the cAMP-regulated Cl^- channel necessary for Cl^- secretion, this perception was reinforced because defective salt and water secretion seemed compatible with the thickened and desiccated sputum that obstructs CF airways. It currently is recognized that surface epithelia from every conducting airway region studied in the adult lung exhibit net absorption of NaCl driven by active Na^+ transport (1,69). Thus, it is unlikely that impaired Cl^- secretion by surface epithelia of proximal airways, as a simple defect, causes CF lung disease. Understanding the role of the CFTR in salt and water physiology of normal mammalian airways requires better characterization of net ion transport in all regions of airways, including thorough definition of all the transepithelial pathways and driving forces present in the system.

The traditional concept of airway epithelial ion transport and surface liquid metabolism is based on early observations by Kilburn (122) and extensive measurements of airway epithelial ion transport over the past 2 decades (1,68,69,117,123). Specifically, isotonic volume absorption is predicted to occur across normal airway surface epithelia, as the volume of airway surface liquid is moved by mucociliary clearance from the large surface area of distal airways to the much smaller surface area of proximal airways (Fig. 1-2, Isotonic (upper) model). This concept implies: 1) that there is bulk flow of airway surface liquid (periciliary fluid) along the longitudinal axis of conducting airways that accompanies the mucociliary clearance of mucus; 2) that the epithelium is relatively water permeable to allow absorptive volume flow; and 3) that the residual airway surface liquid is isotonic. Recently, a fundamentally different concept of the normal physiology of airway surface liquid metabolism has been proposed (124,125). This alternative hy-

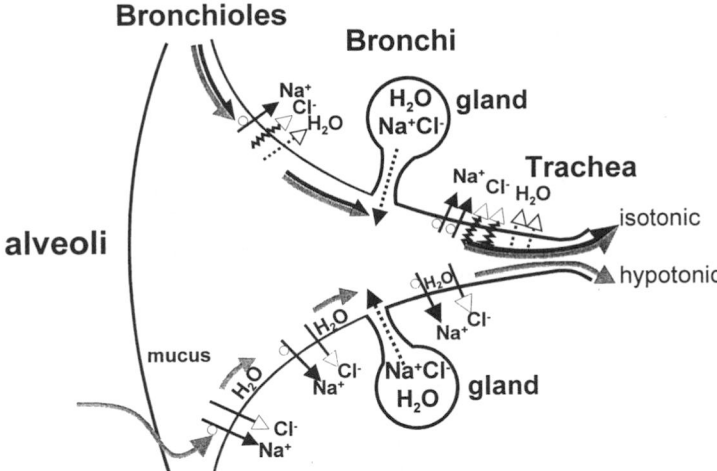

FIG.1–2. Airway surface liquid physiology models. Isotonic model *(top)*: Airway surface liquid (ASL) is proposed to move from distal airways toward the mouth. Na$^+$ driven absorption of NaCl and water regulate the net quantity of ASL and prevent the accumulation of excess quantities on proximal airways. Hypotonic model *(bottom)*: Absorption of NaCl across an epithelium with low water permeability might produce ASL with low salt concentrations. In this model, impaired Cl$^-$ permeability could prevent production of hypotonic ASL.

pothesis suggests that normal airways are like sweat ducts, that is, they maintain ion concentration gradients by absorbing ions but not water (volume), and generate hypotonic airway surface liquid. This alternative concept implies: 1) that only mucus (not bulk flow of periciliary liquid) is moved by mucociliary clearance; and 2) that the epithelium is water impermeable, or other forces (capillarity) retain water in excess of ions on airway surfaces. Recent studies provide strong evidence that isotonic volume absorption is the basal function of airway surface epithelia, rather than maintenance of ion concentration gradients (i.e., hypotonic surface liquid). These data will be discussed in detail.

Sodium Absorptive Path

Na$^+$ absorption is the dominant ion transport pathway of adult mammalian airways (126, 127). The principal transport elements that mediate Na$^+$ absorption have been identified in each (luminal and basolateral) cell membrane. Sodium absorption by airway epithelia is inhibited by luminal amiloride, indicating the

presence of an amiloride-sensitive, conductive step in the luminal cell membrane. Na$^+$ absorption by airways also is sensitive to submucosal ouabain, indicating the role of an ouabain-sensitive Na$^+$-K$^+$-adenosine triphosphatase (ATPase) in the basolateral membrane (Fig. 1–3) (123). Other processes for Na$^+$ entry across the luminal membrane into the cell have been identified in airway epithelia of some species, including Na$^+$-glucose symport (128) and Na$^+$/H$^+$ exchange (129), but these processes are not major routes for Na$^+$ entry into the absorptive path of adult human proximal airway epithelia. Thus, the magnitude of Na$^+$ absorption by proximal airway epithelia is determined primarily by the regulation of the number and open probability of luminal membrane amiloride-sensitive Na$^+$ channels.

The ENaC was cloned in 1993 (130,131). It consists minimally of three related subunits, α-, β-, and γ-ENaCs, which combine to form amiloride-sensitive Na$^+$ channels. As with the identification of the CFTR, cloning the genes for each of the ENaC subunits provided tools for rapid progress in understanding the physiology of amiloride-sensitive Na$^+$ channels in

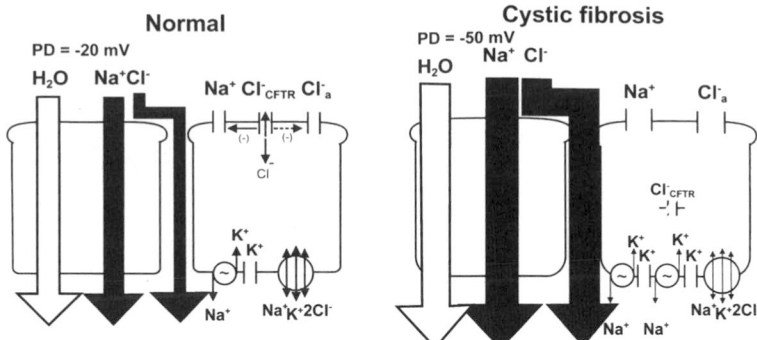

FIG. 1–3. Basal ion transport. Airway epithelial cell models demonstrate the locations of key ion transport proteins. Normal: Na+ enters the cells through amiloride-sensitive epithelial sodium channels (ENaCs) in the apical membrane and is moved across the basolateral membrane by Na+-K+-ATPases. Cl– passes through the paracellular pathway and/or through apical and basolateral Cl– channels (Cl–CFTR, Cl–A, Na+-K+–2Cl–) to maintain electrical neutrality. CF: The apical membrane ENaCs have a greater open probability that leads to increased net Na+ (and Cl–) absorption. PD, potential difference.

airway epithelia. For example, *in situ* hybridization has demonstrated mRNA for each ENaC subunit in airway surface epithelia, although there are some differences in expression level across airway regions, tissues, and species (75,132,133). The importance of these differences is not yet known. Expression of ENaC subunits also is regulated developmentally, increasing acutely in the few days before birth (134). Targeted disruption of the murine α-ENaC gene demonstrated an essential role of ENaC-mediated Na+ absorption in clearing the lungs of fluid at birth (135). Despite such clear-cut demonstrations that ENaCs are present in airways and critical for Na+ absorption, the biophysical properties of airway ENaCs and hormonal regulation of airway epithelial Na+ conductance differ markedly from those of ENaCs in classical salt-conserving epithelia (1,136-138).

Endogenously expressed ENaCs have been characterized by patch clamp in nonairway cells, including rat CCD (139), in M-1 cells (140) and in A6 cells (141). In each of these tissues, amiloride-sensitive channels had a linear slope conductance of 3-8 picoSiemens, slow-gating kinetics at room temperature, mild voltage dependence, and high selectivity for Na+ over K+ (136). These single-channel characteristics were recapitulated by heterologous coexpression of cloned α-, β-, and γ-ENaCs subunits in frog oocytes (142) or in mouse fibroblasts (89). Interestingly, amiloride-sensitive Na+ channels with these hallmarks have been seen only rarely in airway epithelia (143). In most studies of airway ENaCs, a range of single-channel characteristics has been observed (144–147). These properties include slope conductances ranging from 10 to 35 picoSeimens, moderately rapid gating at room temperature, and modest selectivity for Na+ over K+. At present, no molecular or technical basis for these differences is known. Possibilities include the existence of additional ENaC subunits or tissue-specific alternative splicing that leads to ENaC subunits with different characteristics.

The two-step path of Na+ absorption in airway epithelia is the same one that mediates salt absorption in classical salt-conserving epithelia, such as kidney and colon. In these tissues, which maintain homeostasis of volume and composition of extracellular body fluid, the rate of Na+ absorption is regulated tightly through the actions of aldosterone and antidiuretic hormone on expression and function of ENaCs (136). In striking contrast, Na+ absorption by adult mammalian airway epithelia repeatedly has been found to be un-affected by aldosterone and antidiuretic hor-mone (137,138,148,149). This difference may provide an important clue to both the physiologic role of Na^+ absorption by airway surface epithelia and perhaps the physiologic function of the CFTR in airway surface epithelia. The depth and volume of airway surface liquid are believed to play a critical role in efficient propulsion of mucus up and out of the lung. Thus, the volume (and composition) of this liquid compartment is expected to be regulated to optimize defense of the lung by mucociliary clearance (112,150,151). The volume of airway surface liquid in a normal human lung is less than 20 mL, and mucociliary clearance could be compromised if Na^+ absorption by surface epithelia responded to systemic stimuli that govern systemic vascular volume status. In fact, airway ENaCs appear to be shielded from systemic signals that stimulate salt absorption in other ENaC-expressing organs. For example, synthesis of α-ENaC in the lung is not stimulated by physiologic concentrations of mineralocorticoids (149). Moreover, the CFTR appears to directly prevent stimulation of ENaCs by the major pathway for regulation of ENaC function, that is, by vasopressin and cAMP-dependent protein kinase (see previous section on epithelial sodium channels) (84,89). Thus, the Na^+-absorptive pathway in normal airways is active under basal conditions and is not modulated substantially by mechanisms that regulate ENaC function and transcription in other Na^+-absorptive epithelia.

Transepithelial Chloride Conductive Path

In the study of ion transport by airway epithelia, much emphasis has been placed on the role and regulation of Cl^- transport. Fetal lungs, and fetal airway epithelia in particular, secrete Cl^- and liquid that is important for lung development (152–154). However, in the adult, gas-filled lung, the role of epithelial ion transport shifts to maintenance of the small volume of liquid that covers the airway surface. Although the role of Cl^- secretion in this process is not obvious, most adult airway epithelial cells retain the transport elements required for Cl^- secretion. These elements include a Na^+-K^+-ATPase (123), a Na^+-K^+–$2Cl^-$ transporter (155), and K^+ channels (156) in the basolateral membrane, whereas the luminal membrane contains multiple Cl^- conductances (see Fig. 1–3) (157). The basolateral elements operate jointly to drive Cl^- into the cell from the submucosal compartment. If luminal membrane Cl^- conductance is active and if intracellular Cl^- activity exceeds that predicted by the electrochemical equilibrium potential of Cl^- across the apical membrane, Cl^- secretion can occur. However, Cl^- is distributed across the apical membrane at (or near) electrochemical equilibrium (158) and activation of Cl^- conductance in adult surface airway epithelial cells does not cause Cl^- secretion *in situ*. Studies in which Cl^- secretion is measured experimentally routinely use techniques to voltage-clamp the transepithelial membrane potential to zero and usually include amiloride to block Na^+ absorption. Each maneuver hyperpolarizes the luminal cell membrane voltage, thereby increasing the driving force for Cl^- to exit the cell, or be "secreted." Under these conditions, the regulation of luminal membrane Cl^- conductance has been investigated extensively (159). The CFTR is the cAMP-dependent Cl^- conductance of airway epithelial cells. Most airway epithelial cells also secrete Cl^- in response to agonists that raise intracellular Ca^{2+} activity because of activation of a Ca^{2+}-dependent Cl^- conductance, called the alternative Cl^- conductance (Cl-A) (160).

Microelectrode analyses of the luminal and basolateral membranes of human nasal epithelial cells predict the presence of a small Cl^- conductance in the basolateral membrane (158). This conductance has not been characterized, and its molecular identity is unknown. However, the presence of this conductance has several important effects. First, a basolateral Cl^- conductance will depolarize the electrical potential across the basolateral cell membrane, which has the effect of limiting the electrical driving force available to secrete Cl^- across the luminal cell membrane (161). Second, it is in series with the luminal membrane Cl^- conductances and completes a transcellular Cl^-

conductive path that could be used for Cl⁻ to be absorbed as a counter-ion for actively absorbed Na⁺. In summary, there are few—if any—regions of adult, proximal airway surface epithelia in which a driving force for Cl⁻ secretion is known to exist *in vivo*. Consequently, the ability of airway epithelia to secrete Cl⁻ may be important in other regions, such as in submucosal gland acini, or possibly in very small distal airways that have not yet been characterized by electrophysiology.

Paracellular Path

In addition to ion transporters and channels that mediate ion movement across cells, the salt and water physiology of airway surface epithelia is defined critically by the solute and water permeabilities of the paracellular path (162). Studies of freshly excised proximal airway epithelia consistently have detected low to intermediate transepithelial resistances (50–500 ohm.cm²), compared with tight (> 1000 ohm. cm²) or leaky (< 100 ohm.cm²) models of epithelial ion transport. Transepithelial resistance of surface epithelia was found to be apportioned roughly equally between the paracellular and cellular paths by equivalent circuit analyses (163). These results are consistent with other studies that detected permeability of airway epithelia to high molecular weight extracellular markers (164,165). Regional comparisons of airway epithelia reveal a strong tendency for lower transepithelial resistance in smaller, more distal airways (127,161). Thus, surface airway epithelia possess a substantial paracellular path with the properties of free solution.

Water Permeability/Hydraulic Conductivity

The water permeability of airway epithelium has been measured directly, and the reported values are intermediate to high, relative to other barrier epithelia (166,167). The paracellular path in airway epithelia is a route for water flow around cells. In addition, the presence of water channels in airway epithelial cell membranes provides a transcellular path for water to cross the epithelium (166,168–171).The ability of water to cross airway epithelia around and through cells has profound implications for the physiologic function of transepithelial ion transport in airways. If water is free to move down its concentration gradient, as is indicated by the moderately high water permeability of airway epithelia, then ion transport by surface epithelia will not result in steep transepithelial ion activity gradients, but should result in isotonic volume transport (159).

Isotonic Volume Absorption by Normal Airway Surface Epithelium

Basal Na⁺ and Cl⁻ absorption and moderately high permeability to water and extracellular markers are characteristics that predict isotonic absorption of liquid volume by airway surface epithelia under *in vivo* conditions. The process of mucociliary clearance from distal to proximal airways generates a requirement for volume absorption by proximal airway surfaces (122). For example, it is estimated that as much as 1,500 mL of airway surface liquid per day must be absorbed, using estimates of the cross-sectional surface area of small (noncartilaginous) airways, an average periciliary layer depth of 10 µm, and a rate of clearance of 10 mm/minute (69,112,172). Direct measurement of ion fluxes under physiologic (open circuit) conditions in Ussing chambers show that Na⁺ and Cl⁻ are absorbed by proximal airway epithelia at a rate of approximately 1 µeq/cm²/hour (173). As isotonic volume absorption, this is equivalent to approximately 6 to 10 µL/cm²/hour. In the human lung, conducting airways have an aggregate surface area of 30,000 cm². Thus, the rate of active Na⁺ transport is more than sufficient to accommodate the estimated volume required to be absorbed.

It is difficult to experimentally detect volume absorption from the small airway surface liquid compartment present *in vivo*, leading to use of *in vitro* models to assess the volume transport capabilities of airway epithelia. The results obtained are, not surprisingly, dependent on how faithfully the model systems recapitulate *in vivo* function. For example, amiloride-sensitive volume absorption ranging from 2 to 5 $\mu L/cm^2/hour$ was detected in cultured preparations, representative of absorption carried out by freshly excised tissue (see preceeding paragraph) (174). However, cultured preparations with much lower ion transport capacity (175) exhibit volume absorptive flow rates that are very low (~0.1 $\mu L/cm^2/hour$). Whatever the magnitude of the flow rates, a key prediction of isotonic volume absorption is that the ionic composition of surface liquid will be isotonic with extracellular liquid.

Ion Composition

Isotonic absorption of liquid volume by airway surface epithelia predicts that airway surface liquid will be approximately isotonic. Airway surface liquid wicked from beneath the inferior turbinate onto filter paper by a noninvasive technique is isotonic (176). However, using similar sampling procedures through bronchoscope to define bronchial surface liquid ion composition in healthy humans initially suggested that bronchial surface liquid was hypotonic (176–178). However, recent studies in a large number of healthy (and disease control) subjects indicate that apparent hypotonicity in bronchial surface liquid samples arose from collection-induced stimulation of submucosal gland secretion during the sampling period (176). Two different observations support this conclusion. First, it was found that nasal surface liquid, although isotonic at rest, became hypotonic when submucosal glandular secretion was stimulated deliberately. Second, the tonicity of bronchial surface liquid was correlated inversely with the volume of surface liquid that was sampled, with larger volumes presumably reflecting stimulation of bronchial submucosal glands. When estimated osmolarity [double the sum of (Na^+) and (K^+)] was plotted against sample volume (weight), the smallest samples (least stimulated) approached isotonicity. These analyses suggest that submucosal glands are stimulated during bronchoscopic sampling of bronchial surface liquid, and that under baseline conditions, bronchial surface liquid probably is close to isotonic. Current studies are focused on further charac-

terization of the contribution of surface versus submucosal gland epithelia to airway surface liquid metabolism. The results also suggest that submucosal glands are capable of adding hypotonic liquid to the airway surface (see following section on submucosal gland hypothesis).

ABNORMALITIES IN ION TRANSPORT IN CYSTIC FIBROSIS SURFACE AIRWAY EPITHELIA

Overview

Ion transport by CF airway epithelia clearly is abnormal. Both decreased cAMP-dependent Cl^- conductance and increased amiloride-sensitive Na^+ absorption have been demonstrated consistently (1). To understand how these abnormalities lead to CF lung disease, each defect must be considered in the context of overall salt and water transport by airway epithelia. Current concepts are based largely on data from studies of surface epithelia in proximal conducting airways, but characterization of distal (small) airway epithelial function is beginning to emerge.

Sodium Transport

The earliest indication of abnormal ion transport by CF airway epithelia came from the comparison of *in vivo* nasal and bronchial PD in healthy subjects and patients with CF (76,179). The resting electrical potential measured under the inferior turbinate in patients with CF was elevated two- to threefold over normal, and the magnitude of inhibition of the raised potential difference by the Na^+ channel blocker, amiloride, was absolutely and proportionally greater in CF. This fundamental difference between CF and normal was extended rapidly to proximal lower airways (1,76) and, importantly, was found to exist in neonates (180). Thus, raised airway epithelial PD and enhanced amiloride sensitivity are intrinsic properties of CF airway epithelia.

Any doubt regarding the interpretation that the raised amiloride-sensitive PD reflected accelerated Na^+ absorption by CF airway epithelia was eliminated by direct measure of ion fluxes in freshly excised CF nasal epithelia (77). Moreover, microelectrode analyses of freshly excised tissues revealed increased Na$^+$ conductance in the luminal membrane of CF specimens (78). In addition, increased activity of the Na$^+$-absorptive path was detected as increased numbers of ouabain-binding sites in CF airway epithelia (181). This biochemical indication of increased density of Na$^+$-K$^+$-ATPase is predicted by increased Na$^+$ entry into the cell from the luminal solution (see Fig. 1–3) (80,182). This difference between CF and normal recently was extended to lower airway epithelium (183), indicating that abnormally raised Na$^+$ absorption is present in airways of the lower respiratory tract.

Extensive analyses of the permeabilities and ion gradients operative in normal and CF epithelia has been performed on cultured epithelia using microelectrodes (80,158,163,184). These studies determined that Na$^+$ permeability of the apical membrane of CF epithelia was increased by nearly four times greater than normal. Patch clamp of normal and CF-cultured epithelia also identified abnormal behavior of amiloride-sensitive Na$^+$-conducting channels (90,145,185). Those isolated in CF cells were characterized by open probability that was two to three times greater than normal. A substantial body of data, both direct and indirect, supports the notion that Na$^+$ absorption is increased substantially in CF airway epithelia.

Chloride Conductance in Cystic Fibrosis Airway Epithelia

In vivo nasal epithelial PD was first used to compare the Cl$^-$ conductance of normal and CF airway epithelia (179). In normal epithelia, perfusion of the luminal surface with an amiloride-containing Cl$^-$-free solution resulted in a hyperpolarization of transepithelial PD, which was augmented by inclusion of isoproterenol to increase epithelial cAMP (179,186,187). In CF epithelia, there was no hyperpolarization in response to luminal Cl$^-$-free solution and no effect of isoproterenol. These findings also have been extended to lower airways (188,189). The

marked difference in normal and CF responses unambiguously demonstrate that CF airways are devoid of a luminal cAMP-dependent Cl$^-$ conductance. The all-or-none nature of the comparison makes this maneuver the best experimental test to functionally assay for the presence of CFTR (186).

In vivo evidence that CFTR-mediated Cl$^-$ conductance is absent from the luminal membrane has been confirmed by *in vitro* experiments in freshly excised tissues with both ion fluxes (190) and microelectrodes (78) and by numerous studies with cultured epithelia (3,158,160,191–196). Microelectrode analyses revealed further that Cl$^-$ permeability of the CF airway cell luminal membrane is very low at rest, whereas there is a substantial basal Cl$^-$ conductance in unstimulated normal cells (158,163). These results are consistent with earlier *in vivo* PD data, which demonstrated a hyperpolarization of nasal PD in healthy subjects in response to Cl$^-$-free superfusion (179), which is indicative of a basal Cl$^-$ conductance.

Paracellular Path and Hydraulic Conductivity in Cystic Fibrosis Airway Epithelia

The permeability of the paracellular path in normal and CF airway epithelia have not been compared extensively. In the most direct comparison, the electrical shunt resistances of normal and CF-cultured epithelia were compared (163). Direct comparisons of the hydraulic conductivity of normal and CF airway epithelia have not yet been reported. Overall, there currently is no evidence to suggest that normal and CF airway epithelia have markedly different paracellular permeability and/or hydraulic conductivity.

Excessive Isotonic Volume Absorption

Because proximal airway epithelia absorb Na$^+$ and Cl$^-$ under basal conditions and CF epithelia absorb Na$^+$ and Cl$^-$ at an increased rate, it is predicted that CF airway epithelia will absorb volume more rapidly. There have been several attempts to test this hypothesis. Miller et al. described increased volume absorption by cultured CF airway epithelia (174) and by cultured CF tracheal submucosal glands (197). Human bronchial xenografts populated by CF proximal airway cells demonstrated fourfold higher fluid absorption than xenografts populated by normal cells (198). In contrast, Smith et al. (199) found no enhanced volume absorption in CF versus normal cultured epithelia.

Pathogenesis of Cystic Fibrosis Lung Disease: Isotonic Absorption Model

Comparison of the water and solute transport properties of normal and CF airway epithelia suggests that the most dramatic defect resulting from loss of CFTR function is hyperabsorption of salt and water from the airway surfaces (Fig. 1–4, Table 1–1), which would concentrate surface macromolecules, impair mucociliary clearance, and promote bacterial infection. Because of continued salt and water absorption, mucus aggregates that normally are not cleared become progressively dehydrated and refractory to mucociliary transport or cough clearance. Eventually, retained mucus obstructs small airways. Detailed pathology studies of lungs from infants with CF who died of complications of meconium ileus in the 1940s and 1950s detected small airways that were obstructed with mucus plugs in the absence of infection or inflammation (200). Early in life, however, airways of all patients with CF become infected. According to the excessive isotonic volume absorption hypothesis, infection will occur distal to or associated with mucus plugs of small airways. In this scenario, the mucus plugs act as foreign bodies and provide

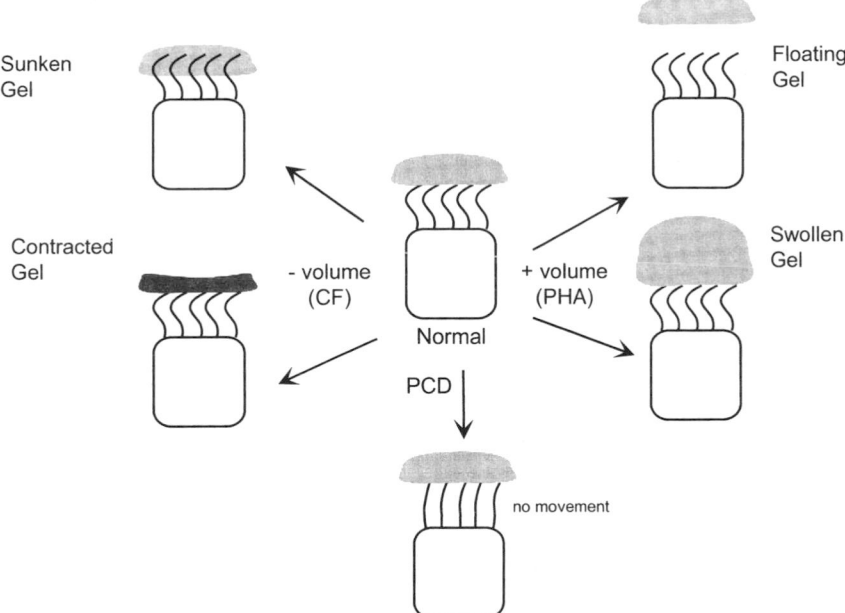

FIG. 1–4. Potential effects of abnormal ion transport on airway mucociliary clearance (MCC). Normal function maintains isotonic airway surface liquid (ASL) adequate for optimal MCC *(center)*. Excess epithelial absorption of ions (and fluid) causes decreased volume of the periciliary fluid *(upper left)*, dehydrated mucus secretions *(lower left)*, or both. These changes impair MCC. Reduced epithelial absorption of ions (and fluid) [e.g., pseudohypoaldosteronism (PHA)] due to loss of function mutations in epithelial Na+ channels (201,202) may increase the volume of periciliary fluid *(upper right)*, increase mucus hydration *(lower right)*, or both. These changes may decrease or increase MCC. Impaired ciliary function due to structural abnormalities (e.g., primary ciliary dyskinesia) impairs MCC independent of ASL volume *(bottom)*. PCD, primary ciliary dyskinesia.

TABLE 1–1. *A comparison of models of airway epithelial salt and water metabolism[a]*

	Isotonic	Hypotonic	
		Sweat duct	Capillary forces
Mucus layer	Yes	Yes	No
Axial surface liquid movement	Yes	No	No
Water permeability	High	Low	High
Volume absorption	Yes	No	Yes/stops
Cl⁻ absorption	Paracellular	Transcellular	Transcellular
Capillary forces	Low	Low	"High"
Na⁺-K⁺–ATPase activity	Upregulated	Downregulated	Downregulated

[a]Essential features that are predicted to distinguish the isotonic, hypotonic sweat duct, and hypotonic capillary force models of airway surface liquid regulation: the presence of a mucus (gel) layer, the movement of the periciliary surface liquid layer toward the mouth, the water permeability of the surface epithelium, the presence of transepithelial water absorption, the path of transepithelial Cl⁻ absorption, the magnitude of periciliary capillary forces, and epithelial cell Na⁺-K⁺–ATPase activity.

a nidus of infection that cannot be killed by local immune response or by antibiotics. Once established, such infections induce an immune response, which contributes substantially to further airway destruction.

Other Hypotheses

Hypotonic Surface Liquid/ Defensin Hypothesis

Recently, a hypothesis was advanced to relate ion transport abnormalities in CF airways to failure of airway surface bacterial defense mechanisms (124,125). Several laboratory studies have reported that airway surface liquid from cultured CF airway cells are deficient in bactericidal activity that is observed in surface liquid in cultures of normal airway cells (125,203). Bactericidal activity of the fluid in contact with CF cells was restored when the solution was made hypotonic. Based on these results, it was speculated that normal airway epithelia, like sweat ducts, absorb Na⁺ and Cl⁻ in excess of water to produce a hypotonic airway surface milieu [see Fig. 1–2, Hypotonic (lower) model, and Table 1–1] that is critical for the bacterial killing activity of several salt-sensitive natural antibiotics. The essential corollaries of this hypothesis are: (1) the CFTR in the apical membrane is rate limiting for Cl⁻ absorption (i.e., there is no paracellular pathway for Cl⁻ absorption); (2) airways are impermeable to water, or some other mechanism

(capillarity) retains water on airway surfaces in excess of ions; and (3) net Na⁺ and Cl⁻ absorption in CF airways will be less than normal. As reviewed previously, each of these projected requirements is not clearly congruent with defined characteristics of normal and CF proximal airway epithelia.

Submucosal Gland Hypothesis

Serous cells in the secretory acini of bronchial submucosal glands have the highest level of CFTR expression in human lungs (24). CF tracheal submucosal glands have dilated ducts, probably from obstruction by macromolecular secretions, and these changes have been observed in the absence of infection (200,204). One proposal is that the deficient CFTR prevents salt and water secretion that normally hydrates glandular mucins and washes them onto the airway surface (205,206). Deficient secretion by CF submucosal glands also would reduce the volume contribution of submucosal gland secretions to airway surface liquid. Further, submucosal gland secretions are rich in lactoferrin, lysozyme and other natural antibiotics (206,207). If the activities of these or other unknown bactericidal compounds arising from glands were diminished in CF airway surface liquid, defense against infection could be diminished (208). However, there are no major alterations in volume output or ion composition in cholinergic-stimulated nasal submucosal gland secretions in subjects with CF, which suggests that non-CFTR pathways may be important in gland secretion in the upper airways (176). This observation implies NaCl absorption across a water impermeable submucosal gland duct, which is congruent with parotid duct function in healthy subjects and those with CF (208). Resolution of these possibilities will require a more detailed understanding of submucosal gland secretions and of the roles of gland ducts in modifying their composition.

NOTE: M.J. Stutts and R.C. Boucher are founding scientists of Inspire Pharmaceuticals, which licensed the patent for aerosolized UTP from the University of North Carolina on March 10, 1995. M.J. Stutts, R.C. Boucher, and the University of North Carolina hold equity in Inspire Pharmaceuticals.

SUMMARY

The function of the CFTR is critical to normal lung defense, but there are two obstacles to deciphering this rather obvious point. First, the CFTR appears to have multiple functions and roles in normal physiology, and a single critical role of the CFTR in preventing lung disease is not obvious. Second, the precise airway region where CF lung disease initiates has not been identified definitively, so it is difficult to isolate a critical function of the normal CFTR that prevents CF lung disease.

Nonetheless, most evidence suggests that excessive absorption of salt and water concentrates macromolecules on airway surfaces and leads to thick, tenacious mucus that is difficult to clear, especially from the smallest airways. Failure to clear bacteria from behind these plugs eventually results in colonization and chronic infection. This initiates a vicious cycle of immune responses that results in more obstruction and eventual damage to airway structures.

Are different hypotheses concerning pathogenesis of CF in the lung incompatible? Not at all. There could be poor clearance because of salt- and water-depleted mucins that obstruct small airways and submucosal glands. Glands also may have deficient capabilities to generate liquid in response to cAMP-signaling stimuli.

Thus, submucosal gland contributions to airway surface liquid may be decreased and/or of abnormal composition. Finally, in the very smallest airways, normal physiology could be different than it is in more proximal airways, and Cl⁻ secretion could play an important role in the genesis of the liquid that normally gets transported up and out of the lung. There is at least some evidence that all of these abnormalities occur; therefore, it is not unreasonable that they each contribute to CF pathogenesis in the lung.

REFERENCES

1. Boucher RC. Human airway ion transport, part 2. *Am J Respir Crit Care Med* 1994;150(2):581–593.
2. Davis PB, Drumm M, Konstan MW. Cystic fibrosis. *Am J Respir Crit Care Med* 1996;154(5):1229–1256.
3. Welsh MJ, Tsui L, Boat TF, et al. Cystic fibrosis. In: Scriver CR, Beaudet AL, Sly WS, et al., eds. *The metabolic and molecular bases of inherited disease,* 7th ed. New York: McGraw-Hill, 1995:3799–3876.
4. Riordan JR, Rommens JM, Kerem B, et al. Identification of the cystic fibrosis gene: cloning and characterization of complementary DNA. *Science* 1989;245 (4922):1066–1073.
5. Anderson MP, Gregory RJ, Thompson S, et al. Demonstration that CFTR is a chloride channel by alteration of its anion selectivity. *Science* 1991;253 (5016):202–205.
6. Bear CE, Li C, Kartner N, et al. Purification and functional reconstitution of the cystic fibrosis transmembrane conductance regulator (CFTR). *Cell* 1992;68(4):809–818.
7. Ferrari M, Cremonesi L. Genotype-phenotype correlation in cystic fibrosis patients. *Ann Biol Clin* 1996; 54(6):235–241.
8. Collins FS. Cystic fibrosis: molecular biology and therapeutic implications. *Science* 1992;256(5058): 774–779.
9. Cutting GR. Genotype defect: its effect on cellular function and phenotypic expression. *Semin Respir Crit Care Med* 1994;15(5):356–363.
10. Tsui LC, Zengerling S, Willard HF, et al. Mapping of the cystic fibrosis locus on chromosome 7. *Cold Spring Harb Symp Quant Biol* 1986;51(Pt 1):325–335.
11. Rommens JM, Iannuzzi MC, Kerem B, et al. Identification of the cystic fibrosis gene: chromosome walking and jumping. *Science* 1989;245(4922):1059–1065.
12. Collins FS. Of needles and haystacks: finding human disease genes by positional cloning. *Clin Res* 1991; 39(4):615–623.
13. Kerem B, Rommens JM, Buchanan JA, et al. Identification of the cystic fibrosis gene: genetic analysis. *Science* 1989;245(4922):1073–1080.
14. Chu C, Trapnell BC, Murtagh JJ Jr, et al. Variable deletion of exon 9 coding sequences in cystic fibrosis transmembrane conductance regulator gene mRNA

transcripts in normal bronchial epithelium. *EMBO J* 1991;10(6):1355–1363.

15. Chu C, Trapnell BC, Curristin S, et al. Genetic basis of variable exon 9 skipping in cystic fibrosis transmembrane conductance regulator mRNA. *Nat Genet* 1993;3(2):151–156.

16. Kiesewetter S, Macek M Jr, Davis C, et al. A mutation in CFTR produces different phenotypes depending on chromosomal background. *Nat Genet* 1993;5(3):274–278.

17. Strong TV, Wilkinson DJ, Mansoura MK, et al. Expression of an abundant alternatively spliced form of the cystic fibrosis transmembrane conductance regulator (CFTR) gene is not associated with a cAMP-activated chloride conductance. *Hum Mol Genet* 1993; 2(3):225–230.

18. Kerem B, Kerem E. The molecular basis for disease variability in cystic fibrosis. *Eur J Hum Genet* 1996; 4(2):65–73.

19. Morales MM, Carroll TP, Morita T, et al. Both the wild type and a functional isoform of CFTR are expressed in kidney. *Am J Physiol* 1996;270(6 Pt 2): F1038–F1048.

20. Horowitz B, Tsung SS, Hart P, et al. Alternative splicing of CFTR Cl⁻ channels in heart. *Am J Physiol* 1993;264(6 Pt 2):H2214–H2220.

21. Vuillaumier S, Dixmeras I, Messai H, et al. Cross-species characterization of the promoter region of the cystic fibrosis transmembrane conductance regulator gene reveals multiple levels of regulation. *Biochem J* 1997;327(3):651–662.

22. Warth JD, Collier ML, Hart P, et al. CFTR chloride channels in human and simian heart. *Cardiovasc Res* 1996;31(4):615–624.

23. McDonald TV, Nghiem PT, Gardner P, et al. Human lymphocytes transcribe the cystic fibrosis transmembrane conductance regulator gene and exhibit CF-defective cAMP-regulated chloride current. *J Biol Chem* 1992;267(5):3242–3248.

24. Engelhardt JF, Yankaskas JR, Ernst SA, et al. Submucosal glands are the predominant site of CFTR expression in human bronchus. *Nat Genet* 1992;2(3): 240–247.

25. Yoshimura K, Nakamura H, Trapnell BC, et al. The cystic fibrosis gene has a "housekeeping"-type promoter and is expressed at low levels in cells of epithelial origin. *J Biol Chem* 1991;266(14):9140–9144.

26. Bargon J, Trapnell BC, Yoshimura K, et al. Expression of the cystic fibrosis transmembrane conductance regulator gene can be regulated by protein kinase C. *J Biol Chem* 1992;267(23):16056–16060.

27. McDonald RA, Matthews RP, Idzerda RL, et al. Basal expression of the cystic fibrosis transmembrane conductance regulator gene is dependent on protein kinase A activity. *Proc Natl Acad Sci U S A* 1995;92(16):7560–7564.

28. Breuer W, Kartner N, Riordan JR, et al. Induction of expression of the cystic fibrosis transmembrane conductance regulator. *J Biol Chem* 1992;267(15): 10465–10469.

29. Matthews RP, McKnight GS. Characterization of the cAMP response element of the cystic fibrosis transmembrane conductance regulator gene promoter. *J Biol Chem* 1996;271(50):31869–31877.

30. Cheng SH, Gregory RJ, Marshall J, et al. Defective intracellular transport and processing of CFTR is the molecular basis of most cystic fibrosis. *Cell* 1990;63 (4):827–834.

31. Chang XB, Hou YX, Jensen TJ, et al. Mapping of cystic fibrosis transmembrane conductance regulator membrane topology by glycosylation site insertion. *J Biol Chem* 1994;269(28):18572–18575.

32. Akabas MH, Kaufmann C, Cook TA, et al. Amino acid residues lining the chloride channel of the cystic fibrosis transmembrane conductance regulator. *J Biol Chem* 1994;269(21):14865–14868.

33. Tabcharani JA, Rommens JM, Hou YX, et al. Multi-ion pore behavior in the CFTR chloride channel. *Nature* 1993;366(6450):79–82.

34. Sheppard DN, Rich DP, Ostedgaard LS, et al. Mutations in CFTR associated with mild-disease-form Cl⁻ channels with altered pore properties. *Nature* 1993; 362(6416):160–164.

35. Sarkadi B, Price EM, Boucher RC, et al. Expression of the human multidrug resistance cDNA in insect cells generates a high activity drug-stimulated membrane ATPase. *J Biol Chem* 1992;267(7):4854–4858.

36. Li C, Ramjeesingh M, Wang W, et al. ATPase activity of the cystic fibrosis transmembrane conductance regulator. *J Biol Chem* 1996;271(45):28463–28468.

37. Quinton PM, Reddy MM. Control of CFTR chloride conductance by ATP levels through non-hydrolytic binding. *Nature* 1992;360(6399):79–81.

38. Gadsby DC, Nairn AC. Regulation of CFTR channel gating. *Trends Biochem Sci* 1994;19(11):513–518.

39. Travis SM, Carson MR, Ries DR, et al. Interaction of nucleotides with membrane-associated cystic fibrosis transmembrane conductance regulator. *J Biol Chem* 1993;268(21):15336–15339.

40. Gunderson KL, Kopito RR. Effects of pyrophosphate and nucleotide analogs suggest a role for ATP hydrolysis in cystic fibrosis transmembrane regulator channel gating. *J Biol Chem* 1994;269(30):19349–19353.

41. Chang X, Tabcharani JA, Hou Y, et al. Protein kinase A (PKA) still activates CFTR chloride channel after mutagenesis of all 10 PKA consensus phosphorylation sites. *J Biol Chem* 1993;268(15):11304–11311.

42. Picciotto MR, Cohn JA, Bertuzzi G, et al. Phosphorylation of the cystic fibrosis transmembrane conductance regulator. *J Biol Chem* 1992;267(18):12742–12752.

43. Rich DP, Gregory RJ, Anderson MP, et al. Effect of deleting the R domain on CFTR-generated chloride channels. *Science* 1991;253(5016):205–207.

44. Seibert FS, Tabcharani JA, Chang XB, et al. cAMP-dependent protein kinase-mediated phosphorylation of cystic fibrosis transmembrane conductance regulator residue Ser-753 and its role in channel activation. *J Biol Chem* 1995;270(5):2158–2162.

45. Ma J, Tasch JE, Tao T, et al. Phosphorylation-dependent block of cystic fibrosis transmembrane conductance regulator chloride channel by exogenous R domain protein. *J Biol Chem* 1996;271(13):7351–7356.

46. Puchelle E, Gaillard D, Ploton D, et al. Differential localization of the cystic fibrosis transmembrane conductance regulator in normal and cystic fibrosis airway epithelium. *Am J Respir Cell Mol Biol* 1992; 7(5):485–491.

47. Kartner N, Augustinas O, Jensen TJ, et al. Mislocalization of DF508 CFTR in cystic fibrosis sweat gland. *Nat Genet* 1992;1(5):321–327.

48. Denning GM, Anderson MP, Amara JF, et al. Processing of mutant cystic fibrosis transmembrane conductance regulator is temperature-sensitive. *Nature* 1992;358(6389):761–764.

49. Lukacs GL, Chang X, Bear C, et al. The delta F508 mutation decreases the stability of cystic fibrosis membrane conductance regulator in the plasma membrane: determination of functional half-lives on transfected cells. *J Biol Chem* 1993;268(29):21592–21598.

50. Logan J, Hiestand D, Daram P, et al. Cystic fibrosis transmembrane conductance regulator mutations that disrupt nucleotide binding. *J Clin Invest* 1994;94(1): 228–236.

51. Brown CR, Hongbrown LQ, Biwersi J, et al. Chemical chaperones correct the mutant phenotype of the delta-F508 cystic fibrosis transmembrane conductance regulator protein. *Cell Stress Chaperones* 1996; 1(2):117–125.

52. Rubenstein RC, Egan ME, Zeitlin PL. In vitro pharmacologic restoration of CFTR-mediated chloride transport with sodium 4-phenylbutyrate in cystic fibrosis epithelial cells containing delta F508-CFTR. *J Clin Invest* 1997;100(10):2457–2465.

53. Rommens JM, Dho S, Bear CE, et al. cAMP-inducible chloride conductance in mouse fibroblast lines stably expressing the human cystic fibrosis transmembrane conductance regulator. *Proc Natl Acad Sci U S A* 1991;88(17):7500–7504.

54. Li C, Ramjeesingh M, Reyes E, et al. The cystic fibrosis mutation (DeltaF508) does not influence the chloride channel activity of CFTR. *Nat Genet* 1993;3(4):311–316.

55. Olsen JC, Johnson LG, Stutts MJ, et al. Correction of the apical membrane chloride permeability defect in polarized cystic fibrosis airway epithelia following retroviral-mediated gene transfer. *Hum Gene Ther* 1992;3(3):253–266.

56. Drumm ML, Pope HA, Cliff WH, et al. Correction of the cystic fibrosis defect in vitro by retrovirus-mediated gene transfer. *Cell* 1990;62(6):1227–1233.

57. Rich DP, Anderson MP, Gregory RJ, et al. Expression of cystic fibrosis transmembrane conductance regulator corrects defective chloride channel regulation in cystic fibrosis airway epithelial cells. *Nature* 1990; 347(6291):358–363.

58. Tabcharani JA, Linsdell P, Hanrahan JW. Halide permeation in wild-type and mutant cystic fibrosis transmembrane conductance regulator chloride channels. *J Gen Physiol* 1997;110(4):341–354.

59. Jia Y, Mathews CJ, Hanrahan JW. Phosphorylation by protein kinase C is required for acute activation of cystic fibrosis transmembrane conductance regulator by protein kinase A. *J Biol Chem* 1997;272(8):4978–4984.

60. Tien XY, Brasitus TA, Kaetzel MA, et al. Activation of the cystic fibrosis transmembrane conductance regulator by cGMP in the human colonic cancer cell line, Caco-2. *J Biol Chem* 1994;269(1):51–54.

61. Fischer H, Machen TE. The tyrosine kinase p60c-src regulates the fast gate of the cystic fibrosis transmembrane conductance regulator chloride channel. *Biophys J* 1996;71(6):3073–3082.

62. Travis SM, Berger HA, Welsh MJ. Protein phosphatase 2C dephosphorylates and inactivates cystic fibrosis transmembrane conductance regulator. *Proc Natl Acad Sci U S A* 1997;94(20):11055–11060.

63. Reddy MM, Quinton PM. Deactivation of CFTR-Cl conductance by endogenous phosphatases in the native sweat duct. *Am J Physiol* 1996;270(2 Pt 1): C474–C480.

64. Becq F, Verrier B, Chang XB, et al. cAMP- and Ca^{2+}-independent activation of cystic fibrosis transmembrane conductance regulator channels by phenylimidazothiazole drugs. *J Biol Chem* 1996;271(27): 16171–16179.

65. Kelley TJ, al-Nakkash L, Cotton CU, et al. Activation of endogenous deltaF508 cystic fibrosis transmembrane conductance regulator by phosphodiesterase inhibition. *J Clin Invest* 1996;98(2):513–520.

66. Weinreich F, Wood PG, Riordan JR, et al. Direct action of genistein on CFTR. *Pflugers Arch* 1997;434 (4):484–491.

67. Cohen BE, Lee G, Jacobson KA, et al. 8-Cyclopentyl-1,3-dipropylxanthine and other xanthines differentially bind to the wild-type and deltaF508 mutant first nucleotide binding fold (NBF-1) domains of the cystic fibrosis transmembrane conductance regulator. *Biochemistry* 1997;36(21):6455–6461.

68. Boucher RC Jr, Bromberg PA, Gatzy JT. Airway transepithelial electric potential in vivo: species and regional differences. *J Appl Physiol* 1980;48(1):169–176.

69. Boucher RC. Human airway ion transport, part 1. *Am J Respir Crit Care Med* 1994;150(1):271–281.

70. Van Scott MR, Hester S, Boucher RC. Ion transport by rabbit nonciliated bronchiolar epithelial cells (Clara cells) in culture. *Proc Natl Acad Sci U S A* 1987;84(15):5496–5500.

71. Van Scott MR, Davis CW, Boucher RC. Na$^+$ and Cl$^-$ transport across rabbit nonciliated bronchiolar epithelial (Clara) cells. *Am J Physiol* 1989;256(4 Pt 1):C893–C901.

72. Ballard ST, Schepens SM, Falcone JC, et al. Regional bioelectric properties of porcine airway epithelium. *J Appl Physiol* 1992;73(5):2021–2027.

73. Ballard ST, Taylor AE. Bioelectric properties of proximal bronchiolar epithelium. *Am J Physiol* 1994; 267(1 Pt 1):L79–L84.

74. Al-Bazzaz JJ. Regulation of Na and Cl transport in sheep distal airways. *Am J Physiol* 1994;267(2 Pt 1): L193–L198.

75. Burch L, Talbot C, Knowles MR, et al. Relative expression of the human epithelial Na$^+$ channel (ENaC) sub-units in normal and cystic fibrosis airways. *Am J Physiol* 1995;269(2 Pt 1):C511–C518.

76. Knowles M, Gatzy J, Boucher R. Increased bioelectric potential difference across respiratory epithelia in cystic fibrosis. *N Engl J Med* 1981;305(25): 1489–1495.

77. Boucher RC, Stutts MJ, Knowles MR, et al. Na$^+$ transport in cystic fibrosis respiratory epithelia: abnormal basal rate and response to adenylate cyclase activation. *J Clin Invest* 1986;78(5):1245–1252.

78. Cotton CU, Stutts MJ, Knowles MR, et al. Abnormal apical cell membrane in cystic fibrosis respiratory

epithelium: an in vitro electrophysiologic analysis. *J Clin Invest* 1987;79(1):80–85.

79. Willumsen NJ, Boucher RC. Transcellular sodium transport in cultured cystic fibrosis human nasal epithelium. *Am J Physiol* 1991;261(2 Pt 1):C332–C341.

80. Boucher RC, Cotton CU, Gatzy JT, et al. Evidence for reduced Cl⁻ and increased Na⁺ permeability in cystic fibrosis human primary cell cultures. *J Physiol (Lond)* 1988;405:77–103.

81. Grubb BR, Vick RN, Boucher RC. Hyperabsorption of Na⁺ and raised Ca²⁺-mediated Cl⁻ secretion in nasal epithelia of CF mice. *Am J Physiol* 1994;266(5 Pt 1):C1478–C1483.

82. Mall M, Hipper A, Greger R, et al. Wild type but not delta F508 CFTR inhibits Na⁺ conductance when coexpressed in *Xenopus* oocytes. *FEBS Lett* 1996;381 (1–2):47–52.

83. Ismailov II, Berdiev BK, Shlyonsky VG, et al. Role of actin in regulation of epithelial sodium channels by CFTR. *Am J Physiol* 1997;272(4 Pt 1):C1077–C1086.

84. Stutts MJ, Canessa CM, Olsen JC, et al. CFTR as a cAMP-dependent regulator of sodium channels. *Science* 1995;269(5225):847–850.

85. Schafer JA, Troutman SL. cAMP mediates the increase in apical membrane Na⁺ conductance produced in rat CCD by vasopressin. *Am J Physiol* 1990;259(5 Pt 2):F823–F831.

86. Marunaka Y, Eaton DC. Effects of vasopressin and cAMP on single amiloride-blockable Na channels. *Am J Physiol* 1991;260(5 Pt 1):C1071–C1084.

87. Ecke D, Bleich M, Greger R. The amiloride inhibitable Na⁻ conductance of rat colonic crypt cells is suppressed by forskolin. *Pflugers Arch* 1996;431 (6):984–986.

88. Letz B, Korbmacher C. cAMP stimulates CFTR-like Cl⁻ channels and inhibits amiloride-sensitive Na⁺ channels in mouse CCD cells. *Am J Physiol* 1997; 272(2 Pt 1):C657–C666.

89. Stutts MJ, Rossier BC, Boucher RC. CFTR inverts PKA-mediated regulation of ENaC single channel kinetics. *J Biol Chem* 1997;272(22):14037–14040.

90. Kunzelmann K, Kathofer S, Greger R. Na⁺ and Cl⁻ conductances in airway epithelial cells: increased Na⁺ conductance in cystic fibrosis. *Pflugers Arch* 1995;431(1):1–9.

91. Ling BN, Zuckerman JB, Lin C, et al. Expression of the cystic fibrosis phenotype in a renal amphibian epithelial cell line. *J Biol Chem* 1997;272(1):594–600.

92. Quinton PM. Missing Cl conductance in cystic fibrosis. *Am J Physiol* 1986;251(4 Pt 1):C649–C652.

93. Welsh MJ, Li M, McCann JD. Activation of normal and cystic fibrosis Cl⁻ channels by voltage, temperature, and trypsin. *J Clin Invest* 1989;84(6):2002–2007.

94. Schoumacher RA, Shoemaker RL, Halm DR, et al. Phosphorylation fails to activate chloride channels from cystic fibrosis airway cells. *Nature* 1987;330 (6150):752–754.

95. Gabriel SE, Clarke LL, Boucher RC, et al. CFTR and outward rectifying chloride channels are distinct proteins with a regulatory relationship. *Nature* 1993;363 (6426):263–268.

96. Egan M, Flotte T, Afione S, et al. Defective regulation of outwardly rectifying Cl⁻ channels by protein kinase A corrected by insertion of CFTR. *Nature* 1992;358(6387):581–584.

97. Ward CL, Krouse ME, Gruenert DC, et al. Cystic fibrosis gene expression is not correlated with rectifying Cl⁻ channels. *Proc Natl Acad Sci U S A* 1991;88 (12):5277–5281.

98. Schwiebert EM, Flotte T, Cutting GR, et al. Both CFTR and outwardly rectifying chloride channels contribute to cAMP-stimulated whole cell chloride currents. *Am J Physiol* 1994;266(5 Pt 1):C1464–C1477.

99. McNicholas CM, Guggino WB, Schwiebert EM, et al. Sensitivity of a renal K⁺ channel (ROMK2) to the inhibitory sulfonylurea compound glibenclamide is enhanced by coexpression with the ATP-binding cassette transporter cystic fibrosis transmembrane regulator. *Proc Natl Acad Sci U S A* 1996;93(15):8083–8088.

100. Gribble FM, Ashfield R, Ammala C, et al. Properties of cloned ATP-sensitive K⁺ currents expressed in Xenopus oocytes. *J Physiol (Lond)* 1997;498(Pt 1): 87–98.

101. Shyng S, Nichols CG. Octameric stoichiometry of the KATP channel complex. *J Gen Physiol* 1997; 110(6):655–664.

102. Mall M, Kunzelmann K, Hipper A, et al. cAMP stimulation of CFTR-expressing Xenopus oocytes activates a chromanol-inhibitable K⁺ conductance. *Pflugers Arch* 1996;432(3):516–522.

103. Yun CH, Oh S, Zizak M, et al. cAMP-mediated inhibition of the epithelial brush border Na⁺/H⁺ exchanger, NHE3, requires an associated regulatory protein. *Proc Natl Acad Sci U S A* 1997;94(7): 3010–3015.

104. Clarke LL, Harline MC. CFTR is required for cAMP inhibition of intestinal Na⁺ absorption in a cystic fibrosis mouse model. *Am J Physiol* 1996;270(2 Pt 1): G259–G267.

105. Sohma Y, Gray MA, Imai Y, et al. A mathematical model of the pancreatic ductal epithelium. *J Membr Biol* 1996;154(1):53–67.

106. Scheele GA, Fukuoka SI, Kern HF, et al. Pancreatic dysfunction in cystic fibrosis occurs as a result of impairments in luminal pH, apical trafficking of zymogen granule membranes, and solubilization of secretory enzymes. *Pancreas* 1996;12(1):1–9.

107. Grubman SA, Perrone RD, Lee DW, et al. Regulation of chloride/bicarbonate exchanger activity by wild-type and mutant CFTR. *Pediatr Pulmonol Suppl* 1997;14:277–278 [Abstract].

108. Devidas S, Guggino WB. The cystic fibrosis transmembrane conductance regulator and ATP. *Curr Opin Cell Biol* 1997;9(4):547–552.

109. Prat AG, Reisin IL, Ausiello DA, et al. Cellular ATP release by the cystic fibrosis transmembrane conductance regulator. *Am J Physiol* 1996;270(2 Pt 1): C538–C545.

110. Schwiebert EM, Egan ME, Hwang T, et al. CFTR regulates outwardly rectifying chloride channels through an autocrine mechanism involving ATP. *Cell* 1995;81(7):1063–1073.

111. Sleigh MA, Blake JR, Liron N. The propulsion of mucus by cilia. *Am Rev Respir Dis* 1988;137(3):726–741.

112. Wanner A, Salathe M, O'Riordan TG. Mucociliary clearance in the airways (state of the art). *Am J Respir Crit Care Med* 1996;154(6 Pt 1):1868–1902.

113. Cantiello HF. Nucleotide transport through the cystic fibrosis transmembrane conductance regulator. *Biosci Rep* 1997;17(2):147–171.

114. Reddy MM, Quinton PM, Haws C, et al. Failure of the cystic fibrosis transmembrane conductance regulator to conduct ATP. *Science* 1996;271(5257):1876–1879.

115. Grygorczyk R, Hanrahan JW. CFTR-independent ATP release from epithelial cells triggered by mechanical stimuli. *Am J Physiol* 1997;272(3 Pt 1): C1058–C1066.

116. Pasyk EA, Foskett JK. Cystic fibrosis transmembrane conductance regulator-associated ATP and adenosine 3'-phosphate 5'-phosphosulfate channels in endoplasmic reticulum and plasma membranes. *J Biol Chem* 1997;272(12):7746–7751.

117. Olver RE, Davis B, Marin MG, et al. Active transport of Na^+ and Cl^- across the canine tracheal epithelium in vitro. *Am Rev Respir Dis* 1975;112(6): 811–815.

118. Widdicombe JH, Welsh MJ, Finkbeiner WE. Cystic fibrosis decreases the apical membrane chloride permeability of monolayers cultured from cells of tracheal epithelium. *Proc Natl Acad Sci U S A* 1985;82: 6167–6171.

119. Marin MG, Davis B, Nadel JA. Effect of acetylcholine on Cl^- and Na^+ fluxes across dog tracheal epithelium in vitro. *Am J Physiol* 1976;231(5 Pt 1): 1546–1549.

120. Widdicombe JH, Welsh MJ. Ion transport by dog tracheal epithelium. *Fed Proc* 39(13):3062–3066, 1980

121. Davis B. Mucous secretion and ion transport in airways. In: Murray JF, Nadel JA, eds. *Textbook of respiratory medicine.* Philadelphia: WB Saunders, 1988:374–388.

122. Kilburn KH. A hypothesis for pulmonary clearance and its implications. *Am Rev Respir Dis* 1968;98(3): 449–463.

123. Widdicombe JH, Ueki IF, Bruderman I, et al. The effects of sodium substitution and ouabain on ion transport by dog tracheal epithelium. *Am Rev Respir Dis* 1979;120(2):385–392.

124. Quinton PM. Viscosity versus composition in airway pathology [editorial]. *Am J Respir Crit Care Med* 1994;149(1):6–7.

125. Smith JJ, Travis SM, Greenberg EP, et al. Cystic fibrosis airway epithelia fail to kill bacteria because of abnormal airway surface fluid. *Cell* 1996;85(2):229–236.

126. Boucher RC, Narvarte J, Cotton C, et al. Sodium absorption in mammalian airways. In: Quinton PM, Martinez JR, Hopfer U, eds. *Fluid and electrolyte abnormalities in exocrine glands in cystic fibrosis.* San Francisco: San Francisco Press Inc, 1982:271–287.

127. Boucher RC, Stutts MJ, Gatzy JT. Regional differences in bioelectric properties and ion flow in excised canine airways. *J Appl Physiol* 1981;51(3): 706–714.

128. Joris L, Quinton PM. Evidence for electrogenic Na-glucose cotransport in tracheal epithelium. *Pflugers Arch* 1989;415(1):118–120.

129. Liedtke CM. Electrolyte transport in the epithelium of pulmonary segments of normal and cystic fibrosis lung. *FASEB J* 1992;6(12):3076–3984.

130. Canessa CM, Horisberger J, Rossier BC. Epithelial sodium channel related to proteins involved in neurodegeneration. *Nature* 1993;361:467–470.

131. Canessa CM, Schild L, Buell G, et al. Amiloride-sensitive epithelial Na^+ channel is made of three homologous subunits. *Nature* 1994;367(6462):463–467.

132. Farman N, Talbot CR, Boucher R, et al. Non-coordinated expression of alpha-, beta-, and gamma-subunit mRNAs of epithelial Na^+ channel along the rat respiratory tract. *Am J Physiol* 1997;272(1 Pt 1): C131–C141.

133. Renard S, Voilley N, Bassilana F, et al. Localization and regulation by steroids of the alpha, beta and gamma subunits of the amiloride-sensitive Na^+ channel in colon, lung and kidney. *Pflugers Arch* 1995; 430(3):299–307.

134. Tchepichev S, Ueda J, Canessa C, et al. Lung epithelial Na channel subunits are differentially regulated during development and by steroids. *Am J Physiol* 1995;269(3 Pt 1):C805–C812.

135. Hummler E, Barker P, Gatzy J, et al. Early death due to defective neonatal lung liquid clearance in alpha ENaC-deficient mice. *Nat Genet* 1996;12(3):325–328.

136. Garty H, Palmer LG. Epithelial sodium channels: function, structure, and regulation. *Physiol Rev* 1997;77(2):359–396.

137. Knowles MR, Gatzy JT, Boucher RC. Aldosterone metabolism and transepithelial potential difference in normal and cystic fibrosis subjects. *Pediatr Res* 1985;19(7):676–679.

138. Boucher RC, Gatzy JT. Characteristics of sodium transport by excised rabbit trachea. *J Appl Physiol* 1983;55:1877–1883.

139. Palmer LG, Frindt G. Amiloride-sensitive Na channels from the apical membrane of the rat cortical collecting tubule. *Proc Natl Acad Sci U S A* 1986;83(8): 2767–2770.

140. Letz B, Ackermann A, Canessa CM, et al. Amiloride-sensitive sodium channels in confluent M-1 mouse cortical collecting duct cells. *J Membr Biol* 1995;148 (2):127–141.

141. Hamilton KL, Eaton DC. Single-channel recordings from two types of amiloride-sensitive epithelial Na^+ channels. *Membr Biochem* 1986;6(2):149–171.

142. Puoti A, May A, Canessa CM, et al. The highly selective low-conductance epithelial Na channel of Xenopus laevis A6 kidney cells. *Am J Physiol* 1995;269(1 Pt 1):C188–C197.

143. Voilley N, Lingueglia E, Champigny G, et al. The lung amiloride-sensitive Na^+ channel: biophysical properties, pharmacology, ontogenesis, and molecular cloning. *Proc Natl Acad Sci U S A* 1994;91(1): 247–251.

144. Marunaka Y. Amiloride-blockable Ca^{2+}-activated Na^+-permeant channels in the fetal distal lung epithelium. *Pflugers Arch* 1996;431(5):748–756.

145. Chinet TC, Fullton JM, Yankaskas JR, et al. Sodium-permeable channels in the apical membrane of human nasal epithelial cells. *Am J Physiol* 1993;265(4 Pt 1):C1050–C1060.

146. Jorissen M, Vereecke J, Carmeliet E, et al. Identification of a voltage- and calcium-dependent non-selective cation channel in cultured adult and fetal human nasal epithelial cells. *Pflugers Arch* 1990;415(5): 617–623.

147. Tohda H, Foskett JK, O'Brodovich H, et al. Cl⁻ regulation of a Ca²⁻-activated nonselective cation channel in beta-agonist-treated fetal distal lung epithelium. *Am J Physiol* 1994;266(1 Pt 1):C104–C109.

148. Davis B, Marin MG, Yee JW, et al. Effect of terbutaline on movement of Cl⁻ and Na⁺ across the trachea of the dog in vitro. *Am Rev Respir Dis* 1979;120(3): 547–552.

149. Champigny G, Voilley N, Lingueglia E, et al. Regulation of expression of the lung amiloride-sensitive Na⁺ channel by steroid hormones. *EMBO J* 1994;13(9): 2177–2181.

150. App EM, Zayas JG, King M. Rheology of mucus and transepithelial potential difference: small airways versus trachea. *Eur Respir J* 1993;6:67–75.

151. Wills PJ, Hall RL, Chan W, et al. Sodium chloride increases the ciliary transportability of cystic fibrosis and bronchiectasis sputum on the mucus-depleted bovine trachea. *J Clin Invest* 1997;99(1):9–13.

152. Ramsden CA, Markiewicz M, Walters DV, et al. Liquid flow across the epithelium of the artificially perfused lung of fetal and postnatal sheep. *J Physiol (Lond)* 1992;448:579–597.

153. Cotton CU, Boucher RC, Gatzy JT. Paths of ion transport across canine fetal tracheal epithelium. *J Appl Physiol* 1988;65(6):2376–2382.

154. Cotton CU, Boucher RC, Gatzy JT. Bioelectric properties and ion transport across excised canine fetal and neonatal airways. *J Appl Physiol* 1988;65(6): 2367–2375.

155. Haas M, Johnson LG, Boucher RC. Regulation of Na-K-Cl cotransport in cultured canine airway epithelia. A (³H)bumetanide binding study. *Am J Physiol* 1990;28(4 Pt 1):C557–C569.

156. McCann JD, Welsh MJ. Basolateral K⁺ channels in airway epithelia: II, role in Cl⁻ secretion and evidence for two types of K⁺ channel. *Am J Physiol* 1990;258 (6 Pt 1):L343–L348.

157. Clarke LL, Burns KA, Bayle J, et al. Sodium and chloride conductive pathways in cultured mouse tracheal epithelium. *Am J Physiol* 1992;263(5 Pt 1): L519–L525.

158. Willumsen NJ, Davis CW, Boucher RC. Intracellular Cl⁻ activity and cellular Cl⁻ pathways in cultured human airway epithelium. *Am J Physiol* 1989;256(5 Pt 1):C1033–C1044.

159. Welsh MJ, Widdicombe JH, Nadel JA. Fluid transport across the canine tracheal epithelium. *J Appl Physiol* 1980;49(5):905–909.

160. Willumsen NJ, Boucher RC. Activation of an apical Cl⁻ conductance by Ca²⁺ ionophores in cystic fibrosis airway epithelia. *Am J Physiol* 1989;256(2 Pt 1): C226–C233.

161. Boucher RC, Larsen EH. Comparison of ion transport by cultured secretory and absorptive canine airway epithelia. *Am J Physiol* 1988;254(4 Pt 1):C535–C547.

162. Novotny JA, Jakobsson E. Computational studies of ion-water flux coupling in the airway epithelium: II, role of specific transport mechanisms. *Am J Physiol* 1996;270(6 Pt 1):C1764–C1772.

163. Willumsen NJ, Boucher RC. Shunt resistance and ion permeabilities in normal and cystic fibrosis airway epithelium. *Am J Physiol* 1989;256(5 Pt 1):C1054–C1063.

164. Ranga V, Powers MA, Padilla M, et al. Effect of allergic bronchoconstriction on airway epithelial permeability to large polar solutes in the guinea pig. *Am Rev Respir Dis* 1983;128(6):1065–1070.

165. Johnson LG, Cheng P, Boucher RC. Albumin absorption by canine bronchial epithelium. *J Appl Physiol* 1989;66(6):2772–2777.

166. Folkesson HG, Matthay MA, Frigeri A, et al. Transepithelial water permeability in microperfused distal airways: evidence for channel-mediated water transport. *J Clin Invest* 1996;97(3):664–671.

167. Widdicombe JH. Fluid transport across airway epithelia. *Ciba Found Symp* 1984;109:109–120.

168. Tanaka M, Inase N, Fushimi K, et al. Induction of aquaporin 3 by corticosteroid in a human airway epithelial cell line. *Am J Physiol* 1997;273(5 Pt 1): L1090–L1095.

169. King LS, Nielsen S, Agre P. Aquaporins in complex tissues: I, developmental patterns in respiratory and glandular tissues of rat. *Am J Physiol* 1997;273(5 Pt 1):C1541–C1548.

170. Nielsen S, King LS, Christensen BM, et al. Aquaporins in complex tissues: II, subcellular distribution in respiratory and glandular tissues of rat. *Am J Physiol* 1997;273(5 Pt 1):C1549–C1561.

171. Umenishi F, Carter EP, Yang B, et al. Sharp increase in rat lung water channel expression in the perinatal period. *Am J Respir Cell Mol Biol* 1996;15(5): 673–679.

172. Widdicombe J. Airway and alveolar permeability and surface liquid thickness: theory. *J Appl Physiol* 1997;82(1):3–12.

173. Knowles M, Murray G, Shallal J, et al. Bioelectric properties and ion flow across excised human bronchi. *J Appl Physiol* 1984;56:868–877.

174. Jiang C, Finkbeiner WE, Widdicombe JH, et al. Altered fluid transport across airway epithelium in cystic fibrosis. *Science* 1993;262(5132):424–427.

175. Smith JJ, Welsh MJ. Fluid and electrolyte transport by cultured human airway epithelia. *J Clin Invest* 1993;91(4):1590–1597.

176. Knowles MR, Robinson JM, Wood RE, et al. Ion composition of airway surface liquid of patients with cystic fibrosis as compared to normal and disease-control subjects. *J Clin Invest* 1997;100(10):2588–2595.

177. Joris L, Quinton PM. Concentration of elements in airway surface fluid. *Med Sci Res* 1987;15:855–856.

178. Joris L, Dab I, Quinton PM. Elemental composition of human airway surface liquid in healthy and diseased airways. *Am Rev Respir Dis* 1993;148(6 Pt 1): 1633–1637.

179. Knowles M, Gatzy J, Boucher R. Relative ion permeability of normal and cystic fibrosis nasal epithelium. *J Clin Invest* 1983;71:1410–1417.

180. Gowen CW, Lawson EE, Gingras-Leatherman J, et al. Increased nasal potential difference and amiloride sensitivity in neonates with cystic fibrosis. *J Pediatr* 1986;108(4):517–521.

181. Stutts MJ, Knowles MR, Gatzy JT, et al. Oxygen consumption and ouabain binding sites in cystic fibrosis nasal epithelium. *Pediatr Res* 1986;20(12): 1316–1320.

182. Pollack LR, Tate EH, Cook JS. Regulation by turnover of Na,K-ATPase in HeLa cells. *Prog Clin Biol Res* 1982;91:71–87.

183. Peckham D, Holland E, Range S, et al. Na+/K+ ATPase in lower airway epithelium from cystic fibrosis and non-cystic-fibrosis lung. *Biochem Biophys Res Commun* 1997;232(2):464–468.

184. Willumsen NJ, Boucher RC. Sodium transport and intracellular sodium activity in cultured human nasal epithelium. *Am J Physiol* 1991;261(2 Pt 1):C319–C331.

185. Chinet TC, Fullton JM, Yankaskas JR, et al. Mechanism of sodium hyperabsorption in cultured cystic fibrosis nasal epithelium: a patch clamp study. *Am J Physiol* 1994;266(4 Pt 1):C1061–C1068.

186. Knowles MR, Paradiso AM, Boucher RC. In vivo nasal potential difference: techniques and protocols for assessing efficacy of gene transfer in cystic fibrosis. *Hum Gene Ther* 1995;6(4):447–457.

187. Middleton PG, Geddes DM, Alton EWFW. Protocols for in vivo measurement of the ion transport defects in cystic fibrosis nasal epithelium. *Eur Respir J* 1994;7:2050–2056.

188. Waltner WE, Boucher RC, Gatzy JT, et al. Pharmacotherapy of airway disease in cystic fibrosis. *Trends Pharmacol Sci* 1987;8:316–320.

189. Alton EWFW, Chadwick SL, Smith SN, et al. Lower airway potential difference measurements in non CF and CF subjects. *Pediatr Pulmonol Suppl* 1996;135:240 [Abstract].

190. Knowles MR, Stutts MJ, Spock A, et al. Abnormal ion permeation through cystic fibrosis respiratory epithelium. *Science* 1983;221(4615):1067–1070.

191. Widdicombe JH, Widdicombe JG. Regulation of human airway surface liquid. *Respir Physiol* 1995;99(1):3–12.

192. Quinton PM. Cystic fibrosis: a disease in electrolyte transport. *FASEB J* 1990;4(10):2709–2717.

193. Willumsen NJ, Davis CW, Boucher RC. Cellular Cl⁻ transport in cultured cystic fibrosis airway epithelium. *Am J Physiol* 1989;256(5 Pt 1):C1045–C1053.

194. Stutts MJ, Cotton CU, Yankaskas JR, et al. Chloride uptake into cultured airway epithelial cells from cystic fibrosis patients and normal individuals. *Proc Natl Acad Sci U S A* 1985;82(19):6677–6681.

195. Yankaskas JR, Knowles MR, Gatzy JT, et al. Persistence of abnormal chloride ion permeability in cystic fibrosis nasal epithelial cells in heterologous culture. *Lancet* 1985;1(8435):954–956.

196. Widdicombe JH. Ion transport by tracheal epithelial cells in culture. *Clin Chest Med* 1986;7(2):299–305.

197. Jiang C, Finkbeiner WE, Widdicombe JH, et al. Fluid transport across cultures of human tracheal glands is altered in cystic fibrosis. *J Physiol (Lond)* 1997;501(3):637–647.

198. Zhang Y, Yankaskas J, Wilson J, et al. In vivo analysis of fluid transport in cystic fibrosis airway epithelia of bronchial xenografts. *Am J Physiol* 1996;270(5 Pt 1):C1326–C1335.

199. Smith JJ, Karp PH, Welsh MJ. Defective fluid transport by cystic fibrosis airway epithelia. *J Clin Invest* 1994;93(3):1307–1311.

200. Zuelzer WW, Newton WA, Jr. The pathogenesis of fibrocystic disease of the pancreas: a study of 36 cases with special reference to the pulmonary lesions. *Pediatrics* 1949;4(1):53–69.

201. Chang SS, Grunder S, Hanukoglu A, Rosler A, Mathew PM, Hanukoglu I, et al. Mutations in subunits of the epithelial sodium channel cause salt wasting with hyperkalaemic acidosis, pseudohypoaldosteronism type 1. *Nat Genet* 1996;12:248–253.

202. Kerem E, Bistrizer T, Hanukoglu A, MacLaughlin E, Boucher RC, Knowles MR. Respiratory disease in patients with the systemic form of pseudohypoaldosteronism type I. *Pediatr Pulmonol Suppl* 1997;14:78–79.

203. Goldman MJ, Anderson GM, Stolzenberg ED, et al. Human beta-defensin-1 is a salt-sensitive antibiotic that is inactivated in cystic fibrosis. *Cell* 1997;88(4):553–560.

204. Sturgess J, Imrie J. Quantitative evaluation of the development of tracheal submucosal glands in infants with cystic fibrosis and control infants. *Am J Pathol* 1982;106(3):303–311.

205. Finkbeiner WE, Shen B, Widdicombe JH. Chloride secretion and function of serous and mucous cells of human airway glands. *Am J Physiol* 1994;267(2 Pt 1):L206–L210.

206. Yamaya M, Finkbeiner WE, Widdicombe JH. Altered ion transport by tracheal glands in cystic fibrosis. *Am J Physiol* 1991;261(6 Pt 1):L491–L494.

207. Raphael GD, Jeney EV, Baraniuk JN, et al. Pathology of rhinitis: lactoferrin and lysozyme in nasal secretions. *J Clin Invest* 1989;84(5):1528–1535.

208. Basbaum CB, Jany B, Finkbeiner WE. The serous cell. *Annu Rev Physiol* 1990;52:97–113.

209. Wine JJ. A sensitive defense: Salt and cystic fibrosis. *Nat Med* 1997;3(5):494–495.

210. Martinez JR. Alterations in salivary gland structure and function in cystic fibrosis. In: Quinton PM, Martinez JR, Hopfer U, eds. *Fluid and electrolyte abnormalities in exocrine glands in cystic fibrosis*. San Francisco: San Francisco Press Inc, 1982:125–142.

Cystic Fibrosis in Adults,
edited by J. R. Yankaskas and M. R. Knowles,
Lippincott–Raven Publishers, Philadelphia, 1999.

2

Genetics, Diagnosis, and Clinical Phenotype

Michael R. Knowles, *Kenneth J. Friedman, and †Lawrence M. Silverman

*Cystic Fibrosis/Pulmonary Research and Treatment Center, Division of Pulmonary and Critical Care Medicine, and *Department of Pathology and Laboratory Medicine, University of North Carolina School of Medicine; and †Department of Pathology and Laboratory Medicine, University of North Carolina Hospitals, Chapel Hill, North Carolina*

Cystic fibrosis (CF) is an autosomal recessive clinical disorder reflecting mutations in a single gene, which is termed the cystic fibrosis transmembrane conductance regulator (CFTR) gene (1–3). More than 750 mutations in the CFTR gene have been described (4,5). The clinical disease expression ("phenotype") is quite variable and relates, in part, to the type of mutation ("genotype").

The goals of this chapter are to describe the genetics of CF and the approach to clinical diagnosis, including molecular concepts. Molecular mechanisms that relate to the dysfunction of the mutated CFTR and different types of mutations and clinical phenotypes will be addressed. Correlations between genotype and phenotype will be discussed to provide an overview of the range of clinical disease from the classic CF phenotype to atypical mild disease. Finally, the concept of genetic testing in families at risk and population-based carrier screening and neonatal testing will be reviewed.

This chapter is not meant to be an exhaustive review of the genetics and molecular mutations in the CFTR; it provides a reference for clinicians who will be faced with the challenge of integrating the clinical spectrum of CF into their clinical practice. For more detailed information, readers are referred to several comprehensive reviews (6–12) and references provided in individual sections of this chapter.

GENETICS: INCIDENCE/ETHNIC DISTRIBUTION

Cystic fibrosis is the most common autosomal recessive fatal disorder in white populations (6,11). Initial epidemiologic surveys in the United States suggested that the incidence was 1 in 1,900 to 2,500 white live births (6,13–15). However, more recent studies of newborn screening suggest a slightly lower incidence of 1 in 3,500 white births (16,17).

The incidence of CF varies greatly by ethnic group (Table 2–1). The incidence in African Americans is much less common (1 in 15,300 live births) than in whites (18,19), although the mutations in African Americans reflect, in part, European/white American/African admixture (20–22). The incidence in Hispanics in the United States is between 1 in 8,000 to 1 in 9,000 (23–25). In Israel, the incidence is approximately 1 in 5,000 (6,26–28). The disorder has been reported in Native Americans and Asians, but at very low rates (4,29,30).

It has been suggested that the high frequency of the mutated CFTR gene in white populations may reflect some form of selective advantage (6,31). Perhaps the most attractive hypothesis was proposed initially by Paul Quinton, that is, CF heterozygotes might be protected against the CFTR-mediated secretory diarrhea induced by cholera toxin (32,33). This hypothesis is unproven, although indirect data from animal studies are consistent, that is, mice

TABLE 2–1. *Incidence of cystic fibrosis in different populations*

Population	Epidemiologic	Newborn screening	References
White (U.S.)	1 in 1900–3700	1 in 3400–3800	13–17
Hispanic (U.S.)	1 in 8,000–9,000	—	4,23–25
African-American	1 in 15,300	—	22
Native American	1 in 40,000	—	29,30
Asian (U.S./England)	1 in 10,000	—	4
White (England)	1 in 2,400–3,000	1 in 2,200–3,200	4,6,142
Israel	1 in 5000	—	4,26–28
Southern Europe	1 in 2,000–4,000	—	66,143

that are heterozygotes for the mutated CF gene are resistant to cholera toxin (34).

Heterozygotes, such as parents of a child with CF, carry a normal CFTR allele and a mutated CFTR allele. These individuals, called carriers, clinically are asymptomatic. Thus, one copy of a normal CFTR gene is sufficient to protect against the disease. The child of two carriers has one chance in four of inheriting a normal CFTR gene from each parent or two chances in four of inheriting one normal and one mutated CFTR gene and being a carrier, or a one-in-four chance of inheriting a mutated CFTR allele from each parent and developing the clinical phenotype of CF (Fig. 2–1).

Children with symptoms of CF have been described since the Middle Ages, but the first comprehensive description did not occur until 1938. The term *cystic fibrosis of the pancreas* was used by Dorothy Anderson to describe the pathologic lesions associated with pancreatic exocrine insufficiency and malabsorption (35). The excessive loss of salt through the sweat glands of children with CF was described by di Sant'Agnese et al. in 1953 (36). This observation led to the use of the sweat test as the clinical laboratory test [sweat chloride (Cl⁻)] to support the clinical diagnosis of CF, which was crucial to the correct clinical classification of patients with the disease (11,37).

DIAGNOSIS

The diagnosis of CF usually is straightforward (38–40). The classic CF phenotype, that is, pulmonary disease, pancreatic exocrine insufficiency, and abnormal sweat gland function, occurs in more than 90% of patients with CF. Even when pancreatic exocrine function is preserved, the sweat test is diagnostic in the majority of cases.

The diagnosis is based on the presence of one or more characteristic phenotypic features (usually pulmonary and gastrointestinal manifestations), plus evidence of CFTR dysfunction [usually raised sweat Cl⁻; or abnormal nasal potential difference (PD)] or CFTR mutations on each allele (Table 2–2) (38–43). Nonclassic phenotypes (e.g., patients with pancreatic ex-

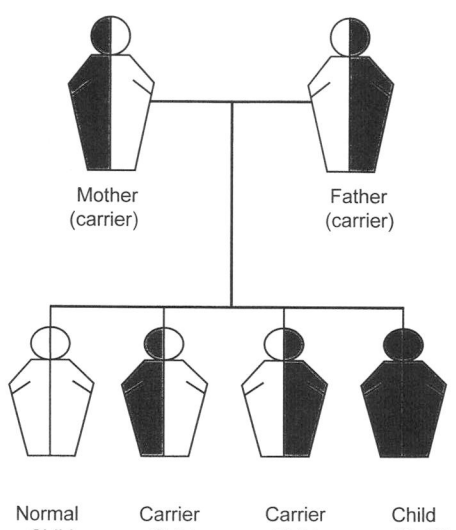

FIG. 2–1. Pattern of inheritance of cystic fibrosis from two carrier parents (shaded half = CF allele; white half = normal allele). The predicted probability is that one in four children is normal, two of four children are carriers, and one in four children inherits a mutated CFTR gene from each parent and has cystic fibrosis.

TABLE 2–2. *Criteria for the diagnosis of cystic fibrosis*

Phenotypic clinical features
  Chronic sinopulmonary disease
    Chronic cough and sputum production
    Persistent infection with characteristic pathogens (*Staph. aureus* and *P. aeruginosa*)
    Airflow obstruction
    Chronic chest radiographic abnormalities
    Sinus disease; nasal polyps
  Gastrointestinal and nutritional abnormalities
    Pancreatic exocrine insufficiency; recurrent pancreatitis
    Meconium ileus; distal intestinal obstruction syndrome (DIOS)
    Focal biliary or multilobar cirrhosis
  Obstructive azoospermia in males
Laboratory evidence of CFTR dysfunction
  Elevated sweat Cl⁻
  Mutation in the CFTR on both alleles
  Characteristic bioelectric abnormalities [nasal potential difference, (PD)] in nasal epithelium *in vivo*

CFTR, cystic fibrosis transmembrane conductance regulator.
Data from references 38–43.

ocrine sufficiency and nondiagnostic sweat Cl⁻ tests) may be more difficult to diagnose and are discussed in more detail in the sections on the pages 34 and 35.

For most individuals with CF, sweat Cl⁻ values clearly are in the diagnostic range (> 60 meq/L) when tested by the pilocarpine iontophoresis method (37–40). Healthy adults may have sweat Cl⁻ values that range up to 60 meq/L, whereas sweat Cl⁻ values in children that range between 40 and 60 meq/L are "indeterminate," and are suggestive of CF and require further study. The sweat Cl⁻ test should be performed under the stringent conditions required by the Cystic Fibrosis Foundation, and as recently reviewed (44,45). Rarely, patients may have a false-positive (elevated) sweat Cl⁻ concentration (Table 2–3), but disorders associated with false-positive sweat Cl⁻ values are relatively uncommon and usually are not confused with CF.

A small percentage of patients with CF (~1%) have sweat Cl⁻ values in the nondiagnostic or normal (< 40 meq/L) range (6,38–40, 45–49). The use of the nasal PD as a diagnostic tool is useful in this select group of patients (40–43). These CF clinical variants will be discussed in more detail see in the sections on pages 34–37.

THE CYSTIC FIBROSIS TRANSMEMBRANE CONDUCTANCE REGULATOR GENE

In 1989, the gene responsible for CF was cloned (1–3). This breakthrough was guided by a positional cloning strategy, which mapped the CFTR gene to the long arm of chromosome

TABLE 2–3. *Diseases other than cystic fibrosis associated with an elevated sweat electrolyte concentration*

Anorexia nervosa	Long-term prostaglandin E₁ infusion
Atopic dermatitis	Mauriac syndrome
Autonomic dysfunction	Mucopolysaccharidosis—type I
Ectodermal dysplasia	Nephrogenic diabetes insipidus
Familial cholestasis (Byler's disease)	Nephrosis
Fucosidosis	Protein–calorie malnutrition
Glucose-6-phosphate dehydrogenase deficiency	Pseudohypoaldosteronism—type I (systemic)
Glycogen storage disease type 1	Untreated adrenal insufficiency
Hypogammaglobulinemia	Untreated hypothyroidism
Klinefelter syndrome	

Data from references 6,44,45,144,145.

7 using DNA markers and linkage analysis. The CFTR gene is large (~250,000 bp) and contains 27 exons. The messenger RNA transcript (~6,129 bp) encodes a protein of 1,480 amino acids. The structure and function of the CFTR gene product is discussed in detail in Chapter 1. Briefly, the CFTR protein contains two halves, each of which consists of six transmembrane-spanning domains, and a consensus sequence for a nucleotide-binding domain. This protein also has an R domain, which links the two halves of the protein. CFTR functions not only as a cyclic adenosine monophosphate (cAMP)-regulated Cl⁻ channel (50,51), but also to regulate other ion channels (52–57) and perhaps contribute to other cellular functions (58–60) (see Chapter 1 for detailed review).

The accumulation of information about genetic mutations in the CFTR and associated clinical phenotypes has been achieved with unprecedented speed. This has been facilitated by the development of a novel approach, that is, the CF Genetic Analysis Consortium, which has been coordinated by Lap-Chee Tsui (4,5,61,62). Almost 100 laboratories have submitted results to the consortium for dissemination to participating investigators. This approach provides a paradigm for rapid accumulation of information about genetic diseases and insights into the relationship between genetic mutations and disease expression.

MUTATIONS IN THE CYSTIC FIBROSIS TRANSMEMBRANE CONDUCTANCE REGULATOR GENE

The most common disease-causing mutation in the CFTR is a three base-pair deletion in exon 10, which results in deletion of the phenylalanine residue at amino acid position 508 (ΔF508). In general terms, the ΔF508 mutation accounts for approximately 66% of the CF chromosomes reported worldwide (4). Application of Hardy–Weinberg equilibrium to the frequency of ΔF508 worldwide indicates that approximately 44% of patients with CF are homozygous for ΔF508, approximately 45% are heterozygous for ΔF508 and a second CFTR mutation, and approximately 11% are compound heterozygotes for two non-ΔF508 alleles.

However, there are striking differences in the proportion of ΔF508 frequency among different ethnic populations (Table 2–4). In general, a high frequency of the ΔF508 mutation (70–80% of chromosomes) is observed in northern Europeans. The ΔF508 mutation is seen with less frequency in southern Europeans (~50–55% of chromosomes), Hispanics in the United States (46% of chromosomes), Ashkenazi Jews (~30% of chromosomes), African Americans (~48% of chromosomes), and Native Americans (< 5% of chromosomes) (4,19,27,63–68). Haplotype analyses of DNA markers indicate that there is a close association of one group of markers with the ΔF508 mutation, which suggests that the ΔF508 allele originated from a single mutation (31,63,69,70).

More than 750 mutations in the CFTR have been reported since the cloning of the CF gene, and the majority of these represent disease-causing mutations. The frequency of common mutations (worldwide) is outlined in Table 2–5. A group of 15 mutations, which includes ΔF508, occurs commonly among white populations and may account for 80% to 90% of the CF alleles in this ethnic group (71).

Some mutations in the CFTR occur at high frequency in specific ethnic groups (Table 2–6). For example, the Ashkenazi Jewish population exhibits the W1282X mutation at a high frequency, and this mutation accounts for approximately half of the mutations in the CFTR in that ethnic group. Indeed, five mutations account for 97% of the mutations in Ashkenazi Jews (28). African Americans have several unique African mutations in the CFTR, and 3120 + 1 G-to-A accounts for 12% of the mutations in African Americans, who should be

TABLE 2–4. *Frequency of ΔF508 mutation in different ethnic groups*

Group	% of CF chromosomes	References
White (worldwide)	66	4
White (N. Europe)	70–80	64,65
White (S. Europe)	50–55	66,67
Hispanic (U.S.)	46	4,23
Jews (Ashkenazi)	30	26–28
African Americans	48	22
Native Americans	< 5	29,30,68

TABLE 2–5. *Frequency of common mutations in the CFTR worldwide*

Mutation	%	Reference[a]
ΔF508	66.0	3
G542X	2.4	146
G551D	1.8	147
W1282X	1.5	148
N1303K	1.2	149
R553X	0.9	147
3849 + 10 kb C-to-T[b]; 621 + 1 G-to-T	0.6	46,150
1717 − 1 G-to-A; 1078 del T	0.5	72,146
711 + 1 G-to-T; R1162X; 1898 + 1 G-to-A	0.4	8,148,151
2789 + 5 G-to-A; R117H[b]	0.3	8,152
G85E; R347P; ΔI507	0.2	146,150,152
A455E[b]; R334W; S549N; G551S[b]	0.1	47,146,147,151

CFTR, cystic fibrosis transmembrane conductance regulator.
Adapted from references 4,6, and 8.
[a]Reference to original descriptions of the mutation.
[b]May be associated with normal or nondiagnostic sweat Cl⁻ value.

tested by a targeted genetic panel (22). Screening Hispanics for mutations in the CFTR by a U.S. white mutation panel identifies only 58% of mutations among Hispanics (23), and a test panel tailored to Southern European mutations has utility for testing Hispanic populations (24,25). Other examples in which ethnic populations exhibit a relatively high frequency of specific mutations include 1078delT in the Celtic population (5.7%) (72) and 394delTT in the Scandinavian/Baltic population (4.9%) (73). Diagnostic laboratories can tailor the mu-

TABLE 2–6. *Frequency of mutations in African-Americans, Ashkenazi Jewish, and Hispanic (U.S.) patients*

Ethnic group	Mutations	% of Chromosomes
African Americans	ΔF508	48.0
	3120 + 1 G-to-A[a]	12.0
	R553X	2.0
	A559T	2.0
	2307insA	2.0
	405 + 3 A-to-C	1.4
	G480C	1.4
	S1255X	1.4
		(total) 70%
Ashkenazi Jews	W1282X	48.0
	ΔF508	30.0
	G542X	12.0
	3849 + 10 kb C-to-T	4.0
	N1303K	3.0
		(total) 97%
Hispanic (U.S.)	ΔF508	46.0
	G542X	5.4
	3849 + 10 kb C-to-T	2.3
	R1162X	1.6
	R334W	1.6
	W1282X	0.8
	R553X	0.8
		(total) 58.5%

Data from references 4, 22–24, 28.
[a]Novel African mutation (22).

tation-testing panels in accordance with the ethnic makeup of their patient base (22,23, 28,74,75). The large number of CF-causing mutations and the rarity of most of these mutations prevents the design of a molecular assay of approximately 100% sensitivity.

TYPES OF CYSTIC FIBROSIS TRANSMEMBRANE CONDUCTANCE REGULATOR MUTATIONS

Mutations in the CFTR gene can be grouped in five general classes (Fig. 2–2), which reflect the biosynthetic pathway and function of the CFTR (8,76). Class I mutations involve defective protein production, which typically reflects mutations with premature termination signals (such as frame-shift mutations caused by insertions or deletions), or nonsense mutations, which create a premature translational stop codon. These mutations also may be associated with unstable (and rapidly degraded) mRNA (77). Class I mutations would be predicted to have no full-length protein and to be the equivalent of a "null" mutation.

Class II mutations reflect defective processing of the CFTR protein, which includes the most common mutation, ΔF508. The ΔF508 mutation is associated with improper folding, which prevents the CFTR from progressing through the biosynthetic pathway to the apical membrane (78). Instead of undergoing full glycosylation, the ΔF508 protein is degraded in the endoplasmic reticulum. The general explanation is that ΔF508 is a "temperature-sensitive" mutant, that is, normal folding does not take place at 37°C (79). *In vitro* studies suggest the ΔF508 mutant normally is folded and processed at lower temperatures (23–30°C) and delivered to the apical membrane, where it exhibits at least partial function as a cAMP-mediated Cl⁻ channel (80–82).

Class III mutations reflect defective regulation of the CFTR Cl⁻ channel. Although these mutated forms of the CFTR are trafficked correctly to the cell membrane, mutations within the nucleotide-binding fold can either impair function dramatically (G551D) or permit some residual Cl⁻ channel activity (G551S) (47,76,82).

Class IV mutations affect the conductive pathway of the channel and alter the ionic conductance of Cl⁻ ions (76,83). Several of these mutations are missense mutations involving arginine residues in the membrane-spanning segment of the channel, including R117H,

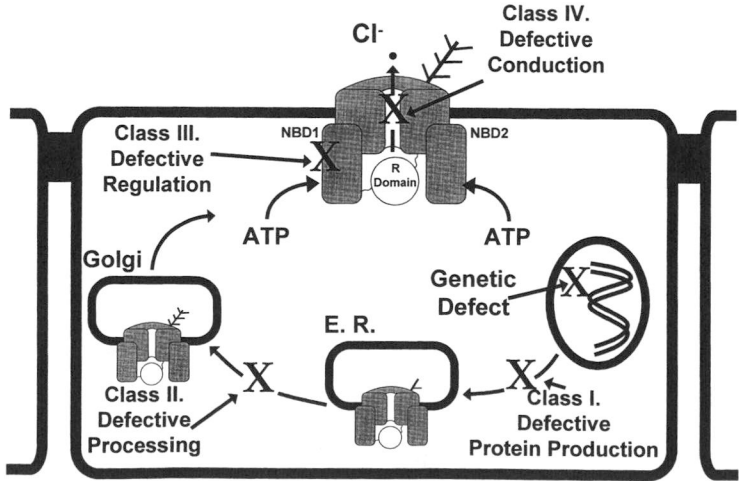

FIG. 2–2. Types of mutations in the CFTR associated with biosynthetic and functional aspects (see text for comments). In addition to the types of mutations (I–IV) depicted in this diagram, mutations that disturb or create splice sites lead to abnormal splicing of the CFTR without change in the genomic coding sequence and are termed type V mutations. (Figure modified from reference 76.)

R334W, and R347P. These alleles are associated with residual Cl⁻ conductive function and, frequently, preservation of pancreatic exocrine function.

Class V mutations disturb or create consensus splice sites and lead to abnormal splicing of the CFTR without alteration of the genomic coding sequence (46,84–86). The magnitude of normal splicing varies by the ability of the splice site mutation to fully block normal splicing. For example, 621 + 1 G > T is associated with no normally spliced mRNA and leads to severe CF (87), whereas 2789 + 5 G-to-A may give as much as 4% to 8% of CFTR mRNA normal splicing and is associated with mild disease (46,49,88–90). Thus, splice mutations may lead to a complete or partial reduction of normal CFTR protein rather than a change in the functional characteristics of the channel.

GENOTYPE/PHENOTYPE CORRELATIONS

General

The relationship between the type of mutation in the CFTR (genotype) and the severity of clinical disease (phenotype) is not clear-cut in most circumstances (6–12). There are many variables that may modify the clinical expression of disease, particularly the lung disease. These variables include genetic factors other than the CFTR, differences in medical treatment, and the influences of environment and exposure to infectious (particularly viral) diseases. However, data have emerged steadily from international studies reported to the CF Consortium, and some insights are beginning to emerge.

Generally, mutations associated with the complete loss of CFTR function as a Cl⁻ channel result in the classic CF clinical phenotype, which includes approximately 85% to 90% of patients with CF. Specifically, these patients have pancreatic exocrine insufficiency at birth (or early in life), a substantial risk of meconium ileus (10–15%) at birth, elevated sweat Cl⁻ values, pulmonary disease of a characteristic type (see Chapter 3), and the absence (or maldevelopment) of the vas deferens in males

(see Chapter 21). These patients typically are diagnosed early in life (< 2 years of age), partially because of maldigestion and failure to thrive, and they have poorer lung function and higher sweat Cl⁻ values than patients with pancreatic sufficiency (91–94). Significant CF-related biliary cirrhosis and portal hypertension may develop in as many as 2% (95) (see Chapter 14). In general, mutations that result in this classic phenotype are classified as nonsense, frame-shift, and amino acid deletions. Also, many (but not all) of the mutations that encode incorrect amino acids yield the severe (pancreatic insufficient) phenotype. For example, the complete loss of CFTR function may be due to nonsense mutations (R553X; class I), abnormal processing of the CFTR to the plasma membrane (ΔF508; class II), or total loss of Cl⁻ channel function even when the CFTR protein is processed successfully to the apical membrane (G551D; class III). Mutations that are associated with the classic CF clinical phenotype (which includes pancreatic insufficiency) are termed "severe." This term is better correlated with the loss of pancreatic exocrine function rather than the status of the pulmonary disease; this concept is fully discussed in the following section (91–94).

Alternatively, mutations with partial preservation of Cl⁻ channel (or other) functions frequently are associated with preservation of pancreatic exocrine function, and occasionally, preservation of sweat gland function. These mutations usually are missense (class III or IV) or splice-type (class V) molecular de-fects. Patients with these mutations almost never have meconium ileus at birth, have less risk for significant cirrhosis or portal hypertension, and tend to be diagnosed later in life (6,93,94–96).

Classic Cystic Fibrosis Clinical Phenotype Associated with ΔF508 (Severe Mutation)

The ΔF508 is the most common mutation causing CF (66% of mutated alleles worldwide), and patients who are homozygous for this mutation have been the most extensively studied group. Studies performed initially in

Toronto clearly demonstrated a high correlation between the presence of the homozygous ΔF508 genotype and pancreatic exocrine insufficiency (91,92). Specifically, more than 99% of these patients produce insufficient pancreatic exocrine enzymes (< 1% of the normal amount of digestive enzymes) for adequate digestion (see Chapter 12). Approximately 15% of the homozygous ΔF508 patients are born with meconium ileus. A small number of these patients have adequate pancreatic exocrine function at birth to prevent malabsorption, but pancreatic exocrine insufficiency most likely will develop in these patients in early childhood (92). The sweat Cl⁻ test is raised uniformly in patients with this mutation, if the test is performed in a CF Foundation quality-controlled laboratory (97,98). The majority of men (> 99%) with this homozygous mutation have obstructive azoospermia and are infertile as a result (99). Specific anatomic changes in the male urogenital tract in this patient group are quite variable (100), but most will have non-palpable vas deferens.

In regard to the pulmonary status of patients homozygous for ΔF508, there is a strikingly broad range of functional status. With the current medical approach to the treatment of pulmonary disease in CF, end-stage lung disease develops in only a few homozygous ΔF508 patients within the first decade of life. At the other end of the spectrum, some of these patients have normal airflow mechanics (FEV_1) into the second and third decades of life (91,93). The broad spectrum of pulmonary disease severity probably reflects many variables, including genetic influences other than the CFTR, environmental and infectious events, and differences in medical treatment. Better definition of key variables to estimate pulmonary outcome currently is being explored in several ongoing research projects.

Other Pancreatic Insufficient (Severe) Mutations

Patients who are heterozygous for the ΔF508 mutation, coupled to another severe mutation, make up part of this category, as do patients who bear two non-ΔF508 severe mutations. For example, mutations projected to have the equivalent of a null effect on CFTR function will cause the classic CF phenotype. The combination of ΔF508/G542X, or G551D/R553X, typically will be associated with the clinical phenotype of pancreatic exocrine insufficiency, raised sweat Cl⁻ values, and other clinical features seen in patients homozygous for ΔF508 (7–11,93,101). Thus, two severe mutations are linked strongly to the presence of pancreatic exocrine insufficiency. However, there is great variability of pulmonary disease severity.

Pancreatic Exocrine Sufficient (Mild) Mutations

It is becoming clear that mutations that are associated with preservation of partial function of the CFTR as a Cl⁻ channel usually are associated with a milder overall clinical phenotype (Table 2–7). The partial preservation of function may reflect a more conservative mutation in one of the transmembrane domains, which preserves some of the Cl⁻ conductive properties of the channel, or low levels of a normal CFTR being produced as a result of leaky (or permissive) splice mutations not associated with any mutation in the CFTR coding sequence (46,47,76,83,84). The clinical phenotype is correlated with the preservation of pancreatic exocrine function, and most of these patients do not have malabsorption (46,47,69, 92,93). It was well recognized even before description of the molecular pathogenesis of CF that patients with preservation of pancreatic exocrine function have better pulmonary functional status and clinical outcome (102). However, it is not known whether this reflects a difference in nutritional status or whether this is a result of the impact of partial CFTR Cl⁻ channel function on other host defense pathways.

Several studies clearly defined that some mutations are associated with preservation of pancreatic function, lower sweat Cl⁻ values, and later age of diagnosis when compared with ΔF508 homozygotes (91–94,96,98). It also was recognized that a single copy of a mild (partial CFTR function) mutation was suffi-

TABLE 2–7. *Clinical disease phenotype associated with some mutations in the CFTR[a]*

Lung disease and pancreatic exocrine insufficiency (PI) "severe"	Lung disease and pancreatic exocrine sufficiency (PS) "mild"	Lung disease, pancreatic exocrine sufficiency (PS), and borderline or normal sweat chlorides	No lung disease, and congenital bilateral absence of the vas deferens (CBAVD)
ΔF508	R117H (5T)[b]	R117H (7T)[b]	R117H (7T)[b]
G542X	3849 + 10 kb C-to-T	3849 + 10 kb C-to-T	D1152H
G551D	2789 + 5 G-to-A	G551S	D1270N
R553X	R334W	D1152H	P67L
W1282X	G85E	A455E	5T
N1303K	G91R		
3905insT	R347P		
1078delT	R347H		
621 + 1 G-to-T	R347L		
1717 − 1 G-to-A	A455E		
ΔI507	Y563N		
R560T	P574H		
S549N	S945L		
3659delC	L1065P		
G480C	D1152H		
	F1286S		

CFTR, cystic fibrosis transmembrane conductance regulator.
Data from references 3,6–9,28,46,47,69,76,89,91–93,115,116,124.
[a]Not inclusive.
[b]Refers to the length of the polythymidine tract in intron 8 (i.e., 5T or 7T or 9T) (69,113).

cient to preserve pancreatic exocrine function. Specifically, patients carrying one severe mutation and one mild mutation are more likely to be pancreatic sufficient (91–93). Mutations associated with pancreatic sufficiency (PS) typically are missense or splice mutations.

Lung Disease and "Severe" and "Mild" Mutations

Although there is clear correlation between pancreatic exocrine status and genotype, the correlation between specific mutations and pulmonary disease severity is less well defined. As a group, patients with mild mutations, that is, those associated with pancreatic sufficiency, are diagnosed at a later age and have later colonization of the airways with *Pseudomonas aeruginosa*, better lung function, and a better prognosis (91–93,96, 103–106). However, milder pulmonary disease has been defined formally with only one specific mild mutation (A455E) (107–109), and preliminary results from a worldwide survey have not definitively linked mild mutations to better lung function (96). One explanation is that the preservation of pancreatic exocrine function, and better nutrition, is the link between mild mutations and better lung function, rather than the partial preservation of CFTR function in pulmonary host defense. Alternatively, current approaches using cross-sectional comparisons of lung function associated with mild versus severe mutations in small, older patient populations may bias against detection of better lung function with mild mutations, that is, that approach may compare the survivors of the severe mutation population to the mild group, which may have had fewer early deaths.

Splice Mutations and Alternative Splicing

Approximately 15% of all monogenic inherited disorders can be attributed to mutations of highly conserved consensus splicing sequences (110). Mutations that modify or create novel splice sites in the CFTR have several interesting effects on the clinical phenotype (46,84). For example, a missense mutation in intron 19 is associated with normal (or nondiagnostic) sweat Cl⁻ values and preservation of pancreatic exocrine function in many patients (50–80%), and normal fertility (i.e., no obstructive azoospermia) in many males (46,88–90,111). This mutation, termed 3849 + 10 kb C-to-T, leads to the creation of a partially active splice site that promotes the insertion of a segment containing an in-frame stop codon between exons 19 and 20 (46). This novel, partially active splice site is associated with normal splicing in 4% to 8% of CFTR transcripts, which presumably is associated with low levels of normal CFTR protein. Thus, this disease-causing mutation reflects low levels of a normal CFTR, rather than reduced function of CFTR transcripts. The mild disease phenotype in patients with this mutation is believed to derive from the partial Cl⁻ channel (and perhaps other cellular) functional activity that is retained. Differential organ involvement in these patients probably reflects, in part, differences in tissue-specific splicing (94).

Another form of altered splicing reflects the influence of a polythymidine tract (contains 5, 7, or 9 thymidines) in intron 8 on the splicing of exon 9. Specifically, more thymidines (7T or 9T) are associated with more efficient, normal splicing of exon 9, whereas fewer thymidines (5T) lead to inefficient splicing of exon 9 (69,112,113). When exon 9 is not spliced into the CFTR, it results in a nonfunctional CFTR Cl⁻ channel (114). Inefficient splicing associated with the 5T allele initially was recognized as modifying disease expression associated with the R117H mutation (discussed in the following section) or the development of congenital bilateral absence of the vas deferens (CBAVD) (69,115, 116). More recently, it has been suggested that the 5T allele may predispose to variable CF phenotypes, including a range of pancreatic and respiratory manifestations (117–122). Differential organ involvement likely reflects, in part, tissue-specific differences in splicing of exon 9 (117,118,123).

R117H Mutation

An interesting story has evolved regarding the R117H mutation and associated different clinical phenotypes. The R117H mutation reduces Cl⁻ channel function as a result of reduced Cl⁻ conductance. However, patients with the R117H mutation may have increased sweat Cl⁻ values and pulmonary disease of substantial severity, or men may present with

congenital bilateral absence of the vas deferens (CBAVD) but no pulmonary disease and normal or borderline sweat Cl⁻ values (69,115, 116,124). We now know that the different clinical phenotypes reflect, in part, whether the R117H mutation occurs in conjunction with a haplotype associated with frequent splicing-out of exon 9 (5T allele) or a haplotype with efficient splice-in of exon 9 (7T or 9T allele) (69). The 5T allele is associated with the highest degree of splice-out of exon 9 and is associated with lung disease in patients with CF when inherited on chromosome 7 with R117H. In contrast, men with R117H with the more common 7T allele more typically exhibit CBAVD without pulmonary disease. We also now recognize that the R117H mutation occurs at 10 times the rate expected in the general population, and some females identified by carrier screening tests have no pulmonary disease and are otherwise asymptomatic despite an R117H/ΔF508 genotype (9,125). Therefore, the R117H (7T) mutation may be associated with only CBAVD in men, or no disease. These data suggest that the R117H mutation occurred on at least two separate occasions in CFTR genes with different chromosomal (polythymidine) backgrounds.

Congenital Bilateral Absence of the Vas Deferens

Obstructive azoospermia is an almost universal phenotype in males with classic CF (100,126). Otherwise healthy men who have CBAVD have a much higher than expected frequency of mutations in the CFTR. As many as 18% of men with CBAVD have two disease-associated mutations in the CFTR, with one of the mutations being mild. An additional 50% to 55% are carriers of a mutation in the CFTR, and the majority of these carriers (up to two thirds) have a 5T allele on the opposite chromosome. In total, 60% to 70% of men with CBAVD have at least one known mutation in the CFTR, and the carrier state for the 5T allele in the remaining 30% to 40% is fivefold higher than in the general population (116,127,128). Although mutations in the CFTR are linked to CBAVD in the majority of cases, extended haplotype analyses suggest that other mechanisms are involved (129,130). Thus, there probably are at least two etiologies for CBAVD, that is, one reflecting mutations in the CFTR gene and the other of an undefined etiology.

Most men with CBAVD and mutations in the CFTR have no evidence of lung disease (131). Even in the absence of pulmonary disease, these men may have elevated sweat Cl⁻ values, which is compatible with an abnormality of CFTR function (124,131). Characterization of nasal epithelial ion transport in men with CBAVD indicates that they have a lower than normal CFTR Cl⁻ conductance in the nasal epithelium and are intermediate between CF and normal (124,132). The long-term pulmonary outcome for these men is not known, and mild lung disease may be present in some cases (116,117,133). It recently has been suggested that the clinical phenotype associated with the 5T allele may be quite variable, and the presence (or absence) of respiratory, gastrointestinal, pancreatic, and urogenital disease may reflect the efficiency of tissue-specific–splicing mechanisms (117,118,123). Currently, the diagnostic criteria for CF would include only those men with CBAVD and evidence of CFTR dysfunction (38,40).

Men with CBAVD are infertile secondary to obstructive azoospermia, but it is possible that microsurgical sperm aspiration techniques and *in vitro* fertilization may be explored in appropriate cases (134,135). Careful genetic counseling should be offered to any men with CBAVD exploring this avenue of reproduction, along with genetic testing of the spouse to better measure the risk of the offspring having classic CF.

GENETIC TESTING FOR MUTATIONS IN THE CYSTIC FIBROSIS TRANSMEMBRANE CONDUCTANCE REGULATOR

General Issues

Since the cloning of the CFTR gene in 1989, genotyping in the clinical setting has advanced from simply testing for ΔF508 to analysis of the most common 6 to 16 mutations, to the recent establishment of a 70 mutation-testing panel (136). Genotyping of patients with CF should be a routine component of standard clinical care. Accurately identifying both CFTR mutations in patients with CF is useful in supporting a clinical diagnosis, as well as providing a straightforward way of testing family members for their carrier status. Additionally, mutation identification in light of the ethnic background of the patients can elucidate the bias in the mutational spectrum often associated with different groups, enabling more effective testing in the future.

Variability in disease presentation is due partially to the nature of the mutant alleles underlying the disease. In the case of patients whose disease is atypical and the diagnosis of CF is problematic, genotyping takes on new significance. There are substantial data in the literature (see Table 2–7) to allow testing for mild mutations. Identification of CFTR mutations in atypical patients can support a CF diagnosis in the absence of the classic CF phenotype. As more individuals carrying mild mutations are identified, physicians ultimately may be able to provide more reliable prognoses for the patients. Unfortunately, in view of the size of the CFTR gene and the large number of mutations identified to date, failure to detect mutations in the CFTR does not disprove a diagnosis of CF.

In addition to the mutation-testing capabilities of the clinical laboratory, several research-based protocols are available. Single-stranded conformational polymorphism (SSCP), denaturing gradient gel electrophoresis (DGGE), heteroduplex analysis (HA), and direct DNA sequencing are different methodologies employed to screen genetic sequences for rare and/or undescribed mutations (137,138). Once such a mutation is identified in a given individual, other atypical patients can be tested for it as well, thereby assessing its prevalence and defining any genotype/phenotype correlations.

Carrier Testing in Cystic Fibrosis Families

It is important to address the high risk of having affected offspring for parents who have a child with CF, namely 1 in 4. Therefore, carrier testing and prenatal diagnosis are important to families at risk. The current genetic screening will provide specific information in the majority of circumstances, which allows for appropriate education and counseling by trained genetic counselors. This allows individuals to examine their reproduction options and define the risk for whether prenatal testing would be appropriate for any specific pregnancy.

Population-Based Carrier Screening and Neonatal Screening

Population-based screening is not recommended in the United States because the sensitivity of the testing will identify less than 90% of carriers (7). There has been extensive discussion about population screening, but the general consensus is that appropriate education and counseling resources are not available to address pertinent reproductive and ethical issues (6). In some ethnic groups, for example, the Ashkenazi Jewish population, screening can be very effective, because five known mutations will identify 97% of carriers (28).

Early reports suggested better outcome for patients with CF detected by nongenetic approaches to neonatal screening (139,140), which prompted pilot studies incorporating genetic screening (141). To date, there is no consistent evidence for the clinical benefit of a diagnosis of CF before symptoms appear, and neonatal screening is not standard.

SUMMARY

The identification of the CF gene has provided the opportunity to define the incidence and demographics of CF in different populations and characterize structure–function relationships of different mutations. The rapid accumulation of information about mutations in the CFTR has been facilitated by the CF Genetic Analysis Consortium, which provides a novel precedent for genetic diseases. Currently, genetic analysis is useful not only for diagnosis of CF, but also for prognosis regarding pancreatic exocrine function. The intensive search for correlations between genotype and clinical phenotype has provided clearer insight into the pathogenesis of pancreatic exocrine insufficiency. Although the impact of different mutations on the severity of lung disease is less clear, emerging clues suggest that more robust approaches will be useful for defining this relationship. Surprising observations emerged from studies of men with CBAVD, which suggest that mutations in the CFTR, and the presence of the 5T allele in intron 8, may contribute to variable expression of clinical disease in the urogenital tract, sweat gland, pancreas, and lungs. Finally, better understanding of the molecular mechanisms of the dysfunction in the CFTR has suggested new approaches to therapy, which currently are being tested (see Chapter 11).

REFERENCES

1. Rommens JM, Iannuzzi MC, Kerem B, et al. Identification of the cystic fibrosis gene: chromosome walking and jumping. *Science* 1989;245(4922):1059–1065.
2. Riordan JR, Rommens JM, Kerem B, et al. Identification of the cystic fibrosis gene: cloning and characterization of complementary DNA. *Science* 1989;245 (4922):1066–1073.
3. Kerem B, Rommens JM, Buchanan JA, et al. Identification of the cystic fibrosis gene: genetic analysis. *Science* 1989;245(4922):1073–1080.
4. [Communicated by] Kazazian HH Jr. Population variation of common cystic fibrosis mutations: the Cystic Fibrosis Genetic Analysis Consortium. *Hum Mutat* 1994;4(3):167–177.
5. *CF Genetic Analysis Consortium.* 1997; http://www.genet.sickkids.on.ca/cftr/.
6. Welsh MJ, Tsui L, Boat TF, et al. Cystic fibrosis. In: Scriver CR, Beaudet AL, Sly WS, et al., eds. *The metabolic and molecular bases of inherited disease.* 7th ed. New York: McGraw-Hill, 1995:3799–3876.
7. Collins FS. Cystic fibrosis: molecular biology and therapeutic implications. *Science* 1992;256(5058): 774–779.
8. Tsui L. The spectrum of cystic fibrosis mutations. *Trends Genet* 1992;8(11):392–398.
9. Cutting GR. Genotype defect: its effect on cellular function and phenotypic expression. *Semin Respir Crit Care Med* 1994;15(5):356–363.
10. Davis PB, Drumm M, Konstan MW. Cystic fibrosis. *Am J Respir Crit Care Med* 1996;154(5):1229–1256.
11. Iannuzzi MC. Cystic fibrosis: genetics. In: Davis PB, ed. *Cystic fibrosis.* New York: Marcel Dekker Inc, 1993:1–27.
12. Dean M, Santis G. Heterogeneity in the severity of cystic fibrosis and the role of CFTR gene mutations. *Hum Genet* 1994;93(4):364–368.
13. Steinberg AG, Brown DC. On the incidence of cystic fibrosis of the pancreas. *Am J Hum Genet* 1960;12 (4):416–424.

14. Kramm ER, Crane MM, Sirkin MG, et al. A cystic fibrosis pilot survey in three New England states. *Am J Public Health* 1962;52(12):2041–2057.

15. Merritt AD, Hanna BL, Todd CW, et al. Incidence and mode of inheritance of cystic fibrosis. *J Lab Clin Med* 1962;60:(6)998–999 [Abstract].

16. Hammond KB, Abman SH, Sokol RJ, et al. Efficacy of statewide neonatal screening for cystic fibrosis by assay of trypsinogen concentrations. *N Engl J Med* 1991;325(11):769–774.

17. Gregg RG, Wilfond BS, Farrell PM, et al. Application of DNA analysis in a population-screening program for neonatal diagnosis of cystic fibrosis (CF): comparison of screening protocols. *Am J Hum Genet* 1993;52(3):616–626.

18. Kulczycki LL, Schauf V. Cystic fibrosis in blacks in Washington, DC: incidence and characteristics. *Am J Dis Child* 1974;127(1):64–67.

19. Hamosh A, FitzSimmons SC, Macek M Jr, et al. Comparison of the clinical manifestations of cystic fibrosis in black and white patients. *J Pediatr* 1998; 132(2):255–259.

20. Estivill X, Scambler PJ, Wainwright BJ, et al. Patterns of polymorphism and linkage disequilibrium for cystic fibrosis. *Genomics* 1987;1(3):257–263.

21. Cutting GR, Antonarakis SE, Buetow KH, et al. Analysis of DNA polymorphism haplotypes linked to the cystic fibrosis locus in North American Black and Caucasian families supports the existence of multiple mutations of the cystic fibrosis gene. *Am J Hum Genet* 1989;44:307–318.

22. Macek M Jr, Mackova A, Hamosh A, et al. Identification of common cystic fibrosis mutations in African-Americans with cystic fibrosis increases the detection rate to 75%. *Am J Hum Genet* 1997;60(5): 1122–1127.

23. Grebe TA, Seltzer WK, DeMarchi J, et al. Genetic analysis of Hispanic individuals with cystic fibrosis. *Am J Hum Genet* 1994;54(3):443–446.

24. Grebe TA, Doane WW, Richter S, et al. A rational approach to cystic fibrosis mutation analysis in Hispanics: reply to Arzimanoglou et al. *Am J Hum Genet* 1996;59(1):269–272.

25. Arzimanoglou II, Tuchman A, Li Z, et al. Cystic fibrosis carrier screening in Hispanics. *Am J Hum Genet* 1995;56(2):544–547.

26. Kerem E, Kalman YM, Yahav Y, et al. Highly variable incidence of cystic fibrosis and different mutation distribution among different Jewish ethnic groups in Israel. *Hum Genet* 1995;96(2):193–197.

27. Lerer I, Cohen S, Chemke M, et al. The frequency of the delta F508 mutation on cystic fibrosis chromosomes in Israeli families: correlation to CF haplotypes in Jewish communities and Arabs. *Hum Genet* 1990;85(4):416–417.

28. Abeliovich D, Lavon IP, Lerer I, et al. Screening for five mutations detects 97% of cystic fibrosis (CF) chromosomes and predicts a carrier frequency of 1:29 in the Jewish Ashkenazi population. *Am J Hum Genet* 1992;51(5):951–956.

29. Grebe TA, Doane WW, Richter S, et al. Mutation analysis of the cystic fibrosis transmembrane regulator gene in Native American populations of the southwest. *Am J Hum Genet* 1992;51(4):736–740.

30. Powers CA, Potter EM, Wessel HU, et al. Cystic fibrosis in Asian Indians. *Arch Pediatr Adolesc Med* 1996;150(5):554–555.

31. Morral N, Bertranpetit J, Estivill X, et al. The origin of the major cystic fibrosis mutation (DeltaF508) in European populations. *Nat Genet* 1994;7(2):169–175.

32. Quinton PM. Abnormalities in electrolyte secretion in cystic fibrosis sweat glands due to decreased anion permeability. In: Quinton PM, Martinez RJ, Hopfer U, eds. *Fluid and electrolyte abnormalities in exocrine glands in cystic fibrosis.* San Francisco: San Francisco Press, 1982:53–76.

33. Quinton PM. What is good about cystic fibrosis? *Curr Biol* 1994;4(8):742–743.

34. Gabriel SE, Brigman KN, Koller BH, et al. Cystic fibrosis heterozygote resistance to cholera toxin in the cystic fibrosis mouse model. *Science* 1994;266 (5182):107–109.

35. Andersen DH. Cystic fibrosis of the pancreas and its relation to celiac disease: a clinical and pathologic study. *Am J Dis Child* 1938;56(2):344–399.

36. di Sant'Agnese PA, Darling RC, Perera GA, et al. Abnormal electrolyte composition of sweat in cystic fibrosis of the pancreas. *Pediatrics* 1953;12(5):549– 563.

37. Gibson LE, Cooke RE. A test for concentration of electrolytes in sweat in cystic fibrosis of the pancreas utilizing pilocarpine by iontophoresis. *Pediatrics* 1959;23(3):545–549.

38. Stern RC. The diagnosis of cystic fibrosis. *N Engl J Med* 1997;336(7):487–491.

39. Wallis C. Diagnosing cystic fibrosis: blood, sweat, and tears. *Arch Dis Child* 1997;76(2):85–88.

40. Rosenstein BJ, Cutting GR. The diagnosis of cystic fibrosis: a consensus statement. *J Pediatr* 1998;132 (4): 589–595.

41. Knowles MR, Paradiso AM, Boucher RC. *In vivo* nasal potential difference: techniques and protocols for assessing efficacy of gene transfer in cystic fibrosis. *Hum Gene Ther* 1995;6(4):447–457.

42. Knowles MR, Gatzy J, Boucher R. Increased bioelectric potential difference across respiratory epithelia in cystic fibrosis. *N Engl J Med* 1981;305:1489–1495.

43. Knowles M, Gatzy J, Boucher R. Relative ion permeability of normal and cystic fibrosis nasal epithelium. *J Clin Invest* 1983;71:1410–1417.

44. National Committee for Clinical Laboratory Standards. *Sweat testing: sample collection and quantitative analysis, approved guideline.* Wayne, PA: National Committee for Clinical Laboratory Standards, 1994; Document C34-A, NCCLS 14(22):C34-A.

45. LeGrys VA. Sweat testing for the diagnosis of cystic fibrosis: practical considerations. *J Pediatr* 1996;129 (6):892–897.

46. Highsmith WE, Burch LH, Zhou Z, et al. A novel mutation in the cystic fibrosis gene in patients with pulmonary disease but normal sweat chloride concentrations. *N Engl J Med* 1994;331(15):974–980.

47. Strong TV, Smit LS, Turpin SV, et al. Cystic fibrosis gene mutation in two sisters with mild disease and normal sweat electrolyte levels. *N Engl J Med* 1991;325(23):1630–1634.

48. Davis PB, Hubbard VS, di Sant'Agnese PA. Low sweat electrolytes in a patient with cystic fibrosis. *Am J Med* 1980;69(4):643–646.

49. Stewart B, Zabner J, Shuber AP, et al. Normal sweat chloride values do not exclude the diagnosis of cystic

fibrosis. *Am J Respir Crit Care Med* 1995;151(3 Pt 1):899–903.

50. Anderson MP, Gregory RJ, Thompson S, et al. Demonstration that CFTR is a chloride channel by alteration of its anion selectivity. *Science* 1991;253 (5016):202–205.

51. Bear CE, Li C, Kartner N, et al. Purification and functional reconstitution of the Cystic Fibrosis Transmembrane Conductance Regulator (CFTR). *Cell* 1992;68(4):809–818.

52. Guggino WB. Outwardly rectifying chloride channels and CF: a divorce and remarriage. *J Bioenerg Biomembr* 1993;25(1):27–35.

53. Stutts MJ, Canessa CM, Olsen JC, et al. CFTR as a cAMP-dependent regulator of sodium channels. *Science* 1995;269:847–850.

54. Mall M, Hipper A, Greger R, et al. Wild type but not delta F508 CFTR inhibits Na+ conductance when coexpressed in *Xenopus* oocytes. *FEBS Lett* 1996;381: 47–52.

55. Ismailov II, Awayda MS, Jovov B, et al. Regulation of epithelial sodium channels by the cystic fibrosis transmembrane conductance regulator. *J Biol Chem* 1996;271(9):4725–4732.

56. Stutts MJ, Rossier BC, Boucher RC. CFTR inverts PKA-mediated regulation of ENaC single channel kinetics. *J Biol Chem* 1997;272:14037–14040.

57. Egan M, Flotte T, Afione S, et al. Defective regulation of outwardly rectifying Cl⁻ channels by protein kinase A corrected by insertion of CFTR. *Nature* 1992;358(6387):581–584.

58. Bradbury NA, Jilling T, Berta G, et al. Regulation of plasma membrane recycling by CFTR. *Science* 1992; 256(5056):530–532.

59. Barasch J, Kiss B, Prince A, et al. Defective acidification of intracellular organelles in cystic fibrosis. *Nature* 1991;352(6330):70–73.

60. Saiman L, Prince A. *Pseudomonas aeruginosa* pili bind to asialoGM1 which is increased on the surface of cystic fibrosis epithelial cells. *J Clin Invest* 1993; 92(4):1875–1880.

61. Worldwide survey of the delta F508 mutation—report from the cystic fibrosis genetic analysis consortium. *Am J Hum Genet* 1990;47(2):354–359.

62. Tsui L. Mutations and sequence variations detected in the cystic fibrosis transmembrane conductance regulator (CFTR) gene: a report from the Cystic Fibrosis Genetic Analysis Consortium. *Hum Mutat* 1992;1(3):197–203.

63. Doerk T, Fislage R, Neumann T, et al. Exon 9 of the CFTR gene: splice site haplotypes and cystic fibrosis mutations. *Hum Genet* 1994;93:67–73.

64. Schwartz M, Johansen HK, Koch C, et al. Frequency of the delta F508 mutation on cystic fibrosis chromosomes in Denmark. *Hum Genet* 1990;85(4):427–428.

65. McIntosh I, Lorenzo ML, Brock DJ. Frequency of delta F508 mutation on cystic fibrosis chromosomes in UK. *Lancet* 1989;2(8676):1404–1405.

66. Estivill X, Chilton M, Casals T, et al. Delta F508 gene deletion in cystic fibrosis in southern Europe. *Lancet* 1989;2(8676):1404.

67. Novelli G, Sangiuolo F, Maceratesi P, et al. The up-to-date molecular genetics of cystic fibrosis. *Biomed Pharmacother* 1994;48(10):455–463.

68. Mercier B, Raguenes O, Estivill X, et al. Complete detection of mutations in cystic fibrosis patients of Native American origin. *Hum Genet* 1994;94(6): 629–632.

69. Kiesewetter S, Macek M Jr, Davis C, et al. A mutation in CFTR produces different phenotypes depending on chromosomal background. *Nat Genet* 1993;5 (3):274–278.

70. Highsmith WE Jr, Chong GL, Orr HT, et al. Frequency of the Delta Phe 508 mutation and correlation with XV.2c/KM-19 haplotypes in an American population of cystic fibrosis patients: results of a collaborative study. *Clin Chem* 1990;36:1741–1746.

71. Cutting GR, Curristin SM, Nash E, et al. Analysis of four diverse population groups indicates that a subset of cystic fibrosis mutations occur in common among Caucasians. *Am J Hum Genet* 1992;50(6):1185–1194.

72. Claustres M, Gerrard B, White MB, et al. A new mutation (1078delT) in exon 7 of the CFTR gene in a southern French adult with cystic fibrosis. *Genomics* 1992;13(3):907–908.

73. Schwartz M, Anvret M, Claustres M, et al. 394de 1TT: a Nordic cystic fibrosis mutation. *Hum Genet* 1994;93(2):157–161.

74. Chillon M, Casals T, Gimenez J, et al. Analysis of the CFTR gene confirms the high genetic heterogeneity of the Spanish population: 43 mutations account for only 78% of CF chromosomes. *Hum Genet* 1994;93 (4):447–451.

75. Tzetis M, Kanavakis E, Antoniadi T, et al. Characterization of more than 85% of cystic fibrosis alleles in the Greek population, including five novel mutations. *Hum Genet* 1997;99(1):121–125.

76. Welsh MJ, Smith AE. Molecular mechanisms of CFTR chloride channel dysfunction in cystic fibrosis. *Cell* 1993;73(7):1251–1254.

77. Hamosh A, Rosenstein BJ, Cutting GR. CFTR nonsense mutations G542X and W1282X associated with severe reduction of CFTR mRNA in nasal epithelial cells. *Hum Mol Genet* 1992;1(7):542–544.

78. Cheng SH, Gregory RJ, Marshall J, et al. Defective intracellular transport and processing of CFTR is the molecular basis of most cystic fibrosis. *Cell* 1990;63 (4):827–834.

79. Denning GM, Anderson MP, Amara JF, et al. Processing of mutant cystic fibrosis transmembrane conductance regulator is temperature-sensitive. *Nature* 1992;358:761–764.

80. Drumm ML, Wilkinson DJ, Smith LS, et al. Chloride conductance expressed by delta F508 and other mutant CFTRs in Xenopus oocytes. *Science* 1991;254 (5039):1797–1799.

81. Li C, Ramjeesingh M, Reyes E, et al. The cystic fibrosis mutation (DeltaF508) does not influence the chloride channel activity of CFTR. *Nat Genet* 1993; 3:311–316.

82. Anderson MP, Welsh MJ. Regulation by ATP and ADP of CFTR chloride channels that contain mutant nucleotide-binding domains. *Science* 1992;257 (5077): 1701–1704.

83. Sheppard DN, Rich DP, Ostedgaard LS, et al. Mutations in CFTR associated with mild-disease-form Cl⁻ channels with altered pore properties. *Nature* 1993; 362(6416):160–164.

84. Highsmith WE, Burch LN, Zhou Z, et al. Identification of a splice site mutation (2789+5 G > A) associated with small amounts of normal CFTR mRNA and mild cystic fibrosis. *Hum Mutat* 1997;9:332–338.

85. Zielenski J, Markiewicz D, Lin S, et al. Skipping of exon 12 as a consequence of a point mutation (1898+5G to T) in the cystic fibrosis transmembrane conductance regulator gene found in a consanguineous Chinese family. *Clin Genet* 1995;47:125–132.

86. Doerk T, Wulbrand U, Tuemmler B. Four novel cystic fibrosis mutations in splice junction sequences affecting the CFTR nucleotide binding folds. *Genomics* 1993;15(3):688–691.

87. Hull J, Shackleton S, Harris A. Abnormal mRNA splicing resulting from three different mutations in the CFTR gene. *Hum Mol Genet* 1993;2(6):689–692.

88. Gilbert F, Li Z, Arzimanoglou II, et al. Clinical spectrum in homozygotes and compound heterozygotes inheriting cystic fibrosis mutation 3849+10kbC > T: significance for geneticists. *Am J Med Genet* 1995;58 (4):356–359.

89. Augarten A, Kerem B, Yahav Y, et al. Mild cystic fibrosis and normal or borderline sweat test in patients with the 3849+10 kb C to T mutation. *Lancet* 1993;342(8862):25–26.

90. Dreyfus DH, Bethel R, Gelfand EW. Cystic fibrosis 3849+10kb C > T mutation associated with severe pulmonary disease and male fertility. *Am J Respir Crit Care Med* 1996;153(2):858–860.

91. Kerem E, Corey M, Kerem B, et al. The relation between genotype and phenotype in cystic fibrosis-analysis of the most common mutation (DF$_{508}$). *N Engl J Med* 1990;323(22):1517–1522.

92. Kristidis P, Bozon D, Corey M, et al. Genetic determination of exocrine pancreatic function in cystic fibrosis. *Am J Hum Genet* 1992;50(6):1178–1184.

93. Hamosh A, Corey M. Correlation between genotype and phenotype in patients with cystic fibrosis: the Cystic Fibrosis Genotype–Phenotype Consortium. *N Engl J Med* 1993;329(18):1308–1313.

94. Kerem E, Kerem B. Genotype-phenotype correlations in cystic fibrosis. *Pediatr Pulmonol* 1996;22(6): 387–395.

95. FitzSimmons SC. *CFF patient registry: 1995 annual report.* Bethesda, MD: Cystic Fibrosis Foundation; 1995.

96. Corey M. Variable phenotypes for nine CFTR mutations associated with pancreatic sufficiency in CF patients: Cystic Fibrosis Genotype–Phenotype Consortium. *Pediatr Pulmonol Suppl* 1996;13:245 [Abstract].

97. Farrell PM, Koscik RE. Sweat chloride concentrations in infants homozygous or heterozygous for F508 cystic fibrosis. *Pediatrics* 1996;97(4):524–528.

98. Wilschanski M, Zielenski J, Markiewicz D, et al. Correlation of sweat chloride concentration with classes of the cystic fibrosis transmembrane conductance regulator gene mutations. *J Pediatr* 1995;127 (5):705–710.

99. Stern RC, Boat TF, Doershuk CF. Obstructive azoospermia as a diagnostic criterion for the cystic fibrosis syndrome. *Lancet* 1982;i(3286):1401–1404.

100. Wilschanski M, Corey M, Durie P, et al. Diversity of reproductive tract abnormalities in men with cystic fibrosis. *JAMA* 1996;276(8):607–608.

101. Rosenstein BJ. Genotype-phenotype correlations in cystic fibrosis. *Lancet* 1994;343(8900):746–747.

102. Gaskin K, Gurevit D, Durie P, et al. Improved respiratory prognosis in patients with cystic fibrosis with normal fat absorption. *J Pediatr* 1982;100:857–862.

103. Hubert D, Bienvenu T, Desmazes-Dufeu N, et al. Genotype–phenotype relationships in a cohort of adult cystic fibrosis patients. *Eur Respir J* 1996;9 (11):2207–2214.

104. Kubesch P, Doerk T, Wulbrand U, et al. Genetic determinants of airways' colonisation with *Pseudomonas aeruginosa* in cystic fibrosis. *Lancet* 1993;341 (8839):189–193.

105. Santis G, Osborne L, Knight R, et al. Genetic influences on pulmonary severity in cystic fibrosis. *Lancet* 1990;335(8684):294.

106. Antinolo G, Borrego S, Gili M, et al. Genotype–phenotype relationship in 12 patients carrying cystic fibrosis mutation R334W. *J Med Genet* 1997;34(2):89–91.

107. Gan KH, Veeze HJ, van den Ouweland AM, et al. A cystic fibrosis mutation associated with mild lung disease. *N Engl J Med* 1995;333(2):95–99.

108. Alton EW. A mild variant of cystic fibrosis. *Thorax* 1996;51 (Suppl 2):S51–S54.

109. Fulmer SB, Schwiebert EM, Morales MM, et al. Two cystic fibrosis transmembrane conductance regulator mutations have different effects on both pulmonary phenotype and regulation of outwardly rectified chloride currents. *Proc Natl Acad Sci U S A* 1995;92 (15):6832–6836.

110. Krawczak M, Reiss J, Cooper DN. The mutational spectrum of single base-pair substitutions in mRNA splice junctions of human genes: causes and consequences. *Hum Genet* 1992;90:41–54.

111. Stern RC, Doershuk CF, Drumm ML. 3849+10 kb C—>T mutation and disease severity in cystic fibrosis. *Lancet* 1995;346(8970):274–276.

112. Chu C, Trapnell BC, Curristin S, et al. Genetic basis of variable exon 9 skipping in cystic fibrosis transmembrane conductance regulator mRNA. *Nat Genet* 1993;3(2):151–156.

113. Chu C, Trapnell BC, Murtagh JJ Jr, et al. Variable deletion of exon 9 coding sequences in cystic fibrosis transmembrane conductance regulator gene mRNA transcripts in normal bronchial epithelium. *EMBO J* 1991;10:1355–1363.

114. Strong TV, Wilkinson DJ, Mansoura MK, et al. Expression of an abundant alternatively spliced form of the cystic fibrosis transmembrane conductance regulator (CFTR) gene is not associated with a cAMP-activated chloride conductance. *Hum Mol Genet* 1993;2(3):225–230.

115. Anguiano A, Oates RD, Amos JA, et al. Congenital bilateral absence of the vas deferens: a primarily genital form of cystic fibrosis. *JAMA* 1992;267(13): 1794–1797.

116. Chillon M, Casals T, Mercier B, et al. Mutations in the cystic fibrosis gene in patients with congenital absence of the vas deferens. *N Engl J Med* 1995;332 (22):1475–1480.

117. Kerem E, Rave-Harel N, Augarten A, et al. A cystic fibrosis transmembrane conductance regulator splice variant with partial penetrance associated with variable cystic fibrosis presentations. *Am J Respir Crit Care Med* 1997;155(6):1914–1920.

118. Rave-Harel N, Kerem E, Nissim-Rafinia M, et al. The molecular basis of partial penetrance of splicing mutations in cystic fibrosis. *Am J Hum Genet* 1997; 60(1):87–94.

119. Pue CA, Noone PG, Friedman KJ, et al. Upper zone bronchiectasis and mucoid *P. aeruginosa* in a patient homozygous for 5T polythymidine tract. *Pediatr Pulmonol Suppl* 1996;13:245 [Abstract].

120. Friedman KJ, Heim RA, Knowles MR, et al. Rapid characterization of the variable length polythymidine tract in the cystic fibrosis (CFTR) gene: association of the 5T allele with selected CFTR mutations and its incidence in atypical sinopulmonary disease. *Hum Mutat* 1997;10(2):108–115.

121. Pignatti PF, Bombieri C, Marigo C, et al. Increased incidence of cystic fibrosis gene mutations in adults with disseminated bronchiectasis. *Hum Mol Genet* 1995;4(4):635–639.

122. Casals T, Bassas L, Ruiz-Romero J, et al. Extensive analysis of 40 infertile patients with congenital absence of the vas deferens: in 50% of cases only one CFTR allele could be detected. *Hum Genet* 1995;95 (2):205–211.

123. Teng H, Jorissen M, Van Poppel H, et al. Increased proportion of exon 9 alternatively spliced CFTR transcripts in vas deferens compared with nasal epithelial cells. *Hum Mol Genet* 1997;6(1):85–90.

124. Osborne LR, Lynch M, Middleton PG, et al. Nasal epithelial ion transport and genetic analysis of infertile men with congenital bilateral absence of the vas deferens. *Hum Mol Genet* 1993;2(10):1605–1609.

125. Handelin BL, Witt D, Skoletsky J, et al. Unexpected prevalence of R117H and G551D CF mutations in a randomly screened population. *Am J Hum Genet* 1992;51(Suppl A218) [Abstract].

126. Kaplan E, Shwachman H, Perlmutter AD, et al. Reproductive failure in males with cystic fibrosis. *N Engl J Med* 1968;279:65–69.

127. Jarvi K, Zielenski J, Wilschanski M, et al. Cystic fibrosis transmembrane conductance regulator and obstructive azoospermia. *Lancet* 1995;345(8964):1578.

128. Zielenski J, Patrizio P, Corey M, et al. CFTR gene variant for patients with congenital absence of vas deferens. *Am J Hum Genet* 1995;57(4):958–960.

129. Rave-Harel N, Madgar I, Goshen R, et al. CFTR haplotype analysis reveals genetic heterogeneity in the etiology of congenital bilateral aplasia of the vas deferens. *Am J Hum Genet* 1995;56(6):1359–1366.

130. Mercier B, Verlingue C, Lissens W, et al. Is congenital bilateral absence of vas deferens a primary form of cystic fibrosis? Analyses of the CFTR gene in 67 patients. *Am J Hum Genet* 1995;56(1):272–277.

131. Colin AA, Sawyer SM, Mickle JE, et al. Pulmonary function and clinical observations in men with congenital bilateral absence of the vas deferens. *Chest* 1996;110(2):440–445.

132. Wilschanski M, Durie P, Ellis L, et al. In vivo electrophysiologic abnormalities of airway epithelium in infertile males with obstructive azoospermia. *Pediatr Pulmonol Suppl* 1996;13:247 [Abstract].

133. Dumur V, Gervais R, Rigot JM, et al. Congenital bilateral absence of the vas deferens (CBAVD) and cystic fibrosis transmembrane regulator (CFTR): correlation between genotype and phenotype. *Hum Genet* 1996;97(1):7–10.

134. Silber SJ, Nagy ZP, Liu J, et al. Conventional in-vitro fertilization versus intracytoplasmic sperm injection for patients requiring microsurgical sperm aspiration. *Hum Reprod* 1994;9(9):1705–1709.

135. Liu J, Lissens W, Silber SJ, et al. Birth after preimplantation diagnosis of the cystic fibrosis delta F508 mutation by polymerase chain reaction in human embryos resulting from intracytoplasmic sperm injection with epididymal sperm. *JAMA* 1994;272:1858–1860.

136. Shuber AP, Michalowsky LA, Nass GS, et al. High throughput parallel analysis of hundreds of patient samples for more than 100 mutations in multiple disease genes. *Hum Mol Genet* 1997;6(3):337–347.

137. Macek M Jr, Mercier B, Mackova A, et al. Sensitivity of the denaturing gradient gel electrophoresis technique in detection of known mutations and novel Asian mutations in the CFTR gene. *Hum Mutat* 1997;9(2):136–147.

138. Glavac D, Dean M. Applications of heteroduplex analysis for mutation detection in disease genes. *Hum Mutat* 1995;6(4):281–287.

139. Wilcken B, Chalmers G. Reduced morbidity in patients with cystic fibrosis detected by neonatal screening. *Lancet* 1985;ii(8468):1319–1321.

140. Bowling F, Cleghorn G, Chester A, et al. Neonatal screening for cystic fibrosis. *Arch Dis Child* 1988;63 (2):196–198.

141. Farrell PM, Mischler EH. Newborn screening for cystic fibrosis: the Cystic Fibrosis Neonatal Screening Study Group. *Adv Pediatr* 1992;39:35–70.

142. Green MR, Weaver LT, Heeley AF, et al. Cystic fibrosis identified by neonatal screening: incidence, genotype, and early natural history. *Arch Dis Child* 1993;68(4):464–467.

143. Gradient of distribution in Europe of the major CF mutation and of its associated haplotype: European Working Group on CF Genetics (EWGCFG). *Hum Genet* 1990;85(4):436–445.

144. Hanukoglu A. Type I pseudohypoaldosteronism includes two clinically and genetically distinct entities with either renal or multiple target organ defects. *J Clin Endocrinol Metab* 1991;73(5):936–944.

145. Hanukoglu A, Bistritzer T, Rakover Y, et al. Pseudohypoaldosteronism with increased sweat and saliva electrolyte values and frequent lower respiratory tract infections mimicking cystic fibrosis. *J Pediatr* 1994;125:752–755.

146. Kerem B, Zielenski J, Markiewicz D, et al. Identification of mutations in regions corresponding to the two putative nucleotide (ATP)-binding folds of the cystic fibrosis gene. *Proc Natl Acad Sci U S A* 1990;87(21):8447–8451.

147. Cutting GR, Kasch LM, Rosenstein BJ, et al. A cluster of cystic fibrosis mutations in the first nucleotide-binding fold of the cystic fibrosis conductance regulator protein. *Nature* 1990;346(6282):366–369.

148. Vidaud M, Fanen P, Martin J, et al. Three point mutations in the CFTR gene in French cystic fibrosis patients: identification by denaturing gradient gel electrophoresis. *Hum Genet* 1990;85(4):446–449.

149. Osborne L, Knight R, Santis G, et al. A mutation in the second nucleotide binding fold of the cystic fibrosis gene. *Am J Hum Genet* 1991;48(3):608–612.

150. Zielenski J, Bozon D, Kerem B, et al. Identification of mutations in exons 1 through 8 of the cystic fibrosis transmembrane conductance regulator (CFTR) gene. *Genomics* 1991;10(1):229–235.

151. Gasparini P, Nunes V, Savoia A, et al. The search for South European cystic fibrosis mutations: identification of two new mutations, four variants, and intronic sequences. *Genomics* 1991;10(1):193–200.

152. Dean M, White MB, Amos J, et al. Multiple mutations in highly conserved residues are found in mildly affected cystic fibrosis patients. *Cell* 1990;61 (5):863–870.

SECTION II

Pulmonary

Cystic Fibrosis in Adults,
edited by J. R. Yankaskas and M. R. Knowles,
Lippincott–Raven Publishers, Philadelphia, 1999.

3

Clinical Pathophysiology and Manifestations of Lung Disease

Pamela B. Davis

Department of Pediatrics, Case Western Reserve University School of Medicine, Cleveland, Ohio

Although patients with cystic fibrosis (CF) have an enormous variety of clinical manifestations, the most important complication is pulmonary disease, because it accounts for more than 90% of the mortality. Some patients appear to have little lung involvement for years, but eventually, chronic obstructive pulmonary disease develops in all patients, which is characterized by relentless progression of bronchiectasis until death (1). In the past 9 years, much information about how the basic defect leads to the pathophysiology of CF lung disease has emerged. This pathophysiologic cascade must be considered because with only symptomatic therapy, the life expectancy in CF has improved from the grim certainty of death in infancy in the 1940s to a current median survival age exceeding 30 years in the United States (Fig. 3–1). Thus, the course of CF lung disease can be modified, and with better understanding of the pathophysiology of this disease, further improvements in outcome can be expected. In this chapter, the pathogenesis of CF lung disease is traced. Many of the topics discussed in this chapter are covered in much more detail in other chapters; however, sufficient information is given in this chapter to allow the reader to follow the flow of the pathophysiologic cascade (Fig. 3–2). Readers are referred to other chapters for greater detail and for more extensive references.

THE BASIC DEFECT

The Cystic Fibrosis Transmembrane Conductance Regulator (CFTR) and Its Mutant Forms

In all families tested thus far, CF is caused by lesions in a single gene located on chromosome 7, region q21–q22 (2). This gene is approximately 250,000 base pairs in length, contains 27 exons, and encodes a protein of 1,480 amino acids, which has a molecular weight of 170,000 daltons, and is called the cystic fibrosis transmembrane conductance regulator, or the CFTR (3). The CFTR is an integral membrane protein, with two regions of six transmembrane loops each (regions referred to as TM6 regions), two intracellular nucleotide-binding folds (NBFs), and an intracellular portion with many consensus phosphorylation sites, called the R domain (4). It is a member of a family of proteins called the ABC family [adenosine triphosphate (ATP)-binding cassette proteins], which includes bacterial transporters for sugars, amino acids, or proteins; the yeast transporter Sterile 6, which transports the a mating factor; and the mammalian multidrug resistance (MDR) protein or P glycoprotein, which transports a variety of hydrophobic drugs, including cancer chemotherapeutic agents, out of the cell. Except for the P glycoprotein, which can transport the chloride ion in addition to larger molecules,

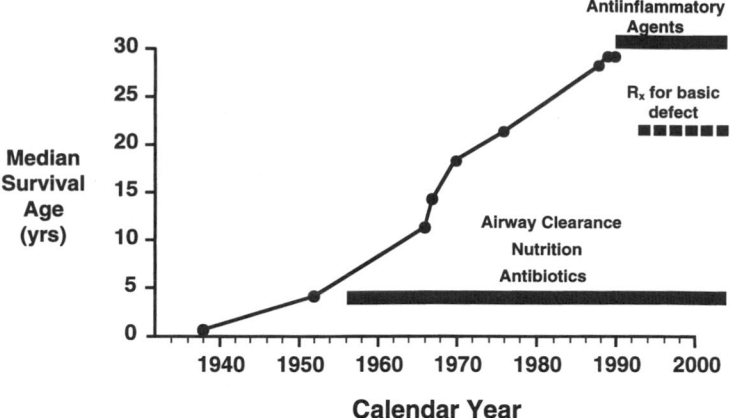

FIG. 3–1. Median survival age for patients with cystic fibrosis in the United States. Therapeutic strategies in extensive use are indicated by the solid bars, and the initiation of clinical trials in a very important therapeutic area are indicated by a broken bar.

members of this family appear to transport complex molecules rather than monovalent ions. In addition, members of this family are transporters, which can pump substrate against a concentration gradient with hydrolysis of one molecule of ATP per molecule of substrate transported. In contrast, the CFTR functions as an ion channel, allowing movement of anions down the electrochemical gradient, and no stoichiometic relationship can be demonstrated between ATP hydrolysis and chloride transport, although ATP binding and hydrolysis and phosphorylation of the R domain are required to open the channel (5). The cDNA encoding CFTR, expressed in CF cells, corrects the phenotypic abnormality of impaired cAMP-dependent chloride secretion (6,7). Over-expression of the wild type—but not CF-mutant—CFTR cDNA in heterologous cells, which ordinarily lack cyclic adenosine mono-

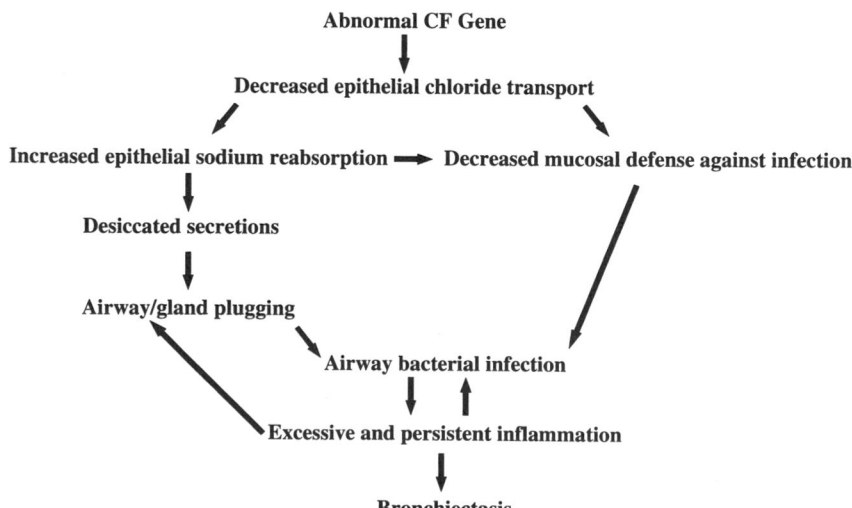

FIG. 3–2. Postulated pathophysiologic cascade for development of the lung disease in patients with cystic fibrosis. See text for details.

phosphate (cAMP)-regulable chloride conductance, produces a cAMP-regulable chloride conductance (8–10). The simplest explanation for these findings is that the CFTR itself is a chloride channel.

Site-directed mutagenesis experiments with the CFTR support the hypothesis that the CFTR is an anion channel. Substitutions of the positively charged amino acid residues in the TM6 regions of the CFTR are among the naturally occurring CF-associated mutations (11), and site-directed mutation of these residues alters the ionic specificity of the chloride conductance (12). Deletion of amino acids #708 to #835 from the R domain allows the channel to open without phosphorylation (13), and when the unphosphorylated R domain (exon 13) peptide is added to CFTR channels, conduction is abolished (14). Finally, purification of the CFTR from a baculovirus expression system followed by insertion into an artificial membrane produces a regulated chloride conductance (15). Therefore, the CFTR itself has channel activity.

More than 750 different mutations in the CFTR have been reported, including nonsense mutations, point mutations, splice site variants, and in-frame deletions. Welsh and Smith (16) classified these mutants into four types. Type I mutants express little or no protein; Type II mutants express protein that is degraded rapidly and fails to reach its intended site of action; Type III and Type IV mutants express protein that reaches the surface of the cell, but either the regulation of the channel (Type III) or the channel itself (Type IV) is defective. Examples of Type I mutants are nonsense mutations (e.g., R553X) for which most transcripts are nonfunctional. Type III and Type IV mutations often are amino acid substitutions for which transcripts are produced and the protein is processed and arrives at the plasma membrane. Some of the Type IV mutations, amino acid substitutions in the transmembrane domains (e.g., R117H), are associated with pancreatic sufficiency and milder phenotype. An additional class of mutations, Type V, splice site variants, has been described. For these mutations, some normal transcripts are produced (e.g., 3849 + 10 KB C to T), so a small amount

of normal CFTR can be expressed, and disease may be mild (17).

The most common CF mutation, ΔF508, is an example of a Type II mutation. This mutation, observed on 70% of all CF chromosomes, deletes three base pairs and eliminates a phenylalanine residue at the 508 position (in the first NBF) (3). Several lines of evidence indicate that this mutant is processed poorly and fails to arrive at the plasma membrane. In COS cells, overexpressed wild-type and mutant CFTRs give different patterns on Western blot analysis (18). Cells transfected with a wild-type CFTR display three bands for the CFTR, which correspond to the unglycosylated, core glycosylated, and fully glycosylated proteins. Moreover, in these cells expressing a wild-type CFTR, protein can be detected at the cell membrane by immunofluorescence. The ΔF508 transfected cells lack the fully glycosylated form of the CFTR, and immunofluorescence studies show only intracellular CFTR. Because core glycosylation is believed to take place in the endoplasmic reticulum but full glycosylation occurs in the Golgi, these data are consistent with the hypothesis that the ΔF508 CFTR never arrives at the Golgi to be glycosylated but is degraded in the endoplasmic reticulum. Recent data indicate that both wild-type and ΔF508 CFTRs bind to p88, a chaperon in the endoplasmic reticulum, but that only the wild type can dissociate readily (19). This binding may be one mechanism by which the ΔF508 CFTR can be retained in the endoplasmic reticulum to be degraded by proteasomes (20,21). Glycosylation per se appears to be merely a marker for passage through the Golgi and is not obligatory for CFTR function. Mutations of the glycosylation sites of CFTR result in a fully functional but nonglycosylated protein (22), and the CFTR produced in Sf9 insect cells, in which full glycosylation fails to occur, forms normal channels (9).

The ΔF508 mutation has some conductive properties (23–25). Other Type II mutations, such as A455E, are clinically mild mutations because the A455E CFTR has normal conductive properties and approximately 5% of it reaches the plasma membrane (26,27). The question arises as to whether improving processing of Type II mutants might confer function on CF cells or whether sufficient protein already reaches the surface of the cell for some of these mutants to allow activation with a sufficiently powerful stimulus. *In vitro* experiments indicate that simply inhibiting proteasomal degradation will not increase the processing of the ΔF508 CFTR, so other strategies must be employed (21). The answers to these questions carry important therapeutic implications. With the gathering evidence that even small amounts of functional CFTR at critical sites may be protective against disease, the capacity to activate the major CF mutants might be of critical clinical importance. This question may need to be addressed in relevant human tissues, rather than in artificial overexpression systems. Indeed, in the COS cell system, even most wild-type CFTR is not glycosylated fully and is found within the cell as well as at the plasma membrane (18). In contrast, immunohistochemistry and confocal microscopy of normal CFTR in human epithelial cells appear to localize protein at or near the plasma membrane (28), and Western blot analysis of many human tissues does not separate an underglycosylated CFTR band [e.g., T84 cells (10), pancreas (28)], even in CF samples [e.g., nasal tissue (29)]. In addition, one study of human airway shows colocalization of the CFTR with apical membrane, not endosomal, markers in both normal and CF samples (30). Even small amounts of a partially functional mutant CFTR may be subject to maximal activation at the plasma membrane for therapeutic purposes.

Regardless, the molecular physiology of the various CF mutations is that there is less apical chloride channel function in the cells in which the CFTR normally is expressed. The molecular physiology fits well with the electrophysiology of CF established several years earlier.

Physiology of the Basic Defect

The physiologic defect in CF was established to be reduced chloride conductance across affected epithelia well before the gene was cloned. This reduced chloride conductance had been demonstrated in CF sweat ducts (31,32), in airway epithelium (33), and in the pancreas, where chloride output into pancreatic juice is impaired (34). The fact that the cloned protein CFTR is indeed a chloride channel regulated by cAMP is entirely consistent with the physiologic results.

In normal airway tissues, chloride secretion occurs in response to many distinct signals, such as increased intracellular cAMP with activation of protein kinase A (PKA), activation of protein kinase C (PKC), increased intracellular free calcium, and, possibly, activation by a purinergic receptor independent of intracellular free calcium. In CF airway cells, chloride secretion occurs normally in response to extracellular ATP or to agents that increase intracellular calcium, but there is no response to agents that increase cAMP content or activate either PKA or PKC (35–43). However, the direct response to PKC is small, and PKC appears to function principally in synergy with PKA (10). These phenomena have been demonstrated in nasal and tracheal epithelial cells in both primary culture and immortalized cell lines (35,44,45), in intact tissues mounted in an Ussing chamber (36), and *in vivo* by measurement of transepithelial potential differences (46). Single-channel studies in cultured cells demonstrate comparable activation of chloride conductances in normal and CF tissues by voltage, temperature, Ca^{++}, and cytoplasmic application of trypsin, but not the catalytic subunit of PKA (47). There are at least two distinct chloride conductances in airway epithelium, one regulated by cAMP, the other by Ca^{++} (48), which may reside in different proteins. The Ca^{++} regulation of chloride conductance in airway cells is mediated by a calcium/calmodulin-dependent protein kinase (49), and the channel is DIDS sensitive, whereas the channel that is impaired in CF is regulated by PKA and is not inhibited by DIDS (50). Chloride conductances stimulated by these two pathways are additive. In intestinal (T84) cells, the cAMP-regulated conductance has a linear current–voltage relationship and shows no time-dependent changes in current during voltage pulses. The Ca^{++}-regulated conductance, activated by calmodulin-dependent kinase II (51), also has a nearly linear current–voltage relationship but activates during depolarizing voltage pulses and is additive with the cAMP-regulated conductance (52). It appears that the primary CF defect is confined to the chloride conductance that (1) is regulated by cAMP and protein kinase A, (2) has linear current–voltage relationship, (3) has permselectivity $Br^- > Cl^- > I^-$, (4) has conductance of less than 30 pS, more in the range of 5 to 10 picoSiemen(pS), and (5) is DIDS insensitive. These properties are similar to the properties reported for the recombinant CFTR expressed in test cell systems. Thus, the physiologic data from CF tissues are consistent with the data derived from artificial systems in which the cDNA for the CFTR is overexpressed: the CF lesion resides in a cAMP-regulable chloride conductance.

Related Ion Transport Abnormalities

Some of the initial electrophysiologic work on the "CF channel," performed in cell-detached patches, characterized this channel as an outward rectifying chloride channel (ORCC). It now appears that such a channel does exist in epithelia and is distinct from the CFTR channel but is regulated by CFTR (53,54). Thus, activation of the ORCC is abnormal in CF. It has been suggested that the CFTR activates the ORCC by regulating release of ATP from the epithelial cell. ATP then acts as an autocrine activator of the ORCC (55,56). Whether the CFTR itself transports ATP remains unclear (57).

Another abnormality that appears to be associated with the CF genotype but does not appear to be related directly to the CFTR mutation is increased amiloride-sensitive sodium transport. Markedly increased sodium reabsorption is observed *in vivo* in patients with CF, *in vitro* in intact CF tissues, and in primary culture remote from the effects of the CF disease, and cannot be explained as an electrophysiologic consequence of the chloride secretion abnormality (58). It is present in all patients with CF from the first days of life and persists in primary culture, and thus is unlikely to be a secondary result of disease. This defect may be of critical clinical importance (59). Recent data indicate that the CFTR directly regulates the amiloride-sensitive sodium channel, known as the epithelial Na channel (ENaC), which is responsible for the amiloride-sensitive sodium reabsorption in airways. The CFTR reduces ENaC activity. In addition, in the absence of CFTR, the ENaC is activated by cAMP; however, in the presence of functional CFTR, the ENaC is inhibited by cAMP (60). Although the exact molecular mechanism for regulation still is being studied, there is a direct relationship between CFTR and ENaC that explains the abnormal sodium reabsorption in CF.

Thus, the basic defect in CF resides in a PKA-regulated chloride channel in the apical plasma membrane of cells in affected epithelia. This defect also appears to contribute to defective regulation of an ORCC, the functional consequences of which are unknown, and to marked increase in amiloride-sensitive sodium reabsorption, which may be important in the pathophysiology of the disease. Other abnormalities in ion transport may result from reduced activity of the CFTR, which may result in abnormalities in bicarbonate and hydrogen ion activity.

The Basic Defect in Airways

Ion Transport In Vivo

The local ionic consequences of elimination of cAMP-regulated chloride conductance probably depend on the availability of other channels and the paracellular pathway. It is difficult to predict the impact of CFTR mutation in airway epithelium, which has multiple channels and "leaky" paracellular pathways. In addition, the CFTR is not abundant in the lung. Even in lung epithelial cells, whether freshly isolated, cultured, or transformed cell lines, it is difficult to demonstrate the mRNA for the CFTR without resorting to amplification by the polymerase chain reaction (PCR) method, although the CF physiologic defect is observed readily. The protein is difficult to demonstrate *in situ* in the lung with antibodies that readily reveal the protein in pancreatic or sweat ducts. Indeed, in the intact upper airway, the most impressive ion transport abnormality is not the impaired chloride conductance, which barely can be detected electrophysiologically under basal conditions (i.e., when there are normal levels of extracellular chloride), but the enormously elevated sodium reabsorption. This threefold elevation in sodium reabsorption is well in excess of what would be predicted from the chloride conductance lesion alone and, therefore, may represent a separate consequence of the CF gene. Moreover, chloride conductance is not absent from the CF apical membrane: chloride ion is secreted in response to ATP or UTP in CF airways *in vivo* and *in vitro*, and the response to these stimuli exceeds the norm (61).

Secondary effects of disease also may affect ion transport. Patients with pancreatic insufficiency have abnormal fatty acid composition of membrane lipids in airway epithelial cells (62). In tissue culture, such an abnormality in fatty acid composition is associated with markedly abnormal paracellular transport, although cellular ion transport pathways appear unaffected (63). Moreover, chronic bacterial infection and massive neutrophilic inflammation in the lung result in bathing of the epithelium in a milieu containing uninhibited elastases, cytokines, eicosanoid mediators, and bacterial products; these agents might affect the expression of the CF defect or the ability of the epithelium to compensate for it. For example, elastase causes separation of the tight junctions between epithelial cells (64) and thus may alter the paracellular transport pathways or allow access of luminal contents to the basolateral epithelial surface. In animals, elastase causes a shift in the airway cell population toward secretory cells. If secretory and ciliated cells differ in their ion transport capabilities, altered cellular distribution might affect the overall ion transport. All these factors also make it difficult to predict *a priori* the functional consequences of mutant CFTR in the airways. Attempts to measure the ionic composition of airway surface liquid in healthy subjects and those with CF have been fraught with difficulty. Collecting mucous secretions and measuring their salt content is inherently unsatisfactory for all the aforementioned reasons.

Collections at bronchoscopy also are subject to the secondary changes previously described, but in one such study, secretions from patients with CF appeared to have considerably elevated chloride content compared with non-CF subjects (65). Attempts to measure the ion composition of airway surface liquid by touching the surface with filter paper and analyzing the ion composition by microanalytic methods suggest that the normal airway surface liquid is hypotonic (66). However, it is difficult to guarantee that even this brief stimulus does not provoke rapid secretory response and somehow alter the system under study. Even these measurements can only be made in the nose and the larger airways, and comparisons between normal and CF airways are subject to the aforementioned caveats. Patients with CF appear to have elevated $[Na^+]$ and $[Cl^-]$ on airway surface liquid compared with controls, but values are comparable to controls with chronic irritation or acute infection (67). A recent review (68) summarizes some of these considerations. However, somehow mutant CFTR must give rise to plugging of glands, tenacious secretions, and Pseudomonas colonization.

Abnormal Properties of Secretions

The abnormal physicochemical properties of CF secretions are striking and give rise to duct obstruction throughout the body. How the chloride transport defect gives rise to the abnormal behavior of macromolecular secretions still is not clear. At the molecular level, abnormal solution properties may be conferred on CF mucins at the moment of secretion. Mucin molecules are stored in highly condensed form in secretory granules. When granule fusion with the plasma membrane occurs, mucin molecules are released, become hydrated, and assume a solution structure. Gasser et al. (69) have shown that secretory granule membranes contain ion transporters that are activated by hormones that promote secretion. They suggest that these transporters are activated with granule fusion, serve to flush out granule contents, probably control the ionic microenvironment into which the macromolecules are first secreted, and thus contribute to the physical chemistry of unfolding of mucins from the condensed to the solution state. If the transporter in the granule membrane is a mutant CFTR, patients with CF may not perform these functions properly. Mucins may assume a different solution conformation, leading to altered rheologic properties.

An alternative—although not mutually exclusive—hypothesis is that the CF defect affects the composition of the macromolecules themselves. Macromolecules secreted by patients with CF differ chemically from those secreted by patients who do not have CF (for a review of the older literature, see reference 70). Even CF airway epithelial cells in culture, remote from infection and inflammation, secrete macromolecules that are more highly sulfated. Abnormalities in sulfate transport or sulfate pool size in airway epithelial cells have been suggested to explain this observation (71). Alternatively, or in addition, posttranslational modifications of macromolecules may be abnormal in CF because of defective acidification of intracellular compartments or aberrant localization of sialyl transferases. In some intracellular compartments, chloride provides the counterion for hydrogen ion when acidification occurs. Compartments that depend on the CFTR to admit chloride ion may not be acidified properly in CF, and the enzymes within them that are most pH sensitive (e.g., sialyl transferases) may not function normally (72). However, confirmatory data for this important idea have not been reported. Direct mislocalization of sialyl transferases, or other explanations, must be sought. Abnormalities in macromolecules notwithstanding, a simple parsimonious hypothesis is that failure to secrete chloride and water into the secretory product alters both the ionic strength of the secretion and the concentration of the macromolecules. If the concentration becomes too high and/or the salt conditions become inappropriate, the macromolecules precipitate, plugging the duct and causing obstructive complications. This hypothesis predicts that secretions that exhibit abnormal physicochemical properties also will have abnormal monovalent ion composition and reduced water content. This hypothesis is consistent with the pathology of the pancreas observed at necropsy (73), and with the reduced water and chloride content of CF pancreatic juice (74). For cervical mucus, water content is reduced and a cervical plug forms (75). In the intestine, inadequate water content of the fecal stream probably leads to high fecal impaction, as occurs in meconium ileus at birth or the syndrome of "distal intestinal obstruction" later in life. This postulate is supported by the example of the CFTR knockout mice, which have as the major cause of death intestinal obstruction, despite nearly normal pancreatic function (76).

In the CF lung, it has been difficult unambiguously to demonstrate alterations in the salt and water content of secretions. The picture in the lung is complicated by infection and inflammation in the majority of patients, epithelial damage, leakage of serum and its solutes across a damaged mucosal barrier, and the influx of massive numbers of phagocytic cells that die in the airways, releasing their contents. All these ancillary events make it difficult to measure the salt and water content of CF secretions, and appropriate controls are difficult to select. However, obstruction of organ passages still occurs. Obstruction of submucosal gland ducts occurs even before infection and inflammation (77,78), and hypertrophy and hyperplasia of the mucus-secreting apparatus also can occur in infants without appreciable evidence of inflammation (79). Because of the difficulties of making the appropriate measurements *in situ*, investigators have turned to model systems *in vitro* to investigate fluid secretion and reabsorption by CF and normal airway epithelial cells. One group clearly demonstrated impaired secretory response from the surface epithelial cells from patients with CF compared with healthy subjects in short-term studies (80) and went on to show that sheets of cells from submucosal glands not only fail to secrete in CF, but they actually reabsorb fluid from the surface liquid (81). Thus, fluid reabsorption by the submucosal glands might further deplete liquid from an already marginally hydrated airway surface because of the defect in surface epithelium. However, other investigators who studied fluid transport over 24 hours failed to demonstrate major differences between normal and CF surface epithelium (82). In such an *in vitro* system, Smith et al. (83) performed experiments that suggest a link between the ion transport defect and the propensity to bacterial infection in CF airways. Primary cultures of CF airway epithelial cells grown with media only on the basolateral side fail to kill bacteria placed on the apical surface, as do normal airway epithelial cells. Both normal and CF airway epithelial cell cultures produce bactericidal factors, but in the ionic environment produced at the apical surface of the CF cultures, this killing activity was inhibited. Separate experiments indicated that the killing activity was inhibited in a hypertonic environment. However, as discussed previously, it is difficult to prove that airway surface liquid in CF at the relevant level of the airway is indeed hypertonic, or even to devise a mechanism by which hypertonicity can be sustained in small airways. Nevertheless, this hypothesis is attractive to explain the initial bacterial colonization.

Other factors may contribute to the propensity to sustain infection. For example, it has been suggested that the CF ion transport abnormalities might cause not only inadequately hydrated secretions but also reduced periciliary fluid, leading to ciliary dysfunction. Impaired mucociliary clearance predisposes to infection of the airways and bronchiectasis (e.g., as it does in patients with ciliary dyskinesia syndrome). However, this probably is not the only explanation for bronchial infection in CF. If impaired mucociliary clearance were the primary pathophysiologic mechanism for development of the CF lung disease, direct measurements of mucociliary clearance should consistently demonstrate impairment, and they do not (84,85). Moreover, in patients with ciliary dyskinesia syndrome, lower zone bronchiectasis develops (as opposed to upper zone in CF), the infecting organism often is not *Pseudomonas aeruginosa*, and infections are controlled more easily by antibiotic therapy than in CF (86).

Expression Pattern of the Cystic Fibrosis Transmembrane Conductance Regulator in the Lung

There are additional problems in relating the CF basic defect to disease in the airways. Much of the elegant ion transport work has been done in the upper airways, yet the CF disease appears, at least by pulmonary function testing, to begin in the small airways. The pattern of ion transport probably differs at different levels of the airway. The total surface area of the airways diminishes markedly distally to proximally, yet the airways are lined with fluid at all levels, and clearance is upward toward the mouth. Thus, fluid reabsorption must occur as secretions are cleared. Therefore, because water itself is not transported in the lung, but rather passively follows ionic gradients, ion transport must differ at different levels of the lung. In support of this idea, the normal transepithelial potential difference across the airways is greatest in the nose and the proximal lung, and less in the distal lung (46). In addition, in animal airway epithelial cells in culture, ion transport pathways differ in cells from different airway levels (87). We know little about the consequences of the CF lesion for the ion transport pathways in the distal airways.

Recent data on the distribution of CFTR protein and mRNA in the lung in adults and during development are confusing if one attempts to relate the amount of CFTR expression to the presumed site and timing of disease. Although there are no obvious histologic abnormalities in the lung at birth in CF in the absence of infection, with the possible exception of the submucosal gland ducts, the CFTR in the fetal lung is more abundant than it is in the adult lung, and its distribution extends to the terminal bronchioles and alveoli. As development proceeds, distal expression diminishes and expression in proximal airways persists (88,89). However, during fetal life, the CFTR appears to be absent from the glands, the only site of histologic abnormality (90). In older patients, CFTR is most abundant in a few cells studding the submucosal gland ducts, abundant in the serous cells of the submucosal glands, sparse in surface epithelium of the large- and medium-sized airways, and very difficult to detect at all in alveoli and terminal bronchioles (90–92). However, *in vitro*, CFTR function can be demonstrated when presence of protein or mRNA cannot, so it is possible that functional CFTR is active in areas of the lung with little or no demonstrable protein or mRNA. In addition, the mere presence of the protein or mRNA may not imply that a channel is functional in that tissue, although this has not been shown for the CFTR. It also is possible that the presumed early disease in small airways in CF is a consequence of something separate from the basic defect, such as tropism of the initial infecting agents (e.g., viruses) for this site. The very early appearance of inflammatory mediators in the bronchoalveolar lavage fluid of infants with CF identified by neonatal screening lends some support to this suggestion.

SECONDARY CONSEQUENCES OF DISEASE

Pulmonary Infection and Inflammation

Bacterial infection is a hallmark of CF and occurs early in life. Whether the lung is primed by viral infection or precisely which bacteria occur first is not completely clear. Recent data from bronchoalveolar lavage of infants diagnosed by newborn screening indicate that even many asymptomatic infants harbor bacteria in their lungs, and even some of those who do not have bacteria in the lung display evidence of inflammation, including an excess of neutrophils in the bronchoalveolar lavage and the chemotactic cytokine interleukin (IL)-8 (93–95). Whether these inflammatory cells and mediators are the residual of earlier infection, as seems likely, or the result of some more fundamental derangement in CF, such as abnormalities in cytokine production or regulation, has not been determined. Nevertheless, bacter-

ial infection and its inflammatory consequences occur much earlier than previously thought, and they may be present even in the absence of signs or symptoms. Studies of viral infections in older children suggest that such infections are no more frequent in patients with CF than in their unaffected siblings, although they may produce more worrisome symptoms, and patients with more frequent viral infections may have more rapid decline in pulmonary function (96). Bacterial infection, however, is quite different. Although patients with CF do not have increased prevalence of bacterial infection outside the respiratory tract, chronic bacterial infection of the sinuses and bronchi regularly develop, sometimes with *Staphylococcus aureus*, intermittent *Hemophilus influenzae*, and usually, *P. aeruginosa*. The bacteria that infect CF lungs are unusual. Although patients with bronchiectasis of other etiologies harbor *Staph. aureus, H. influenzae*, and occasionally *P. aeruginosa,* in the lungs of patients with CF, *P. aeruginosa* are remarkably frequent, and particular serotypes predominate (97). One possible explanation for this phenomenon is that patients with CF, clustered in centers for care, infect each other (98,99). Arguments against this suggestion include: data that show that many patients harbor *P. aeruginosa* at their initial presentation to centers for care; even siblings living together do not necessarily have the same serotypes (100); and study of *P. aeruginosa* in summer camp does not support person-to-person transmission (101). An alternative explanation is that there is a particularly hospitable environment in the lungs of patients with CF for *P. aeruginosa.*

It is a tenet of infection pathogenesis that adherence precedes infection. In patients with CF, colonization of the mouth by Pseudomonas is much more dense than in healthy subjects. Fibronectin, and possibly other protective molecules, are destroyed by proteases in the mouths of patients with CF, and once *P. aeruginosa* are established in the mouth, they could provide a constant infectious "seed" for the lower airways (102). Chronic sinus infection also may seed below, but we still are left with the problem of the predilection of infection for the upper airways. In addition, Pseudomonas adhere in greater numbers to CF airway epithelial cells, particularly ΔF508 homozygotes, than to normal airway cells (103,104). This greater adherence has been related to the presence of increased amounts of asialoGM1, a receptor for Pseudomonas, on the surface of CF cells (105). Another hypothesis to explain the predilection of Pseudomonas for CF recently has been advanced. This hypothesis is based on the observation that Pseudomonas are taken up less avidly by CF airway epithelial cells than by normal cells. In this case, the clearance mechanism for Pseudomonas is postulated to be uptake of the bacteria by the epithelial cell and subsequent sloughing of the cell for clearance in the mucociliary escalator (106). Regardless, at least 60% of all patients with CF are reported to have *P. aeruginosa* in their respiratory cultures, and the prevalence increases with age (107).

Once *P. aeruginosa* gains a foothold in the CF lung, it is not controlled by neutrophil phagocytosis and killing, as it is in the healthy host, yet a systemic defect in neutrophil function has not been demonstrated. This persistence may be due in part to the acquisition of a mucoid phenotype *in vivo*. The development of mucoidy, unusual in other disease states but observed at other sites in patients with CF (such as intestinal flora) (108), may defend the bacteria against opsonization, phagocytosis, and killing (109). In addition, neutrophils at the site of inflammation are subject to modification by the local environment. The massive neutrophilic infiltration of CF lungs allows for the release of neutrophil elastase, which overwhelms the antiproteases of the lung and, uninhibited, destroys the C3b receptor (CR1) on neutrophils (110). In addition, the C3bi opsonin is destroyed by neutrophil elastase (111). The complement opsonin-receptor system, the main opsonophagocytic system used by neutrophils for Pseudomonas, is thereby crippled in the CF lung. At the same time, proteases in the CF lung cleave immunoglobulin G (IgG) antibodies to Pseudomonas, leaving Fab fragments able to bind to Pseudomonas but lacking

the Fc recognition signal for macrophages (112). Antibody-mediated phagocytosis predominates in the macrophage's handling of Pseudomonas. Thus, both of the major phagocytic systems of the lung are crippled by proteases, and infection can be sustained. The persistence of bacteria in the lung further stimulates the inflammatory response, and a vicious cycle is set in motion.

Bacterial chemoattractants are only part of the milieu in the CF lung that establishes the persistent neutrophilic infiltration. Activated neutrophils themselves produce a panoply of chemoattractants, including leukotriene B_4 (LTB$_4$), which sustain the neutrophilic infiltration. Airway epithelial cells and inflammatory cells may secrete IL-8. Pseudomonas products (113,114) are potent neutrophil attractants. IL-8 secretion is stimulated in epithelial cells by elastase. Breach of the mucosal barrier allows transudation and a ready source of complement, and C5a also is produced. All these factors continue to recruit massive numbers of neutrophils into the CF airway. These neutrophils are ineffective in destroying the resident bacteria but cause considerable damage.

Uninhibited neutrophil elastase, present in substantial quantities even in patients mildly affected with CF, is a potent stimulus for macromolecule secretion by cultured airway epithelial cells (114), and in experimental animals, a single intratracheal instillation of elastase results in permanent mucosecretory differentiation in rodents (115). Thus, hypertrophy and hyperplasia of the mucus-secreting apparatus, as well as increased secretion, is promoted by neutrophil products. As the neutrophils die in the airway, they release massive quantities of DNA, which contributes substantially to the viscosity and tenacity of CF sputum. The enzymes released from neutrophils, including elastase, cathepsins, and others, contribute to the destruction of the fabric of the airway wall and the development of bronchiectasis. Because true emphysema and loss of elastic recoil are rare in CF, it is presumed that there is relatively little destruction of the alveoli and interstitium around them by neutrophil elastase.

The cytokine cascades that are activated in the CF lung are only beginning to be described. However, IL-8 appears to be an early feature of the CF airways disease, appearing in bronchoalveolar lavage samples from even asymptomatic infants. The exact source of IL-8 is not established because macrophages, neutrophils, and epithelial cells all can produce it, and increased number of neutrophils also are observed in the CF bronchoalveolar lavage of infants (93–95). However, the epithelial cell also appears to be an important source of IL-8 in CF airways, and the mRNA for this cytokine also is upregulated dramatically in these cells. Concomitantly, there is a decrease in the mRNA and protein for IL-10, a cytokine that modulates the inflammatory response. In the bronchoalveolar lavage fluid from CF airways, the concentration of all proinflammatory cytokines tested [tumor necrosis factor (TNF)-α, IL-1, IL-6, IL-8] is elevated: IL-10 concentration is reduced markedly (116,117). The inflammatory environment in the CF lung is characterized by increases in all the proinflammatory cytokines and reduction in the antiinflammatory cytokine. Whether early inversion of the IL-8/IL-10 ratio is a consequence of the CF genetic defect or of other factors has not yet been established.

Pathophysiology of Airways Disease

The result of the underlying CF abnormalities, in addition to the persistent infection and inflammation, is obstruction to airflow and ultimately lung damage. Obstruction to airflow in CF is caused largely by the compromise of the airway lumen, primarily by mucous secretions, inflammatory exudate, and sloughed epithelial lining cells, rather than by loss of elastic recoil, the major mechanism of reduced airflow in emphysema. Airway plugging is especially striking in end-stage disease, and at postmortem examination, tenacious mucus and pus may appear to fill every orifice. Obstruction also is increased by thickening of the airway wall by mucosal edema (as a result of inflammation) and by space-occupying hypertrophy of the mucus-secreting apparatus. In-

flammation surely plays a role in increased gland bulk (in animal models, even a single instillation of neutrophil elastase causes long-lasting secretory metaplasia), but pulmonary secretory cell increase can be seen even in the absence of inflammation in patients with CF (79), and hypertrophy of mucus-secreting structures is common in uninflamed sites in patients with CF, such as the intestinal wall.

Airway Reactivity

Increase in airway smooth muscle and increased airway reactivity also may contribute to obstruction in CF. Whether airway reactivity is a consequence of the CF gene, whether it develops as a secondary consequence of lung infection, inflammation, and progressive airways disease (118–122), or whether it is present in some patients as a genetic trait independent of CF or a consequence of allergy has not been established clearly. Difficulties inherent in the assessment of airway reactivity in the face of disease have complicated studies of the phenomenon. Airway reactivity cannot be defined by improvement in pulmonary function with bronchodilator administration, but must be assessed by the bronchoconstrictor response to provocation. Even these tests are ambiguous, for accurate administration of the provocative stimulus is difficult in patients with lung disease: the challenge from exercise or cold air depends on minute ventilation, which may be reduced (and variable) in patients with disease, and distribution and penetration to the target receptors of a pharmacologic stimulus, such as histamine or methacholine, is irregular and variable in patients with inflammation and infection. Therefore, it is not surprising that different provocative agents may not identify the same patients as reactive, or that the same patient responds differently to the same provocation at different times (123). Nevertheless, most studies of airway reactivity in patients with CF demonstrate increased cross-sectional prevalence of airway reactivity. The proportion of reactive subjects ranges from 0% to 68% and averages approximately 40% (124–133). In some studies, airway reactivity is most prevalent in patients with the most severe lung disease, probably because the degree of bronchoconstriction required to achieve the target change in flow is smaller for those with smaller baseline flows. However, the prevalence of reactivity to histamine is 40% among patients with near-normal baseline forced expiratory volume in 1 second (FEV_1) (128), so severe disease is not required for airway reactivity in CF.

In non-CF patient populations, increased airway reactivity is familial (134–136). Therefore, evaluation of the disease-free parents of patients with CF may provide information inaccessible from the patients themselves. Unselected parents of children with CF have higher prevalence of wheeze and dyspnea compared with controls on a standardized questionnaire (137), but the possibility that these parents are particularly sensitized to respiratory symptoms cannot be excluded. Indeed, parents of children with CF who had normal baseline pulmonary function and who took no medication displayed no greater airway reactivity to either methacholine (54 subjects) or cold air (44 subjects) than age-matched controls (138). Although the selection criteria for this population—which excluded subjects undergoing treatment for lung disease—biased the study against a positive result, these data argue that a single gene for CF, by itself, probably does not predispose to airway reactivity.

Atopy

If patients with CF are atopic, they might be predisposed to increased airway reactivity on this basis. When one assembles data from earlier studies (for summary, see reference 139), one finds that approximately two thirds of patients with CF have at least one positive skin test and 40% have elevated serum immunoglobulin E (IgE) levels. Skin test reactivity is most prevalent against fungi such as Aspergillus, and reactivity to nonfungal allergens is not increased significantly (140). Most studies show that the families of patients with CF with elevated IgE levels do not have increased prevalence of high IgE level or skin test reactivity, and atopy in the parents does not predict atopy in their children with CF, as it does in unaffected siblings (141). Taken together, these data suggest that there is not an increased inborn tendency to allergy in patients with CF, but patients become reactive to some allergens because of continuous exposure.

However, some patients with CF are clearly allergic. Although cross-sectional studies have given conflicting results on the question of whether allergic patients have more severe lung disease, Wilmott and coworkers (142) studied 117 patients prospectively in longitudinal fashion and found that patients with CF who are allergic do not have a more severe course than patients with CF who are not allergic. Thus, symptomatic atopy and allergy occur in patients with CF and should be treated, but they probably are not a consequence of the CF gene and do not compromise longevity.

Bronchiectasis

Bronchiectasis also contributes to obstruction to airflow. As the airway wall is destroyed, it becomes floppy and prone to collapse under conditions of high flow. Air trapping increases, and small airways eventually collapse even at flows generated by tidal breathing. The destruction of the airway wall presumably results mostly from the action of lysosomal enzymes derived from neutrophils in CF airways. Accompanying the destruction of the airway wall is a dramatic increase in the volume of the bronchial circulation. Distention of the bronchial vessels may further compromise the airway lumen. These vessels are vulnerable to breakage, and as in other forms of bronchiectasis, patients with CF regularly suffer minor hemoptysis. Some 8% to 10% of patients, as they get older, have massive bronchial bleeding (1).

All the accompanying effects of bronchiectasis develop in patients with CF. Clubbing develops in nearly all patients, and hypertrophic pulmonary osteoarthropathy develops in a few, with periosteal elevation in the distal long bones, warmth and tenderness over these sites, and effusions in adjacent joints (1).

In patients with chronic obstructive pulmonary disease who do not have CF, a major mechanism of airflow reduction is the loss of elastic recoil due to destruction of the alveolar walls, presumably due to the action over time of uninhibited elastase on the walls of the gas exchange units, which leads to alveolar simplification and increase in the alveolar airspace (i.e., anatomic emphysema). However, true emphysema is rare in CF. Patients with CF who die before 2 years of age have no emphysema demonstrated at postmortem, and even patients who survive into adulthood have less than 10% of the lung involved in emphysematous changes, if any of the lung is involved at all (143). These findings emphasize that CF is more a disease of the conducting airways than of the gas exchange units. The microscopic pathology of the CF lung resembles that of bronchiectasis from other causes (144). Airway wall thickening, persistent neutrophilic infiltration, plugging of small and large airways with mucus, inflammatory cells, and bacteria, microabscesses, sometimes ulceration of the mucosa, dilation of airways, and enlarged tortuous bronchial arteries contrast with the relatively well-preserved alveolar architecture.

Pulmonary Function

All these factors conspire to affect the function of the lung. Although rare, early in the course of the lung disease, a restrictive or mixed restrictive–obstructive pattern of pulmonary function may be evident in a few adults (1), but the majority of patients with CF develop an obstructive pattern on pulmonary function testing.

Pulmonary function testing in patients with CF requires care. Lung volumes should be determined by plethysmography because helium dilution or measurements on chest roentgenograms seriously underestimate lung volumes (145). In addition, the variability in pulmonary function tests in patients with CF is much greater than it is in healthy subjects (146,147). The variability is greatest in the youngest subjects. When age is controlled, variability is similar in mildly and severely obstructed patients. Therefore, age and learning effect may be important, but despite the extensive practice of most patients with CF with pulmonary func-

tion tests compared with controls, variability is still approximately twice that of healthy subjects.

Early changes in pulmonary function are the rule rather than the exception. Only 9 of 28 infants with CF in Israel in the first year of life had normal S_{Gaw} at the initial presentation, although thoracic gas volumes and V_{max} functional residual capacity (FRC) usually were within the normal range. Seventeen of these 28 infants, including 5 with initially normal test results, had repeated studies; most deteriorated. Only two infants' pulmonary function remained in the normal range, but two infants who previously had abnormal test results improved to normal (148). Therefore, CF affects pulmonary function very early in life, and the tendency to deteriorate is evident even then. Data from the Cleveland Cystic Fibrosis Center database show that at the earliest age at which reliable routine pulmonary function tests can be obtained (5–7 years), mean residual volume/total lung capacity (RV/TLC) already is abnormal in patients with CF, more so in girls than in boys (P. Byard, personal communication, 1994).

For patients able to perform routine pulmonary function tests, the most sensitive tests for airways obstruction in CF are the RV/TLC ratio and the instantaneous flows at low lung volumes (149,150). As a stand-in for instantaneous flows, the $FEF_{25\%-75\%}$ displays excellent sensitivity. Other, more complex tests, such as closing volume, slope of Phase III of single-breath nitrogen washout, volume of isoflow for air and heliox mixtures, or frequency dependence of dynamic compliance are more complex to obtain and/or difficult for children to perform, yet afford no advantages in sensitivity (151–153). Early abnormalities in these test results suggest that small airways disease develops early in the course of CF.

As the lung disease progresses, the RV/TLC ratio increases and the $FEF_{25\%-75\%}$ decreases (153). The FEV_1 starts to decrease and the ratio of the FEV_1 to the forced vital capacity (FEV_1/FVC) decreases. As in adult chronic obstructive pulmonary disease, the FEV_1 in CF is correlated with subsequent survival (154).

However, the pattern of change in pulmonary function over time differs from patient to patient (155,156). In some patients, linear decline is evident; in others, a stepwise decrease with long plateaus is the pattern; still others maintain near-normal function for years and then rapidly deteriorate. Studies of adults with CF, a special select population of survivors, may present a picture of a less severe pulmonary disease. Although as many as 10% to 15% of adults have entirely normal pulmonary function (1,155), it should be noted that patients must have survived until adulthood even to be included in such a tally.

Gas Exchange

Increased alveolar–arterial oxygen gradient may be an early indicator of lung disease (157), but as the obstructive disease progresses, frank hypoxemia develops. Although there is a general correlation between the degree of hypoxemia and measures of airways obstruction, spirometric parameters cannot predict the need for supplemental oxygen (158). The mismatch of ventilation and perfusion is evident in reduced diffusing capacity for carbon monoxide (1,159), but this test usually offers no clinical insight beyond the measurement of arterial oxygen and carbon dioxide tensions. Arterial oxygen tension often diminishes in patients with CF during exercise, sleep, or assumption of the supine position. Postural hypoxemia is most prominent in those with mild to moderate disease. Patients with severe disease actually may improve arterial oxygenation with the redistribution of blood flow that the supine position affords (160). However, during sleep, the most profound desaturation occurs in the most severely ill patients. The greatest desaturation with exercise also occurs in the most severely obstructed patients (161). Patients with mild airways obstruction actually may improve the arterial oxygen tension with exercise because of recruitment of little-used ventilatory units and the mild bronchodilation of the catecholamines released during exercise. If exercise is limited in patients with CF, it usually is limited by ventilation, not by cardiac factors or conditioning.

Hypercapnia develops relatively late in the course of the lung disease of patients with CF. It occurs at lower FEV_1 than in patients with chronic obstructive pulmonary disease (157). End-tidal carbon dioxide (CO_2) increases with exercise, as in healthy subjects, and thus may present difficulties for patients who already have hypercarbia (162).

Patients with CF endure many of the consequences of chronic hypoxemia and hypercarbia. Increased muscularization of the pulmonary vasculature and right-sided cardiac hypertrophy are observed in CF and are more prevalent the greater the degree of hypoxemia. In general, patients with arterial oxygen pressure (P_aO_2) less than 50 torr can be expected to have cor pulmonale (163,164). Frank right heart failure is a grim prognostic indicator (164). However, another expected consequence of hypoxemia, polycythemia, is rare in patients with CF. This failure of physiologic adjustment probably results from a number of factors. There probably is inadequate erythropoietin response in patients with CF (165). However, even if erythrocyte mass increases, blood volume also increases as disease progresses. Some patients are iron deficient and cannot respond on that basis.

Chest Roentgenogram

Early in the course of CF lung disease, the chest roentgenogram may be normal, and even some adults have normal chest x-rays. However, abnormalities of the chest roentgenogram usually occur early in the course of the disease, and persist. In one series of adults with CF, no patient with abnormal pulmonary function had a normal chest roentgenogram, so x-ray changes precede detectable abnormalities in pulmonary function (1). Although children with CF may display hyperinflation as the first roentgenographic change, in adults, hyperinflation invariably is accompanied by increased interstitial markings. Although patients with CF occasionally may develop episodes of pneumonia, ordinarily the early changes in lung markings do not display an alveolar pattern. In all age groups, there is a tendency for the initial abnormalities to appear in the upper lobes, and more frequently on the right than on the left. The reason for this predilection is unclear. As the disease progresses, the increased interstitial markings progress into a cystic–bronchiectatic pattern. Tram tracks (parallel lines representing thickening of the walls of a bronchus seen in longitudinal section) and cystic changes (from saccular bronchiectasis) become evident. Segmental or subsegmental atelectasis is intermittent and often asymptomatic. Lobar atelectasis may occur. These changes may progress so that in the central regions, dense markings are evident, and in more distal regions of the lung, especially the upper lobes, thin-walled cysts that appear to extend to the surface of the lung are evident. Fluid-filled cysts may empty spontaneously. Pneumothorax is observed with increasing frequency in older patients. Hyperinflation persists, with low flat diaphragms and increased retrocardiac airspace, and chest deformities, especially kyphosis, may develop. Underlying these abnormalities is advanced saccular bronchiectasis, usually worse in the upper lobes. Later in the course of CF, there may be little correspondence between radiologic abnormalities and acute clinical changes. Severe deterioration in functional status, gas exchange, and pulmonary function may occur in the absence of progression of x-ray changes.

More recent data from thin-section computed tomography (CT) scans of the chest confirm this progression of lung disease inferred from the plain films. However, because CT is much more sensitive, structural abnormalities are identified by this technique before they can be detected on plain chest radiographs (166). Cylindrical, followed by saccular bronchiectasis, in the upper lobes first but eventually in all areas of the lung, is identified on CT scan. Early changes are the thickening of airway walls, even before the dilation of the lumen is evident (167). Although the bronchiectasis of CF tends to be more extensive, involving all areas of the lung, than the changes in bronchiectasis of other etiologies, there are no pathognomonic features for CF evident on thin-section CT (168). Figure 3–3 provides an illustration of bronchiectasis in CF.

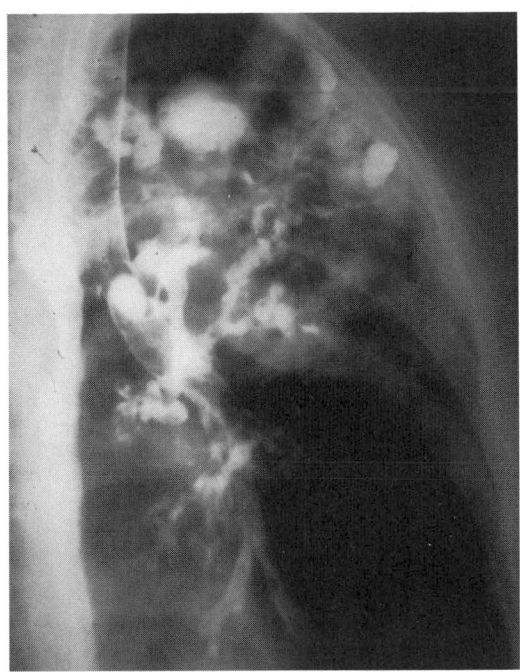

FIG. 3–3. Bronchogram from an adult patient with cystic fibrosis. Bronchi in the lower lobe illustrate cylindrical bronchiectasis and patchy distribution of dye characteristic of retained secretions. Upper lobes show saccular bronchiectasis, both central and peripheral, with massive dilation of the airways even out to the surface of the pleura.

Factors That Influence Pulmonary Function and Survival

Because most patients die a respiratory death, the pulmonary status is a strong predictor of survival in patients with CF. The best independent predictor of survival has been, in several studies, the FEV_1. Thus, factors that affect the FEV_1 are expected to influence survival in patients with CF. These factors, and appropriate interventions, are summarized in Table 3–1.

Patients who have pancreatic sufficiency have at least one copy of genes with specific CF mutations that have been termed "mild," and thus clearly have a different genetic lesion compared with patients with pancreatic insufficiency (3,169). At the same time, pancreatic-sufficient patients have better pulmonary function at any given age and longer survival (170).

TABLE 3–1. *Factors influencing survival in cystic fibrosis*

Factor	Mechanism	Interventions/comments
Pancreatic sufficiency	? Milder genetic lesion with greater residual CFTR function ? Better nutrition	Vigorous nutritional repletion
Gender	Unknown	Gender gap narrowing

Infecting organisms
  mucoid *P. aeruginosa*
  B. cepacia
	Not certain	Cohorting of patients to to prevent *B. cepacia* transmission
		Vigorous antibiotic therapy

Fitness	Unknown	Recommend physical exercise
Treatment	Reducing lung damage	Nutrition Antimicrobial therapy Airway clearance Antiinflammatory therapy Center care

CFTR, cystic fibrosis transmembrane conductance regulator.

It is not clear whether the milder lung disease can be ascribed to the milder genetic lesion or whether it is attributable to better nutrition (because pancreatic sufficient patients have normal levels of fat-soluble vitamins and normal fatty acid composition of membrane lipids, in contrast to pancreatic insufficient patients). The distinction between genetic and nutritional causes for the milder pulmonary disease may be important because if the difference derives from nutrition, vigorous supplementation of pancreatic insufficient patients may be useful.

Gender affects survival in CF. In the U.S. national registry data, male median survival age is approximately 30 years and female median survival age is 25 years (169). The reasons for this difference are not clear, but they probably cannot be attributed entirely to the hormonal changes that occur with puberty because the survival difference is apparent in the first decade of life. This gender difference has been noted for years, is consistent in the United States and Canada, and is demonstrable in longitudinal data from a single large U.S. center (Cleveland), as well as in the cross-sectional data reported to the registry. In some areas of the world where overall CF survival is poorer, the gender difference is less evident. The gender difference is somewhat surprising because girls have better canalization of growth than boys (171) and because for most other airways

diseases, boys seem to fare more poorly than girls (172,173). One possible explanation is that girls seem to acquire mucoid *P. aeruginosa* at an earlier age than boys (174). Although the negative impact of this organism on the rate of change of pulmonary function is comparable in boys and girls, the earlier acquisition by girls may account in part for the modest survival difference.

The infecting organisms in the lung of patients with CF have strong influence on survival. Survival is better in patients with CF without *P. aeruginosa* than in patients with this organism (142). Although some cross-sectional studies have not been able to demonstrate increased decline in pulmonary function in colonized as opposed to uncolonized patients, subsequent studies provide some explanation for this result. Detailed longitudinal examination of the data from the Cleveland center demonstrates that acquisition of nonmucoid *P. aeruginosa* is not associated with acceleration of rate of decline of pulmonary function, but acquisition of the mucoid phenotype of this organism is associated with significant increase in the rate of decline. Thus, studies in which patients infected with nonmucoid strains were considered together with patients who were infected with mucoid strains would dilute the effect of the mucoid organism on decline of pulmonary function and may fail to detect an effect of

Pseudomonas at all. Patients who acquire the mucoid phenotype before the age of 6 years have substantially higher mortality than patients who acquire it later (174). Acquisition of *Burkholderia cepacia* clearly is associated with increased mortality, particularly in the first year, and with increased rate of deterioration of pulmonary function, particularly in females (175).

An interesting independent variable that strongly affects survival is fitness. A 10-year study of patients with CF who were evaluated for fitness at the outset and then followed showed that only two independent variables contributed to survival—presence or absence of *P. cepacia* and the degree of fitness. In this analysis, even FEV_1 did not contribute independently to survival (176).

Treatment clearly influences survival; the symptomatic care that has evolved in the last 30 years improved the median survival age from less than 10 to more than 30 years. Although infants identified in screening programs and entered into treatment programs appear to do better than historical controls who came to treatment only when symptomatic, the definitive study of this question currently is in progress in Wisconsin. Care in CF centers around the world appears to confer an advantage compared with care outside of organized centers (177).

Prospects for Modifying the Course of the Lung Disease in Cystic Fibrosis

The complexity of the CF disease and the multiple factors that affect the pathophysiology of the lung disease and therefore survival do complicate the clinical picture, but at the same time, they afford many opportunities for intervention. It would seem that therapies directed at the basic defect afford the best hope for definitive treatment, but should they prove impractical or ineffective for those already ill, interruption of the pathophysiologic cascade at multiple points also may be effective.

The collection of patients with CF into centers has allowed systematic observations on the clinical syndrome to be made, rapid dissemination of new ideas and therapies, and availability of well-characterized patients for research purposes. All of these results have been tremendously valuable for CF therapeutics. Quite likely it was the institution of aggressive treatment protocols based on the principles of attention to nutrition, pulmonary mucus clearance, and vigorous treatment of pulmonary infection 30 years ago that raised the median survival age of patients with CF into the mid 20s in the most aggressive centers. Over the years, other centers have adopted this aggressive approach to treatment, and gradually, the median survival nationwide has come to approximate that in the most aggressive centers (see Fig. 3–1) (178). However, in those centers that 30 years ago achieved routine survival into adulthood, the recent rate of improvement has been slow, despite the introduction of new and more potent anti-Pseudomonal antibiotics, innovations in mucus clearance, and advances in the ability to normalize nutrition. Median survival ages in the mid 30s may be what is achievable with current conventional therapy, and entirely new approaches may be required to push survival even higher. Several new approaches are in various stages of clinical testing now. For example, the strategy of inhibition of the inflammatory response with "broad-spectrum" antiinflammatory agents such as ibuprofen, has been demonstrated in a 4-year controlled clinical trial to slow the progression of the CF lung disease, especially in younger patients with good to excellent pulmonary function (179). This strategy currently is in use clinically, and its impact on overall CF survival remains to be determined. More specific interventions in the vicious cycle of infection and inflammation, such as antiproteases, may be of help. Ultimately, strategies that strike at the basic defect, such as means of activating mutant forms of CFTR or introducing a normal gene into the airways, or activating alternative pathways for chloride secretion while inhibiting the excessive sodium reabsorption may be the best bet.

SUMMARY

The genetic lesion in CF occurs in a protein that functions as a cAMP-regulable chloride channel and is expressed in airway epithelial cells (as well as many other epithelia). In the lung, the direct consequence of this lesion is failure of the cAMP-regulated chloride secretion at the apical surface of the epithelium. A secondary consequence is elevated sodium reabsorption and elevated amiloride-sensitive transepithelial potential differences, particularly in the upper airways. Together, these ion transport abnormalities may lead to desiccated secretions and impaired mucociliary clearance. In addition, the CF lesion somehow predisposes to bacterial colonization of the airways, most frequently with *P. aeruginosa*. Once established, the infection and the inflammation it provokes are self-sustaining, mostly because of the crippling effects of uninhibited proteases on opsonophagocytosis of Pseudomonas. Destruction of the airway wall, mucus hypersecretion, and the wearing systemic effects of chronic inflammation combine to create progressive obstructive pulmonary disease, bronchiectasis, and ultimately death from respiratory insufficiency. This pathophysiologic process may be susceptible to intervention at any level, but it stands to reason that correction of the defect at the gene or the protein level has the most appeal and the greatest promise. However, once the vicious cycle of infection and inflammation is established, it may continue even if the initiating stimulus is removed. It may be prudent, therefore, to design strategies for intervention in CF directed not only at the basic defect but also at interrupting the cycle of infection and inflammation.

REFERENCES

1. diSant'Agnese PA, Davis PB. Cystic fibrosis in adults: 75 cases and a review of 232 cases in the literature. *Am J Med* 1979;66(1):121–132.
2. Rommens JM, Iannuzzi MC, Kerem B, et al. Identification of the cystic fibrosis gene: chromosome walking and jumping. *Science* 1989;245(4922):1059–1065.
3. Kerem B, Rommens JM, Buchanan JA, et al. Identification of the cystic fibrosis gene: genetic analysis. *Science* 1989;245(4922):1073–1080.
4. Riordan JR, Rommens JM, Kerem B, et al. Identification of the cystic fibrosis gene: cloning and characterization of complementary DNA. *Science* 1989;245 (4922):1066–1073.
5. Anderson MP, Berger HA, Rich DP, et al. Nucleotide triphosphates are required to open the CFTR chloride channel. *Cell* 1991;67(4):775–784.
6. Rich DP, Anderson MP, Gregory RJ, et al. Expression of cystic fibrosis transmembrane conductance regulator corrects defective chloride channel regulation in cystic fibrosis airway epithelial cells. *Nature* 1990; 347(629):358–363.
7. Drumm ML, Pope HA, Cliff WH, et al. Correction of the cystic fibrosis defect *in vitro* by retrovirus-mediated gene transfer. *Cell* 1990;62(6):1227–1233.
8. Anderson MP, Rich DP, Gregory RJ, et al. Generation of cAMP-activated chloride currents by expression of CFTR. *Science* 1991;251(4994):679–682.
9. Kartner N, Hanrahan JW, Jensen TJ, et al. Expression of the cystic fibrosis gene in non-epithelial invertebrate cells produces a regulated anion conductance. *Cell* 1991;64(4):681–691.
10. Tabcharani JA, Chang X-B, Riordan JR, et al. Phosphorylation-regulated Cl− channel in CHO cells stably expressing the cystic fibrosis gene. *Nature* 1991; 352(6336):628–631.
11. Dean M, White MB, Amos J, et al. Multiple mutations in highly conserved residues are found in mildly affected cystic fibrosis patients. *Cell* 1990;61 (5):863–870.
12. Anderson MP, Gregory RJ, Thompson S, et al. Demonstration that CFTR is a chloride channel by alteration of its anion selectivity. *Science* 1991;253 (5016):202–205.
13. Rich DP, Gregory RJ, Anderson MP, et al. Effect of deleting the R domain on CFTR-generated chloride channels. *Science* 1991;253(5016):205–207.
14. Perez A, Risma KA, Eckman EA, et al. Overexpression of R domain eliminates cAMP stimulated chloride secretion in 9/HTEo- cells in culture. *Am J Physiol* 1996;271(*Lung Cell Mol Physiol* 15):L85–L92.
15. Bear CE, Li C, Kartner N, et al. Purification and functional reconstitution of the cystic fibrosis transmembrane conductance regulator (CFTR). *Cell* 1992;68 (4):809–818.
16. Welsh MJ, Smith AE. Molecular mechanisms of CFTR chloride channel dysfunction in cystic fibrosis. *Cell* 1993;73(7):1251–1254.
17. Highsmith WE, Burch LH, Zhou Z, et al. A novel mutation in the cystic fibrosis gene in patients with pulmonary disease but normal sweat chloride concentrations. *N Engl J Med* 1994;331:974–980.
18. Cheng SH, Gregory RJ, Marshall J, et al. Defective intracellular transport and processing of CFTR is the molecular basis of most cystic fibrosis. *Cell* 1990;63 (4):827–834.
19. Pind S, Riordan JR, Williams DB. Participation of the endoplasmic reticulum chaperone calnexin (p88, IP90) in the biogenesis of the cystic fibrosis transmembrane conductance regulator. *J Biol Chem* 1994; 269(17):12784–12788.
20. Jensen TJ, Loo MA, Pind S, et al. Multiple proteolytic systems, including the proteasome, contribute to CFTR processing. *Cell* 1995;83:129–135.
21. Ward CL, Omura S, Kopito RR. Degradation of CFTR by the ubiquitin-proteasome pathway. *Cell* 1995;83:121–127.
22. Gregory RJ, Rich DP, Cheng SH, et al. Maturation and function of cystic fibrosis transmembrane con-

ductance regulator variants bearing mutations in putative nucleotide-binding domains 1 and 2. *Mol Cell Biol* 1991;11(8)3886–3893.

23. Drumm ML, Wilkinson DJ, Smit LS, et al. Chloride conductance expressed by ΔF508 and other mutant CFTRs in *Xenopus oocytes. Science* 1991;254(5039): 1797–1799.

24. Li C, Ramjeesingh M, Reyes E, et al. The cystic fibrosis mutation (ΔF508) does not influence the chloride channel activity of CFTR. *Nature Genet* 1993;3 (4):311–316.

25. Sherry AM, Cuppoletti J, Malinowska DH. Differential acidic pH sensitivity of ΔF508 CFTR Cl⁻ channel activity in lipid bilayers. *Am J Physiol* 1994;266 (3 Pt 1):C870–C875.

26. Gan KH, Veeze HJ, van den Ouweland AM, et al. A cystic fibrosis mutation associated with mild lung disease. *N Engl J Med* 1995;333(2):95–99.

27. Sheppard DN, Ostedgaard LS, Winter MC, et al. Mechanism of dysfunction of two nucleotide binding domain mutations in cystic fibrosis transmembrane conductance regulator that are associated with pancreatic sufficiency. *EMBO J* 1995;14:876–883.

28. Marino CR, Matovcik LM, Gorelick S, et al. Localization of the cystic fibrosis transmembrane conductance regulator in pancreas. *J Clin Invest* 1991;88(2): 712–716.

29. Zeitlin PL, Crawrod I, Lu L, et al. CFTR protein expression in primary and cultured epithelia. *Proc Natl Acad Sci U S A* 1992;89(120):344–347.

30. Sarkadi B, Bauzon D, Huckle WR, et al. Biochemical characterization of the cystic fibrosis transmembrane conductance regulator in normal and cystic fibrosis epithelial cells. *J Biol Chem* 1992;267(3):2087–2095.

31. Quinton PM. Chloride impermeability in cystic fibrosis. *Nature* 1983;301:421–422.

32. Quinton PM. Missing Cl conductance in cystic fibrosis. *Am J Physiol* 1986;251(4 Pt 1):C649–C652.

33. Knowles MR, Stutts MJ, Spock A, et al. Abnormal ion permeation through cystic fibrosis respiratory epithelium. *Science 1983;*221:1067–1070.

34. Kopelman H, Corey M, Gaskin K, et al. Impaired chloride secretion, as well as bicarbonate secretion, underlies the fluid secretory defect in cystic fibrosis of the pancreas. *Gastroenterology* 1988;95(2):349– 355.

35. Frizzell RA, Rechkemmer G, Shoemaker RL. Altered regulation of airway epithelial cell chloride channels in cystic fibrosis. *Science* 1986;233:558–560.

36. Boucher RC, Cheng EHC, Paradiso AM, et al. Chloride secretory response of cystic fibrosis human airway epithelia: preservation of calcium but not protein kinase C⁻ and A⁻ dependent mechanisms. *J Clin Invest* 1989;84(5):1424–1431.

37. Willumsen NJ, Boucher RC. Activation of an apical Cl⁻ conductance by Ca²⁺ ionophores in cystic fibrosis airway epithelia. *Am J Physiol* 1989;256(2 Pt 1): C226–C233.

38. Li M, McCann JD, Liedtke CM, et al. Cyclic AMP-dependent protein kinase opens chloride channels in normal but not cystic fibrosis airway epithelium. *Nature* 1988;331(6154):358–360.

39. Li M, McCann JD, Anderson MP, et al. Regulation of chloride channels by protein kinase C in normal and cystic fibrosis airway epithelia. *Science* 1989;244 (4910):1353–1356.

40. Schoumacher RA, Shoemaker RL, Halm DR, et al. Phosphorylation fails to activate chloride channels from cystic fibrosis airway cells. *Nature* 1987;330 (6150):752–754.

41. Hwang T-C, Lu L, Zeitlin PL, et al. Cl⁻ channels in CF: lack of activation by protein kinase C and cAMP-dependent protein kinase. *Science* 1989;244 (4910):1351–1356.

42. Widdicombe JH. Cystic fibrosis and β-adrenergic response of airway epithelial cell cultures. *Am J Physiol* 1986;251(4142):R818–R822.

43. Mason SJ, Paradiso AM, Boucher RC. Regulation of transepithelial ion transport and intracellular calcium by extracellular ATP in human normal and cystic fibrosis airway epithelium. *Br J Pharmacol* 1991;103 (3):1649–1656.

44. Yankaskas JR, Knowles MR, Gatzy JT, et al. Persistence of abnormal chloride ion permeability in cystic fibrosis nasal epithelial cells in heterologous culture. *Lancet* 1985;I(8435):954–956.

45. Jetten AM, Yankaskas JR, Stutts MJ, et al. Persistence of abnormal chloride conductance regulation in transformed cystic fibrosis epithelia. *Science* 1989; 244(4911):1472–1475.

46. Knowles MJ, Gatzy J, Boucher R. Increased bioelectric potential difference across respiratory epithelia in cystic fibrosis. *N Engl J Med* 1981;305(25):1489–1495.

47. Welsh MJ, Li M, McCann JD. Activation of normal and cystic fibrosis Cl⁻ channels by voltage, temperature, and trypsin. *J Clin Invest* 1989;84(6):2002–2007.

48. Anderson MP, Welsh MJ. Calcium and cAMP activate different chloride channels in the apical membrane of normal and cystic fibrosis epithelia. *Proc Natl Acad Sci U S A* 1991;88(14):6003–6007.

49. Wagner JA, Cozens AL, Schulman H, et al. Activation of chloride channels in normal and cystic fibrosis airway epithelial cells by multifunctional calcium/calmodulin-dependent protein kinase. *Nature* 1991;349(6312):793–796.

50. Widdicombe JH, Wine JJ. The basic defect in cystic fibrosis. *Trends Biochem Sci* 1991;16(12):474–477.

51. Worrell RT, Frizzell RA. CaMKII mediates stimulation of chloride conductance by calcium in T84 cells. *Am J Physiol* 1991;260(4 Pt 1):C877–C882.

52. Cliff WH, Frizzell RA. Separate Cl⁻ conductances activated by cAMP and Ca²⁺ in Cl⁻-secreting epithelial cells. *Proc Natl Acad Sci U S A* 1990;87(13): 4956–4960.

53. Egan M, Flotte T, Afione S, et al. Defective regulation of outwardly rectifying Cl⁻ channels by protein kinase A corrected by insertion of CFTR. *Nature* 1992;358(6387):581–584.

54. Guggino WB. Outwardly rectifying chloride channels and CF: a divorce and remarriage. *J Bioenerg Biomembr* 1993;25(1):27–35.

55. Schwiebert EM, Egan ME, Hwang T-H, et al. CFTR regulates outwardly rectifying chloride channels through an autocrine mechanism involving ATP. *Cell* 1995;81:1063–1073.

56. Gabriel SE, Clarke LL, Boucher RC, et al. CFTR and outward rectifying chloride channels are distinct proteins with a regulatory relationship. *Nature* 1993; 363:263–268.

57. Reddy MM, Quinton PM, Haws C, et al. Failure of the cystic fibrosis transmembrane conductance regulator to conduct ATP. *Science* 1996;271:1876–1879.

58. Boucher RC, Stutts MJ, Knowles MR, et al. Na⁺ transport in cystic fibrosis respiratory epithelia: abnormal basal rate and response to adenylate cyclase activation. *J Clin Invest* 1986;78(5):1245–1252.

59. Knowles MR, Church NL, Waltner WE, et al. A pilot study of aerosolized amiloride for the treatment of lung disease in cystic fibrosis. *N Engl J Med* 1990;322(14):1189–1194.

60. Stutts MJ, Canessa CM, Olsen JC, et al. CFTR as a cAMP-dependent regulator of sodium channels. *Science* 1995;269:847–850.

61. Knowles MR, Clarke LL, Boucher RC. Activation by extracellular nucleotides of chloride secretion in the airway epithelia of patients with cystic fibrosis. *N Engl J Med* 1991;325:533–538.

62. Alpert S, Walenga R, Kramer C, et al. Fatty acid content of airway epithelial cells from CF and non-CF subjects. *Pediatr Pulmonol Suppl* 1990;5:230 (abstract).

63. Liedtke CM, Alpert SE. Ion transport properties and fatty acid (FA) profiles in cultured rabbit airway epithelial cell (AEC). *FASEB J* 1991;5(6)A1761 (abstract).

64. Chung Y, Kercsmar CM, Davis PB. Ferret tracheal epithelial cells grown *in vitro* are resistant to lethal injury by activated neutrophils. *Am J Respir Cell Mol Biol* 1991;5(2):125–132.

65. Gilljam H, Ellin A, Strandvik B. Increased bronchial chloride concentration in cystic fibrosis. *Scand J Clin Lab Invest* 1989;49:121–124.

66. Joris L, Quinton PM. Concentration of elements in airway surface fluid. *Med Sci Res* 1987;15:855–856.

67. Joris L, Dab I, Quinton PM. Elemental composition of human airway surface fluid in healthy and diseased airways. *Am Rev Respir Dis* 1993;148:1633–1637.

68. Boucher RC. State of the art: human airway ion transport. *Am J Respir Crit Care Med* 1994;150:271–281.

69. Gasser KW, DiDomenico J, Hopfer U. Secretagogues activate chloride transport pathways in pancreatic zymogen granules. *Am J Physiol* 1988;254(1 Pt 1): G93–G99.

70. diSant'Agnese PA, Davis PB. Research in cystic fibrosis. *N Engl J Med* 1976;295(10):481–485, 534–541, 597–602.

71. Cheng PW, Boat TF, Cranfill K, et al. Increased sulfation of glycoconjugates by cultured nasal epithelial cells from patients with cystic fibrosis. *J Clin Invest* 1989;84:68–72.

72. Barasch J, Kiss B, Prince A. Defective acidification of intracellular organelles in cystic fibrosis. *Nature* 1991;353:70–73.

73. Sturgess JM. Structural and developmental abnormalities of the exocrine pancreas in cystic fibrosis. *J Pediatr Gastroenterol Nutr* 1984;3(Suppl 1):S55–S66.

74. Kopelman H, Durie P, Gaskin K, et al. Pancreatic fluid secretion and protein hyperconcentration in cystic fibrosis. *N Engl J Med* 1985;312:329–334.

75. Kopito LE, Kosasky HJ, Shwachman H. Water and electrolytes in cervical mucus from patients with cystic fibrosis. *Fertil Steril* 1973;24(7):512–516.

76. Gabriel SE, Brigman KN, Koller BH, et al. Cystic fibrosis heterozygote resistance to cholera toxin in the cystic fibrosis mouse model. *Science* 1994;266: 107–109.

77. Sturgess J, Imrie J. Quantitative evaluation of the development of tracheal submucosal glands in infants with cystic fibrosis and control infants. *Am J Pathol* 1982;106:303–311.

78. Oppenheimer EH. Tracheal and bronchial mucous glands and epithelium in infants with cystic fibrosis and controls. *Cystic Fibrosis Club* 1978;19:2 (abstract).

79. Zuelzer WW, Newton WA Jr. The pathogenesis of fibrocystic disease of the pancreas: a study of 36 cases with special reference to the pulmonary lesions. *Pediatrics* 1949;4:53–69.

80. Jiang CW, Finkbeiner WE, Widdicombe JH, et al. Altered fluid transport across airway epithelium in cystic fibrosis. *Science* 1993;262:424–427.

81. Jiang CW, Finkbeiner WE, Widdicombe JH, et al. Active fluid transport across cultures of human tracheobronchial glands (HTG) in cystic fibrosis. *Pediatr Pulmonol* 1993;suppl 9:208.

82. Smith JJ, Karp PH, Welsh MJ. Defective fluid transport by cystic fibrosis airway epithelia. *J Clin Invest* 1994;93:1307–1311.

83. Smith JJ, Travis SM, Greenberg EP, et al. Cystic fibrosis airway epithelia fail to kill bacteria because of abnormal airway surface fluid. *Cell* 1996;85:229–236.

84. Wood RE, Wanner A, Hirsch J, et al. Tracheal mucociliary transport in patients with cystic fibrosis and its stimulation by terbutaline. *Am Rev Respir Dis* 1975;111(6):733–738.

85. Yeates DB, Sturgess JM, Kahn SR, et al. Mucociliary transport in trachea of patients with cystic fibrosis. *Arch Dis Child* 1976;51(1)28–33.

86. Afzelius BA, Mossberg B. Immotile cilia syndrome (primary ciliary dyskinesia), including Kartagener Syndrome. In: Scriver CR, Beaudet AL, Sly WS, Valle D, eds. *The metabolic basis of inherited disease.* New York: McGraw Hill Information Services, 1995:3943–3954.

87. Boucher RC, Larsen EH. Comparison of ion transport by cultured secretory and absorptive canine airway epithelia. *Am J Physiol* 1988;254(4 Part 1) :C535–C547.

88. Tizzano EF, O'Brodovich H, Chitayat D, et al. Regional expression of CFTR in developing human respiratory tissues. *Am J Respir Cell Mol Biol* 1994;10 (4):355–362.

89. McGrath SA, Basu A, Zeitlin PL. Cystic fibrosis gene and protein expression during fetal lung development. *Am J Respir Cell Mol Biol* 1993;8(2):201–208.

90. Engelhardt JF, Yankaskas JR, Ernst SA, et al. Submucosal glands are the predominant site of CFTR expression in the human bronchus. *Nature Genet* 1992; 2(3):240–248.

91. Jacquot J, Puchelle E, Hinnrasky J, et al. Localization of the cystic fibrosis transmembrane conductance regulator in airway secretory glands. *Eur Respir J* 1993;6(2):169–176.

92. Crawford I, Maloney PC, Zeitlin PL, et al. Immunocytochemical localization of the cystic fibrosis gene product CFTR. *Proc Natl Acad Sci U S A* 1991;88 (20):9262–9266.

93. Khan TZ, Wagener JS, Bost T, et al. Early pulmonary inflammation in infants with cystic fibrosis. *Am J Respir Crit Care Med* 1995;151:1075–1082.

94. Armstrong DS, Grimwood K, Carzino R, et al. Lower respiratory infection and inflammation in infants with newly diagnosed cystic fibrosis. *BMJ* 1995;310: 1571–1572.

95. Cantin A. Cystic fibrosis lung inflammation: early, sustained, and severe. *Am J Respir Crit Care Med* 1995;151:939–941.

96. Wang EEL, Prober CG, Manson B, et al. Association of respiratory viral infections with pulmonary deterioration in patients with cystic fibrosis. *N Engl J Med* 1984;311(26):1653–1653.

97. Zierdt CH, Williams RL. Serotyping of *Pseudomonas aeruginosa* isolates from patients with cystic fibrosis of the pancreas. *J Clin Microbiol* 1975;1 (6):521–526.

98. Pedersen SS, Jensen T, Pressler T, et al. Does centralized treatment of cystic fibrosis increase the risk of *Pseudomonas aeruginosa* infection? *Acta Paediatr Scand* 1986;75:840–845.

99. Pedersen SS, Koch C, Hoiby N, et al. An epidemic spread of multiresistant Pseudomonas aeruginosa in a cystic fibrosis centre. *J Antimicrob Chemother* 1986;17(4):505–516.

100. Laraya-Cuasay LR, Cundy KR, Huang NN. *Pseudomonas* carrier rats of patients with cystic fibrosis and of members of their families. *J Pediatr* 1976;89:23–26.

101. Speert DP, Lawton D, Damm S. Communicability of *Pseudomonas aeruginosa* in a cystic fibrosis summer camp. *J Pediatr* 1982;101(2):227–228.

102. Woods DE, Bass JA, Johanson Jr WG, et al. Role of adherence in the pathogenesis of *Pseudomonas aeruginosa* lung infection in cystic fibrosis. *Infect Immunol* 1980;30:694–699.

103. Saiman L, Cacalano G, Gruenert D, Prince A. Comparison of adherence of *Pseudomonas aeruginosa* to respiratory epithelial cells from cystic fibrosis patients and healthy subjects. *Infect Immun* 1992; 60:2808–2814.

104. Zar H, Saiman L, Quittell L, et al. Binding of *Pseudomonas aeruginosa* to respiratory epithelial cells from patients with various mutations in the cystic fibrosis transmembrane regulator. *J Pediatr* 1995;126: 230–233.

105. Imundo L, Barasch J, Prince A, et al. Cystic fibrosis epithelial cells have a receptor for pathogenic bacteria on their apical surface. *Proc Natl Acad Sci U S A* 1995;92:3019–3023.

106. Pier GB, Grout M, Zaidi TS, et al. Role of mutant CFTR in hypersusceptibility of cystic fibrosis patients to lung infections. *Science* 1996;271:64–67.

107. Fitzsimmons SC. The changing epidemiology of cystic fibrosis. *J Pediatr* 1993;122:1–9.

108. Macone AB, Pier GP, Pennington JE, et al. Mucoid *Escherichia coli* in cystic fibrosis. *N Engl J Med* 1981;304:1445–1449.

109. May TB, Shinabarger D, Maharaj R, et al. Alginate synthesis by *Pseudomonas aeruginosa*: a key pathogenic factor in chronic pulmonary infections of cystic fibrosis patients. *Clin Microbiol Rev* 1991;4(2): 191–206.

110. Berger M, Sorensen RU, Tosi MF, et al. Complement receptor expression on neutrophils at an inflammatory site, the *Pseudomonas*-infected lung in cystic fibrosis. *J Clin Invest* 1989;84:1302–1313.

111. Tosi MF, Zakem H, Berger M. Neutrophil elastase cleaves C3bi on opsonized pseudomonas as well as CR1 on neutrophils to create a functionally important opsonin receptor mismatch. *J Clin Invest* 1990;86(1): 300–308.

112. Fick RB Jr., Naegel GP, Matthay RA, et al. Cystic fibrosis pseudomonas opsonins: inhibitory nature in an *in vitro* phagocytic assay. *J Clin Invest* 1981;68(4): 899–914.

113. DiMango E, Zar HJ, Bryan R, et al. Diverse *Pseudomonas aeruginosa* gene products stimulate respiratory epithelial cells to produce interleukin-8. *J Clin Invest* 1995;96:2204–2210.

114. Kim KC, Nassiri J, Brody JS. Mechanisms of airway goblet cell mucin release: studies with cultured tracheal surface epithelial cells. *Am J Respir Cell Mol Biol* 1989;1(2):137–143.

115. Christensen TG, Breuer R, Hornstra LJ, et al. An ultrastructural study of the response of hamster bronchial epithelium to human neutrophil elastase. *Exp Lung Res* 1987;13(3):279–297.

116. Bonfield TL, Panuska JR, Konstan MW, et al. Inflammatory cytokines in cystic fibrosis lungs. *Am J Respir Crit Care Med* 1995;152:2111–2118.

117. Bonfield TL, Konstan MW, Burfeind P, et al. Normal bronchial epithelial cells constitutively produce the anti-inflammatory cytokine interleukin-10, which is downregulated in cystic fibrosis. *Am J Respir Cell Mol Biol* 1995;13:257–261.

118. Woolcock AJ. Therapies to control airway inflammation of asthma. *Eur J Respir Dis Suppl* 1986;147: 166–174.

119. Laitinen LA, Heino M, Laitinen A. Damage of the airway epithelium and bronchial reactivity in patients with asthma. *Am Rev Respir Dis* 1985;131(4):599–606.

120. Busse WW. The contribution of viral respiratory infections to the pathogenesis of airway hyperreactivity. *Chest* 1988;93(5):1076–1082.

121. Jenkins CR, Breslin ABX. Upper respiratory tract infections and airway reactivity in normal and asthmatic subjects. *Am Rev Respir Dis* 1984;130(5):879–883.

122. Empey DW, Laitinen LA, Jacobs L, et al. Mechanisms of bronchial hyperreactivity in normal subjects after upper respiratory tract infections. *Am Rev Respir Dis* 1976;113(2):131–139.

123. Holzer FJ, Olinsky A, Phelan PD. Variability of airways hyperreactivity and allergy in cystic fibrosis. *Arch Dis Child* 1981;56(6):455–459.

124. Rothstein RJ, Pinney MA, Buckley JM, et al. Evaluation of reactive airway disease in atopic cystic fibrosis patients. *J Allergy Clin Immunol* 1974;53(2): 100–101 (abstract).

125. Mitchell I, Corey M, Woenne R, et al. Bronchial hyperreactivity in cystic fibrosis and asthma. *J Pediatr* 1978;93(5):744–748.

126. Haluszka J, Scislicki A. Bronchial liability in children suffering from some diseases of the bronchi. *Respiration* 1975;32(3):217–226.

127. Mellis CM, Levison H. Bronchial reactivity in cystic fibrosis. *Pediatrics* 1978;61(3):446–450.

128. Van Asperen P, Mellis CM, South RT, et al. Bronchial reactivity in cystic fibrosis with normal pulmonary function. *Am J Dis Child* 1981;135(9):815–819.

129. Price JF, Weller PH, Harper SA, et al. Bronchial provocation tests in cystic fibrosis. *Monogr Paediatr* 1979;10:123–124.

130. Day G, Mearns MB. Bronchial lability in cystic fibrosis. *Arch Dis Child* 1973;48(5):355–359.
131. Tobin MJ, Maguire O, Reen D, et al. Atopy and bronchial reactivity in older patients with cystic fibrosis. *Thorax* 1980;35(11):807–813.
132. Silverman M, Hobbs FDR, Gordon IRS, et al. Cystic fibrosis, atopy, and airways lability. *Arch Dis Chil* 1978;53(11):873–877.
133. Skorecki K, Levison H, Crozier DN. Bronchial lability in cystic fibrosis. *Acta Paediatr Scand* 1976;65 (1):39–44.
134. Konig P, Godfrey S. Exercise-induced bronchial lability and atopic status of families of infants with wheezy bronchitis. *Arch Dis Child* 1973;48(12):942–46.
135. Konig P, Godfrey S. Prevalence of exercise-induced bronchial lability in families of children with asthma. *Arch Dis Child* 1984;48(7):513–518.
136. Townley R, Bewtra A. Airway reactivity to methacholine in asthma family members and twins. In: Spector LL, ed. *Provocative challenge procedures: bronchial, oral, nasal, and exercise.* Vol. 1. Boca Raton: CRC Press, 1983.
137. Byard J, Davis PB. Pulmonary function in obligate heterozygotes for cystic fibrosis. *Am Rev Respir Dis* 1988;138(2):312–316.
138. Davis PB, Byard PJ. Heterozygotes for cystic fibrosis: models for study of airway and autonomic reactivity. *J Appl Physiol* 1989;66(5):2124–2128.
139. Davis PB. Airway responsiveness and atopy in cystic fibrosis. In: Weiss ST, Sparrow D, eds. *Airway responsiveness and allergy in the development of chronic lung disease.* New York: Raven Press, 1989.
140. Moss RB. Immunology of cystic fibrosis: immunity, immunodeficiency and hypersensitivity. In: Lloyd-Still JD, ed. *Textbook of cystic fibrosis.* Boston: John Wright/PSG, 1983:109–151.
141. Reen DJ, Carson J, Maguire O, et al. Atopy and cystic fibrosis: a study of CF sibling pairs and their families. *Clin Allergy* 1981;11(6):571–577.
142. Wilmott RW, Tyson SL, Matthew DJ. Cystic fibrosis survival rates: the influence of allergy and *Pseudomonas aeruginosa.* *Am J Dis Child* 1985;139(7):669–671.
143. Bedrossian CWM, Greenberg SD, Singer DB, et al. The lung in cystic fibrosis: a quantitative study including prevalence of pathologic findings among different age groups. *Hum Pathol* 1976;7(2):195–204.
144. Tomashefski JF Jr., Abramowsky CR, Dahms BB. The pathology of cystic fibrosis. In: Davis PB, ed. *Cystic fibrosis.* New York: Marcel Dekker Inc, 1993:435–489.
145. Cutrera R, Helms P. Retrospective estimation of values for total lung capacity by plethysmography, helium gas dilution, and chest radiography in patients with cystic fibrosis. *Thorax* 1988;43(11):931–932.
146. Nickerson BG, Lemen RJ, Gerdes CB, et al. Within-subject variability and percent change for significance of spirometry in normal subjects and in patients with cystic fibrosis. *Am Rev Respir Dis* 1980;122(6):859–866.
147. Cooper PJ, Robertson CF, Hudson IL, et al. Variability of pulmonary function tests in cystic fibrosis. *Pediatr Pulmonol* 1990;8(1):16–22.
148. Beardsmore CS, Bar-Yashay E, Maayan C, et al. Lung function in infants with cystic fibrosis. *Thorax* 1988;43(7):545–551.
149. Zapletal A, Motoyama EK, Gibson LE, et al. Pulmonary mechanics in asthma and cystic fibrosis. *Pediatrics* 1971;48(1):64–72.
150. Cooper DM, Doron I, Mansell AL, et al. The relative sensitivity of closing volume in children with asthma and cystic fibrosis. *Am Rev Respir Dis* 1974;109(5):519–524.
151. Lutchen KR, Habib RH, Dorkin HL, et al. Respiratory impedance and multibreath N_2 washout in healthy, asthmatic, and cystic fibrosis subjects. *J Appl Physiol* 1990;68(5):2139–2149.
152. Mansell A, Dubrawsky C, Levison H, et al. Lung elastic recoil in cystic fibrosis. *Am Rev Respir Dis* 1974;109(2):190–197.
153. Landau LI, Phelan PD. The spectrum of cystic fibrosis: a study of pulmonary mechanics in 46 patients. *Am Rev Respir Dis* 1973;108(3):593–602.
154. Wagener JS, Taussig LM, Burrows B, et al. Comparison of lung function and survival patterns between cystic fibrosis and emphysema or chronic bronchitis patients. In: Sturgess JM, ed. *Proceedings of the 8th international congress on cystic fibrosis.* Toronto, Canada: Canadian Cystic Fibrosis Foundation, 1980.
155. Fink RJ, Doershuk CF, Tucker AS, et al. Pulmonary function and morbidity in 40 adult patients with cystic fibrosis. *Chest* 1978;74(6):643–647.
156. Corey ML. Longitudinal studies in cystic fibrosis. In: Sturgess JM, ed. *Perspectives in cystic fibrosis: proceedings of the 8th international congress on cystic fibrosis.* Toronto, Canada: Canadian Cystic Fibrosis Foundation, 1980.
157. Lamarre A, Reilly BJ, Bryan AC, et al. Early detection of pulmonary function abnormalities in cystic fibrosis. *Pediatrics* 1972;50(2):291–298.
158. Desmond KJ, Coates AL, Beaudry PH. Relationship between the partial pressure of arterial oxygen and airflow limitation in children with cystic fibrosis. *Can Med Assoc J* 1984;131(4)325–326.
159. Cotton DJ, Graham BL, Mink JT, et al. Reduction of the single breath CO diffusing capacity in cystic fibrosis. *Chest* 1985;87(2):217–222.
160. Stokes DC, Wohl MEB, Khaw KT, et al. Postural hypoxemia in cystic fibrosis. *Chest* 1985;87(6):785–789.
161. Marcus CL, Bader D, Stabile MW, et al. Supplemental oxygen and exercise performance in patients with cystic fibrosis with severe pulmonary disease. *Chest* 1992;101(1):52–57.
162. Coates AL. Oxygen therapy, exercise, and cystic fibrosis (editorial). *Chest* 1992;101(1):2–4.
163. Moss AJ, Harper WH, Dooley RR, et al. Cor pulmonale in cystic fibrosis of the pancreas. *J Pediatr* 1965;67(5):797–807.
164. Stern RC, Borkat G, Hirshfeld SS, et al. Heart failure in cystic fibrosis: treatment and prognosis of cor pulmonale with failure of the right side of the heart. *Am J Dis Child* 1980;134(3):267–272.
165. Vichinsky EP, Pennathur-Das R, Nickerson B, et al. Inadequate erythroid response to hypoxia in cystic fibrosis. *J Pediatr* 1984;105(1):15–21.
166. Grum CM, Lynch JP III. Chest radiographic findings in cystic fibrosis. *Semin Respir Infect* 1992;7(3):193–209.

167. Santis G, Hodson ME, Strickland B. High resolution computed tomography in adult cystic fibrosis patients with mild lung disease. *Clin Radiol* 1991; 44:20–22.

168. Reiff DB, Wells AU, Carr DH, et al. CT findings in bronchiectasis: limited value in distinguishing between idiopathic and specific types. *Am J Roentgenol* 1995;165(2):261–267.

169. Correlation between genotype and phenotype in patients with cystic fibrosis: the Cystic Fibrosis Genotype–Phenotype Consortium. *N Engl J Med* 1993;329 (18)1308–1313.

170. Gaskin K, Gurwitz D, Durie P, et al. Improved respiratory prognosis in patients with cystic fibrosis with normal fat absorption. *J Pediatr* 1982;100(6):857–862.

171. Byard PJ. The adolescent growth spurt in children with cystic fibrosis. *Ann Hum Biol* 1994;21(3):229–240.

172. Sears MR, Burrows B, Flannery EM, et al. Relation between airway responsiveness and serum IgE in children with asthma and in apparently normal children. *N Engl J Med* 1991;325(15):1067–1071.

173. Schwartz J, Gold D, Dockery DW, et al. Predictors of asthma and persistent wheeze in a national sample of children in the United States: association with social class, perinatal events and race. *Am Rev Respir Dis* 1990;142(3):555–562.

174. Demko CA, Byard PJ, Davis PB. Gender differences in cystic fibrosis: *Pseudomonas aeruginosa* infection. *J Clin Epidemiol* 1994;48(8):1041–1049.

175. Lewin LO, Byard PJ, Davis PB. Effect of *Pseudomonas cepacia* colonization on survival and pulmonary function of cystic fibrosis patients. *J Clin Epidemiol* 1990;43(12):125–131.

176. Nixon PA, Orenstein DM, Kelsey SF, et al. The prognostic value of exercise testing in patients with cystic fibrosis. *N Engl J Med* 1992;327(25):1785–1788.

177. Walters S, Britton J, Hodson ME. Hospital care for adults with cystic fibrosis: an overview and comparison between special cystic fibrosis clinics and general clinics using a patient questionnaire. *Thorax* 1994;49(4):300–306.

178. Kerem E, Reisman J, Corey M, et al. Prediction of mortality in patients with cystic fibrosis. *N Engl J Med* 1992;326(18):1187–1191.

179. Konstan MW, Byard PJ, Hoppel CL, et al. Effect of high-dose ibuprofen in patients with cystic fibrosis. *N Engl J Med* 1995;332:848–854.

Cystic Fibrosis in Adults,
edited by J. R. Yankaskas and M. R. Knowles,
Lippincott–Raven Publishers, Philadelphia, 1999.

4

Airway Secretions

Margaret W. Leigh

*Division of Pulmonary Medicine and Allergy, Department of Pediatrics, University of North
Carolina School of Medicine, Chapel Hill, North Carolina*

Normal airway surfaces are lined with a thin layer of secretions composed primarily of water, ions, and mucins, as well as a number of minor constituents including glycosaminoglycans, proteins, lipids, and DNA. This surface fluid is believed to be divided into a periciliary fluid layer through which cilia beat freely and an overlying mucus gel layer that entraps particles to be transported cephalad by coordinated ciliary movement. The volume and viscoelastic properties of the mucus gel influence the efficiency of mucociliary clearance. Mucins, also known as mucous glycoproteins, are believed to be the major determinant of the viscoelastic properties, although other components may interact with mucins to modify these properties.

Cystic fibrosis (CF) is characterized by thick, inspissated mucus in a variety of epithelia-lined passages, including the respiratory tract, pancreatic ducts, hepatobiliary tracts, and intestinal lumens. The occurrence of mucus plugging in uninfected regions, such as the pancreatic and hepatobiliary ducts, suggests that alterations in mucus may be mediated by processes other than infection and inflammation. Small mucus plugs have been recovered in bronchoalveolar lavage fluid from infants with CF, even in the absence of coexisting infection, suggesting that CF airway secretions are altered by influences other than infection and inflammation. Early research efforts attempted to define CF-associated abnormalities in mucins, and more recent efforts have explored links between altered cystic fibrosis transmembrane conductance regulator (CFTR) function and alterations in mucins, specifically, their hydration, glycosylation, and gene expression. The complexity and heterogeneity of mucins have confounded these efforts. To date, no distinct CF-associated abnormalities have been defined, although a number of possibilities have been suggested.

Cystic fibrosis patients with chronic airway infections expectorate large volumes of sputum that characteristically is thick and viscous. After a course of antibiotics, the sputum thins and decreases in volume, suggesting that chronic infection and inflammation influence properties of airway secretions. Proposed influences of infection and inflammation include increased volume of mucin secretion and increased concentrations of other components, such as DNA and actin, that alter the viscoelastic properties of the mucus gel and impair clearance. An intriguing aspect of CF lung disease is the chronic colonization of airways with bacterial pathogens, particularly *Pseudomonas aeruginosa* and *Staphylococcus aureus*. A major research focus has centered on potential alterations in CF airway secretions that may impair clearance of these organisms. The role of altered CFTR function in establishing and sustaining these alterations in airway secretion composition and quantity is not well defined. Studies of early pathogenesis of CF lung disease are critical to our understanding of these interrelating influences on airway secretions.

This chapter reviews the function, composition, and viscoelastic properties of normal airway mucus as well as alterations in CF mucus that may contribute to mucus plugging and bacterial colonization of the airways. Emphasis is placed on the structure and physicochemical properties of mucins. The structure and regulation of secretory sources (submucosal glands and goblet cells in the bronchi and Clara cells in the bronchioles) from normal and CF airways are described. Finally, potential influences of a mutated CFTR and/or chronic inflammation on airway secretions are discussed.

NORMAL AIRWAY MUCUS

General

Nomenclature and Definitions

Mucus is a viscoelastic gel-like material covering epithelial surfaces including the respiratory, gastrointestinal, and reproductive tracts. The mucus lining these surfaces forms a protective barrier between the external environment and the underlying epithelial layer. In the respiratory tract, inhaled particles and bacteria are entrapped in the mucus that then is cleared from the airways by mucociliary transport or by coughing. Normal respiratory tract mucus contains secretory products from goblet cells, submucosal glands, Clara cells, and alveolar cells. In the presence of injury or infection, airway mucus also may contain substantial amounts of serum transudate and inflammatory cell products. Sputum contains expectorated mucus mixed with varying amounts of saliva, a watery fluid secreted by the salivary glands (parotid glands and submaxillary glands). The composition and properties of saliva are very different from airway mucus; therefore, analytic studies must minimize contamination of airway mucus samples with saliva.

The adjective *mucous* has been used loosely to refer to anything pertaining to or resembling mucus, that is, mucous secretions, mucous glycoproteins, mucous membranes, mucous glands, mucous cells. To avoid confusion, use of the term *mucous* is minimized in this chapter and more specific terms are used. The noun *mucus* is used instead of the term *mucous secretions* and includes all components of airway surface liquid. Additionally, *mucins* is used instead of *mucous glycoproteins*, *airway epithelium* instead of *mucous membranes*, and *submucosal glands* instead of *mucous glands*. The term *mucous cell* is used to identify a specific cell type in submucosal gland that contains large electron-lucent granules and secretes mucins.

Composition

The small volume of the airway lining fluid layer in healthy subjects limits our ability to selectively sample and analyze surface fluid composition. Each approach to sampling lower airways is complicated by contamination or artifactual alteration of secretion. Expectorated samples are contaminated with saliva. If the mouth is bypassed using an endotracheal tube, tracheostomy, or bronchoscope, these foreign objects may stimulate sensory nerves in the airways and promote glandular secretion, thereby altering the fluid quantity and composition. The volume of mucus production measured by continuous tracheal aspiration in patients who underwent laryngectomy and tracheostomy is 0.2 to 0.5 mL/kg of body weight per day (1); however, this approach most likely overestimates secretion because these airways undoubtedly are irritated by instrumentation and exposure to particulates that would have been filtered by an intact upper airway. Early composition studies using expectorated secretions from laryngectomized healthy subjects or patients with chronic bronchitis demonstrated that the major component of airway secretion is water, accounting for 95% of airway mucus by weight; the solids content includes 2% to 3% proteins and glycoproteins, 1% lipids, and 1% minerals (2). Another approach to collecting airway surface liquid from healthy subjects is the application of preweighed filter paper onto the tracheal or bronchial surface under direct bronchoscopic observation (3,4). By comparing the wet and dry weights with the preapplication weight of the filter paper, the water content in healthy individuals has been estimated at 91% to 93% (3,4).

Definitive characterization of the components of airway secretions has been complicated by several factors. First, composition may vary with location in the tracheobronchial tree because of differences in distribution of secretory sources. Although goblet cells and submucosal glands are the primary sources in the trachea and bronchi, bronchioles have no submucosal glands and the predominant secretory cell is the Clara cell. Bronchiolar secretions most likely contain more surfactant and other products arising from the alveoli than tracheal and bronchial secretions. Second, composition may vary with age because of developmental changes in the distribution of secretory cells and types of secretory products. Third, composition may change with stimulation or injury to airways, such as exposure to pollutants or infectious agents that recruit inflammatory cells (and their products) into the airway. Fourth, composition varies with species, thereby limiting the usefulness of animal models. Fifth, airway secretions contain variable amounts of cellular debris and inhaled particles depending on environmental conditions. Finally, purification and biochemical characterization of mucins and other components require large volumes of airway secretions that are not available at baseline conditions. Studies to characterize these secretions have used different modifications of methods for collection, solubilization, fractionation, and biochemical characterization. Not surprisingly, the results of these analyses have not been uniform. For example, a few studies suggest that mucins are minor constituents in normal airway secretions (5–7) whereas most other studies identify mucins as the major macromolecular component that is primarily responsible for the viscoelastic properties of airway secretions under normal conditions.

Mucin-Type Glycoproteins

Structure

Mucin-type glycoproteins are heterogeneous, high-molecular weight glycoconjugates consisting of a peptide core with multiple (typically several hundred) sugar side chains (Fig. 4–1). The greatest challenge in characterizing mucins is their extensive heterogeneity and complexity. The size (M_r) of airway mucins varies with estimates ranging from 1.8×10^6 to 44×10^6 kD (8). The peptide core varies in length (estimates range from 100 to 600 kDa), and the sugar side chains vary in number, length (typically 1 to 20 sugars/side chain), and branching pattern as well as content of the acidic moieties, sialic acid, and sulfate (8). Characteristically, the sugar side chains of mucin-type glycoproteins are attached by *O*-glycosidic linkages between *N*-acetylgalactosamine in the sugar side chain and serine or threonine in the peptide core. Repulsion of negative charges in adjacent sugar chains is believed to influence molecular structure, resulting in a rigid, "bottle-brush" conformation of mucin molecules (9,10). The overall composition of respiratory mucins is 70% to 80% carbohydrate, 20% protein, and 2% to 7% sulfate (11,12).

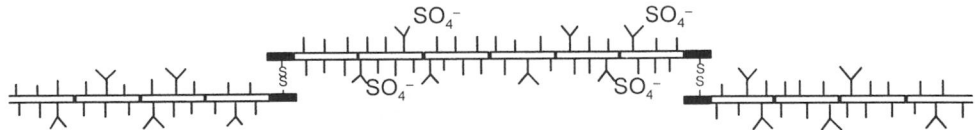

FIG. 4–1. Structure of a mucin-type glycoprotein. This schematic diagram shows a mucin molecule in the center that is linked to two adjacent mucin molecules by disulfide bonds. Attached to the peptide core of each molecule are multiple sugar side chains of various sizes and branching patterns. The central portion of the peptide core containing tandem repeats of amino acid sequences (indicated by open blocks) is heavily glycosylated, but the flanking regions (indicated by the closed blocks) are not glycosylated. The nonglycosylated regions contain cysteine residues that allow for disulfide bonds between the ends of adjacent molecules, resulting in long cords of mucin molecules. SO_4^-, sulfate.

The central portion of the peptide core is composed of tandem repeats of amino acid sequences that are rich in potential glycosylation sites, serine, and threonine (13,14). Serine and threonine account for 40% to 50% of the total amino acids in mucins; other prevalent amino acids are proline, alanine, and, in some cases, glycine. A sugar side chain is linked to every third or fourth amino acid in the central portion of the peptide core. The unique sequences flanking the central portion contain cysteine residues that are believed to link the large mucin molecules through disulfide bonds (14). These intermolecular bonds influence the rigidity of the mucus gel.

Mucin Genes

Our knowledge about mucin genes encoding the protein core is evolving. Currently, nine human mucin genes have been identified and cloned to some degree (Table 4–1) (14–16). Although one of these mucins (MUC1) is membrane associated, most are secreted mucins. For all of these mucin genes, a major portion consists of tandem repeats of variable lengths, encoding peptide sequences of 8 to 169 amino acids. For the presently cloned mucin genes, there is no apparent pattern to the sequence or length of the tandem repeats; however, all are enriched with sequences encoding serine and threonine. The secreted mucins have cysteine-rich domains located in the amino terminal region and carboxy terminal region; homology of these cysteine-rich domains with von Willebrand's factor (17,18) has led to speculation

that these regions are important for packaging and oligomerization of mucins, as has been described for von Willebrand's factor (17). Human mucin genes expressed in airways include MUC2, MUC3, MUC4, and MUC5, although the distribution and extent of expression vary. MUC5 is highly expressed in airways and in colon and pancreatic adenocarcinoma cell lines (19). A number of clones and sequences have been reported for MUC5, including MUC5AC and MUC5B. MUC4 is expressed fairly equally in the lung, the small intestine, the colon, the stomach, and the cervix. MUC3 is expressed more strongly in the intestine than in the lung. MUC2 is expressed predominantly in the small intestine and the colon, but it may be expressed in diseased airways (20). One area of active investigation is regulation of mucin gene expression, with particular emphasis on mechanisms by which inflammatory mediators and bacterial products may modulate mucin gene expression.

Mucin Glycosylation

The five sugars found in mucin oligosaccharide chains are L-fucose (Fuc), D-galactose (Gal), D-*N*-acetylgalactosamine (GalNAc), D-*N*-acetylglucosamine (GlcNAc), and sialic acid, also known as neuraminic acid (NeuAc); mucins contain little or no mannose (prevalent in serum and membrane glycoproteins that have N-glycosidic linkages) or uronic acid (prevalent in proteoglycans). The sugar side chains have a variable length and branching pattern. The extent of microheterogeneity of the mucin sugar side chains exceeds that of

Table 4–1. *Sequences of tandem repeats of cloned human mucin genes*

MUC1	GSTAPPAHGVTSAPDTRPAP (20 aa)
MUC2	PTTTPITTTTTVTPTPTPTGTQT (23 aa)
MUC3	HSTPSFTSSITTTETTS (17 aa)
MUC4	TSSASTGHATPLPVTD (16 aa)
MUC5AC	TTSTTSAP (8 aa)
MUC5B	SSTPGTAHTLTVLTTTATTPTATGSTATP (29 aa)
MUC6	SPFSSTGPMTATSFQTTTTYPTPSHPQTTLPTHVPPFSTSLVTPSTG-TVITPTHAQMATSASIHSTPTGTIPPPTTLKATGSTHTAPPMTPTTS-GTSQAHSSFSTAKTSTSHSHTSSTHHPEVTPTSTTTITPNPTSTGTS-TPVAHTTSATSSRLPTPFTTHSPPTGS (169 aa)
MUC7	TTAAPPTPSATTPAPPSSSAPPE (23 aa)
MUC8	TSCPRPLQEGTPGSRAAHALSRRGHRVHELPTSSPGGDTGF (41 aa)

other molecules. For example, more than 35 different oligosaccharides have been identified by nuclear magnetic resonance (NMR) analysis of airway mucins, excluding a large number of long (containing more than 8 sugars) and sulfated chains (21). The sugar structures have been categorized according to their location in the sugar chain into three distinct groups—core, backbone, and peripheral structures (Fig. 4–2) (8,21,22). The core structures define the sugar linkages between the one to two sugars that may be adjacent to the *N*-acetylgalactosamine that is linked to serine or threonine in the peptide core. For respiratory mucins, four core structures have been defined: core 1, Galβ1–3 GalNAcα-O-Ser/Thr; core 2, Galβ 1–3 (GlcNA cβ1–6)GalNAcα-O-Ser/Thr; core 3, GlcNA cβ 1–3GalNAcα-O-Ser/Thr; core4, GlcNAc β1–3 (GlcNAcβ1–6)-GalNAcα-O-Ser/Thr (Fig. 4–3). The backbone structures are those sugar linkages adjacent to the core structures (Fig. 4–4). The peripheral structures attached to core and backbone structures may be simple and short or long and complex. These sugar structures may be antigenic (e.g., blood group determinants) or serve as binding sites for bacteria such as *P. aeruginosa* (23) and viruses such as influenza virus (24).

Mucin Sulfation

Some of the sugar chains are sulfated, specifically the relatively long oligosaccharide chains containing seven or more sugars (25). Sulfation of the mucin molecule, catalyzed by the enzyme sulfotransferase, occurs at the trans-Golgi membranes when glycosylation is almost complete (26). The activated sulfate donor, 3-phospho-5-phosphoadenosylsulfate (PAPS), enters the Golgi by a specific transporter (27). PAPS is formed from inorganic sulfate by two sequential reactions catalyzed by adenosine triphosphate (ATP) sulfurylase and adenosine 5-phosphosulfate kinase that consume two ATP molecules (28–30). The activated sulfate donor may be degraded by sulfatases. A number of factors may influence the relative sulfation of mucins, including availability of inorganic sulfate, enzymes for activation of sulfate, sulfotransferase, and the sugar acceptor on the mucin molecule.

Mucin Synthesis

Synthesis of mucins is a complex process with different stages occurring in different organelles. The peptide core (apomucin) is

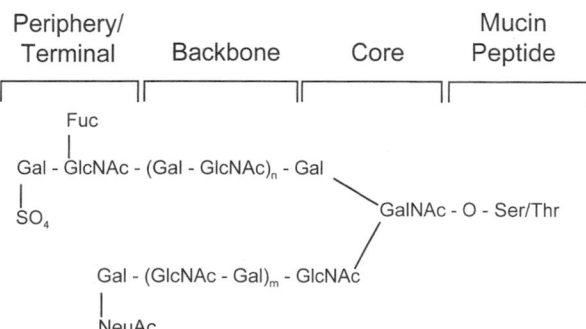

FIG. 4–2. Structure of carbohydrate side chains in mucins. The carbohydrate side chains may be divided into three regions: core, backbone, and terminal regions. The carbohydrate side chains are linked to the mucin peptide through an O-glycosidic linkage between *N*-acetylgalactosamine (GalNAc) and either serine (Ser) or threonine (Thr) in the mucin peptide. The core region of the carbohydrate side chain includes the *N*-acetylgalactosamine linked to the peptide region as well as the one or two sugars linked this *N*-acetylgalactosamine. The backbone structures consist of disaccharide units containing galactose (Gal) and *N*-acetylglucosamine (GlcNAc). These backbone structures link the cores with the terminal regions that may contain sialic acid (NeuAc), fucose (Fuc) and sulfate (SO₄).

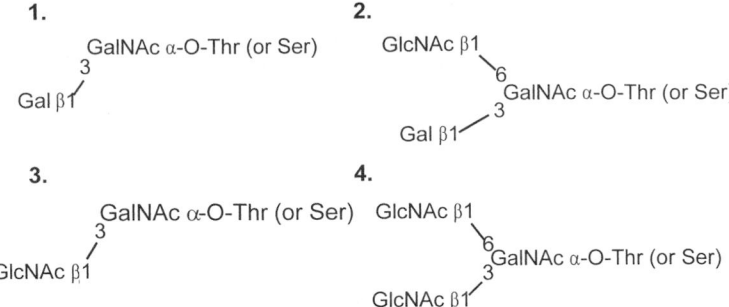

FIG. 4–3. Structure of carbohydrate core regions in respiratory mucins. Each core structure includes the *N*-acetylgalactosamine (GalNAc) linked to the mucin peptide and the one or two sugars attached to this GalNAc. The four core structures identified in mucins recovered from the respiratory tract are shown above. The sugars that may be attached to GalNAc are galactose (Gal) or *N*-acetylglucosamine (GlcNAc) in the linkages shown above. Additional core sugars and linkages have been identified in mucins from other sources.

synthesized in the rough endoplasmic reticulum and then is glycosylated in the Golgi apparatus. Addition of the first sugar, *N*-acetylgalactosamine, is catalyzed by mucin peptide: αGalNAc transferase, an enzyme associated with cis-Golgi membranes (31,32). Each additional sugar is added one by one to the growing oligosaccharide chains by a stepwise transfer that is catalyzed by a specific glycosyltransferase (33). The final structure and length of each oligosaccharide chain is variable, depending on the sequence of additions and specific

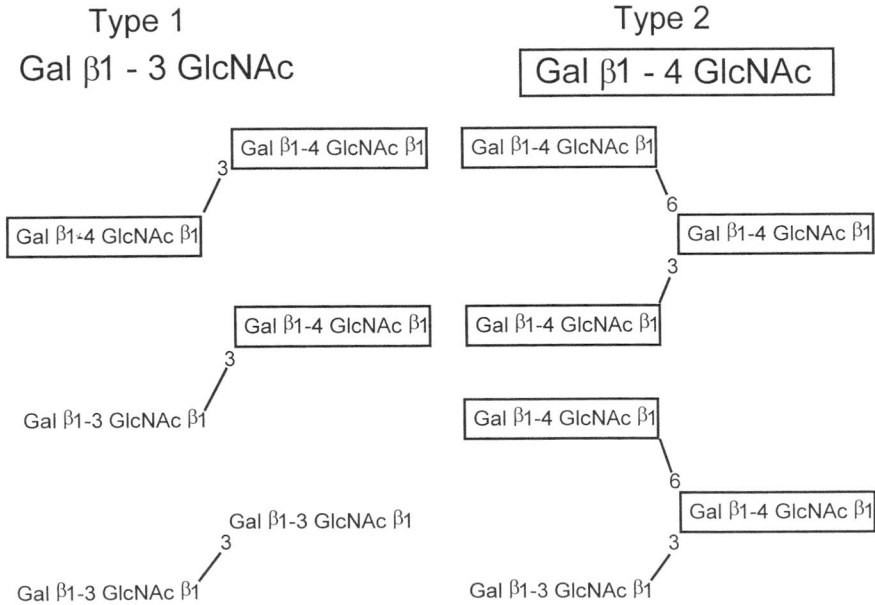

FIG. 4–4. Structure of carbohydrate backbone regions in respiratory tract mucins. Backbone structures consist of disaccharide units containing galactose (Gal) and *N*-acetylglucosamine (GlcNAc). These sugars may have a 1–3 linkage (type 1) or a 1–4 linkage (type 2). Five examples of backbone structures incorporating these two types of chain are shown above.

linkages of the sugars. Addition of sulfate is catalyzed by sulfotransferase as described previously. Most of the posttranslational modification of mucin molecules occurs in the *trans*-Golgi, where most of the glycosyltransferases and sulfotransferase are located.

Mucin Packaging and Secretion

Newly synthesized mucin molecules are packaged in a compact, condensed form within the granules of secretory cells. As aforementioned, the amino and carboxy terminal regions of mucin molecules contain regions that are homologous with von Willebrand's factor, suggesting that these regions may promote dimerization of mucin molecules in a head to tail linkage, as seen for von Willebrand's factor (17). This dimerization of molecules may be important for compact packaging of mucins into secretory granules. In addition, divalent cations are believed to influence the compact packaging of these polyionic mucin molecules within these granules. Calcium ion has been proposed as one of the key ions involved because studies have demonstrated that calcium is concentrated within the granules (relative to cytosol) (34,35), can alter mucin conformation (36,37), and participates in cross-linking of mucin molecules (37–39). Secretion of mucin has been characterized as a rapid, almost explosive expansion of the secretory granules as they are released at the apical membrane (40,41). Secretory granules typically are released by exocytosis, a process that involves fusion of the granule membrane with the apical plasma membrane. This fusion of membranes is believed to be accompanied by a rapid influx of ions and water into the granule that results in rapid expansion and hydration of the mucin that is secreted at the apical surface (41). The chloride ion has been proposed as a critical ion for mucin granule exocytosis (41) and for pancreatic zymogen and parotid granule exocytosis (42,43). By one proposal, sodium ions displace calcium ions that are shielding the polyionic charges, thereby altering interactions between mucin molecules, resulting in expansion of the mucin gel (41). This proposed influ-ence of ions on mucin packaging, secretion, and conformation could have important implications for CF, and conceivably could link the ion transport defect with alterations in mucus.

Other Components

Although mucins are believed to be the major component influencing the viscoelastic properties of normal airway mucus, a number of other components (Table 4–2) have been identified that may influence mucociliary clearance and other defense mechanisms in the airways. Some of these other products could influence the pathogenesis of CF lung disease.

Glycosaminoglycans

Glycosaminoglycans (GAGs) are a specific class of glycoconjugates that includes hyaluronic acid, heparan sulfate, keratan sulfate, and chondroitin sulfates A, B, and C (44). These glycoconjugates consist of polyionic, polysaccharide chains of variable length. Except for keratan sulfate, the polysaccharide chains consist of repeating disaccharide units containing either uronic acid or iduronic acid linked to a hexosamine sugar (GalNAc or GlcNAc). Proteoglycans consist of GAGs linked to peptides. Early studies of airway secretions did not evaluate glycosaminoglycan or proteo-

TABLE 4–2. *Components of airway mucus*

Components influencing mucus clearance
Major
Mucins
Minor
Glycosaminoglycans
Lipids
Lysozyme
Proline-rich proteins (PRPs)
Serum proteins (transudate)
Components influencing microbe killing
Lysozyme
Lactoferrin
Defensins
Immunoglobulins—IgG, IgA, secretory IgA
Components influencing inflammation
Secretory leukocyte proteinase inhibitor (SLPI)
α_1-proteinase inhibitor
Clara cell 10-kD protein

glycan content; however, more recent studies suggest that substantial amounts of these glycoconjugates may be present in airway mucus, particularly in inflamed airways. Hyaluronic acid has been found in asthmatic sputum, accounting for 2% to 3% of the dry weight (45). Hyaluronic acid, chondroitin sulfate, and dermatan sulfate have been identified but not quantitated in airway aspirates from smokers (5), and chondroitin sulfate has been recovered from sputum samples from patients with chronic bronchitis and CF (46). The source of GAGs in inflamed airways has not been defined clearly. GAGs may arise from inflammatory cells or from goblet cells and/or submucosal glands. *In vitro* studies have shown that human and canine airway mucosa (6), bovine tracheal serous cells (47), and canine tracheal epithelial cells (48) release glycoconjugates with proteoglycan characteristics. It is not clear whether these glycoconjugates are released from secretory granules. At least some of the proteoglycans are incorporated into the glycocalyx, coating the surface of epithelial cells (Fig. 4–5), and may be released from the surface glycocalyx by protease exposure (48).

Lipids

Variable amounts of lipids have been identified in airway secretions. Relatively larger amounts of lipids have been recovered in inflamed airways (49), although the source has not been defined. In lavaged secretions from dogs (7) and humans (5), most of the lipids are neutral lipids with components of phospholipids and glycolipids. Studies of intestinal secretions have identified lipids that are bound covalently to mucins (50); however, this association has not been confirmed in airway secretions. Possible sources of lipids include alveolar surfactant, lipids released or secreted by airway epithelial cells, and lipid components of cell membranes that are shed from disrupted cells.

Components Influencing Microbe Killing

Several components in airway surface fluid have antimicrobial properties. Lysozyme (muramidase) is a bacteriolytic enzyme that hydrolyzes bacterial cell wall glycans. Sources of human lung lysozyme include serous cells

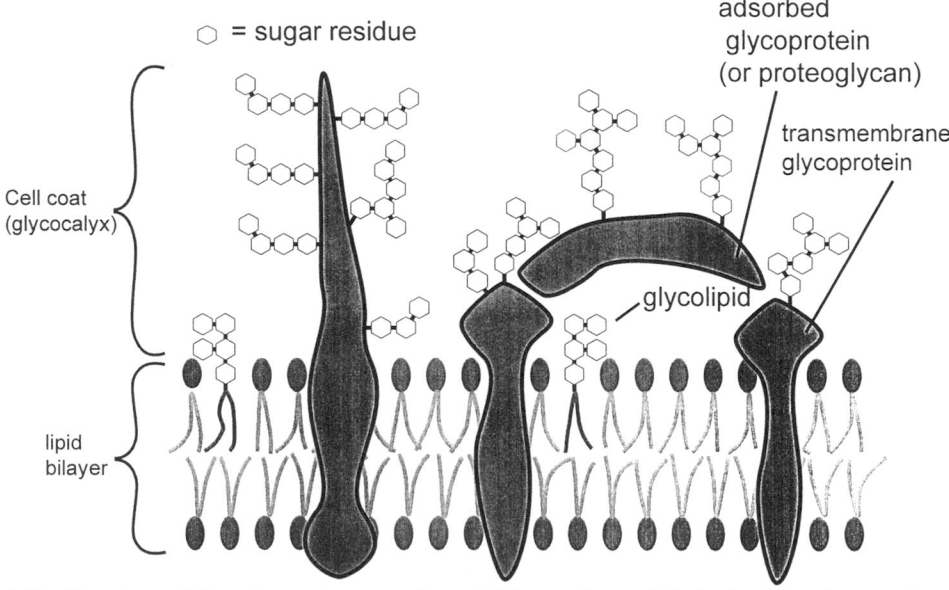

FIG. 4–5. Structure of the glycocalyx or cell coat. The surface of biological membranes is coated with a carbohydrate rich surface containing intrinsic membrane glycolipids and glycoproteins as well as adsorbed glycoproteins and proteoglycans. The glycocalyx may be released, at least in part, by exposure to proteases. (Modified from Alberts B, Bray D, Lewis J, Martin R, Roberts K, Watson JD, eds. *Molecular biology of the cell*. NewYork: Garland Publishing, 1983:284.)

of submucosal glands, alveolar macrophages, neutrophils, and, to a lesser extent, airway surface epithelial cells (51–53). In the presence of chronic airway infection and inflammation, concentrations of lysozyme in bronchoalveolar fluid may be seven- to eightfold greater than those in normal airways (54). Lactoferrin, originally isolated from milk, is present in a variety of secretions, including airway secretions. The sources for lung lactoferrin include serous cells of the submucosal glands and activated neutrophils (55,56). The antimicrobial properties of lactoferrin are attributable to its ability to bind and sequester iron normally available to iron dependent bacteria. In addition, lactoferrin has antiviral activity (57). As with lysozyme, the concentration of lactoferrin is increased in bronchoalveolar lavage from patients with chronic bronchitis (54). Defensins are a family of small antimicrobial peptides that have been recovered from a variety of sites within different animal species (58). One of the defensins, human β-defensin-1 (hBD-1), is expressed in airway epithelium from trachea to alveoli (59). hBD-1 has a broad range of antimicrobial activity against gram-negative organisms, including *Escherichia coli* and *P. aeruginosa* (59).

Airway secretions contain immunoglobulins that play an important role in controlling airway infection. Secretory immunoglobulin A (sIgA) is a complex of secretory component with dimeric IgA. This complex is formed in the airway epithelial cells and secreted into the airway lumen. IgA is synthesized in plasma cells and linked by a small peptide (J-chain) to form a dimer that interacts with an IgA receptor on the basolateral membrane of the airway epithelial cell. This complex undergoes endocytosis, is transported to the apical surface in small vesicles, and then is discharged as sIgA after proteolytic cleavage of the secretory component. Secretory component protects sIgA from proteinases in airway surface fluid. Approximately 50% of IgA in airway secretions is sIgA (60). Serum immunoglobulins (IgG and IgA) move across the vascular-airway barrier as transudates. In patients with chronic airway inflammation, the concentration of serum proteins, including immunoglobulins, in airway secretions is increased (61–63), suggesting that inflammation increases the leakiness of the vascular-airway barrier.

Other Proteins

Airway secretions contain a number of other proteins in small concentrations that may influence inflammation or mucus viscosity. The secretory leukocyte proteinase inhibitor (SLPI) is a 12-kD protein that is present in sputum, saliva, and nasal secretions (64) and is believed to arise from serous cells of submucosal glands and Clara cells (52,65). This small antiproteinase inhibits activity of neutrophil elastase and cathepsin G. The other major antiproteinase in airway secretions is an α_1-proteinase inhibitor, a serum protein that moves across the vascular-airway barrier as a transudate. Proline-rich proteins (PRPs) are a family of peptides that are present in airway secretions and are believed to arise from serous cells in submucosal glands (66). The function of PRPs has not been defined; basic PRPs may interact with acidic mucins and thereby influence mucus viscosity (67). Clara cell 10-kD protein is found in bronchoalveolar lavage, as well as Clara cells, and is believed to have antiinflammatory properties based on its ability to inhibit phospholipase A_2 (68,69). Bronchoalveolar lavage fluid also contains surfactant-associated proteins that are believed to interact with surfactant to enhance the low surface tension properties of the alveolar lining fluid. Four surfactant-associated proteins (SPA, SPB, SPC, and SPD) have been described. Although all are synthesized in alveolar type II cells, three (SPA, SPB, and SPC) have been identified in epithelial cells of the nonciliated terminal bronchioles, and one (SPB) has been identified in gland cells (70–72). Conceivably, the surfactant-associated proteins may interact with the mucus in distal airways and influence adhesiveness of mucus (see below). A number of serum proteins can be detected in airway secretions that filter across the vascular-airway barrier, especially in inflamed airways (61–63).

Mucus Rheology

Mucus is cleared from the airways by mucociliary clearance and cough. The efficiency of both of these defense mechanisms depends on the physical properties of the mucus gel, which possesses some of the characteristics of a viscous liquid (e.g., molasses) and some of the characteristics of an elastic solid (e.g., a rubber band). The viscous properties of mucus gel reflect its resistance to flow. The elastic properties reflect the gel's capacity to store energy when a force is applied to move it so that it recoils when the force is removed. These viscoelastic or rheologic properties of mucus are determined by the interactions between the large molecules in airway secretions. Interactions between mucin molecules are believed to be the primary determinants of mucus viscoelastic properties. Mucin molecules have polyionic properties attributable to the sulfate and sialic acid moieties in the sugar side chains. Repulsion of negative charges in the adjacent sugar chains is believed to result in the rigid, linear structure of these molecules (9,10). Disulfide binding between the nonglycosylated ends of the mucin molecules can result in very long chains of rigid mucin molecules. These long chains of highly charged mucin molecules form a tangled network that is believed to be the primary structure of the mucus gel. The polyionic properties of mucin suggest that hydration of this gel should be determined by a Donnan principle in which pH, ionic, and polyionic compositions of airway surface fluid are major determinants of mucus gel swelling (73). Other mucus components may interact with mucins to influence the rigidity and elasticity of mucus. Many of these interactions are not permanent and can be rearranged when pressure or force is applied to the mucus gel. When a low-shear force is applied, these molecular interactions are preserved, and the mucus gel behaves more like an elastic solid. However, when a high-shear force is applied, molecular interactions are disrupted and the mucus gel behaves more like a viscous liquid.

Measurement of the viscoelastic properties of mucus is complicated because the mucus gel may be altered or deformed during collection, transport, or analysis, resulting in inaccurate measurements. Present methods for characterizing viscoelastic properties include controlled shear rate rheometers (74,75), magnetic rheometers (76), and the double capillary apparatus (77). The dynamic nature of mucus viscoelasticity has been demonstrated by oscillatory testing in which the mucus is subjected to a periodic force (stress) while the resultant strain is monitored. The viscoelastic properties of mucus determine the lag of strain behind stress oscillations. For purely elastic substances, there is no lag, but for purely viscous substances, the phase lag is 90°. For mucus, the lag phase is between 0° and 90°, and the tangent of the phase lag (tangent δ) is the ratio of viscosity to elasticity. Although elasticity remains relatively stable at varying frequencies, viscosity decreases as the frequency of oscillation increases because of the shear forces on the mucus network. Therefore, tangent δ also decreases as the frequency of oscillations increases.

The forces on airway mucus are different during cough and during mucociliary clearance. During mucociliary clearance, the mucus gel is subjected to lower shear forces than during cough; therefore, King proposes that low shear-rate viscoelastic measurements are more predictive of effects on mucociliary clearance and high-shear-rate viscoelasticity measurements are more predictive of effects on cough clearance (78). Although viscosity and elasticity of the mucus gel influence both mucociliary clearance and cough clearance, the relative importance of these properties for the two clearance mechanisms varies. A low viscosity/elasticity ratio (tangent δ) measured at low-shear force reflects an elastic gel that is optimal for mucociliary clearance; however, a high viscosity/elasticity ratio (tangent δ) at high-shear force is optimal for cough clearance. The effects of these physical properties on mucociliary clearance and cough clearance have been assessed *in vitro* using different models. The mucus-depleted frog palate (79) and the mucus-depleted bovine trachea (80) have been used to assess mucocilary clearance, and a simulated cough machine (81) has been used to assess cough clearance of mucus from different sources and conditions.

Two additional properties of a mucus gel that may influence clearance are adhesiveness and spinnability. Mucus adhesiveness is its ability to adhere to the underlying epithelium. Several approaches have been used to measure adhesiveness, the force required to separate mucus from a solid surface (82,83). These studies demonstrate that mucus adhesiveness is dependent on surface tension, wetability, and hydration (83–85). Decreased phospholipid content in airway secretions appears to increase surface tension and adhesiveness and thereby impair clearance (84,85). Mucus spinnability is its ability to form a thread when stretched. Measurement of spinnability is performed by stretching mucus at a defined rate in a Filancemeter until the mucus thread breaks and then measuring the distance at which the thread breaks (86). This property is believed to reflect the length of mucin chains; disruption of disulfide bonds in mucin chains with N-acetylcysteine decreases spinnability (87). Even though spinnability does not correlate with viscoelasticity measures, it does correlate directly with mucociliary clearance (88) and inversely with cough clearance (89).

ABNORMAL PROPERTIES OF AIRWAY MUCUS IN CYSTIC FIBROSIS

An early manifestation of CF lung disease is chronic cough that is productive of tenacious sputum. Early in life, airways are colonized with bacteria such as *S. aureus, Haemophilus influenzae,* and *P. aeruginosa.* These findings have led to speculation that airway secretions are abnormal in CF. Specific abnormalities that have been proposed are altered viscoelastic properties of mucus, enhanced bacterial adherence to airway mucus, and impaired bacterial killing by antimicrobial factors in airway mucus.

Altered Viscoelastic Properties of Cystic Fibrosis Airway Mucus

One of the early names for CF was mucoviscidosis, reflecting the abnormally thick and viscous sputum found in these patients. Some studies have shown that increased sputum vis-cosity correlates with the degree of infection and severity of disease (90,91). For several decades, investigators have attempted to characterize differences in the composition of CF secretions that may explain the altered viscosity of CF sputum. A number of factors may contribute to the altered viscoelastic properties of CF airway secretions, including dehydration of secretions, alterations in mucins, and increased concentrations of other components, such as glycosaminoglycans, lysozyme, lipids, DNA, and actin, in inflamed CF airways.

Dehydration of Secretions

Studies as early as 1959 demonstrated that the relative water content of expectorated secretions and bronchoscopic aspirates from patients with CF was less than that in healthy subjects and in patients with bronchiectasis (87% to 89% water in patients with CF vs. 91% to 95% water in patients with bronchiectasis and healthy subjects) (2–4,90,92). This relative dehydration of CF secretions could reflect decreased water content or increased solid content of the secretions. At these concentrations, a relatively small change in water content is reflected in a large change in solid content. For example, a decrease in water content from 95% to 90% would reflect a doubling of the solid content (from 5% to 10%). Conceivably, the relative dehydration of CF secretions could impair mucociliary clearance by two mechanisms. Increased absorption of water may decrease the periciliary fluid depth to a level that impairs free "sweeping" of the cilia (Fig. 4–6). In addition, dehydration may alter the viscoelastic properties by concentrating mucin molecules and thereby promoting disulfide bonding and other interactions between adjacent mucin molecules and other mucus components.

As discussed previously, hydration of the polyionic mucin gel is believed to follow Donnan equilibrium principles suggesting that pH, ions, and divalent cations in airway surface fluid may influence mucin gel swelling (35,75) and perhaps its viscoelastic properties. Consistent with this model, a recent study showed that

Normal   Cystic Fibrosis

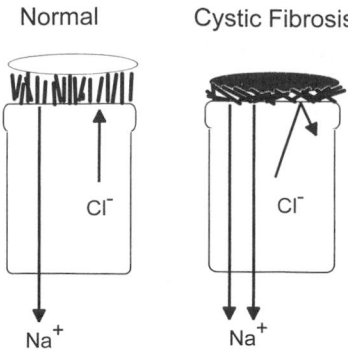

FIG. 4–6. Potential effect of altered water content in CF secretions. The relative dehydration of CF airway secretions is believed to arise from altered ion and water transport across the surface membranes of airway epithelial cells. The normal secretion of chloride ions and absorption of sodium ions is disrupted in CF. Along the ciliated epithelium, a proper balance of ion and water transport may be critical for maintaining the depth of the periciliary fluid layer. If this periciliary fluid layer is too shallow, then the overlying mucus layer may become entangled in the cilia and thereby impair clearance.

increasing the sodium content of CF sputum improved its transportability in the mucus-depleted bovine trachea model (93). This observation suggests that mucus salinity may be a more important determinant of mucus clearance than water content alone and could link altered clearance of CF mucus with the basic defect in ion transport.

Alterations in Mucins

For several decades, investigators have focused on characterizing differences in CF mucins that may explain the altered viscosity of CF sputum. As discussed below, the hypertrophy of submucosal glands and the hyperplasia of goblet cells in CF airways suggests that an increased volume of mucin may be secreted. In addition, early studies suggested a number of compositional differences in CF mucins, including increased fucose content and decreased sialic acid content (94,95). However, subsequent studies identified no alterations in the fu-

cose and sialic acid content (96–98). Another possibility is that sugar linkages may be different in CF, resulting in different terminal structures in the sugar side chains. Comparisons of sugar content and linkages in mucins from different subjects are difficult because of the extensive microheterogeneity in the oligosaccharide side chains of mucin molecules; to date, no consistent differences in sugar content or linkages have been identified in CF mucins. One alteration that has been demonstrated by a variety of approaches is increased sulfation of CF respiratory mucins (25,97–101). Studies of expectorated sputum from patients with CF demonstrated that the level of mucin sulfation increased with the severity of disease (102), suggesting that chronic infection and inflammation influence sulfation. However, when isolated from inflammatory influences, primary cultures of CF nasal epithelial cells continue to secrete mucins that are more highly sulfated than those from non-CF nasal cells (101), suggesting that altered sulfation may result from the basic defect in CF. Recent studies suggest that sulfate uptake and distribution in airway epithelial cells may be linked to that of chloride via a heteroexchanger (103). This linkage of sulfate and chloride distribution ultimately could interrelate the increased sulfation of mucins with the basic defect in chloride secretion. Another possible explanation for the increased sulfation of cystic fibrosis mucins is that altered trafficking of the mutated CFTR in CF could increase the membrane potential in the Golgi and thereby favor accumulation of PAPS (the activated sulfate donor) in the Golgi and increase sulfation of glycoproteins (104). Further studies are needed to define the mechanism(s) promoting sulfation of mucins in patients with CF. Analysis of sulfated oligosaccharides purified from sputum of a patient with CF has identified long, branched chains containing an average of 160 to 200 sugar residues; many of these side chains contain varying amounts of a repeating oligosaccharide sequence with sulfate linked to the 6 position of galactose and possibly N-acetylglucosamine residues (105). Presumably, these long sugar side chains increase the rigidity of the mucin molecule and the gel that contains these rigid and highly charged molecules.

Increased Concentrations of Other Components in Purulent Secretions

Inflammation alters the composition of airway mucus. A number of components, including glycosaminoglycans, lipids, lysozyme, proteinases, DNA, and actin, have been recovered in higher concentrations from inflamed airways than from uninflamed airways. Each of these components could influence the physical properties of the mucus gel. Several glycosaminoglycans, including hyaluronic acid, chondroitin sulfate, and dermatan sulfate, are more abundant in sputum from patients with chronic bronchitis and CF (5,45,46). These highly charged macromolecules can form gels and therefore could influence the physical properties of the mucus gel. The lipid content in CF sputum is approximately three times greater than that in mucus from uninfected laryngectomized individuals (49). Interestingly, the various lipids in airway secretions have different effects on the physical properties of the mucus gel. For example, neutral lipids and glycosphingolipids increase viscosity, but phosphatidylcholine and phosphotidylglycerol decrease adhesiveness of airway mucus (85,106). Levels of lysozyme are increased in lower airway secretions from patients with chronic obstructive lung diseases, including CF (107–109). Lysozyme, a cationic molecule, interacts with polyionic mucin molecules (110); therefore, in high concentrations, lysozyme could increase viscosity of airway mucus. Inflamed airways contain high concentrations of proteases released from neutrophils, mast cells, and bacteria that may partially degrade mucin by hydrolysis of the nonglycosylated regions of the peptide (111–113), resulting in a decrease in mucus viscosity.

DNA and actin are believed to have a substantial influence on the physical properties of CF mucus. Purulent airway secretions from patients with CF contain high concentrations of DNA (114,115) believed to arise from degenerating polymorphonuclear neutrophils. Large, polymerized, polyanionic DNA molecules interact with polyionic mucin molecules and increase the viscosity of the mucus gel (Fig. 4–7). Enzymatic depolymerization of DNA by DNase I reduces the viscosity of purulent CF

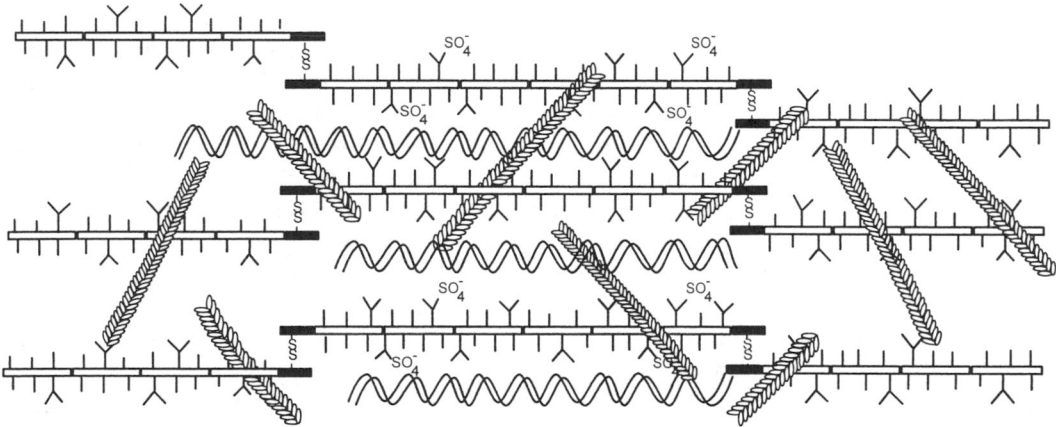

FIG. 4–7. Postulated structure of purulent airway mucus containing mucin, DNA, and actin. Mucin molecules are shown in the same configuration as in Figure 4–1. DNA (designated by the double helix) and actin (designated by long strands of leaflets) are present in purulent airway secretions. Both DNA and mucin are large, rigid, polyionic molecules; presumably, ionic forces influence orientation of DNA molecules within the mucin gel. Filamentous actin can form large rigid filaments; presumably, these filaments become entangled in the mucus gel in a random orientation. SO_4^-, sulfate.

sputum (116). However, DNase treatment does not alter *in vitro* transportability of sputum recovered from patients with bronchiectasis who do not have CF (117). A specific interaction between CF mucins and DNA has been suggested by studies showing a marked increase in viscosity and elasticity after addition of DNA to purified CF mucins but no change in rheologic properties after addition of DNA to purified mucins from patients with bronchitis (118). In addition to DNA, purulent CF sputum contains large amounts of actin (119) that is believed to arise from degenerating neutrophils. Filamentous actin forms long protease-resistant filaments that become entangled in the mucus gel (Fig. 4–7), adding rigidity to the gel; severing actin filaments by addition of gelsolin reduces the viscosity of CF sputum (119).

Bacterial Adherence to Cystic Fibrosis Airway Mucus

Inhaled particles, including bacteria, may impact first on the mucus layer lining the airways. Airway mucins contain a number of terminal sugar structures that serve as specific receptors for microorganisms, such as influenza virus (24). Attachment of microorganisms to receptors in mucins may further impede access to the underlying epithelium. In CF, chronic colonization of airways with *P. aeruginosa* led to speculation that this bacteria may bind more avidly to CF epithelial cells and/or CF mucus that to normal cells or mucus. Several studies have demonstrated that Pseudomonas organisms bind more avidly to CF airway cells than to normal airway cells and that this binding is more apparent with certain genotypes, such as ΔF508 (120,121). The Pseudomonas component important for binding to epithelial cells is pilin (122). Recent studies have shown that the specific pilin receptor for Pseudomonas binding on epithelial cells, asialoGM1 (a ganglioside component of the cell membrane containing the sugar sequence GalNAcβ1–4Gal), is more prevalent on CF cells than normal airway cells (123). Evidence for increased binding to CF mucus is not characterized as well as for airway cells, even though terminal sugars in

mucins serve as receptors for a variety of microorganisms. Most pathologic sections of CF airways demonstrate Pseudomonas organisms within the airway lumen instead of attached to the epithelial surface (124). This observation suggests that either these organisms become entrapped in the mucus without access to the epithelial surface or that organisms that attach to the epithelial surface are immediately ingested or killed. Using different approaches, a number of studies have suggested that *P. aeruginosa* binds more avidly to CF mucins than to normal mucins (125–128). However, the link between increased binding and alteration in carbohydrate structure of CF mucins has not been identified. Studies of Pseudomonas binding to mucins suggest that pilin is not involved (129,130). However, several strains of *P. aeruginosa* bind to respiratory and intestinal mucins (131,132) by a process that is nonspecific, that is, it is lacking a specific ligand-receptor interaction (131). A related organism, *Burkholderia cepacia* (previously known as *Pseudomonas cepacia*), binds specifically to mucins (133) by *B. cepacia* mucin-binding adhesin (134).

Impaired Function of Antimicrobial Factors in Cystic Fibrosis Mucus

Airway secretions contain a number of antimicrobial factors, including lysozyme, lactoferrin, and defensins. Levels of lysozyme and lactoferrin are increased in lower airway secretions from patients with chronic obstructive lung diseases, including CF (107–109). Lysozyme is bactericidal for a number of bacterial pathogens in the lung, including *Streptococcus pneumoniae* (135); however, lysozyme does not appear to be bactericidal for mucoid and nonmucoid strains of *P. aeruginosa* or *S. aureus* (136). Lactoferrin appears to be hydrolyzed by Pseudomonas elastase and/or neutrophil elastase and therefore may have limited activity in chronically infected CF airways (137).

Recent studies suggest that normal and CF epithelial cells secrete other antimicrobial peptides (defensins) that are capable of killing *P. aeruginosa* at low salt concentrations (138).

The recently identified human β defensin-1 (hBD-1) is salt sensitive and may be inactivated in CF (59). Human β defensin-2 (DEFB2) is also expressed in airway epithelia (139) and may contribute to early CF pathogenesis. These observations provide a potential link between the CF basic defect in ion transport and colonization of airways with *P. aeruginosa*.

THE SECRETORY APPARATUS IN AIRWAYS

The major secretory structures in the airways are goblet cells and submucosal glands that secrete mucins and other high molecular weight glycoconjugates, as well as Clara cells in the bronchioles. Pathologic features of CF include alterations in submucosal glands and in prevalence of goblet cells, as discussed below; however, little is known about changes in Clara cells. Some of the pathologic changes in CF are similar to those present in chronic bronchitis or bronchiectasis, suggesting that these changes may be secondary to chronic inflammation. However, the area of highest expression of the CFTR within the airways is in the serous tubules of submucosal glands (with some expression also in the gland ducts) (140), suggesting a possible link between the basic defect and gland pathology.

Structure and Function of Secretory Structures

Goblet Cells

Goblet cells in the airway epithelium, like their counterparts in the intestinal tract, are recognized by their goblet shape when filled with secretory granules. Goblet cells account for up to 15% of the cells in surface epithelium (141), but an increased prevalence occurs with airway disease (142). The histochemical stain, Alcian blue–periodic acid-Schiff (AB-PAS), has been used to characterize mucin-containing granules in secretory cells. PAS reacts with the vicinal hydroxyls in glycoconjugates to produce a magenta color (143). Mucins are glycosylated heavily with sugars containing these vicinal hydroxyls and therefore stain intensely with PAS. Alcian blue binds to acidic moieties, specifically sialic acid and sulfate, in glycoconjugates (143). The prevalence of acidic moieties in mucins varies; consequently, the intensity of Alcian blue staining varies. The combined staining with Alcian blue and PAS can be used to differentiate glycoconjugates containing relatively few acidic moieties (stain magenta with only a slight blue tint) from those containing abundant acidic moieties (stain blue-purple color). The glycoconjugates stained with AB-PAS include mucin-type glycoproteins and proteoglycans. In mature tracheobronchial epithelium, goblet cell granules stain blue-purple with AB-PAS, consistent with acidic mucins.

The mechanism(s) and control of airway goblet cell secretion is less well defined than that for intestinal goblet cell secretion. Most goblet cell secretion occurs by exocytosis of secretory granules, but some stimulated release may occur by an apocrine process in which the apical portion of the goblet cell, including granules and cytoplasm, is expelled. Regulation of goblet cell secretion is not completely defined. Recent studies suggest that ATP may be important for physiologic control of goblet cell secretion (144,145). Other agents known to enhance goblet cell secretion include neutrophil elastase and cathepsin G (146), bacterial proteases (147), platelet-activating factor (PAF) (148), serum (149), and tobacco smoke (150).

Submucosal Glands

In humans, submucosal glands are found in the cartilaginous airways, typically located in the submucosal space between the surface epithelium and underlying cartilage. These glands are complex structures containing multiple acini that open into tubules that drain into a collecting duct that opens to the airway surface (151). The secretory cell types in submucosal glands are mucous cells containing electron-lucent granules and serous cells containing electron-dense secretory granules (152). Mucous cells secrete mucin-type glycoproteins; serous cells secrete lysozyme, lactoferrin, SLPI, proline-rich proteins, and proteoglycans (153). Typically, mucous cells react with both Alcian blue and PAS, resulting in a blue-purple staining pattern similar to goblet cells in the surface epithelium, but serous cells react only with PAS, resulting in a magenta color. Often, mucous cells and serous cells are segregated into different acini. The submucosal gland duct is ciliated at its opening and appears to be a continuation of the airway surface epithelium. However, the epithelium of the collecting duct consists of tall columnar cells with abundant mitochondria and is believed to control the ion and water content of submucosal gland secretions (151,152). This arrangement allows for hydration of the gel formed by the secreted mucin-type glycoproteins and proteoglycans. Surrounding the glands is a semicontinuous layer of myoepithelial cells that contract and "squeeze" tubules during active gland secretion (154).

Regulation of submucosal gland secretion, unlike goblet cell secretion, involves neural pathways. The most completely studied mechanism for regulation of submucosal gland secretion is the cholinergic neural pathway. Postganglionic parasympathetic efferent nerve endings are apparent in submucosal glands (155,156). Submucosal gland secretion is increased by direct stimulation of the vagus nerve or its branches (157,158). In addition, parasympathomimetic agents such as acetylcholine, methacholine, and pilocarpine stimulate gland secretion in tracheal explants (159–161). Cholinergic antagonists, such as atropine, block gland secretion in response to vagal stimulation or cholinergic agonists. Although cholinergic fibers are most prevalent, submucosal glands also contain adrenergic and nonadrenergic, noncholinergic (NANC) nerve fibers (162,163). The role of these neural pathways in regulation of human submucosal gland secretion is undefined. Interestingly, β-adrenergic agents promote gland secretion in some animal species but not in humans (160,161). Vasoactive intestinal peptide (VIP), one of the neuropeptides associated with NANC fibers, inhibits baseline and methacholine-induced gland secretions in humans but has a stimulatory effect in many animal species (164).

Other Airway Epithelial Cells

Other airway epithelial cells synthesize and release products into the airway lumen. Clara cells, found in the bronchioles of humans, are secretory cells that often project into the airway lumen and contain abundant smooth endoplasmic reticulum and apical, membrane-bound, electron-dense granules (165). Most of the proteins secreted by Clara cells have a low molecular weight (6,000 to 10,000Da). The Clara cell 10-kDa protein is specific for Clara cells (166), appears to be a counterpart of rabbit uteroglobulin (167), and is believed to have antiinflammatory properties (168). In addition, SLPI has been identified within Clara cells and is believed to protect against protease destruction of the lung (169). Little is known about the regulation of Clara cell secretion. Although these cells secrete antiinflammatory products that could play an important protective role in chronic airway diseases such as CF, no studies to date have compared Clara cells from patients with CF with those from non-CF subjects.

A number of other secretory products, such as secretory IgA, arachidonic acid metabolites, cytokines, and lipids are released by airway epithelium, but the specific cell source has not been defined. Some studies suggest that airway epithelium secretes factors that inhibit airway smooth muscle contraction (170) and submucosal gland secretion (171) because removal of epithelium promotes increased airway tone and gland secretion, respectively. Conceivably, loss of airway surface epithelium from acute or chronic bronchitis could decrease the concentrations of these epithelium-derived relaxing factors, resulting in bronchoconstriction and increased gland secretion.

CHANGES IN SECRETORY STRUCTURES IN CYSTIC FIBROSIS

Submucosal gland size has been assessed semiquantitatively by the Reid index, a ratio of gland thickness to bronchial wall thickness (172). Enlarged airway submucosal glands (Reid index > 0.6) are apparent in chronic diseases such as chronic bronchitis (172) and CF (173,174). One of the earliest pathologic findings in the lungs of patients with CF is gland hypertrophy (174). However, the size of submucosal glands in newborn infants with CF does not differ from matched controls (175), suggesting that the stimuli that promote gland growth are not present during the fetal period but become activated early in the disease process. Submucosal gland hypertrophy involves not only gland growth but also invasion into the submucosal matrix. Recent studies suggest that metalloproteinases and plasminogen activators degrade extracellular matrix, enabling enlarging glands to invade the submucosal region (176–178). In an animal model of infection-associated gland hypertrophy (e.g., *Mycoplasma pulmonis*-infected rat), tracheal concentrations of collagenase and a urokinase-like plasminogen activator increase during the period of gland enlargement (179). Gland growth also involves cell proliferation. In hypertrophied CF submucosal glands, the prevalence of proliferating cells is increased compared with that in nonhypertrophied glands from non-CF subjects (180). Presumably, inflammatory mediators and cytokines influence cell proliferation and expression of the matrix-degrading enzymes to promote gland hypertrophy in chronically infected CF airways. The enlarged submucosal glands in CF airways contain a larger volume of stored secretory product than normal glands. As a result, CF submucosal glands secrete more than normal airways when stimulated. Conceivably, chronically infected CF airways contain a number of inflammatory mediators and other stimuli that will promote gland secretion. The specific role of the inflammatory cell mediators and bacterial products in CF airways on regulation of gland secretion has not been defined, although neutrophil proteases appear to stimulate gland secretion (181,182).

One characteristic feature of CF submucosal glands that is apparent even before hypertrophy is dilatation of the gland lumina (183). This dilatation could result from an increased rate of secretion by the mucous and serous cells and/or from plugging of the lumina by ab-

normally thick mucus secretions. Engelhardt et al. demonstrated that the predominant site of the CFTR in non-CF bronchi is the submucosal gland, particularly at the apical surface of cells in ducts and serous tubules; however, in airways from patients with CF with the ΔF508/ΔF508 genotype, no CFTR protein was detectable in either ducts or serous cells (140). Bioelectric studies of submucosal glands in culture suggest active chloride ion secretion (184) through CFTR-like channels (185) in normal airways; however, chloride ion secretion is limited in CF gland cells (186). This reduced chloride ion secretion by CF gland cells could lead to dehydrated, viscous secretions that could obstruct gland ducts, leading to ductal dilatation and limiting net secretion from glands.

In CF airways, goblet cells may play a role in altered secretions. Two typical pathologic findings in CF airways are goblet cell hyperplasia (increase in goblet cell prevalence) and goblet cell metaplasia (extension of goblet cells into bronchioles where they usually do not occur). This increased number of goblet cells could account for an increase in baseline secretion, assuming that the basal regulation is unchanged. Studies of nasal and tracheobronchial tissues have shown that baseline degranulation of single goblet cells from CF subjects is not different from those obtained from non-CF subjects (187). Additionally, regulation of goblet cell secretion by ATP in CF airway tissues does not differ from non-CF tissues (187). However, CF airways contain a number of inflammatory mediators and factors, such as neutrophil elastase, cathepsin G, bacterial proteases, and serum proteins that are known to promote goblet cell secretion. The combination of increased prevalence of goblet cells and mediators that stimulate goblet cell secretion in CF airways could result in a substantial increase in secretions derived from goblet cells.

SUMMARY

Normal airway secretions are not adequately characterized, and our knowledge of their source and composition is limited by sampling artifacts and analytic techniques. Airway secretions in CF have markedly increased quantity and viscosity, but the causes of these abnormalities have not been established clearly. Altered CFTR protein expression or function due to CF gene mutations clearly change epithelial permeability and ion transport. The finding of abnormal mucus plugs in uninfected airways of infants with CF suggests that these ion transport abnormalities alter airway secretions and cause the obstruction before chronic infection and inflammation. However, a direct link of CF mutations to abnormal synthesis or secretion of mucin or other mucus components has not been established.

A number of hypothetical links between CF mutations and abnormal secretions have been examined. Abnormal CFTR function in the Golgi apparatus and other organelles may alter sialylation, sulfation, or other posttranslational modifications of mucins (104). Subtle structural abnormalities could lead to abnormal binding of *P. aeruginosa, B. cepacia*, or other bacteria that characteristically infect CF airways. Alternatively, changes in synthesis, secretion, or activity of epithelial-derived antibacterial molecules (59,138) may predispose patients with CF to chronic airway infection and inflammation. These in turn lead to the submucosal gland hypertrophy, goblet cell hyperplasia, and goblet cell metaplasia that typify CF. Further studies are needed to define these potential influences of altered CFTR on airway secretions.

Most studies have examined mucus from patients with CF with chronic bacterial colonization of the airways where effects of the primary defect in the CFTR are difficult to distinguish from the effects of chronic inflammation. Secondary effects of chronic infection and inflammation, as seen in CF and chronic bronchitis, impact on mucus volume and clearance. Inflammatory mediators and bacterial products promote mucus secretion from goblet cells and glands. In addition, DNA and actin released from degenerating airway neutrophils in the airways become enmeshed in the mucus, thereby altering its viscoelastic properties and impairing mucus clearance by cough or mucociliary clearance. These effects of infection and inflammation have a major impact on the progression of obstructive airway disease in CF. Present therapeutic strategies include antimicrobial, antiinflammatory, and mucolytic (DNase) approaches to counter the effects of infection and inflammation. With these approaches, the progression of lung disease may be slowed but not interrupted.

A full understanding of the link between CF mutations, abnormal airway secretions, and bacterial colonization will require studies to identify the effects of normal and mutated CFTRs on cellular functions, including the synthesis and secretion of mucin and other constituents of airway secretions. Studies of airway secretions in infants with CF are needed to characterize the relative roles of ion transport defects, alterations in mucins, and alterations in inflammatory responses in the early pathogenesis of CF lung disease before infection. A better definition of the link(s) between the basic defect in the CFTR and abnormal airway secretions in CF may elucidate therapeutic approaches to prevent the development of CF lung disease.

REFERENCES

1. Toremaln NG. The daily amount of tracheobronchial secretions in man, a method for continuous tracheal aspiration in laryngectomized and tracheostomized patients. *Acta Otolaryngol (Stockh)* 1960;158(Suppl): 43–53.
2. Matthews LM, Spector S, Lemm J, Potter JL. Studies on pulmonary secretion. *Am Rev Respir Dis* 1963;88: 199–204.
3. Boucher RC. Human airway ion transport: part one. *Am J Respir Crit Care Med* 1994;150:271–281.
4. Boucher RC. Human airway ion transport: part two. *Am J Respir Crit Care Med* 1994;150:581–593.
5. Bhaskar KR, O'Sullivan DD, Seltzer J, Rossing TH, Drazen JM, Reid LM. Density gradient study of bronchial mucus aspirates from healthy volunteers (smokers and nonsmokers) and from patients with tracheostomy. *Exp Lung Res* 1985;9:289–308.
6. Bhaskar KR, O'Sullivan DD, Opaskar-Hincman H, Reid LM, Coles SJ. Density gradient analysis of secretions produced in vitro by human and canine airway mucosa: identification of lipids and proteoglycans in such secretions. *Exp Lung Res* 1986;10:401–422.
7. Bhaskar KR, Drazen JM, O'Sullivan DD, Scanlon PM, Reid LM. Transition from normal to hypersecretory bronchial mucus in a canine model of bronchitis: changes in yield and composition. *Exp Lung Res* 1988;14:101–120.

8. Roussel P, Lamblin G, Lhermitte M, et al. The complexity of mucins. *Biochimie* 1988;70:1471–1482.

9. Lamblin G, Lhermitle M, Degand P, et al. Chemical and physical properties of human bronchial mucous glycoproteins. *Biochimie* 1979;61:23–43.

10. Rose MC, Voter WA, Brown CF, et al. Structural features of human tracheobronchial mucin glycoprotein. *Biochem J* 1984;222:371–377.

11. Boat TF, Cheng P-W. Biochemistry of airway mucus secretions. *Fed Proc* 1980;39:3067–3074.

12. Lamblin G, Aubert J-P, Perini JM, et al. Human respiratory mucins. *Eur Respir J* 1992;5:247–256.

13. Aubert J-P, Porchet N, Crepin M, et al. Evidence for different human tracheobronchial mucin peptides deduced from nucleotide cDNA sequences. *Am J Respir Cell Mol Biol* 1991;5:178–185.

14. Gum JR. Mucin genes and the proteins they encode: structure, diversity, and regulation. *Am J Respir Cell Mol Biol* 1992;7:557–564.

15. Gendler SJ, Spicer AP. Epithelial mucin genes. *Annu Rev Physiol* 1995;57:607–634.

16. Shankar V, Gilmore MS, Elkins RC, Sachdev GP. A novel human mucin cDNA encodes a protein with unique tandem repeat organization. *Biochem J* 1994;300:295–298.

17. Gum JR, Hicks JW, Toribara NW, Siddiki B, Kim YS. Molecular cloning of human intestinal mucin (MUC2) cDNA. *J Biol Chem* 1994;269(4):2440–2446.

18. Meerzaman D, Charles P, Daskal E, Polymeropoulos MH, Martin BM, Rose MC. Cloning and analysis of cDNA encoding a major airway glycoprotein, human tracheobronchial mucin (MUC5). *J Biol Chem* 1994;269:12932–12939.

19. Voynow JA, Rose MC. Quantitation of mucin mRNA in respiratory and intestinal epithelial cells. *Am J Respir Cell Mol Biol* 1994;11:742–750.

20. Jany BH, Gallup MW, Yan P-S, Gum JR, Kim YS, Basbaum CB. Human bronchus and intestine express the same mucin gene. *J Clin Invest* 1991;87:77–82.

21. Klein A, Lamblin G, Lhermitte M, et al. Primary structure of neutral oligosaccharides derived from respiratory mucus glycoproteins of a patient suffering from bronchiectasis, determined by combination of 500MHz H-NMR spectroscopy and quantitative sugar analysis. *Eur J Biochem* 1988;171:631–642.

22. Lamblin G, Lhermitte M, Klein A, et al. The carbohydrate diversity of human respiratory mucins: A protection of the underlying mucosa? *Am Rev Respir Dis* 1991;144:S19–S24.

23. Ramphal R, Carnoy C, Fievre S, et al. *Pseudomonas aeruginosa* recognizes carbohydrate chains containing type 1 (Galb1–3GlcNAc) or type 2 (Galb1–4GlcNAc) disaccharide units. *Infect Immunol* 1991;59:700–704.

24. Higa HH, Rogers GN, Paulson JC. Influenza virus hemagglutinins differentiate between receptor determinants bearing *N*-acetyl, *N*-glycolyl, and *N*,O-diacetylneuraminic acid. *Virology* 1985;144:279–282.

25. Roussel P, Lamblin G, Degand P, et al. Heterogeneity of the carbohydrate chains of sulfated bronchial glycoproteins isolated from a patient suffering from cystic fibrosis. *J Biol Chem* 1975;250:2114–2122.

26. Hirschberg CB, Snider MD. Topography of glycosylation in the rough endoplasmic reticulum and Golgi apparatus. *Ann Rev Biochem* 1987;56:63–87.

27. Schwarz JK, Capasso JM, Hirschberg CB. Translocation of adenosine3-phosphate 5-phosphosulfate into rat liver Golgi vesicles. *J Biol Chem* 1984;259:3554–3559.

28. Carter SR, Slomiany A, Gwazdzinski K, Lau YH, Slomiany BL. Enzymatic sulfation of mucus glycoprotein in gastric mucosa: effect of ethanol. *J Biol Chem* 1988;263:11977–11984.

29. Renosto F, Seubert PA, Segel IH. Adenosine 5-phospho-sulfate from Penicillium chrysogenum: purification and kinetic characterization. *J Biol Chem* 1984;259:2113–2123.

30. Renosto F, Martin RL, Segel IH. ATP sulfurylase from Penicillium chrysogenum: molecular basis of the sigmoidal velocity curves induced by sulfhydryl group modification. *J Biol Chem* 1987;262:16279–16288.

31. Roth J. Cytochemical localization of terminal *N*-acetyl-*D*-galactosamine residues in cellular compartments of intestinal goblet cells: implications for the topology of *O*-glycosylation. *J Cell Biol* 1984;98:399–406.

32. Abeijon C, Hirschberg CB, Subcellular site of synthesis of the *N*-acetylgalactosamine (a1–0) serine (or threonine) linkage in rat liver. *J Biol Chem* 1987;262:4153–4159.

33. Schachter H. In: Horowitz MI, Pigman W, eds. *The glycoconjugates.* Vol III. New York: Academic Press, 1978:87–181.

34. Roomans GM, Euler AM, von Muller RM, Gillijman H. X-ray microanalysis of goblet cells in bronchial epithelium of patients with cystic fibrosis. *J Submicrosc Cytol Pathol* 1986;18:613–615.

35. Verdugo P, Deyrup-Olsen I, Aitken M, Villalon MJ, Johnson D. Molecular mechanisms of mucin secretion: I, the role of intragranular charge shielding. *J Dent Res* 1987;66:506–508.

36. Varma BK, Demers, A, Jamieson AM, Blackwell J, Jentoft N. Light scattering studies of the effect of Ca^{2+} on the structure of porcine submaxillary mucin. *Biopolymers* 1990;29:441–448.

37. Steiner CA, Litt M, Nossal R. Effect of Ca^{2+} on the structure and rheology of canine tracheal mucin. *Biorheology* 1984;21:235–253.

38. Marriott C, Shih CK, Litt M. Changes in the gel properties of tracheal mucus induced by divalent cations. *Biorheology* 1979;16:331–337.

39. Mian N, Kent PW. Role of directional Ca^{2+} effect on reduced viscosities of mucus secretions from chicken trachea in vitro. *Biochim Biophys Acta* 1986;883:486–495.

40. Verdugo P. Goblet cells, secretion and mucogenesis. *Annu Rev Physiol* 1990;52:157–176.

41. Verdugo P. Mucin exocytosis. *Am Rev Respir Dis* 1991;144:S33–S37.

42. Gasser KW, DiDomenico J, Hopfer U. Secretagogues activate chloride transport pathways in pancreatic zymogen granules. *Am J Physiol* 1988;254:G93–G99.

43. Gasser K, Hopfer U. Chloride transport across the membrane of parotid secretory granules. Am J Physiol 1990;259:C413–C420.

44. Hascall VC. Proteoglycans: structure and function. In: Ginsburg V, Robbin P, eds. *Biology of carbohydrates.* Vol. 1. New York: Wiley, 1981:1–49.

45. Sahu S, Lynn WS. Hyaluronic acid in the pulmonary secretions of patients with asthma. *Biochem J* 1978; 173:565–568.

46. Rahmoune H, Lamblin G, Lafitte J, Galabert C, Filliat M, Roussel P. Chondroitin sulfate in sputum from patients with cystic fibrosis and chronic bronchitis. *Am J Respir Cell Mol Biol* 1991;5:315–320.

47. Paul A, Picard J, Mergey D, Veissiere D, Finkbeiner WE, Basbaum CB. Glycoconjugates secreted by bovine tracheal serous cells in culture. *Arch Biochem Biophys* 1988;260:75–84.

48. Varsano S, Basbaum CB, Forsberg LS, Borson DB, Caughey G, Nadel JA. Dog tracheal epithelial cells in culture synthesize sulfated macromolecular glycoconjugates and release them from the cell surface upon exposure to extracellular proteases. *Exp Lung Res* 1987;13:157–184.

49. Matthews LM, Spector S, Lemm J, Potter JL. Studies on pulmonary secretions. *Am Rev Respir Dis* 1963; 88:199–204.

50. Slomiany A, Slomiany BL, Witas H, Aono M, Newman LJ. Isolation of fatty acids covalently bound to the gastric mucus glycoprotein of normal and cystic fibrosis patients. *Biochem Biophys Res Commun* 1983;113:286–293.

51. Spicer SS, Frayser R, Virella G, Hall BJ. Immunocytochemical localization of lysozymes in respiratory and other tissues. *Lab Invest* 1977;36:282–295.

52. Konstan MW, Cheng PW, Sherman JM, Thomassen MJ, Wood RE, Boat TF. Human lung lysozyme: sources and properties. *Am Rev Respir Dis* 1981;123: 120–124.

53. Franken C, Meijer CJLM, Dijkman JH. Tissue distribution of antileukoprotease and lysozyme in humans. *J Histochem Cytochem* 1989;37:493–498.

54. Thompson AB, Bohling T, Payvandi F, Rennard SI. Lower respiratory tract lactoferrin and lysozyme arise primarily in airways and are elevated in association with chronic bronchitis. *J Lab Clin Med* 1990; 115:148–158.

55. Bowes D, Clark AE, Corrin B. Ultrastructural localization of lactoferrin and glycoprotein in human bronchial glands. *Thorax* 1981;36:108–111.

56. Briggs RC, Glass WF, Montiel MM, Hnilica LS. Lactoferrin: nuclear localization in the human neutrophilic granulocyte. *J Histochem Cytochem* 1981; 29:1128–1136.

57. Harmsen MC, Swart PJ, de Bethune MP, et al. Antiviral effects of plasma and milk proteins: lactoferrin shows potent activity against both human immunodeficiency virus and human cytomegalovirus replication in vitro. *J Infect Dis* 1995;172:380–388.

58. Ganz T, Lehrer RI. Defensins. *Pharmacol Ther* 1995;66:191–205.

59. Goldman MJ, Anderson GM, Stolzenberg ED, Kari UP, Zasloff M, Wilson JM. Human β-defensin-1 is a salt-sensitive antibiotic in lung that is inactivated in cystic fibrosis. *Cell* 1997;88:553–560.

60. Stockley RA, Afford SC, Burnette D. Assessment of 7S and 11S immunoglobulin A in sputum. *Am Rev Respir Dis* 1980;22:959–964.

61. Brogan TD, Ryley HC, Neale L, Yassa J. Soluble proteins of bronchopulmonary secretions from patients with cystic fibrosis, asthma and bronchitis. *Thorax* 1975;36:72–79.

62. Stockley RA, Mistry M, Bradwell AR, Burnet. A study of plasma proteins in the sol phase of sputum from patients with chronic bronchitis. *Thorax* 1979;34:777–782.

63. Stockley RA. Measurement of soluble proteins in lung secretions. *Thorax* 1984;39:241–247.

64. Kramps JA, Franken C, Dijkman JH. ELISA for quantitative measurement of low molecular weight bronchial protease inhibitor in human sputum. *Am Rev Respir Dis* 1984;129:959–963.

65. Basbaum CB, Jany B, Finkbeiner WE. The serous cell. *Annu Rev Physiol* 1990;52:97–113.

66. Warner TF, Azen EA. Proline-rich proteins are present in serous cells of submucosal glands in the respiratory tract. *Am Rev Respir Dis* 130:115–118, 1984.

67. Bailleul V, Richet C, Hayem A, Degand P. Properties rheologiques des secretions bronchiques: mise en evidence et role de polypeptides riches en proline (PRP). *Clin Chim Acta* 1977;74:115–123.

68. Singh G, Katyal SL. Pulmonary proteins as cell-specific markers. *Exp Lung Res* 1991;17:245–253.

69. Bedetti CD, Singh J, Singh G, Katyal SL, Wong-Chong ML. Ultrastructural localization of rat Clara cell 10KD secretory protein by immuno-gold technique using polyclonal and monoclonal antibodies. *J Histochem Cytochem* 1987;35:789–794.

70. Phelps DS, Floros J. Localization of surfactant synthesis in human lung by in situ hybridization. *Am Rev Respir Dis* 1988;137:939–942.

71. Khoor A, Gray ME, Hull WM, Whitsett JA, Stahlman MT. Developmental expression of SP-A and SP-A mRNA in the proximal and distal respiratory epithelium in the human fetus and newborn. *J Histochem Cytochem* 1993;41:1311–1319.

72. Khoor A, Stahlman MT, Gray ME, Whitsett JA. Temporal-spatial distribution of SP-B and SP-C proteins and mRNAs in developing respiratory epithelium of human lung. *J Histochem Cytochem* 1994;42:1187–1199.

73. Tam PY, Verdugo P. Control of mucus hydration as a Donnan equilibrium process. *Nature* 1981;292:340–342.

74. Braga, PC. Sinusoidal oscillation method. In: Braga PC, Allegra L, eds. *Methods in bronchial mucology*. New York: Raven Press, 1988:63–71.

75. Davis SS. Mathematical description. In: Braga PC, Allegra L, eds. *Methods in bronchial mucology*. New York: Raven Press, 1988:33–49.

76. King M. Magnetic microrheometer. In: Braga PC, Allegra L, eds. *Methods in bronchial mucology*. New York: Raven Press, 1988:73–83.

77. Kim CS. Capillary type viscometer. In: Braga PC, Allegra L, eds. *Methods in bronchial mucology*. New York: Raven Press, 1988:93–103.

78. King M. Role of mucus viscoelasticity in cough clearance. *Biorheology* 1987;24:589–597.

79. Rubin BK, Ramirez O, King M. The mucus depleted frog palate as a model for the study of mucociliary clearance. *J Appl Physiol* 1990;69:424–429.

80. Wills PJ, Garcia Suarez MJ, Rutman A, Wilson R, Cole PJ. The ciliary transportability of sputum is slow on the mucus-depleted bovine trachea. *Am J Respir Crit Care Med* 1995;151:1255–1258.

81. Agarwal M, King M, Rubin BK, Shulka JB. Mucus transport in a miniaturized simulated cough machine:

effect of constriction and serous layer simulant. *Biorheology* 1989;26:977–988.

82. Puchelle E, Zahm JM, Jacquot J, Plotkowski C, Duvivier C. A simple technique for measuring adhesion tension properties of human bronchial secretions. *Eur J Respir Dis* 1987;71(Suppl 153):281.

83. Rubin BK, Ramirez O, King M. The role of mucus rheology and transport in neonatal respiratory distress syndrome and the effect of surfactant therapy. *Chest* 1992;101:1080–1085.

84. Girod S, Galabert C, Pierrot D, et al. Role of phospholipid lining on respiratory mucus clearance by cough. *J Appl Physiol* 1991;71:2262–2266.

85. Girod S, Galabert C, Lecuirre A, Zahm JM, Puchelle E. Phospholipid composition and surface-active properties of tracheobronchial secretions from patients with cystic fibrosis and chronic obstructive pulmonary diseases. *Pediatr Pulmonol* 1992;13:22–27.

86. Zahm JM, Puchelle E, Duvivier C, Didelon J. Spinability of respiratory mucus. Validation of a new apparatus: the Filancemeter. *Bull Eur Physiopathol Respir* 1986;22:609–613.

87. Dasgupta B, King M. Reduction in viscoelasticity in cystic fibrosis sputum in vitro using combined treatment with nacystelyn and rhDNase. *Pediatr Pulmonol* 1996;22:161–166.

88. Puchelle E, Zahm JM, Duvivier C. Spinability of bronchial mucus: relationship with viscoelasticity and mucus transport properties. *Biorheology* 1987;20:239–249.

89. King M, Zahm JM, Pierrot D, Vaquez-Girod S, Puchelle E. The role of mucus gel viscosity, spinability, and adhesive properties in clearance by simulated cough. *Biorheology* 1989;26:737–745.

90. Feather EA, Russell G. Sputum viscosity and pulmonary function in cystic fibrosis. *Arch Dis Child* 1970;45:807–808.

91. Puchelle E, Jacquot J, Beck G, Zahm JM, Galabert C. Rheological and transport properties of airway secretions in cystic fibrosis: relationships with the degree of infection and severity of the disease. *Eur J Clin Invest* 1985;15:389–394.

92. Chernick WS, Barbero GJ. Composition of tracheobronchial secretions in cystic fibrosis of the pancreas and bronchiectasis, *Pediatrics* 1959;24:739–745.

93. Wills PJ, Hall RL, Chan W, Cole PJ. Sodium chloride increases the transportability of cystic fibrosis and bronchiectasis sputum on mucus-depleted bovine trachea. *J Clin Invest* 1997;99:9–13.

94. Dische Z, di Sant'Agnese P, Pallavicini C, et al. Composition of mucoprotein fractions from duodenal fluid of patients with cystic fibrosis of the pancreas and from controls. *Pediatrics* 1959;24:74–91.

95. Chernick WS, Barbero GJ. Studies on human tracheobronchial and submaxillary secretions in normal and pathophysiological conditions. *Ann N Y Acad Sci* 1963;106:755–756.

96. Menguy R, Masters VF, Desbaillets L. Salivary mucins of patients with cystic fibrosis: composition and susceptibility to degradation by salivary glycosidases. *Gastroenterology* 1970;59:257–264.

97. Boat TF, Cheng PW, Iyer R, et al. Human respiratory tract secretions: Mucous glycoproteins of nonpurulent tracheobronchial secretions and sputum of pa-

tients with bronchitis and cystic fibrosis. *Arch Biochem Biophys* 1976;177:95–104.

98. Boat TF, Cheng PW, Wood RE, et al. Tracheobronchial mucus secretion in vivo and in vitro by epithelial tissues from cystic fibrosis and control subjects. *Mod Probl Paediatr* 1976;19:141–152.

99. Boat TF, Kleinerman JI, Carlson DM, et al. Human respiratory tract secretions: mucous glycoproteins secreted by cultured nasal polyp epithelium from subjects with allergic rhinitis and with cystic fibrosis. *Am Rev Respir Dis* 1974;110:428–441.

100. Frates RC, Kaizu T, Last JA. Mucus glycoproteins secreted by respiratory epithelial tissue from cystic fibrosis patients. *Pediatr Res* 1983;17:30–34.

101. Cheng P-W, Boat TF, Cranfill K, et al. Increased sulfation of glycoconjugates by cultured nasal epithelial cells from patients with cystic fibrosis. *J Clin Invest* 1989;84:68–72.

102. Chace KV, Leahy DS, Martin R, et al. Respiratory mucous secretions in patients with cystic fibrosis: relationship between levels of highly sulfated mucin component and severity of the disease. *Clin Chim Acta* 1983;132:143–155.

103. Mohapatra NK, Cheng P-W, Parker JC, et al. Sulfate concentrations and transport in human bronchial epithelial cells. *Am J Physiol* 1993;264:C1231–C1237.

104. Barasch J, Al-Awqati Q. Defective acidification of the biosynthetic pathway in cystic fibrosis. *J Cell Sci Suppl* 1993;17:229–233.

105. Sangadala S, Bhat UR, Mendicino J. Structures of high molecular weight sulfated oligosaccharides in human tracheal mucin glycoproteins. *Mol Cell Biochem* 1993;126:37–47.

106. Girod S, Zahm JM, Plotkowski C, Beck G, Puchelle E. Role of the physicochemical properties of mucus in the protection of the respiratory epithelium. *Eur Respir J* 1992;5:477–487.

107. Gawel J, Rudnik J, Pryjma J, et al. Protein in bronchial secretion of children with chronic obstructive pulmonary diseases: I, relation to clinical diagnosis. *Scand J Respir Dis* 1979;60:63–68.

108. Kotlar HK, Harbitz O, Jenssen AO, Smidsrod O. Quantitation of proteins in sputum from patients with chronic obstructive lung disease: II, determination of albumin, transferrin, alpha-1 acid glycoprotein, IgG, IgM, lysozyme and C3-complement factor. *Eur J Respir Dis* 1980;61:233–239.

109. Harbitz O, Jennsen AO, Smidsrod O. Lysozyme and lactoferrin in sputum from patients with chronic obstructive pulmonary disease. *Eur J Respir Dis* 1984;65:512–520.

110. Creeth JM, Bridge JL, Horton JR. An interaction between lysozyme and mucus glycoproteins. *Biochem J* 1982;181:717–724.

111. Rose MC, Brown JZ, Jacoby WS, Lynn B, Kaufman B. Biochemical properties of tracheobronchial mucins from cystic fibrosis and non-cystic fibrosis individuals. *Pediatr Res* 1987;22:545–551.

112. Poncz L, Jentoft N, Ho M, Dearborn D. Kinetics of proteolysis of hog gastric mucin by human neutrophil elastase and *Pseudomonas* elastase. *Infect Immunol* 1986;56:703–704.

113. Gupta R, Jentoft N. Structural studies of mucins from cystic fibrosis and control patients. *J Biol Chem* 1992;267:3160–3167.

114. Chernick WS, Barbero GJ. Composition of tracheo-bronchial secretions in cystic fibrosis of the pancreas and bronchiectasis. *Pediatrics* 1959;24:739–745.

115. Potter JL, Spector S, Matthews LW, et al. Studies on pulmonary secretions: III, the nucleic acids in whole pulmonary secretions from patients with cystic fibrosis, bronchiectasis and laryngectomy. *Am Rev Respir Dis* 1969;99:909–916.

116. Shak S, Capon DJ, Hellniss R, et al. Recombinant human DNase I reduces viscosity of cystic fibrosis sputum. *Proc Natl Acad Sci U S A* 1990;87:9188–9192.

117. Wills PJ, Wodehouse T, Corkery K, Mallon K, Wilson R, Cole PJ. Short-term recombinant human DNase in bronchiectasis: effect on clinical state and in vitro sputum transportability. *Am J Respir Crit Care Med* 1996;154:413–417.

118. Lethem MI, James SL, Marriott C. The role of mucous glycoproteins in the rheologic properties of cystic fibrosis sputum. *Am Rev Respir Dis* 1990;142:1053–1058–971.

119. Vasconcellos CA, Allen PG, Wohl ME, Drazen JM, Jamney PA, Stossel TP. Reduction in viscosity of cystic fibrosis sputum by gelsolin. *Science* 1994;263:969–971.

120. Prince A. Comparison of *Pseudomonas aeruginosa* binding to normal and CF respiratory epithelial cells. *J Clin Invest Suppl* 1991;6:138.

121. Zar H, Saiman L, Quittell L, et al. Binding of *Pseudomonas aeruginosa* to respiratory epithelial cells from patients with various mutations in the cystic fibrosis transmembrane regulator. *J Pediatr* 1995;126:230–233.

122. Irvin RT, Doig P, Lee KK, et al. Characterization of the *Pseudomonas aeruginosa* pilus adhesin: confirmation that the pilin structural protein subunit contains a human epithelial cell-binding domain. *Infect Immunol* 1989;57:3720–3726.

123. Imundo L, Barasch J, Prince A, et al. Cystic fibrosis cells have a receptor for pathogenic bacteria on their apical surface. *Proc Natl Acad Sci U S A* 1995;92:3019–3023.

124. Baltimore RS, Christie CDC, Smith GJW. Immunohistopathologic localization of *Pseudomonas aeruginosa* in lungs from patients with cystic fibrosis. *Am Rev Respir Dis* 1989;140:1650–1661.

125. Devaraj N, Sheykhanazari M, Warren WS, Bhavanandan VP. Differential binding of *Pseudomonas aeruginosa* to normal and cystic fibrosis tracheobronchial mucins. *Glycobiology* 1994;4:307–316.

126. Carnoy C, Ramphal R, Scharfman A, Houdret N, et al. Altered carbohydrate composition of salivary mucins from patients with cystic fibrosis and the adhesion of *Pseudomonas aeruginosa*. *Am J Respir Cell Mol Biol* 1993;9:323–334.

127. Komiyama K, Habbick BF, Tumber SK. Role of sialic acid in saliva-mediated aggregation of *Pseudomonas aeruginosa* isolated from cystic fibrosis. *Infect Immunol* 1987;55:2364–2369.

128. Nelson JW, Tredgett MW, Sheehan JK, et al. Mucinophilic and chemotactic properties of Pseudomonas aeruginosa in relation to pulmonary colonization in cystic fibrosis. *Infect Immunol* 1990;58:1489–1495.

129. Paranchych W, Sastry PA, Drake D et al. *Pseudomonas pili*: studies on antigenic determinants and mammalian cell receptors. *Antibiot Chemother* 1985;36:49–57.

130. Ramphal R, Koo L, Ishimoto KS, et al. Adhesion of *Pseudomonas aeruginosa* pilin-deficient mutants to mucin. *Infect Immunol* 1991;59:1307–1311.

131. Sajjan U, Reisman J, Doig P, et al. Binding of nonmucoid *Pseudomonas aeruginosa* to normal human intestinal mucin and respiratory mucin from patients with cystic fibrosis. *J Clin Invest* 1992;89:657–665.

132. Reddy MS. Human tracheobronchial mucin: purification and binding to *Pseudomonas aeruginosa*. *Infect Immunol* 1992;60:1530–1535.

133. Sajjan U, Corey M, Karmali M, Forstner J. Binding of *Pseudomonas cepacia* to normal human intestinal mucin and respiratory mucin from patients with cystic fibrosis. *J Clin Invest* 1992;89:648–656.

134. Sajjan SU, Forstner JF. Identification of the mucin-binding adhesin of *P. cepacia* isolated from patients with cystic fibrosis. *Infect Immunol* 1992;60:1434–1440.

135. Coonrod JD, Varble R, Yoneda K. Mechanism of killing of pneumococci by lysozyme. *J Infect Dis* 1991;164:527–532.

136. Hughes WT, Koblin BA, Rosenstein BJ. Lysozyme activity in cystic fibrosis. Pediatr Res 1982;16:874–876.

137. Britigan BE, Hayek MB, Doebbeling BN, Fick RB. Transferrin and lactoferrin undergo proteolytic cleavage in pseudomonas-infected lungs of patients with cystic fibrosis. *Infect Immunol* 1993;61:5049–5055.

138. Smith JJ, Travis SM, Greenberg EP, Welsh MJ. Cystic fibrosis airway epithelia fail to kill bacteria because of abnormal airway surface fluid. *Cell* 1996;85:229–236.

139. Harder J, Siebert R, Zhang Y, Matthiesen P, Christophers E, Schlegelberger B, Schroder JM,. Mapping of the gene encoding human beta-defensin-2 (DEFB2) to chromosome region 8p22-p23.1. *Genomics* 1997;46(3):472–475.

140. Engelhardt JF, Yankaskas JR, Ernst SA, et al. Submucosal glands are the predominant site of CFTR expression in the human bronchus. *Nat Genet* 1992;2:240–248.

141. Rhodin JA. The ciliated cell: ultrastructure and function in human tracheal mucosa. *Am Rev Respir Dis* 1966;93(Suppl):1–15.

142. Ellefsen P, Tos M. Goblet cells in human trachea: quantitative studies of a pathological biopsy material. *Arch Otolaryngol* 1972;95:547–555.

143. Spicer SS, Schulte BA, Chakrin LW. Ultrastructural and histochemical observations of respiratory epithelium and glands. *Exp Lung Res* 1983;4:137–156.

144. Kim KC, Lee BC. P2 purinoceptor regulation of mucin release by airway goblet cells in primary culture. *Br J Pharmacol* 1991;103:1053–1056.

145. Davis CW, Dowell ML, Lethem M, et al. Goblet cell degranulation in isolated canine tracheal epithelium: response to exogenous ATP, ADP and adenosine. *Am J Physiol* 1992;262:C1313–1323.

146. Kim KC, Nassiri J, Brody JS. Mechanisms of airway goblet cell mucin release; studies with cultured tracheal surface epithelial cells. *Am J Respir Cell Mol Biol* 1989;1:137–143.

147. Klinger JD, Tandler B, Liedke CM, et al. Proteinases of *Pseudomonas aeruginosa* evoke mucin release by tracheal epithelium. *J Clin Invest* 1984; 74:1669–1678.

148. Rieves RD, Goff J, Wu T, et al. Airway epithelial cell mucin release: immunologic quantitation and response to platelet-activating factor. *Am J Respir Cell Mol Biol* 1992;6:158–167.

149. Boat TF, Polony I, Cheng PW. Mucin release from rabbit tracheal epithelium in response to sera from normal and cystic fibrosis subjects. *Pediatr Res* 1982;16:792–797.

150. Kuo HP, Rohde JA, Barnes PJ, et al. Cigarette smoke-induced airway goblet cell secretion; dose dependent differential nerve activation. *Am J Physiol* 1992;263:L161–167.

151. Meyrick B, Sturgess JM, Reid L. A reconstruction of the duct system and secretory tubules of the human bronchial submucosal gland. *Thorax* 1969;24: 729–736.

152. Meyrick B, Reid L. Ultrastructure of cells in human bronchial submucosal glands. *J Anat* 1970;107:281–299.

153. Basbaum CB, Jany B, Finkbeiner WE. The serous cell. *Annu Rev Physiol* 1990;52:97–113.

154. Shimura S, Sasaki T, Sasaki H, et al. Contractility of isolated single submucosal gland from trachea. *J Appl Physiol* 1986;60:1237–1247.

155. Partanen M, Laitinen A, Hervonen A, et al. Catecholamine- and acetylcholinesterase-containing nerves in human lower respiratory tract. *Histochemistry* 1982; 76:175–188.

156. Meyrick B, Reid L. Ultrastructure of cells in human bronchial submucosal glands. *J Anat* 1970;107: 281–299.

157. Davis B, Marin MG, Fischer S, et al. New method for study of canine mucous gland secretion in vivo: cholinergic regulation. *Am Rev Respir Dis* 1976;113: (4 Part 2):257 (abstract).

158. Ueki I, German VF, Nadel JA. Micropipette measurement of airway submucosal gland secretion; autonomic effects. *Am Rev Respir Dis* 1980;121:351–357.

159. Chakrin LW, Baker AP, Christian P, et al. Effect of cholinergic stimulation on the release of macromolecules by canine trachea, in vitro. *Am Rev Respir Dis* 1973;108:69–76.

160. Boat TF, Kleinerman JI. Human respiratory tract secretions: 2, effect of cholinergic and adrenergic agents on in vitro release of protein and mucous glycoprotein. *Chest* 1975;67:32S–34S.

161. Shelhamer JH, Marom Z, Kaliner M. Immunologic and neuropharmacologic stimulation of mucous glycoprotein release from human airways in vitro. J Clin Invest 1980;66:1400–1408.

162. Laitinen A, Partanen M, Hervonen A, et al. Electron microscopic study on the innervation of the human lower respiratory tract. Evidence of adrenergic nerves. Eur J Respir Dis 1985;67:209–215.

163. Dey RD, Shannon WA, Said SI. Localization of VIP-immunoreactive nerves in airways and pulmonary vessels of dogs, cats and human subjects. Cell Tissue Res 1981;220:231–238.

164. Coles SJ, Bhaskar KR, O'Sullivan DD, et al. Airway mucus: composition and regulation of its secretion by neuropeptides in vitro. In: *Mucus and mucosa: Ciba Foundation symposium 109.* London: Pitman, 1984:40–60.

165. Plopper CG, Hill LH, Mariassy AT, et al. Ultrastructure of the non-ciliated bronchiolar epithelial (Clara) cell of mammalian lung: a study of man with comparison of 15 mammalian species. *Exp Lung Res* 1980; 1:171–180.

166. Singh G, Katyal SL, Wong-Chong ML. A quantitative assay for a Clara cell-specific protein and its application in the study of development of pulmonary airways in the rat. *Pediatr Res* 1986;20:802–805.

167. Mantile G, Miele L, Cordella-Miele E, et al. Human Clara cell 10-kDa protein is the counterpart of rabbit uteroglobin. *J Biol Chem* 1993;268:20343–20351.

168. Miele L, Cordella-Miele E, Mukherjee AB. Uteroglobin: structure, molecular biology, and new perspectives on its function as a phospholipase A2 inhibitor. *Endocr Rev* 1987;8:474–491.

169. DeWalter R, Willems LNA, VanMuijen, et al. Ultrastructural localization of bronchial antileukoprotease in central and peripheral human airways by a gold-labeling technique using monoclonal antibodies. *Am Rev Respir Dis* 1986;133:882–890.

170. Farmer SG, Hay DWP. Airway epithelial modulation of smooth-muscle function: the evidence for epithelium-derived inhibitory factor. In: Farmer SG, Hay DWP, eds. *The airway epithelium.* New York: Marcel Dekker Inc, 1991:437–483.

171. Sasaki T, Shimura S, Sasaki H, et al. Effect of epithelium on mucus secretion from feline tracheal submucosal glands. *J Appl Physiol* 1989;66:764–770.

172. Reid L. Measurement of the bronchial mucous gland layer: a diagnostic yardstick in chronic bronchitis. *Thorax* 1960;15:132–141.

173. Bedrossian CWM, Greenberg SD, Singer DB, et al. The lung in cystic fibrosis: a quantitative study including prevalence of pathologic findings among different age groups. *Hum Pathol* 1976;7:195–204.

174. Lamb L, Reid L. The tracheobronchial submucosal glands in cystic fibrosis: a qualitative and quantitative histochemical study. *Br J Dis Chest* 1972;66: 239–247.

175. Chow CW, Landau LI, Taussig LM. Bronchial mucous glands in the newborn with cystic fibrosis. *Eur J Pediatr* 1982;139:240–243.

176. Infeld MD, Brennan JA, Davis PB. Human fetal lung fibroblasts promote invasion of the extracellular matrix by normal human tracheobronchial epithelial cells in vitro: a model of early airway gland development. *Am J Respir Cell Mol Biol* 1993;8:69–76.

177. Tournier JM, Polette M, Hinnrasky J, Beck J, Werb Z, Basbaum C. Expression of gelatinase A, a mediator of extracellular matrix remodeling, by tracheal gland serous cells in culture and in vivo. *J Biol Chem* 1994;269:25454–25464.

178. Lim M, Elfman F, Dohrman A, Cunha G, Basbaum C. Upregulation of the 72-kDa type IV collagenase in epithelial and stromal cells during rat tracheal gland morphogenesis. *Devel Biol* 1995;171:521–530.

179. Lim M, Bowden J, McDonald D, et al. Analysis of metalloproteinases and plasminogen activators in tracheal gland development and hypertrophy. *Pediatr Pulmonol Suppl* 1993;9:252 (abstract).

180. Leigh MW, Kylander J, Yankaskas JR, Boucher RC. Cell proliferation in bronchial epithelium and submucosal glands of cystic fibrosis patients. *Am J Respir Cell Mol Biol* 1995;12:605–612.

181. Fahy JV, Schuster A, Ueki I, et al. Mucus secretion in bronchiectasis: the role of neutrophil proteases. *Am Rev Respir Dis* 1992;146:1430–1433.

182. Schuster A, Ueki I, Nadel JA. Neutrophil elastase stimulates tracheal gland secretion that is inhibited by ICI 200,355. *Am J Physiol* 1992;262:L86–L91.

183. Sturgess J, Imrie J. Quantitative evaluation of the development of tracheal submucosal glands in infants with cystic fibrosis and control infants. *Am J Pathol* 1982;106:303–311.

184. Yamaya M, Finkbeiner WE, Widdicombe JH. Ion transport by cultures of human tracheobronchial submucosal glands. *Am J Physiol* 1991;261:L485–L490.

185. Becq F, Merten MD, Voelckel MA, et al. Characterization of cAMP dependent CFTR-chloride channels in human tracheal glands. *FEBS Lett* 1993; 321:73–78.

186. Yamaya M, Finkbeiner WE, Widdicombe JH. Altered ion transport by tracheal glands in cystic fibrosis. *Am J Physiol* 1991;261:L491–L494.

187. Lethem MI, Dowell ML, Van Scott M, et al. Nucleotide regulation of goblet cells in human airway epithelial explants: normal exocytosis in cystic fibrosis. *Am J Respir Cell Mol Biol* 1993;9:315–322.

Cystic Fibrosis in Adults,
edited by J. R. Yankaskas and M. R. Knowles,
Lippincott–Raven Publishers, Philadelphia, 1999.

5

Microbiology of Cystic Fibrosis Lung Disease

Peter H. Gilligan

*Clinical Microbiology–Immunology, University of North Carolina Hospitals, and
Departments of Microbiology-Immunology and Pathology, University of
North Carolina School of Medicine, Chapel Hill, North Carolina*

The genetic defects found in patients with cystic fibrosis (CF) cause their airways to be coated with thick, tenacious secretions, resulting in diminished mucociliary clearance. This creates an ideal environment for chronic lung infection. These lung infections, which lead to cardiopulmonary failure, are responsible for greater than 90% of deaths in adults with CF (1).

Chronic lung infections in patients with CF are characterized as a series of acute pulmonary exacerbations interspersed with varying periods of relative well-being. Signs and symptoms of an acute pulmonary exacerbation are an increasingly severe cough, increased volume and purulence of sputum, dyspnea, low-grade fever, weight loss, rising leukocyte count, and declining pulmonary function. Aggressive intravenous antimicrobial therapy in the early stages can frequently abrogate the clinical symptoms. However, postexacerbation pulmonary function frequently does not return to preexisting levels despite aggressive therapy. As the number of pulmonary exacerbations increases, lung function continues its inextricable decline. Antimicrobial therapy becomes less effective as the microbes chronically infecting these patients become increasingly resistant due to antimicrobial pressure (2).

Over the past 40 years, improving antimicrobial therapy and clinical management have resulted in impressive gains in the median survival time in patients with CF. Nevertheless, the grim reality is that more than 50% of patients with CF will die before their 31st birthday from the effect of underlying lung infection. What is particularly frustrating is that the agents responsible for chronic infection and death are well known to the physicians, nurses, microbiologists, respiratory therapists, pharmacists, and in many instances, the patients and their families. Interestingly, there are three bacterial species, *Staphylococcus aureus*, *Pseudomonas aeruginosa*, and *Burkholderia cepacia*, that appear to be especially well adapted to cause chronic lung infection in patients with CF (3). Although impressive gains have been made in our understanding of the organisms and the mechanism by which they damage the lung and evade both the patient's and physician's attempts to eradicate them, we have not yet found ways to reliably prevent or cure chronic lung infections in the vast majority of patients with CF . The organisms most frequently encountered in the lungs of adult patients with CF are listed in Table 5–1. In this chapter, we summarize what we have learned thus far concerning these specially adapted killers, with an emphasis on the agents most likely to be encountered in adults with CF.

STAPHYLOCOCCUS AUREUS

Staph. aureus are gram-positive cocci that can be found as a component of the microbiota of the skin and nares in healthy individuals. It is usually the initial etiology of chronic lung

TABLE 5–1. *Agents chronically infecting the respiratory tract of patients with cystic fibrosis*

Organism	Onset of infection	% of adult CF patients infected	Contribution to lung damage
Staphylococcus aureus	Early childhood	18–26	Moderate
Pseudomonas aeruginosa	Childhood to adolescence	79–80	Major
Burkholderia cepacia	Adolescence to adult	6	Little to major
Mycobacterium not tuberculosis	Adolescence to adult	0.4[a]	Unknown
Aspergillus sp.	Adolescence to adult	5–8	Unknown
Stenotrophomonas maltophilia	Adolescence to adult	1.8	No evidence
Burkholderia gladioli and *pickettii*	Adolescence to adult	<1	Unknown
Alcaligenes xylosoxidans	Adolescence to adult	<1	No evidence

[a]Actual prevalence may be higher. See "*Mycobacterium* sp.," p.108.
Data from 1990 and 1993 CF Patient Registry (U.S. Cystic Fibrosis Foundation, Rockville, MD).

disease in patients with CF. In the preantibiotic era, it was the leading cause of death due to infection in these patients.

Pathogenesis

The initial events that lead to infection with *Staph. aureus* are not well understood. Some evidence exists that *Staph. aureus* infection is preceded by infection by common respiratory viruses such as respiratory syncytial (RSV) or the parainfluenza viruses. Since infants with CF have the same numbers and type of viral respiratory infections as their non-CF siblings (3) and respiratory viruses such as influenza are known to predispose non-CF patients to bacterial lung infection especially with *Staph. aureus* the theory of viral infection "setting up" the CF lung for *Staph. aureus* chronic infection is appealing (3). However, no data from large, longitudinal natural history studies of viral infections in patients with CF currently exist to support this popular hypothesis.

Most successful pulmonary pathogens have developed two characteristic strategies to adhere to respiratory epithelium and to evade the immune system. The precise mechanisms by which *Staph. aureus* evades the immune system and establishes chronic infection in patients with CF are not understood. *Staph. aureus* produces a number of factors, including protein A, leukocidin, capsule, and lipase (4,5), that may interfere with normal phagocytic cell function. Inhibition of phagocytic function coupled with

decreased mucociliary clearance due to the dehydrated, viscous secretions seen in CF may partially explain the ability of *Staph. aureus* to cause chronic infection in CF populations.

Another important factor in establishing chronic lung infection is the ability of this organism to adhere to respiratory epithelium. Studies have shown that *Staph. aureus* binds equally well to CF and non-CF respiratory epithelial cells. However, isolates recovered from the airway of patients with CF showed a higher level of respiratory cell adherence than those recovered from the airway of non-CF patients. These data suggest that factors within the CF lung lead to selection of more highly adherent *Staph. aureus* strains (6).

Once chronic infection with *Staph. aureus* is established, there are three potential microbiologic outcomes. One is the eradication of the organism by antimicrobial therapy. The number of patients in which this occurs is unknown. A second possible outcome is eradication of the organism followed by reinfection with a second strain of *Staph. aureus*. This second strain may also be eradicated and lead to infection with a third strain and so on. The third and most common scenario based on molecular epidemiology studies is a cycle of exacerbation, treatment, and remission, with a reduction in numbers of organisms resulting in a period of well-being, increasing organism load leading to another acute exacerbation due to the same strain of *Staph. aureus* (7,8). These repeated pulmonary exacerbations chronicle inflammatory events in the lung that result in further lung damage and an accompanying slow decline in pulmonary function. Lung tissue damaged by *Staph. aureus* infection may provide a nidus for *P. aeruginosa* infection that frequently follows chronic *Staph. aureus* infection. Chronic co-infection with these two organisms may also occur.

The emergence of *P. aeruginosa* as the primary pulmonary pathogen in adolescent and adult patients with CF especially after months to years of prior chronic infection with *Staph. aureus,* makes it difficult to determine the exact role of *Staph. aureus* in the fatal lung failure suffered by most current patients with CF. However, most clinicians continue to treat *Staph. aureus* aggressively, either acutely or with prophylactic oral agents.

Antimicrobial Susceptibility

The development of the antistaphylococcal penicillins, which include oxacillin, nafcillin, and dicloxacillin, has significantly contributed to the dramatic increase in the life expectancy experienced by patients with CF over the past 50 years. Resistance to these antimicrobials has remained very low (< 5%) for many years. However, recent experience at the University of North Carolina suggests that resistance to the antistaphylococcal penicillins is on the rise. Between September 1994 and August 1996, 27 of 259 patients with CF infected with *Staph. aureus* had strains resistant to the antistaphylococcal penicillins (7). Oxacillin-resistant strains of *Staph. aureus* were more frequently seen in patients with CF older than 15 years of age. Approximately half were chronically infected. Molecular epidemiology studies suggest that patients with CF can obtain these organisms while hospitalized or from other patients with CF.

Resistance to antistaphylococcal penicillins is almost always due to modifications in the organism's penicillin-binding proteins. As a result of these modifications, beta-lactam antimicrobials can no longer bind to kill these organisms. Organisms resistant to the antistaphylococcal penicillins via modification of penicillin-binding proteins (also called oxacillin-resistant *Staph. aureus*) are resistant to all beta-lactam antimicrobials, including all penicillin, cephalosporin, monobactam (aztreonam), carbapenem (imipenem), and penicillin-beta-lactamase inhibitor combination antimicrobials. In addition, these oxacillin-resistant *Staph. aureus* strains show varying degrees of resistance to the following antimicrobials: erythromycin, chloramphenicol, tetracycline, clindamycin, gentamicin, and tobramycin.

The organism may remain susceptible only to ciprofloxacin, trimethoprim/sulfamethoxazole, and/or vancomycin. Resistance to both ciprofloxacin (a quinolone antimicrobial that inhibits DNA gyrase activity) and trimethoprim/sulfamethoxazole may develop following oral therapy with these agents, especially when these antibiotics are used prophylactically over extended periods (weeks to months). For example, in 39 patients with CF infected with *Staph. aureus* who were receiving trimethoprim/sulfamethoxazole (TMP/SMX) prophylactically, 20 harbored *Staph. aureus* strains that were resistant to this antimicrobial. Patients who harbored TMP/SMX-resistant strains had received an average of 30 months of TMP/SMX prophylaxis versus 11 months for those patients with sensitive strains. In TMP/SMX-resistant *Staph. aureus* isolates, the organism is able to take up thymidine from its environment, circumventing the pathway blocked by TMP/SMX. Sensitive isolates are unable to take up thymidine (9).

The majority of *Staph. aureus* isolates continue to be susceptible to several oral anti-microbial agents. How much longer agents such as clindamycin, dicloxacillin, cephalexin, and TMP/ SMX will continue to be effective against *Staph. aureus* strains recovered from patients with CF is unclear. What is clear is that resistance to these agents is increasing and few oral antistaphylococcal agents are on the horizon. This may mean that, like *P. aeruginosa,* only agents administered intravenously or by aerosol will be effective against *Staph. aureus.*

Laboratory Detection

Accurate detection of *Staph. aureus* from the respiratory secretions of patients with CF requires the use of a selective medium (mannitol salts agar) for two reasons. First, the high salt content of this medium inhibits the growth of most other organisms present in these secretions. Second, this medium supports the growth of thymidine dependent (TMP/SMX-resistant) *Staph. aureus* isolates while these isolates grow poorly or not at all on other commonly used media. Because of the increasing importance of oxacillin resistance in *Staph. aureus*, all isolates should be screened for oxacillin resistance using an oxacillin screening plate. This plate containing 6 µg/mL oxacillin and 2% sodium chloride (NaCl) has been shown to be the most accurate method for detecting oxacillin resistance.

PSEUDOMONAS AERUGINOSA

General Characteristics

P. aeruginosa is the most important infectious agent in chronic lung infection in adult patients with CF (1,2). The organism is a motile, aerobic, gram-negative rod that is ubiquitous in nature. It has a predilection for aqueous environments in the home, clinic, and inpatient settings. The organisms can be found in sinks, tap water, shower heads, whirlpool baths, respiratory therapy equipment such as nebulizers, and on the surface of fresh fruits and vegetables. Not surprisingly, molecular epidemiology studies using a genotyping method called pulse field gel electrophoresis (PFGE) suggest that most patients become infected from environmental sources rather than via person-to-person spread (10–12). Most patients are infected with their own genetically unique strain (clone or genotype) of *P. aeruginosa*. Infection with these unique strains can continue for months to years. Some patients may be intermittently infected with other genotypes, but long-term co-infection with multiple genotypes is not common. Siblings may be infected by the same genotype, but this probably reflects exposure to common environmental sources rather than person-to-person spread. Small groups of unrelated patients have also been found to be infected chronically with the same genotype.

(10–12) Distinguishing person-to-person spread from exposure to a common environmental source is difficult because of the ubiquity of this organism in the locations shared by patients with CF such as clinics, inpatient rooms and wards, and a variety of social settings.

Pathogenesis

P. aeruginosa appears to be especially adapted for survival in the unusual physiologic environment found in the CF lung. In nature, this organism is motile and piliated and has a planktonic mode of growth. Phenotypically, it is serum resistant, has a smooth lipopolysaccharide, and produces a variety of virulence factors, including two proteases, alkaline protease, and elastase, which appears to play an important role in pathogenesis of chronic CF airway disease. The environmental form of the organism that is believed to be responsible for initiating chronic infection in the airway of patients with CF (13,14).

Pili are responsible for the initial adherence of *P. aeruginosa* to the respiratory epithelium of patients with CF (14). Once adherent, the organism evolves to a form adapted for survival in the CF lung. This is known as the "mucoid" form of *P. aeruginosa* (Fig. 5–1). Mucoid *P. aeruginosa* strains produce a thick layer of an exopolysaccharide called alginate. Alginate is a polymer composed of acetylated D-mannuronic acid and L-guluronic acid. Mucoid strains vary significantly from the original, infecting wild-type strains. These mucoid strains have a rough lipopolysaccharide, are serum sensitive, frequently are nonmotile, and grow as microcolonies in the airways (Fig. 5–2) (13,15).

Infection with mucoid strains of *P. aeruginosa* is a hallmark of CF lung disease in adults. Up to 80% of adults with CF are chronically infected with this organism (1). In contrast, patients with other forms of chronic lung disease, such as patients with chronic obstructive pulmonary disease with chronic bronchitis, rarely are infected with the mucoid form of this organism. Much of the capability of mucoid *P. aeruginosa* to cause chronic lung infection can be attributed to the alginate surround-

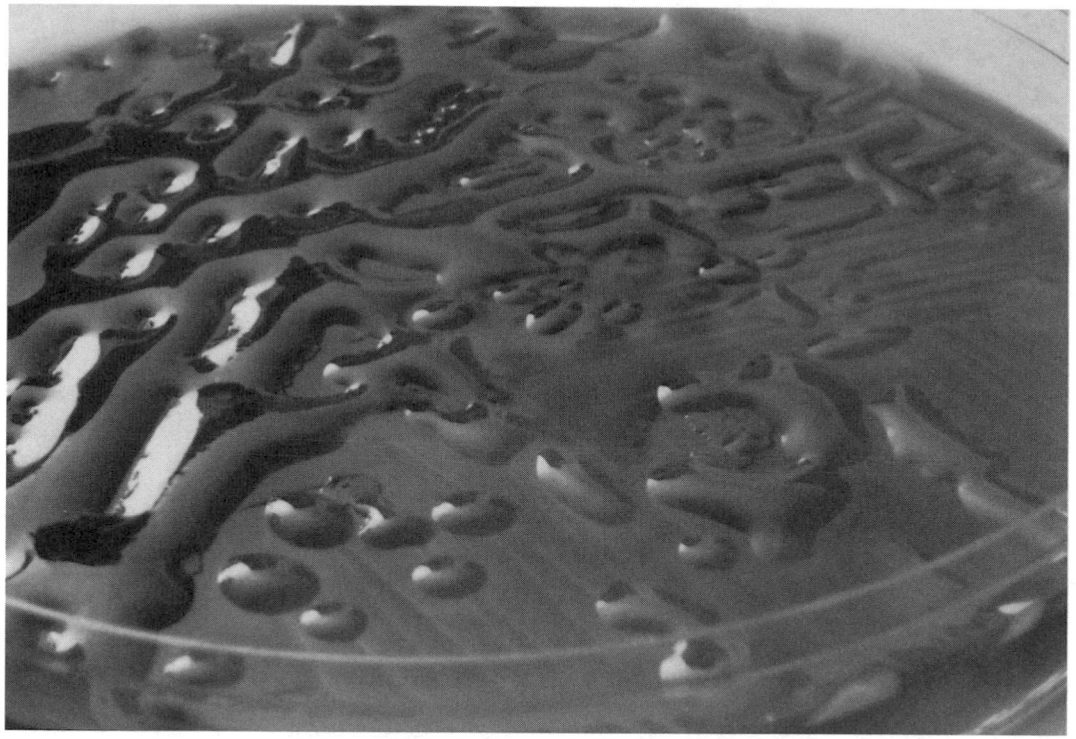

FIG. 5–1. Mucoid colonies of mucoid *P. aeruginosa* on MacConkey agar.

ing these organisms. Mucoid *P. aeruginosa* grow as microcolonies, that is, biofilms of alginate in which pseudomonads are embedded (see Fig. 5–2). This microcolony form of growth is thought to be important in the organism's adherence to epithelial cells in the airway and in making the organisms refractory to mucociliary clearance. It is believed to protect the organism from antimicrobials and toxic, reactive intermediates produced by leukocytes (15–17). A small subpopulation of adult patients with CF never becomes chronically infected with mucoid *P. aeruginosa*. Pier and colleagues (18) have shown that these patients possess opsonophagocytic antibodies for the alginate polysaccharide. *P. aeruginosa* infected patients with CF also had opsonophagocytic antibodies, but they were not directed against alginate. These data suggest that alginate also protects these strains of *P. aeruginosa* from phagocytosis.

The conversion to the mucoid form of growth has been the object of intense study at the molecular level. It is now clear that many strains of *P. aeruginosa* are capable of producing alginate, and that the production of alginate is under tight genetic control. The signal(s) that result in the "turning on" of the genes for alginate production are not understood. Several factors, including osmolarity, nitrogen, and phosphate starvation, have been postulated as triggers for the production of alginate (15,16).

Alginate production is regulated by genes that control the transcription of the alginate biosynthetic gene cluster. Transcription of AlgD gene, the first gene in this cluster, is highly regulated. This gene encodes the enzyme, GDP-mannose dehydrogenase, which catalyzes the oxidation of GDP-mannose to GDP-mannuronic acid. This unidirectional step is critical in alginate biosynthesis because it shunts GDP-mannose from the production of the oligosaccharide portion of lipopolysaccharide to alginate production. This shunting in mucoid strains explains the conversion of the lipopolysaccharide from smooth to rough (15).

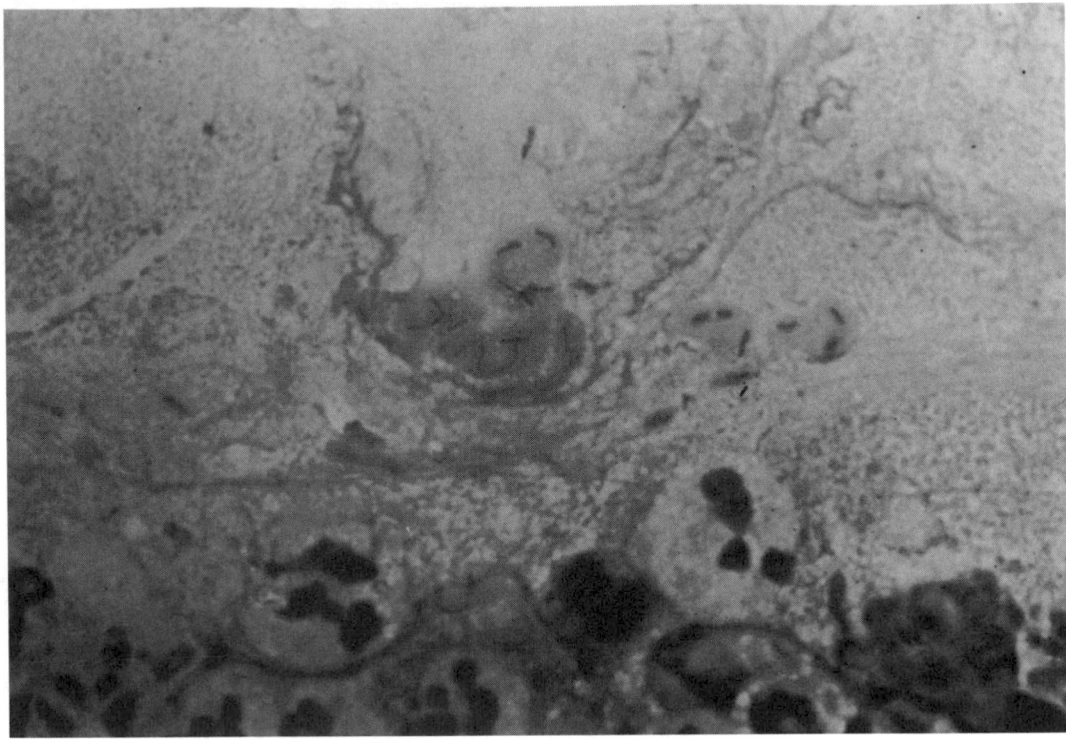

FIG. 5–2. Gram stain of sputum from a CF patient infected with mucoid *P. aeruginosa*. Note microcolonies composed of rod-shaped organisms embedded in alginate gel.

The transcription of AlgD is under the control of the products of two other genes, AlgR and AlgU. Both gene products must be produced for the transcription of the AlgD gene and the other alginate biosynthetic genes to occur. AlgU is under negative regulation by the product of two other genes, muc A and B. Mutation in muc A or B results in the biosynthesis of alginate whereas mutation in AlgU results in reversion of mucoid to nonmucoid strains (15, 16,19–21). How environmental factors affect the transcription of these regulatory genes is not yet understood.

In addition to alginate, proteases produced by *P. aeruginosa* also are believed to be important in the maintenance of chronic infection. These proteases have the capacity to degrade antiprotease inhibitors, complement components, immunoglobulin A (IgA), IgG, and gamma-interferon (14,22). Degradation of antibodies and complement by these proteases results in reduced opsonization and thus protection from

phagocytosis of mucoid *P. aeruginosa* during chronic infection.

Lung damage in patients with CF chronically infected with mucoid *P. aeruginosa* is a two-fold process. First, microcolonies of the mucoid variant produce virulence factors, such as proteases, exotoxins A, and hemolysins which cause localized tissue damage and increased mucus production (14,22). This localized damage results in an inflammatory response, which is believed to play a primary role in the lung damage seen in patients with CF. Phagocytes, unable to efficiently engulf mucoid *P. aeruginosa*, release a variety of toxic molecules into the airways, including elastase, toxic oxygen metabolites, and bioactive lipids. Because the *P. aeruginosa* proteases have degraded considerable quantities of various antiprotease inhibitors in the lung, significant tissue damage can result from the release of neutrophil-derived elastase. It is the action of human neutrophil elastase that is believed to be responsible for much of the tissue destruction that occurs in the CF lung during chronic infection. The formation of immune complexes containing pseudomonal antigens may enhance the inflammatory response in the lung, further exacerbating inflammation-associated lung damage (14,22,23).

Pulmonary exacerbation in patients chronically infected with mucoid *P. aeruginosa* is clinically similar to that already described for *Staph. aureus.* During *P. aeruginosa*–associated pulmonary exacerbation, both immune complex and exoenzyme levels increase in respiratory secretions (14,23,24). Increases in these two factors is accompanied by increased inflammation, mucus production, and lung damage, as evidenced by declining pulmonary function. Organism load is frequently high during acute exacerbation, with 10^7–10^9 cfu/mL present in the patient's respiratory secretions. The large number of degrading bacterial, neutrophil, and tissue cells increase the DNA content and thus the viscosity of the already thick, tenacious secretions in the patient's airway. Increasing levels of these secretions may block or "plug" the bronchioles, adversely affecting air exchange. As a result, treatment for pulmonary exacerbation requires strategies to both clear the airways of these secretions and reduce the organism-induced inflammation (14,23). Strategies for clearance of the airway secretions are beyond the scope of this chapter and are discussed in Chapter 7. The focus in this chapter is on problems encountered when using antimicrobial therapy to reduce *P. aeruginosa* organism load in CF airways.

Response to Antimicrobial Agents

Once established, mucoid *P. aeruginosa* is almost always impossible to eradicate. Antimicrobial trials have shown that *P. aeruginosa* levels in sputum at the beginning of intravenous antimicrobial therapy may be as high as 10^9 cfu/mL of sputum. Organism count may drop to undetectable levels at the conclusion of antimicrobial therapy. Alternatively, the reduction in organism load may be more modest, perhaps 10^2- to 10^4-fold. In some patients, the organism load may remain unchanged (25). However, all three groups of patients may show clinical improvement by such measures as reduction in leukyte count and decreased cough and sputum production. In the first scenario, where the organism burden is markedly reduced, understanding the improvement in clinical well-being is intuitive. However, when the organism load is reduced only modestly reduced or not at all, it is difficult to reconcile the clinical improvement with the lack of microbiologic response. This observation has been used by some to justify a nihilistic approach to antimicrobial therapy in patients with CF or to implicate more difficult-to-detect microbes, such as anaerobes or *Legionella pneumophila* as potential causes of pulmonary exacerbation. However, antimicrobial therapy may act not only by killing microbes directly, but it also may act by inhibiting the production of pseudomonal virulence factors. Sublethal concentrations of both the aminoglycosides (gentamicin and tobramycin) and ciprofloxacin have been shown to inhibit the production of various Pseudomonas virulence factors, including the proteases (25,26). Because increasing exoenzyme levels have been associated with pulmonary exacerbation, clinical improvement in patients whose organism burden remains unchanged is likely the result of decreased virulence factor production. Declining virulence factor production should, in turn, result in reduced levels of inflammation and improving lung function.

Antimicrobial therapy slows but rarely prevents the decline in pulmonary function caused by chronic pseudomonal lung infection. After the cessation of antimicrobial therapy for acute exacerbations, organism load may return to previous levels within a matter of weeks to months. Molecular analyses of these organisms indicate that the patient usually has the same organism before and after therapy (12,27). During the time immediately following antimicrobial therapy, the patient may have a period of comparative well-being followed by another decline requiring another round of antimicrobial therapy.

Antimicrobial Resistance

Despite continuous improvements in antimicrobial therapy for *P. aeruginosa*, antimicrobial resistance continues to be a major problem. When *P. aeruginosa* is first isolated from a patient with CF it is usually susceptible to a wide array of bactericidal, antipseudomonal antimicrobials, including the antipseudomonal penicillins, piperacillin, piperacillin-tazobactam (a beta-lactamase inhibitor), ticarcillin, ticarcillin-clavulanate, mezlocillin, ceftazidime (an antipseudomonal cephalosporin), imipenem (a carbapenem), aminoglycosides, and ciprofloxacin. As patients receive multiple courses of antimicrobial therapy, resistance to one or more classes of antimicrobial may develop. It is not unusual for a adult with CF who has received many antimicrobial courses to be infected with *P. aeruginosa* isolates resistant to all available antimicrobial agents. Patients with such isolates frequently have a grim prognosis.

P. aeruginosa can develop antimicrobial resistance either by acquisition of resistance genes via gene transfer or by mutation. Molecular epidemiology studies suggest that mutation to a resistant phenotype is the most common manner by which *P. aeruginosa* develops resistance (27). Figure 5–3 is a schematic of how antimicrobial resistant clones may be selected in the airways of patients with CF, which usually evolves in the following manner. A chronic lung infection with *P. aeruginosa* is treated with antimicrobials. Constantly ongoing are bacterial mutational events. Most mutations that occur in this population either are lethal, killing the bacteria in which they occur, or are silent, causing no phenotypic change in the organism. Occasionally, a mutation, rather than being silent or lethal, will result in a *selective advantage*. Such a mutation, for example, might produce a change in a bacterium, allowing it to survive the presence of antimicrobial agent. Most other pseudomonal organisms are killed. This bacterium then will multiply and produce a "resistant clone," which may become the predominant isolate in the lung during antimicrobial therapy. Susceptible strains also may survive while protected from antimicrobials by alginate that surrounds them (28) or while they are sequestered in areas of the lung into which the antimicrobial cannot penetrate in sufficient concentration to kill them. When antimicrobial therapy is halted, two events may occur. First, if the mutation puts the resistant clone at a selective disadvantage in the absence of antimicrobials, the pseudomonal population may undergo *reversion* to a sensitive population, only to have resistant clones again selected by the next round of antimicrobial therapy (Fig. 5–3). Alternatively, the mutant-resistant clone may become part of a mixed population of sensitive and resistant isolates in the lung. As soon as antibiotic pressure is applied, *selection* of the resistant clone will proceed quickly (see Fig. 5–3). During further antimicrobial courses of therapy, this resistant clone may become the predominant pseudomonal isolate. If alternative antimicrobials are used, mutation to resistance followed by selection and expansion of a clone resistance to both the initial and alternative antimicrobial may occur. With sufficient selective pressure due to multiple treatment courses with a variety of antimicrobial agents, resistance to all these antimicrobials may eventually arise.

The mechanisms by which *P. aeruginosa* develops resistance to various antipseudomonal antimicrobials is fairly well understood (Table 5–2). Both chromosomal mutation and plasmid acquisition play a role in the expression of resistance. All *P. aeruginosa* strains possess a chromosomally encoded, inducible beta-lactamase.

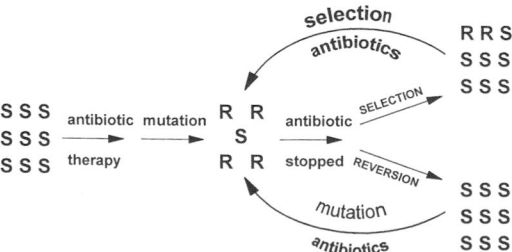

FIG. 5–3. Mechanisms for evolution of antibiotic resistance in *Pseudomonas* organisms. S represents an antibiotic susceptible *Pseudomonas* isolate. R represents an antibiotic resistant *Pseudomonas* isolate.

TABLE 5–2. *Mechanisms of resistance to antipseudomonal antimicrobials in* Pseudomonas aeruginosa

Agent	Mode of resistance acquisition	Resistance mechanism
Beta-lactams (penicillins, cephalosporins)	Chromosomal mutation	Hyperproduction of chromosomal encoded beta-lactamase (cephalosporinase)
		Modification of porin proteins
		Modification of penicillin-binding proteins
		Active efflux of drug
	Plasmid encoded	Constitutive beta-lactamase production (penicillinase)
Imipenem	Chromosomal mutation	Modification of porin proteins
		Active efflux of drug
Aminoglycosides	Chromosomal mutation	Modification of lipopolysaccharide
		Modification of ribosomal target site
	Plasmid encoded	Aminoglycoside inactivating enzymes
Ciprofloxacin	Chromosomal mutation	Modification of DNA gyrase
		Modification of porin proteins
		Active efflux of drug

This enzyme is usually produced at only low, clinically insignificant levels in the presence of an inducer. However, mutation in the beta-lactamase regulatory genes can result in high-level, constitutive production of this enzyme, which is most active against cephalosporins. Plasmid-encoded beta-lactamases are constitutively produced and have penicillinase activity. They are most active against the antipseudomonal penicillins such as piperacillin (29).

In addition to beta-lactam resistance due to beta-lactamase production, mutation can result in modification of penicillin-binding proteins, porin proteins, and overproduction of efflux proteins (30–32). Modification of penicillin-binding proteins may alter the ability of beta-lactams to bind to their target. Porin proteins are molecules in the outer membrane of gram-negative organisms that act as "gates" through which larger molecules must pass to enter the cell. Modification in these molecules result in

decreased permeability of beta-lactams and other antimicrobials into the periplasmic space.

Efflux or export proteins have recently been recognized as having an important role in the intrinsic resistance of *P. aeruginosa* (32–34). It is postulated that proteins in the cytoplasmic membrane "pump" antimicrobials out of the cytoplasm into their periplasmic space in an energy-dependent manner (32). Antimicrobials in the periplasmic space are then pumped out of the periplasmic space to outside the cell via another efflux protein located in the outer membrane. This mechanism is believed to play a role in the resistance of *P. aeruginosa* to tetracycline, chloramphenicol, quinolones, and beta-lactam antimicrobials (34–36). Mutation in regulatory genes for efflux protein synthesis leads to increased expression of these proteins and may result in increased resistance to antimicrobials of several different classes. For example, fluoroquinolone-resistant mutants also are resistant to a variety of beta-lactam antimicrobials (34). Resistance to antimicrobials with different mechanisms of actions is known as *cross-resistance*. Cross-resistance of beta-lactams and quinolones in *P. aeruginosa* has developed during monotherapy with quinolones (37).

Nikaido (38) has coined the term *pleiotropic resistance* to describe antimicrobial resistance mechanisms acting together and resulting in clinical resistance. In beta-lactam antimicrobials, beta-lactamase production, reduction in permeability of the antimicrobial, modification in penicillin-binding proteins, and activation of efflux of antimicrobials may act in concert in a variety of combinations to produce *P. aeruginosa* isolates much more resistant to beta-lactam antimicrobials than those that would be present if only one of the resistance mechanisms was operable.

Imipenem, a carbapenem antimicrobial, is not degraded by the beta-lactamase usually produced by *P. aeruginosa*. Resistance in this antimicrobial is probably pleiotropic, with decreased permeability into the cell due to modification of porin proteins (31) coupled with increased efflux from the cell. The role of modification of penicillin-binding protein in resistance to this agent has not been defined.

In a recent study of ciprofloxacin resistance following monotherapy, approximately one third of the resistance seen was due to mutation in the antimicrobial target, DNA gyrase. In the other two thirds, the resistance mechanism was not determined but modification in porin proteins coupled with active efflux of the drug from the cell would be a distinct possibility (39).

Several mechanisms of aminoglycoside resistance for *P. aeruginosa* have been recognized. Plasmids have been found in *P. aeruginosa* strains that encode several different enzymes that can inactivate these antimicrobials. However, aminoglycoside resistance in *P. aeruginosa* isolated in patients with CF is probably due to selection of resistance mutants as a result of persistent antimicrobial pressure. Resistance in this setting is caused by to either ribosomal modification or modification in lipopolysaccharide such that the antimicrobial

may no longer bind to and thus penetrate through the outer membrane of this organism.

Certain strategies are used to try to prevent the evolution of multidrug resistance. First, single agents rarely are used for the treatment of acute pulmonary exacerbations because of the risk for the rapid emergence of resistant clones. Rather, a combination of two bactericidal agents, a beta-lactam antimicrobial (penicillins, cephalosporins, or carbapenems) and an aminoglycoside (gentamicin, tobramycin, netilmicin, and amikacin) typically are used to treat CF pulmonary exacerbations. Beta-lactams inhibit cell wall synthesis, and aminoglycosides inhibit protein synthesis. The rationale for combination therapy is that mutants resistant to one antimicrobial will be killed by the other agent provided that the antimicrobials' mechanisms of action are sufficiently different so that a single mutation will not lead to resistance to both agents. In fact, mutation may occur such that both antimicrobials may become inactive. Fortunately, this cross-resistance between aminoglycosides and beta-lactams is rare. Second, the combination of beta-lactams and aminoglycosides often shows synergy, that is, the combination of two antimicrobials kill the organism much more rapidly and efficiently than would be predicted by the individual killing capacity of each individual agent.

Ciprofloxacin and beta-lactam antimicrobials are another antimicrobial combination that can be effective against *P. aeruginosa*. This combination may be particularly useful in aminoglycoside-resistant *P. aeruginosa* strains. Cross-resistance due to increased expression of export proteins may occur more frequently with this combination of antimicrobials.

The use of combinations of beta-lactams against *P. aeruginosa* should be avoided. The reason for the prohibition is that certain beta-lactams (imipenem) are potent inducers of beta-lactamase production in *P. aeruginosa*. This induction of beta-lactamase production would negate the benefit of combination therapy because most other beta-lactams would be inactivated, although imipenem is not degraded by the chromosomally encoded inducible beta-lactamase.

Another approach to treat chronic pseudomonal lung infections is to use aerosolized tobramycin. The rationale is that tobramycin, a potent antipseudomonal drug, would be highly toxic if given intravenously at doses necessary to reach sufficient endobronchial concentrations to kill *P. aeruginosa*. Aerosolized tobramycin attains much higher concentrations in the airways, without systemic toxicity, than obtained by the intravenous route. Aerosolized tobramycin may lead to better killing of these organisms. Preliminary studies suggest that the emergence of tobramycin resistance was no greater in patients receiving aerosolized tobramycin versus the control population, and that the therapy was safe and efficacious. It should be emphasized that this treatment modality is probably best used as maintenance therapy between pulmonary exacerbations rather than as primary therapy during exacerbations (40).

Oral ciprofloxacin has been recommended for intermittent therapy of pseudomonal infections. The problem with this therapy, as with any monotherapy, is that resistance can develop (see Fig. 5-3). Fortunately, once antimicrobial therapy is stopped, the organism frequently reverts to susceptibility (41).

Laboratory Detection and Susceptibility Testing

The laboratory diagnosis of *P. aeruginosa* infection in adult patients with CF is easily accomplished. Almost all adults with chronic *P. aeruginosa* infection can produce sputum. This organism can be recovered from sputum or other respiratory secretions on a variety of media, and multiple colonial morphotypes of *P. aeruginosa* are frequently observed. Molecular epidemiologic studies have shown that these different morphotypes often are of the same genotype. The important issues that confront the microbiology laboratory staff when determining the antimicrobial susceptibility of *P. aeruginosa* recovered from patients with CF is how to approach susceptibility testing when multiple morphotypes are isolated, and how frequently susceptibility testing should be performed. Testing multiple morphotypes each time a respiratory specimen is obtained for culture is an extremely laborious and expensive process. One approach to testing multiple morphotypes is to combine the different morphotypes into a single susceptibility test. The rationale here is that these organisms usually belong to the same genotype and should show the same susceptibility pattern. Unfortunately, susceptibility may vary among members of the same genotype because of differential expression of resistance mechanisms. This approach is not as efficient at detection of resistance as testing each individual morphotype (42).

The problem of testing morphotypes individually is that as many as four to six may be observed. In a hospitalized patient or a patient often seen for an exacerbation from whom respiratory secretions are frequently sent for culture and susceptibility testing, testing multiple morphotypes each time a specimen is submitted for culture can become exceedingly expensive. Resistance in *P. aeruginosa* is primarily the result of mutation and selection. This process is not a rapid one. It may require days to weeks of antimicrobial therapy for resistance to emerge. Therefore, less frequent antimicrobial testing of all morphotypes may be a cost efficient approach. Currently, our laboratory performs susceptibility testing on *P. aeruginosa* recovered from outpatients at 3-month intervals. *P. aeruginosa* isolates from inpatients are tested from the initial specimen and then only on request for the remainder of the hospital admission. Frequency of susceptibility testing is different for CF lung transplant patients in the immediate posttransplant period. These isolates are tested every third day until the patient's discharge. Postdischarge, transplant patients follow the same testing strategy as all other patients with CF.

Four other issues should be addressed when discussing susceptibility testing of *P. aeruginosa* recovered from patients with CF. First, automated susceptibility systems currently used in many clinical laboratories have not been adequately evaluated to determine their accuracy in detecting resistance in the mucoid morphotypes of *P. aeruginosa*. Disc diffusion susceptibility testing is more reliable for this organism and should be performed. Second, susceptibility test results are based on achievable serum concentration of various antimicrobials. The concentration reached in airways is frequently a fraction of that found in the bloodstream. Susceptibility results should be interpreted taking this factor into account. Third, tobramycin levels 20- to 50-fold higher than serum levels are frequently reached in the airway after aerosolization (40). Therefore, *P. aeruginosa* reported to be tobramycin resistant based on standard susceptibility testing may be susceptible to the concentration reached in the airway by aerosolization. Therefore, special susceptibility testing on "resistant" *P. aeruginosa* isolates should be performed in patients receiving aerosolized tobramycin. Some type of MIC testing at 50 μg/mL and 100 μg/mL tobramycin concentrations should be done. Fourth, combination therapy, typically a beta-lactam and an aminoglycoside, almost always is used in therapy. Standard susceptibility testing done by either disc diffusion or MIC determination may not be helpful in determining the best combination of beta-lactam and aminoglycoside to use especially if the *P. aeruginosa* isolates are resistant to multiple beta-lactams and aminoglycosides. Synergy testing where combinations of beta-lactams and aminoglycosides are tested may reveal combinations that may be more active *in vitro* than when either of the combinations is tested individually (43).

Despite aggressive antimicrobial and supportive therapies, these therapeutic modalities eventually fail and the patient succumbs to his or her chronic *P. aeruginosa* infection. Because of the observation that a subpopulation of patients with CF never develop chronic mucoid *P. aeruginosa* infection because of their ability to make opsonophagocytic antibodies to alginate (18), an alginate vaccine is under development for use in patients with CF. Preliminary studies looking at the safety and efficacy of this vaccine to elicit opsonic antibodies to this antigen in non-CF individuals are promising (44). Trials in patients with CF are needed to evaluate this novel vaccine. Other *P. aeruginosa* vaccines evaluated in patients with CF directed against several other antigens were not efficacious.

BURKHOLDERIA CEPACIA

General Characteristics

In the early 1980s, a third bacterium, *Burkholderia* (formerly *Pseudomonas*) *cepacia* was recognized at three separate CF centers as a potentially important respiratory pathogen in adults with CF (45–47). This organism, like *P. aeruginosa*, is an aerobic, gram-negative rod that is ubiquitous in nature and is found in water and soil. It was first recognized as a phytopathogen and later seen as a cause of iatrogenic and pseudoinfections associated with contaminated disinfectants and intravenous solutions (3). This organism is generally quite resistant to antimicrobials, even before exposure to repeated antimicrobial courses.

Case-controlled studies at CF centers showed that the population of patients infected with *B. cepacia* had higher morbidity (as measured by decline in pulmonary function) and mortality than controls (45,46). The patients who became infected with *B. cepacia* tended to have poorer lung function prior to infection than the control population. Interestingly, patients infected with the organism appeared to follow three very different disease courses. One group of approximately 20% of the patients infected with *B. cepacia* had what is now called the "cepacia syndrome." Once infected, these patients deteriorate rapidly, often dying in weeks to a few months. They may be bacteremic, a finding almost never seen with other organisms that chronically infect the CF lung. At autopsy, multiple abscesses could be seen. This pathologic picture is similar to that seen with melioidosis, a pulmonary disease caused by the closely related organism, *Burkholderia pseudomallei* (48). The second group of patients did not have as dramatic a disease course, but rather had a continuing decline in their lung function eventually resulting in death. Because many of these patients were concurrently infected with *P. aeruginosa*, the contribution of *B. cepacia* to their continuing decline is not clear (46). The third group of patients, many of whom are infected in childhood, may carry the organism for extended periods of time with apparently no adverse outcome. The seeming arbitrariness of the type of disease course seen with *B. cepacia* where some patients rapidly deteriorate and die while others are apparently unaffected has led to great concern about this organism in the CF community. Much of this concern is due to lack of understanding of both the epidemiology and virulence of this organism. Recent studies have shed considerable light in both of these areas.

Epidemiology

Soon after the recognition that *B. cepacia* was a threat to the CF population, some CF centers began to cohort their patients who were infected with this organism. This was done because of concern that this organism was spread from person to person. This supposition was supported by two observations. First, sibling pairs frequently were infected. Second, this organism was rarely found in the patients' environment, making common source outbreaks less likely (49). Cohorting as a policy appeared to be successful as incidence of *B. cepacia* declined in centers where this policy was implemented (46), but the question of person-to-person spread had not been resolved. The answer to this question awaited the development of highly discriminatory, reliable, and reproducible epidemiologic typing systems.

Over the past few years, two genotyping systems, ribotyping and pulse field gel electrophoresis (PFGE), have been applied to the study of *B. cepacia* molecular epidemiology (50–52). Using these techniques, it was learned that the epidemiology of this organism was complex. In one CF center, there was a highly transmissible strain of *B. cepacia* that had spread transcontinentally from Canada to the United Kingdom (52,53). Transmission was believed to occur when patients from a Canadian center where the highly transmissible strain was being disseminated attended a CF summer camp with individuals from the United Kingdom. An individual from the United Kingdom became infected and carried this organism back to a UK CF center where other patients were infected and several developed the "cepacia syndrome" and died. This highly transmissible strain subsequently was spread to other UK centers (54,55). Other studies indicate that this same strain spread to another CF center in Canada (56). However, not all *B. cepacia* strains are highly transmissible. In one center, several patients with CF infected with *B. cepacia* were found to have genetically unique strains suggesting that cross infection had not occurred and that these patients most likely obtained their organism from the environment (51).

The recognition that *B. cepacia* is transmissible has led the CF community to institute strong measures to stop its spread, including the withdrawal of support by the US Cystic Fibrosis Foundation for summer camp programs for patients with CF (57); the cohorting at some CF centers of all patients with CF who are *B. cepacia* positive patients with CF from noninfected patients with CF; and at some centers, the exclusion of these individuals as lung transplant candidates (58). Because the CF community is socially tight-knit, these exclusionary practices have been psychologically devastating to some *B. cepacia*-infected patients who may be counseled not to socialize with their friends. This becomes particularly problematic in relationships between individuals with CF where only one of the couple is infected, and in households with CF siblings where only one of the individuals is infected. These problems highlight the need for greater understanding of the exact mode of transmission of this organism from person to person, the pathogenesis of this organism, and the importance of accurately distinguishing *B. cepacia* from *B. gladioli* and *B. pickettii*; organisms closely related biochemically but not as pathogenic as *B. cepacia* (48,59).

Pathogenesis

The pathogenesis of *B. cepacia* is poorly understood, especially the difference between infection in patients who have a rapidly fatal course and those whose infection is less aggressive. Unlike *P. aeruginosa*, *B. cepacia* is relatively avirulent in animal models of chronic lung infection, although a recent study in a CF mouse model suggests that this organism may cause pneumonia in these genetically altered animals. These data should be interpreted with caution because high inoculum was needed to induce infection and organism burdens were very low (60). The organism produces both protease and lipase. The protease that is related immunologically to *P. aeruginosa* elastase can cause bronchopneumonia when purified enzyme is instilled directly into rat lungs (61). Purified lipase at very high concentration (2.5 to 20 μg/mL) inhibits rat alveolar macrophage function (62). However, it is doubtful that such high lipase levels would be reached in the human lung. Whether this enzyme can cause dysfunction of lung surfactant in patients with CF has not been investigated.

Recent studies have greatly increased our understanding of factors involved in the adherence of *B. cepacia*. Differences in the adherence may explain the transmissibility of certain strains of *B. cepacia*. All CF *B. cepacia* isolates examined to date possess two different pili. All strains of *B. cepacia* isolates from patients with CF express a mesh pili (53,63). The role of mesh pili in adherence is not clear, but mesh pili form a mat linking other *B. cepacia* bacteria, which may explain why colonies of this organism recovered from patients with CF adhere to the surface of agar plates. It may also form groups of bacteria similar to the microcolonies seen with mucoid *P. aeruginosa*.

A second pilus has been found on the surface of epidemic strains of *B. cepacia*. This pilus is called a cable pilus (52,53,63). This pilus is unusually long (2 to 4 μm) and has a braided, cable-like appearance. It is found embedded in the mat formed by the mesh-like pili and can become entangled with cable-like pili from other bacteria, again forming a microcolony type structure. An adhesive subunit is dispersed at intervals along the surface of the cable pilus rather than being found just at the tip of the pilus. This type of structure is believed to enhance its binding to mucus in the CF airway. Cable pili have been found only on organisms from two CF centers that had epidemic spread of these organisms among their patients with CF (52). It is believed that the transmissibility of these strains is due to the presence of cable pili on their cell surface.

Other CF *B. cepacia* isolates not associated with the epidemic strain possess a second pilus different from the cable pilus. This pilus has been designated as a filamentous pilus. It, too, is embedded in the mesh pili mat. Its function in adherence has not been determined (53,63).

These observations begin to explain differences in transmissibility of *B. cepacia*. Strains possessing cable pili appear to be transmissible while strains without cable pili may be less transmissable or nontransmissible. Whether strains with cable pili are more virulent remains to be determined. Molecular techniques that would allow the detection of strains with cable pili might allow a more rational and kind approach to patient segregation based on the real threat of transmission of this organism rather than an assumed one.

Antimicrobial Resistance

Like *P. aeruginosa*, *B. cepacia* is impossible to eradicate with antimicrobial therapy once chronic infection has been established (2). This organism is even more resistant to antimicrobials than *P. aeruginosa*. When first recovered, the organisms may be sensitive to anti-pseudomonal beta-lactam antimicrobials, including ceftazidime, piperacillin, and imipenem, in addition to trimethoprim/sulfamethoxazole, and chloramphenicol. The organism is resistant to all aminoglycosides, a mainstay of anti-*P. aeruginosa* therapy, with MIC values greater than 500 μg/mL making even aerosolized aminoglycosides of little value. The organism is also resistant to ciprofloxacin and colistin (another agent aerosolized to control multidrug-resistant *P. aeruginosa*). Once exposed to an antimicrobial, the organism quickly develops resistance, probably because of modification in the outer cell envelope such that antimicrobials can no longer enter the bacterium. As a result, it is not unusual to find isolates that are resistant to all available antimicrobials.

Studies have shown that patients with *B. cepacia*-associated pulmonary exacerbation, like those with *P. aeruginosa*, may show clinical benefit from combinations of beta-lactams and aminoglycosides. Unlike *P. aeruginosa*, beta-lactams and aminoglycosides do not show synergistic antimicrobial activity against *B. cepacia*. Aminoglycoside MIC levels suggest that *B. cepacia* does not penetrate into the bacterium, making it highly unlikely that the benefit of this therapy is due to suppression of the synthesis of virulence factors. Because the study that claimed a benefit of the beta-lactam and aminoglycoside combination for *B. cepacia* exacerbation was small and had several confounding factors, these data should be interpreted with caution (64). However, the reality is that there often are no alternative therapeutic choices to manage this multidrug-resistant organism.

There is one unconventional approach to the treatment of *B. cepacia* that may prove to be useful. *In vitro* studies have shown that the combination of amiloride and tobramycin is active against *B. cepacia* at concentrations achievable in the airways by aerosolization of both agents (65). This therapeutic approach has not been systematically studied.

Laboratory Isolation and Identification

One of the most demanding aspects of the laboratory diagnosis of bacterial lung infection in patients with CF is the isolation and identification of *B. cepacia*. The isolation of *B. cepacia* is complicated in two ways. First, the organism is somewhat slow growing, requiring 48 to 72 hours of incubation before colonies are visible. Second, other organisms are usually abundant in respiratory secretions of patients with CF. In particular, mucoid *P. aeruginosa*, when present in the respiratory secretions of patients coinfected with *B. cepacia*, will frequently obscure the growth of *B. cepacia*, making its recovery extremely difficult.

To ensure consistent and accurate recovery of *B. cepacia*, two selective media, PC and OFPBL agar have been developed (66,67). In a survey sponsored by the U.S. Cystic Fybrosis Foundation to assess the capability of laboratories to recover *B. cepacia* from mock sputum specimens, 14 of 15 laboratories (93%) using these two special media were able to recover this organism, whereas only 22 of 100 laboratories could recover it using other types of selective media. Of these 100 laboratories, 75 agreed to repeat the survey using one of the *B. cepacia*–selective media. On retesting, 73 (97%) laboratories were successful at isolating this organism (68). Other studies have confirmed that these two media are reliable for the recovery of *B. cepacia* (66,67).

These media also allow the growth of two other closely related *Burkholderia* sp., *B. gladioli*, and *B. pickettii*. *B. gladioli* is particularly problematic on OFPBL because it can produce a bright yellow pigment (59). This pigment production can be confused with lactose oxidation, a trait used to separate *B. cepacia* from other organisms on this medium. Differentiation of these three organisms by biochemical means can be very difficult, especially when *B. cepacia* strains are either lactose oxidation or lysine decarboxylase negative, two biochemical traits that reliably differentiate *B. cepacia* from these other two organisms (48). Many laboratories use commercial systems to identify *B. cepacia*. These systems lack accuracy because they may incorrectly identify *B. cepacia* as an organism other than *B. cepacia*. In addition, they may identify both *B. pickettii* and *B. gladioli* as *B. cepacia* (69). Because of this, laboratories using commercial systems should confirm the identity of all isolates designated as belonging to the genus *Burkholderia* by submitting the isolates to reference laboratories for confirmation in view of the social and medical consequences for a patient identified as being *B. cepacia* positive.

Because of the difficulties encountered with phenotypic characterization of *Burkholderia* sp., molecular methods have been developed for detection of *B. cepacia* (70,71). Using sophisticated bacterial cell protein analysis and DNA–DNA hybridization, *B. cepacia* can be divided into four different genetic groups called *genomovars* (71). One of these, designated genomovar III, has been associated with the cepacia syndrome and includes the highly transmissible strain of *B. cepacia* that has been spread from North America to Europe (52). The other genomovars appear to be less likely to cause the cepacia syndrome, but the numbers of isolates analyzed in this manner are small. However, these data suggest a difference in virulence among different strains of *B. cepacia*. The current means of identifying genomovar III organisms is only available in the research laboratory. Simpler molecular techniques such as polymerase chain reaction (PCR) will need to be developed to differentiate *B. cepacia* into its different genomovars before large-scale epidemiologic studies can be done to determine whether there are specific virulent and nonvirulent genomovars.

Susceptibility testing of *B. cepacia* is typically done by disc-diffusion, although microbroth MIC determination may also work. Because of its slow growth, susceptibility plates may require incubation for as long as 48 hours before zones of inhibition are visible. Automated susceptibility systems are not accurate in determining antimicrobial susceptibility for these slow growing organisms and should not be used.

One final issue concerning *B. cepacia* that should be addressed is the problem of this organism in candidates for lung transplantation. In many lung transplant centers, infection with *B. cepacia* is a reason for exclusion from the transplant list. The rationale for this is based on two observations. First, the isolates are frequently resistant to all known antimicrobials. Because the transplanted lung will frequently become infected with the same organism that was in the recipient's original lung (51), there will be no antimicrobial that might be effective especially if the patient becomes bacteremic. Second, experience at one CF center that transplanted *B. cepacia* infected patients was abysmal (72). Fifteen patients were infected with *B. cepacia* posttransplant, 5 of whom were nosocomially infected. Seven died within a year of transplant (4 within a month) of *B. cepacia* pneumonia. These patients were trans-

planted at the Canadian center known to have patients infected with the highly transmissible strain of *B. cepacia* belonging to genomovar III. However, the strains from the transplant patients have not been available for study. This abysmal experience is in contrast to the experience at two other centers. In one, two of eight patients infected with *B. cepacia* died soon after transplant because of *B. cepacia* pneumonia and bacteremia. Other patients have done well and several are free of *B. cepacia* infection (73). In another larger series, 3 of 14 patients with *B. cepacia* died of infection within 2 weeks of transplantation. Otherwise, posttransplant survival was the same for patients with *B. cepacia* versus those infected with *P. aeruginosa* (58). These data support the idea that there may be differences in virulence among *B. cepacia* strains. Until virulent *B. cepacia* can be distinguished from seemingly nonvirulent strains of *B. cepacia* by determining genomovars or by detecting virulence markers, individual centers will need to decide their policy concerning transplantation of *B. cepacia* positive patients.

Other *Burkholderia* sp.

Two species of *Burkholderia* that are genetically similar to *B. cepacia* are *B. pickettii* and *B. gladioli*. There are no data available that suggest that *B. pickettii* plays any role in pulmonary deterioration in patients with CF. The initial report on the recovery of *B. gladioli* from the respiratory secretions of patients with CF suggested that this organism was nonpathogenic (59). Subsequent reports suggest (74,75) that *B. gladioli* can cause pulmonary exacerbation and even death in patients with CF. These data should be viewed cautiously, however, because of the problems in actually identifying *B. gladioli* and the lack of supporting animal model data. Further study is required to determine the role of *B. gladioli* in CF lung disease.

Mycobacterium sp.

Mycobacterium tuberculosis is rarely recovered from the lungs of patients with CF and as such is not considered an important pathogen in these patients. The situation is less clear with the nontuberculous mycobacteria. The U.S. Cystic Fibrosis Foundation reported that in 1993, 0.4% of adults with CF were infected/colonized with nontuberculous mycobacteria (NTM). This is almost surely an underestimation because of the difficulty of recovering NTM from CF respiratory secretions because of overgrowth of mycobacterial cultures by mucoid *P. aeruginosa* (76). When mycobacterial culture techniques are used that suppress *P. aeruginosa* growth, colonization/infection rates of as high as 20% have been reported (77). The organisms recovered are primarily *Mycobacterium avium* complex (MAC) with a small number of *Mycobacterium fortuitum* and *Mycobacterium abscessus* isolates.

A multicenter study sponsored by the U.S. Cystic Fibrosis Foundation is currently being done to answer questions concerning the role of NTM in CF lung disease (78). Preliminary data on 745 patients show that 94 (13%) are colonized/infected with NTM (79). The case control portion of the study, now under way, should give more information on the pathogenic role of these organisms in lung disease in patients with CF. Currently, it is very difficult to determine whether if these organisms are nothing more than harmless saprophytes or whether they are playing an active role in these patient's lung disease. At least in some patients, these organisms do appear to have a pathogenic role, and patients may benefit from aggressive antimycobacterial therapy (77). In addition, some centers exclude patients infected/colonized with NTM as transplant candidates because of the difficulty in treating infections with these multidrug-resistant organisms. Until further data are obtained, the role of NTM in the lung disease of patients with CF will remain unclear.

Other Bacteria

Stenotrophomonas (formerly *Xanthomonas*) *maltophilia* and *Alcaligenes xylosoxidans* are glucose nonfermenting gram negative rods whose natural habitat is water and soil (80). Both are well recognized as causes of nosocomial pneumonia in intubated patients. They are being seen with increasing frequency in adults with CF, especially patients who have received repeated courses of antimicrobials. *S. maltophilia* is highly resistant to most antimicrobials. It produces a beta-lactamase that degrades imipenem resulting in uniform resistance to this agent. In the intensive care unit setting, *S. maltophilia* is selected for by imipenem use. In a series of 16 patients with CF with *S. maltophilia*, aerosolized antimicrobial therapy rather than imipenem use was associated with colonization/infection (81). When first isolated from patients with CF, its antimicrobial sensitivity is quite similar to that seen with *B. cepacia*, except that *S. maltophilia* may also be sensitive to ticarcillin/clavulanate and minocycline, to which *B. cepacia* will usually be resistant. When susceptible, a combination of minocycline, trimethoprim/sulfamethoxazole and ticarcillin/clavulanate has been suggested for use with immunocompromised patients (82). The effectiveness of this combination in patients with CF with *S. maltophilia* infection is not known. Like *B. cepacia*, *S. maltophilia* can quickly develop resistance and it, too, can become resistant to all available antimicrobial agents. Unlike *B. cepacia*, *S. maltophilia* appears to be relatively avirulent in patients with CF (83). Which role, if any, *S. maltophilia* and *A. xylosoxidans* play in CF lung disease is currently unknown.

Haemophilus influenzae has been recognized as an important pathogen in the early stages of chronic lung infection in patients with CF. Using quantitative culture techniques and a selective medium, it was found in the sputum of 30% of adult patients in one series (84). However, many of these patients also were infected with *P. aeruginosa* making it difficult to determine which role, if any, *H. influenzae* has in pulmonary exacerbations in adults. It responds well to oral antimicrobial agents, such as augmentin, cefuroxime, ciprofloxacin, or doxycycline (85). Many strains produce beta-lactamases that inactivate amoxicillin and piperacillin. Such strains are easily detected in the laboratory by beta-lactamase testing, which should be done routinely on all *H. influenzae* isolates.

Bronchoscopically obtained specimens are optimal for the detection of anaerobes in the lung. Sputum specimens are of no value in anaerobic organism detection because they can be heavily contaminated as they pass through the oropharynx by the resident anaerobic flora. Bronchoscopy is rarely done in patients with CF, except in lung transplant recipients. At least in this selected population, anaerobes have not been reported to play a role in respiratory infection, but whether these specimens are routinely and appropriately cultured for anaerobic bacteria is not clear. It must be emphasized that these lungs are genetically non-CF tissue, so this population—which is also heavily immunosuppressed—is not reflective of the general CF population. Anaerobic culture of thoracotomy obtained CF lung tissue showed that a small percentage of patients had anaerobes present (3). However, these patients had *P. aeruginosa* present as well, suggesting a minor or no role for anaerobes in CF lung disease.

Legionella pneumophila has also been implicated in pulmonary exacerbation in patients with CF. This observation was based on serologic survey data (3). Subsequently, it was shown that *P. aeruginosa* shared common antigens with *L. pneumophila,* indicating that this serologic response could be due to cross-reactions with *P. aeruginosa*. These data call into doubt the role of *L. pneumophila* in CF lung disease. Recently, a urine antigen detection test has been developed which is both highly sensitive and specific for *L. pneumophila* serogroup 1, the most commonly isolated *Legionella* species. This test may be useful in the diagnosis of legionella in patients with CF if in fact this organism has a role in CF lung disease.

Fungi

Aspergillus sp., especially *Aspergillus fumigatus* is frequently cultured from respiratory secretions of adults with CF. Although the most serious manifestation of *Aspergillus* infection, invasive disease, is rare in patients with CF, allergic bronchopulmonary aspergillosis (ABPA) may occur in as many as 5% to 15% of adult patients with CF (86).

A. fumigatus is the species of *Aspergillus* most frequently associated with ABPA. However, the finding of this organism in sputum and the presence of IgE, IgA, IgG antiaspergillus antibody can occur in patients with CF without ABPA. Diagnosis of ABPA is made on the basis of both clinical and laboratory criteria. These criteria include the presence of asthma, pulmonary infiltrates, central bronchiectasis, positive immediate skin reactivity to *A. fumigatus*, peripheral blood eosinophilia, serum IgE levels of greater than 1,000 µg/mL, and elevated serum IgE and IgG levels of anti-*A. fumigatus* antibodies. This disease is controlled by corticosteroid therapy. Antifungal therapy has not been shown to be effective (86).

In one study, *Aspergillus* sp. have been reported to be present in a high proportion of pretransplant sputa of lung transplant recipients (73). In this group of patients, no invasive aspergillus infections were reported posttransplant. Other transplant centers have reported invasive aspergillosis after lung transplantation, with high mortality (87,88). Whether patients with CF colonized with *Aspergillus* sp. should be transplanted is currently controversial.

Candida sp. can frequently be found in the sputum of adults with CF . This is not surprising since these patients have received multiple antimicrobial courses, a factor that is well known to result in oropharyngeal colonization with this organism. There are no data that indicate that *Candida* sp. play a role in CF lung disease. *Candida* bacteremia has been reported in patients with CF in association with implantable, intravascular devices (89). This problem may become more frequent with increasing use of home intravenous antimicrobial therapy and nutritional support.

Pneumocystis carinii has recently been reclassified as a fungi. This organism is only of concern in CF lung transplant recipients because of their immunosuppression. These patients typically receive lifetime pneumocystis prophylaxis posttransplant. As a result, this organism has not been a problem in this group of patients (73,87,88). Other than transplant recipients, this organism is not of concern in adults with CF who typically are immunocompetent.

Viruses

The study of viral infections in adults with CF is hampered by a lack of nonculture techniques adequate for detecting viruses in respiratory secretions. Consequently, little information is available on the role of respiratory viruses in adult CF lung disease. Case reports have shown that influenza A virus can be associated with severe pulmonary deterioration in adults with CF (90). These data emphasize the importance of influenza vaccination for this patient population. A rapid enzyme immunoabsorbent assay is now commercially available for the direct detection of influenza A virus. This test may be of value in determining the role of this virus in adult CF pulmonary exacerbation. Determination of the role of other respiratory viruses in this disease process awaits the development of rapid, accurate detection methods.

As with all transplant recipients, cytomegalovirus (CMV) is an important cause of post-transplant infection in CF lung transplant recipients. The ideal situation is to match donors and recipients on the basis of their CMV serostatus. This is important because seronegative recipients who receive lungs from seropositive donors are much more likely to develop severe CMV disease than matched donors and recipients (91). However, this is not always possible because of the scarcity of lung donors. As a result, seronegative patients receiving seropositive lungs receive prophylactic ganciclovir and hyperimmune CMV globulin (73,87,88). Nevertheless, rates of CMV pneumonia in these patients are high. In one series, 27 of 44 patients had 44 courses of CMV disease. Only three were judged to have serious CMV pneumonia, one of whom died (73).

CONCLUSION

Chronic lung infection remains the most important cause of early death in patients with CF. Although the organisms responsible for much of the lung damage in these patients, *Staph. aureus*, *P. aeruginosa*, and *B. cepacia*,

are well known, strategies have not yet been developed to eliminate these organisms from CF airways. Antimicrobial therapy has contributed to an impressive extension in life span in patients with CF. However, antimicrobial resistance continues to be a major problem with *P. aeruginosa* and *B. cepacia* and may be emerging as an important problem in *Staph. aureus*. Alternate therapies are needed that focus on the cellular defect seen in CF airways. Pharmacologic approaches to reverse the defect at the epithelial cell surface are in their infancy. Vaccines targeted at the alginate virulence factor of *P. aeruginosa* appear promising but require extensive clinical evaluation in the CF population. Lung replacement via transplant is currently an extraordinarily expensive therapy available to only a fraction of those who might benefit. The great promise of gene therapy appears years from fruition.

As patients with CF live longer in part because of improving new antimicrobial and adjunct therapies, new organisms are emerging as potential threats. NTM and *S. maltophilia* are highly resistant to antimicrobial therapy. They also appear to be of low virulence, but case control studies are not yet available to confirm this impression. Our understanding of the contribution of viral agents in CF pulmonary exacerbation is minimal, although it is clear that CMV is an important pathogen in CF lung transplant recipients.

Until therapies are developed that reverse the basic cellular defect, patients with CF will continue to die much too soon from the ravages of chronic lung infection.

REFERENCES

1. Fitzsimmons SC. The changing epidemiology of cystic fibrosis. *J Pediatr* 1993;122(1):1–9.
2. Knowles MR, Gilligan PH, Boucher RC. Cystic fibrosis. In: Mandell GL, et al, ed. *Principles and practices of infectious disease.* New York: Churchill Livingstone, 1995.
3. Gilligan PH. Microbiology of airway disease in patients with cystic fibrosis. *Clin Microbiol Rev* 1991;4(1):35–51.
4. Marks MI. Clinical significance of *Staphylococcus aureus* in cystic fibrosis. *Infection* 1990;18(1):53–56.
5. Rollof J, Branconier JH, Soderstrom C, et al. Interference of *Staphylococcus aureus* lipase with human

granulocyte function. *Eur J Clin Microbiol Infect Dis* 1988;7(4):505–510.

6. Schwab UE, Wold AE, Carson JH, et al. Increased adherence of *Staphylococcus aureus* from cystic fibrosis lungs to airway epithelial cells. *Am Rev Respir Dis* 1993;148(2):365–369.

7. Gilligan P, Jordan M, Wait K, et al. Oxacillin resistant *Staphylococcus aureus* in patients with cystic fibrosis. *Pediatr Pulmonol Suppl* 1996;13:297.

8. Branger C, Gardye C, Lambert-Zechovsky N. Persistence of *Staphylococcus aureus* strains among cystic fibrosis patients over extended periods of time. *J Med Microbiol* 1996;45(3):294–301.

9. Gilligan PH, Gage PA, Welch DF, et al. Prevalence of thymidine-dependent *Staphylococcus aureus* in patients with cystic fibrosis. *J Clin Microbiol* 1987;25(7):1258–1261.

10. Boukadida J, De Montalembert M, Lenoir G, et al. Molecular epidemiology of chronic pulmonary colonization by *Pseudomonas aeruginosa* in cystic fibrosis. *J Med Microbiol* 1993;38(1):29–33.

11. Romling U, Feidler B, Bosshammer J, et al. Epidemiology of chronic *Pseudomonas aeruginosa* infections in cystic fibrosis. *J Infect Dis* 1994;170(6):1616–1621.

12. Struelens MJ, Schwam V, DePlano A, et al. Genome macrorestriction analysis of diversity and variability of *Pseudomonas aeruginosa* strains infecting cystic fibrosis patients. *J Clin Microbiol* 1993;31(9):2320–2326.

13. Mahenthiralingam E, Campbell ME, Speert DP. Non motility and phagocytic resistance of *Pseudomonas aeruginosa* isolates from chronically colonized patients with cystic fibrosis. *Infect Immunol* 1994;62(2):596–605.

14. Fick RB Jr., Sonoda F, Hornick DB. Emergence and persistence of *Pseudomonas aeruginosa* in the cystic fibrosis airway. *Semin Respir Infect* 1992;7(3):168–178.

15. May TB, Charkrabarty AM. *Pseudomonas aeruginosa*: genes and enzymes of alginate synthesis. *Trends Microbiol* 1994;2(5):151–157.

16. Deretic V, Schurr MJ, Boucher JC, et al. Conversion of *Pseudomonas aeruginosa* to mucoidy in cystic fibrosis: environmental stress and regulation of bacterial virulence by alternative sigma factors. *J Bacteriol* 1994;176(10):2773–2780.

17. Lam J, Chan R, Lam K, et al. Production of mucoid microcolonies by *Pseudomonas aeruginosa* within infected lungs in cystic fibrosis. *Infect Immunol* 1980; 28(2):546–556.

18. Pier GB, Saunders JM, Ames P, et al. Opsonophagocytic killing antibody of *Pseudomonas aeruginosa* mucoid exopolysaccharide in older non-colonized patients with cystic fibrosis. *N Engl J Med* 1987;317 (13):793–798.

19. Martin DW, Schurr MJ, Yu H, et al. Analysis of promoters controlled by the putative sigma factor AlgU regulating conversion to mucoidy in *Pseudomonas aeruginosa*: relationship to sigma E and stress response. *J Bacteriol* 1994;176(21):6688–6696.

20. Schurr MJ, Martin DW, Mudd MH, et al. Gene cluster controlling conversion to alginate-overproducing phenotype in *Pseudomonas aeruginosa*: functional analysis in a heterologous host and role in the instability of mucoidy. *J Bacteriol* 1994;176(11):3375–3382.

21. Xie ZH, Hershberger CD, Shankar S, et al. Sigma factor-anti-sigma factor interaction in alginate synthesis: inhibition of AlgT by MucA. *J Bacteriol* 1996;178 (16):4990–4996.

22. Suter S. The role of bacterial proteases in the pathogenesis of cystic fibrosis. *Am J Respir Crit Care Med* 1994;150(6, Part 2):S118–S122.

23. Moss RB. Cystic fibrosis: pathogenesis, pulmonary infection, and treatment. *Clin Infect Dis* 1995;21(4): 839–851.

24. Grimwood K, Semple RA, Rabin HR, et al. Elevated exoenzyme expression by *Pseudomonas aeruginosa* is correlated with exacerbations of lung disease in cystic fibrosis. *Pediatr Pulmonol* 1993;15(3):135–139.

25. Grimwood K, To M, Rabin HR, et al. Inhibition of *Pseudomonas aeruginosa* exoenzyme expression by subinhibitory antibiotic concentrations. *Antimicrob Agents Chemother* 1989;33(1):41–47.

26. Grimwood K, To M, Rabin HR, et al. Subinhibitory antibiotics reduce *Pseudomonas aeruginosa* tissue injury in the rat lung model. *J Antimicrob Chermother* 1989;24(6):937–945.

27. Bingen E, Denamur E, Picard B et al. Molecular epidemiological analysis of *Pseudomonas aeruginosa* strains causing failure of antibiotic therapy in cystic fibrosis patients. *Eur J Clin Microbiol Infect Dis* 1992;11(5):432–437.

28. Anwar H, Strap JL, Costerton JW. Establishment of aging biofilms: possible mechanism of bacterial resistance to antimicrobial therapy. *Antimicrob Agents Chemother* 1992;36(7):1347–1351.

29. Zabner R, Quinn JP. Antimicrobials in cystic fibrosis: emergence of resistance and implications for treatment. *Semin Respir Infect* 1992;7(3):210–217.

30. Godfrey AJ, Bryan LE, Rabin HR. Beta-lactam-resistant *Pseudomonas aeruginosa* with modified penicillin-binding proteins emerging during cystic fibrosis treatment. *Antimicrob Agents Chemother* 1981;19(5): 705–711.

31. Yoneyama H, Nakae T. Mechanism of efficient elimination of protein D2 in outer membrane of imipenem-resistant *Pseudomonas aeruginosa*. *Antimicrob Agents Chemother* 1993;37(11):2385–2390.

32. Nikaido H. Prevention of drug access to bacterial targets: permeability barriers and active efflux. *Science* 1994;264(5157):382–388.

33. Poole K, Krebes K, McNally C, et al. Multiple antibiotic resistance in *Pseudomonas aeruginosa:* evidence for involvement of an efflux operon. *J Bacteriol* 1993;175(22):7363–7372.

34. Masuda N, Sakagawa E, Ohya S. Outer membrane proteins responsible for multiple drug resistance in *Pseudomonas aeruginosa*. *Antimicrob Agents Chemother* 1995;39(3):645–649.

35. Li X-Z, Ma D, Livermore DM et al. Role of efflux pump(s) in intrinsic resistance of *Pseudomonas aeruginosa*: active efflux as a contributing factor to beta-lactam resistance. *Antimicrob Agents Chemother* 1994;38(8):1742–1752.

36. Li X-Z, Livermore DM, Nikaido H. Role of efflux pump(s) in intrinsic resistance of *Pseudomonas aeruginosa:* resistance to tetracycline, chloramphenicol, and norfloxacin. *Antimicrob Agents Chemother* 1994;38 (8):1732–1741.

37. Aubert G, Pozzetto B, Dorche G. Emergence of quinolone-imipenem cross-resistance in *Pseudomonas aeruginosa* after fluoroquinolone therapy. *J Antimicrob Chemother* 1992;29(3):307–312.

38. Nikaido H. Outer membrane barrier as a mechanism of antimicrobial resistance. *Antimicrob Agents Chemother* 1989;33(11):1831–1836.

39. Kureishi A, Diver JM, Beckthold B, et al. Cloning and nucleotide sequence of *Pseudomonas aeruginosa* DNA gyrase gyrA gene from strain PA01 and quinolone-resistant clinical isolates. *Antimicrob Agents Chemother* 1994;38(9):1944–1952.

40. Ramsey BW, Dorkin HL, Eisenberg JD, et al. Efficacy of aerosolized tobramycin in patients with cystic fibrosis. *N Engl J Med* 1993;328(24):1740–1746.

41. Diver JM, Schollaardt T, Rabin HR, et al. Persistence mechanisms in *Pseudomonas aeruginosa* from cystic fibrosis patients undergoing ciprofloxacin therapy. *Antimicrob Agents Chemother* 1991;35(8):1538–1546.

42. Morlin GL, Hedges DL, Smith AL, et al. Accuracy and cost of antibiotic susceptibility testing of mixed morphotypes of *Pseudomonas aeruginosa*. *J Clin Microbiol* 1994;32(4):1027–1030.

43. Weiss K, LaPointe JR. Routine susceptibility testing of four antibiotic combinations for improvement of laboratory guide to therapy of cystic fibrosis infections caused by *Pseudomonas aeruginosa*. *Antimicrob Agents Chemother* 1995;39(11):2411–2414.

44. Pier GB, DesJardin D, Grout M, et al. Human immune response to *Pseudomonas aeruginosa* mucoid exopolysaccharide (alginate) vaccine. *Infect Immunol* 1994;62(9):3972–3979.

45. Tablan OC, Chorba TL, Schidlow DV, et al. *Pseudomonas cepacia* colonization in patients with cystic fibrosis: risk factors and clinical outcome. *J Pediatr* 1985;107(3):382–387.

46. Lewin LO, Byard PJ, Davis PB. Effect of *Pseudomonas cepacia* colonization on survival and pulmonary function of cystic fibrosis patients. *J Clin Epidemiol* 1990;43(2):125–131.

47. Isles A, Maclusky I, Corey M, et al. *Pseudomonas cepacia* infection in cystic fibrosis: an emerging problem. J Pediatr 1984;104(2):206–210.

48. Gilligan PH. *Pseudomonas* and *Burkholderia*. In: Murray PR, Baron EJ, Pfaller MA, et al., eds.: *Manual of Clinical Microbiology*. 6th ed. Washington, DC: ASM Press, 1995.

49. Hardy KA, McGowan KL, Fisher MC, et al. *Pseudomonas cepacia* in the hospital setting: lack of transmission between cystic fibrosis patients. *J Pediatr* 1986;109(1):51–54.

50. Fisher MC, LiPuma JJ, Dasen SE, et al. Source of *Pseudomonas cepacia*: ribotyping of isolates from patients and from the environment. *J Pediatr* 1993; 123(5):745–747.

51. Steinbach S, Sun L, Jiang R-Z, et al. Transmissibility of *Pseudomonas cepacia* infection in clinic patients and lung transplant recipients with cystic fibrosis. *N Engl J Med* 1994;331(15):981–987.

52. Sun L, Jiang R-Z, Steinbach S. et al. The emergence of a highly transmissible lineage of Cbl+ *Pseudomonas (Burkholderia) cepacia* causing CF centre epidemics in North America and Britain. *Nature Med* 1995;7(7): 661–666.

53. Goldstein R, Sun L, Jiang R-Z, et al. Structurally variant classes of pilus appendage fibers co-expressed from *Burkholderia (Pseudomonas) cepacia*. *J Bacteriol* 1995;177(4):1039–1052.

54. Govan JRW, Brown PH, Maddison J, et al. Evidence for transmission of *Pseudomonas cepacia* by social contact. *Lancet* 1993;342(8862):15–19.

55. Pitt TL, Kaufmann ME, Patel PS, et al. Type characterisation and antibiotic susceptibility of *Burkholderia (Pseudomonas) cepacia* isolates from patients with cystic fibrosis in the United Kingdom and the Republic of Ireland. *J Med Microbiol* 1996;44(2): 203–210.

56. Johnson WM, Tyler SD, Rozee KR. Linkage analysis of geographic and clinical clusters in *Pseudomonas cepacia* infections by multilocus enzyme electrophoresis and ribotyping. *J Clin Microbiol* 1994;32 (4):924–930.

57. Pegues DA, Carson LA, Tablan OC, et al. Acquisition of *Pseudomonas cepacia* at summer camps for patients with cystic fibrosis. *J Pediatr* 1994;124(5, Part 1):694–702.

58. Egan JJ, McNeil K, Bookless B, et al. Post-transplantation survival of cystic fibrosis patients infected with *Pseudomonas cepacia*. *Lancet* 1994;344(8921):552–553.

59. Christenson JC, Welch DF, Mukwaya G et al. Recovery of *Pseudomonas gladioli* from respiratory tract specimens of patients with cystic fibrosis. *J Clin Microbiol* 1989;27(2):270–273.

60. Davidson DJ, Dorin JR, McLachlan G, et al. Lung disease in the cystic fibrosis mouse exposed to bacterial pathogens. *Nature Genet* 1995;9(4):351–357.

61. Kooi C, Cox A, Darling P, et al. Neutralizing monoclonal antibodies to extracellular *Pseudomonas cepacia* protease. *Infect Immunol* 1994;62(7):2811–2817.

62. Straus DC, Lonon MK, Hutson JC. Inhibition of rat alveolar macrophage phagocytic function by a *Pseudomonas cepacia* lipase. *J Med Microbiol* 1992;37 (5):335–340.

63. Sajjan US, Sun L, Goldstein R, et al. Cable (Cb1) type II pili of cystic fibrosis-associated *Burkholderia (Pseudomonas) cepacia*: nucleotide sequence of the cblA major subunit pilin gene and novel morphology of the assembled appendage fibers. *J Bacteriol* 1995; 177(4):1030–1038.

64. Peckham D, Crouch S, Humphreys H, et al. Effect of antibiotic treatment on inflammatory markers and lung function in cystic fibrosis patients with *Pseudomonas cepacia*. *Thorax* 1994;49(8):803–807.

65. Cohn RC, Jacobs M, Aronoff SC. *In vitro* activity of amiloride combined with tobramycin against *Pseudomonas* isolates from patients with cystic fibrosis. *Antimicrob Agents Chemother* 1988;32(3): 395–396.

66. Gilligan PH, Gage PA, Bradshaw LM, et al. Isolation medium for the recovery of *Pseudomonas cepacia* from respiratory secretions of patients with cystic fibrosis. *J Clin Microbiol* 1985;22(1):5–8.

67. Welch DF, Muszynski MJ, Pai CH, et al. Selective and differential medium for recovery of *Pseudomonas cepacia* from the respiratory tracts of patients with cystic fibrosis. *J Clin Microbiol* 1987;25(9):1730–1734.

68. Tablan OC, Carson LA, Cusick LB, et al. Laboratory proficiency test results on use of selective media for isolating *Pseudomonas cepacia* from simulated spu-

tum specimens of patients with cystic fibrosis. *J Clin Microbiol* 1987;25(3):485–487.

69. Kiska DL, Kerr A, Jones MC, et al. Evaluation of four commercial identification systems for glucose nonfermenters from cystic fibrosis patients. *J Clin Microbiol* 1996;34(4):886–891.

70. Campbell PW 3rd, Phillip JA 3rd, Heidecker GJ, et al. Detection of *Pseudomonas (Burkholderia) cepacia* using PCR. *Pediatr Pulmonol* 1995;20(1):44–49.

71. Kollberg H, Vandamme P. Analysis of genomovars of *Burkholderia cepacia*: a helpful epidemiologic and prognostic tool? *Pediatr Pulmonol Suppl* 1996;13:297.

72. Snell GI, de Hoyos A, Krajden M, et al. *Pseudomonas cepacia* in lung transplant recipients with cystic fibrosis. *Chest* 1993;103(2):466–471.

73. Egan TM, Detterbeck FC, Mill MR et al. Improved results of lung transplantation for patients with cystic fibrosis. *J Thorac Cardiovasc Surg* 1995;109(2):224–235.

74. Simpson IN, Finlay J, Winstanley DJ, et al. Multiresistance isolates possessing characteristics of both *Burkholderia (Pseudomonas) cepacia* and *Burkholderia gladioli* from patients with cystic fibrosis. *J Antimicrob Chemother* 1994;34(3):355–361.

75. Wilsher ML, Kolbe, Morris AJ, et al. Nosocomial acquisition of *Burkholderia gladioli* with fatal outcome in patients with cystic fibrosis. *Am J Respir Crit Care Med* 1996;153(4):A 705.

76. Whittier S, Hopfer RL, Knowles MR, et al. Improved recovery of mycobacteria from respiratory secretions of patients with cystic fibrosis. *J Clin Microbiol* 1993;31(4):861–864.

77. Kilby JM, Gilligan PH, Yankaskas JR et al. Nontuberculous mycobacteria in adults with cystic fibrosis. *Chest* 1992;102(1):70–75.

78. Olivier KN, Thiede SG, NTM in CF Study Group. Nontuberculous mycobacteria in the adult patient with CF: colonizers or pathogens? *Pediatr Pulmonol Suppl* 1994; 10:176–177 (abstract).

79. Jones BJ, Faiz AR, Gilbert RE, et al. Multicenter investigation of nontuberculous mycobacteria in patients with cystic fibrosis. *Pediatr Pulmonol Suppl* 1995;12:248.

80. von Graevenitz A. *Acinetobacter, Alcaligenes, Moraxella*, and other non-fermentative gram negative bacteria. In: Murray PR, Baron EJ, Pfaller MA, et al., eds. *Manual of Clinical Microbiology*. 6th ed. Washington DC: ASM Press, 1995

81. Ballestero S, Virseda I, Escobar H, et al. *Stenotrophomonas maltophilia* in cystic fibrosis patients. *Eur J Clin Microbiol Infect Dis* 1995;14(8):728–729.

82. Vartivarian S, Anaissie E, Bodey G, et al. A changing pattern of susceptibility of *Xanthomonas maltophilia* to antimicrobial agents: implications for therapy. *Antimicrob Agents Chemother* 1994;38(3):624–627.

83. Gladman G, Connor PJ, Williams RF, et al. Controlled studies of *Pseudomonas cepacia* and *Pseudomonas maltophilia* in cystic fibrosis. *Arch Dis Child* 1992;67(2):192–195.

84. Bilton D, Pye A, Johnson MM, et al. The isolation and characterization of non-typeable *Haemophilus influenzae* from the sputum of adult cystic fibrosis patients. *Eur Respir J* 1995;8(6):948–957.

85. Rayner RJ, Hiller EJ, Ispahani P, et al. Haemophilus infection in cystic fibrosis. *Arch Dis Child* 1990;65(3):225–258.

86. Knutsen AP, Slavin RG. Allergic bronchopulmonary mycosis complicating cystic fibrosis. *Semin Respir Infect* 1992;7(3):179–192.

87. Paradis IL, Williams P. Infection after lung transplantation. *Semin Respir Infect* 1993;8(3):207–215.

88. Kramer MR, Marshall SE, Starnes VA, et al. Infectious complications in heart-lung transplantation: analysis of 200 episodes. *Arch Intern Med* 1993;153(17):2010–2016.

89. Fahy JV, Keoghan MT, Crummy EJ, et al. Bacteraemia and fungaemia in adults with cystic fibrosis. *J Infect* 1991;22(3):241–245.

90. Conway SP, Simmonds EJ, Littlewood JM. Acute severe deterioration in cystic fibrosis associated with influenza A virus infection. *Thorax* 1992;47(2):112–114.

91. Armitage JM, Kurland G, Michaels M, et al. Critical issues in pediatric lung transplantation. *J Thorac Cardiovasc Surg* 1995;109(1):60–65.

Cystic Fibrosis in Adults,
edited by J. R. Yankaskas and M. R. Knowles,
Lippincott–Raven Publishers, Philadelphia, 1999.

6

Immunopathogenesis of Cystic Fibrosis Lung Disease

Melvin Berger and *Michael W. Konstan

*Department of Immunology and Allergy, Rainbow Babies and Children's Hospital, and *Department of Pediatrics and Cystic Fibrosis Center, Case Western Reserve University School of Medicine, Cleveland, Ohio*

Despite recent progress in understanding the ion transport abnormalities in cystic fibrosis (CF), the link between the CF basic defect and the establishment of chronic Pseudomonas infection in the CF lung remains unknown. The bulk of the evidence suggests that this infection is related intimately to the development of a chronic, destructive inflammatory response that still accounts for the majority of the morbidity and almost all of the mortality in CF. Studies in babies diagnosed by neonatal screening suggest that both Pseudomonas infection and inflammation begin in infancy (1–4). Thus, it seems likely that the development of Pseudomonas infection is related specifically to the basic defect in CF, but the actual connection remains undefined (see below). In most patients with CF, the clinical course is manifest as a slowly progressive chronic bronchitis that is punctuated intermittently by acute exacerbations. Results from bronchoalveolar lavage (BAL) studies of stable patients with mild disease show that microorganisms, inflammatory cells, and their destructive products are present even when the patients are relatively asymptomatic (5), and that inflammation actually may be present without apparent infection (2–4,6). Thus, three processes—airway obstruction, chronic endobronchial infection, and inflammation—interact continuously for the patient's entire lifetime and ultimately destroy the lung. Although patients with CF have intrinsically normal immune sys-

tems and do not demonstrate any increased susceptibility to infection outside of the respiratory tract, they are unable to eradicate the chronic Pseudomonas infection, at least partially because of unique adaptations of the organisms in the CF lung. The resulting inflammatory response to this infection is excessive; it not only damages the lung, but it contributes to the hypersecretory state that causes airway obstruction, and it directly interferes with local host defense mechanisms. Thus, a vicious cycle is set up that ultimately results in severe bronchiectasis, progressive destruction of the lung, and death.

Once this vicious cycle has been established, even correction of the basic defect by gene therapy may not be able to fully halt the progressive lung damage. Thus, for most patients, continuous efforts to reduce the burden of infecting organisms and ameliorate the effects of the inflammatory response remain mainstays of daily treatment. Thus, understanding the interaction between infection and inflammation is a critical basis for rational therapy aimed at retarding the progression of CF lung disease.

THE IMMUNE SYSTEM IN PATIENTS WITH CYSTIC FIBROSIS

The increased susceptibility of patients with CF to respiratory infection has prompted many investigators to search for an immune defect in CF, but no primary systemic immune defect has been identified. Although the gene for the cystic fibrosis transmembrane conductance regulator (CFTR) is expressed in lymphocytes (see below), functional consequences of CFTR mutations in lymphoid cells have not been documented. Lymphocyte subsets (7–9) and proliferative responses to mitogens and standard test antigens generally are normal (7,10). The lack of increased susceptibility to protozoans or other opportunistic infections and the observation that delayed hypersensitivity skin tests usually are normal (7) suggest that cell-mediated immunity is intact *in vivo* as well. Although peripheral blood cells of patients with advanced disease may have decreased proliferative responses to Pseudomonas antigens (10), this improves after antibiotic treatment (10). Thus, like the ineffective antibody responses (see below), this is likely to be a secondary effect of chronic infection and/or excessive antigenic stimulation rather than a primary defect. Reports that T-cells of patients with CF have decreased activity in regulating immunoglobulin synthesis *in vitro* (8,9) primarily may reflect decreased *in vitro* stimulation of the B-cells rather than T-cell deficits per se. Similar decreased *in vitro* stimulation of B-cells has been reported in many other conditions in which there is polyclonal B-cell activation *in vivo*, such as systemic lupus erythematosus (SLE) (11), and probably is the result of prior activation of B-cell precursors due to chronic antigenic stimulation.

The major role of T-cells in defense against bacterial infection is the production of cytokines, including γ-interferon, which increase intracellular killing by macrophages and regulate B-cell responses. Deficient cytotoxic activity of CF T-cells has been reported, but this has not been confirmed and its significance is not clear (8). There have been reports that T-cells are capable of killing Pseudomonas directly and can transfer immunity against Pseudomonas to naive mice (12,13). However, other reports showing little difference in the severity or immunopathology of chronic *Pseudomonas aeruginosa* infection in athymic rats compared with normal rats (14) raise doubts about the importance of T-cells in this infection

in vivo. Increased production of lipopolysaccharide-induced cytokines by macrophages in the CF lung also is mainly secondary to chronic stimulation by antigens, immune complexes, and lipopolysaccharides (LPS) (15).

Despite their continuous carriage of large burdens of bacteria, patients with CF usually are afebrile. Laboratory indices such as the leukocyte count and erythrocyte sedimentation rate usually are normal, except in severe exacerbations. This probably is because the infection usually is restricted to the airway lumen, with minimal invasion into the parenchyma or bloodstream. Nevertheless, because organisms are continuously present and there is an ongoing local inflammatory response with release of inflammatory mediators and subsequent tissue damage, this should be considered chronic "infection," not harmless "colonization." Elevation of the C-reactive protein (CRP) may be a sensitive indicator of impending pulmonary exacerbation; severe episodes may include fever in addition to increased cough and marked increase in the purulence of the sputum. However, even the CRP returns to normal when the acute episode resolves (16), except in severely infected patients (16,17). Elevated levels of neutrophil elastase/α_1–protease inhibitor complexes are found in most patients' plasma and probably are formed when free elastase from the airways diffuses into pulmonary capillaries. The concentration of these complexes in plasma also increases during exacerbations and decreases after antibiotic treatment (17–20) and may be one of the most sensitive noninvasive measures of the amount of ongoing inflammation in the lung. Progressive hyperglobulinemia is seen in most patients (21), probably reflecting prolonged, excessive antigenic exposure and the effects of interleukin-6 (IL-6) produced in the lung (15). Despite the persistent burden of organisms in the lung, bacteremia and/or hematogenous metastatic infection is rare except as a preterminal event (22,23). This is consistent with reports of normal reticuloendothelial clearance in CF (24). The detection of circulating immune complexes varies with the sensitivity of the assay employed, but these may increase as the burden of infection becomes severe. High concentrations of circulating immune complexes and/or clinical manifestations of immune complex deposition in tissues usually are late observations that carry a poor prognosis (25–27). Like bacteremia or metastatic infection, this most likely indicates that the burden of microorganisms in the lung is out of control and that the normal clearance mechanisms are overwhelmed.

Defense against bacterial infection usually is considered the responsibility of the phagocytic defense system, which consists of the phagocytes—neutrophils and macrophages—and the opsonins—antibodies and complements. Despite extensive analysis, no characteristic defect in chemotactic, phagocytic, or microbicidal activity ever has been identified in the peripheral blood neutrophils or monocytes of CF patients (28). Indeed, the lack of an increased incidence of infection outside of the respiratory tract and the predominance of neutrophils in CF sputum and BAL samples confirm that neutrophil migration is normal *in vivo* as well. Similarly, phagocytosis and killing of organisms other than Pseudomonas by CF blood monocytes and alveolar macrophages also has been found to be normal (29–33). Serum complement levels and functional activity generally are normal in CF (24,29,34), although levels may decrease because of consumption in some cases (27,34). Alternative and classical complement components are found in normal bronchial secretions (35,36), and the reports that Pseudomonas in CF sputum are coated with C3 fragments (37) and that the concentration of C3c in CF sputum correlates with *P. aeruginosa* infection (38) suggest that complement activation occurs as expected *in situ*.

Cystic Fibrosis Transmembrane Conductance Regulator Expression in Lymphocytes: Lack of Immunologic Effects

Although CF generally is considered to be a disease of epithelial cells, several investigators have detected CFTR transcripts and/or Cl⁻ conductances characteristic of CFTR in lymphocytes and blood monocytes (39–44). The CFTR transcripts in these types of cells are present in 200- to 1,000-fold lower numbers than in T-84 cells (39,40). Although defects in cyclic adenosine monophosphate (cAMP)-dependent Cl⁻ conductance in CF lymphocytes have been reported (41,42), these studies have not included assays of immunologic functions or detailed analyses of signal transduction or secretory pathways. Thus, it is not clear how altered Cl⁻ permeability might impact on lymphocyte activation or effector functions. Interestingly, the "transporter for antigen presentation" protein (TAP), a membrane channel through which peptide fragments of degraded antigens are transported for binding to major histocompatibility complex (MHC) molecules, is a member of the adenosine triphosphate (ATP)-binding cassette family and is quite homologous with CFTR (45). It is not clear whether CFTR serves this function or affects this homologue, but CF lymphocytes do not share the immunologic phenotype of murine cells that lack this antigen transporter, which fail to express class I MHC antigens on their surface.

There are a few reports of phenomena in monocytes that might relate to the CF basic defect or to ion transport abnormalities. For example, monocytes from patients with CF and obligate heterozygotes release increased amounts of O_2^- when they adhere to plastic surfaces or in response to certain lectins (46). The signal transduction pathway for this effect and its relevance *in vivo* are unknown, but the response to other stimuli is normal. An interesting report that monocyte-derived macrophages from patients with CF produce more tumor necrosis factor (TNF) in response to LPS than similar cells from controls could reflect a secondary effect of chronic LPS exposure, but the fact that the CF cells were less sensitive to inhibition by amiloride than normal cells suggests that further investigation of ion transport abnormalities may be warranted (47).

Most reports of altered immunologic function *in vitro* of cells from patients with CF have shown that the "defects" are more severe in patients with advanced disease, are reversible with antibiotic treatment, and/or are found only in the presence of autologous serum. Thus, these observations are more likely results of the chronic antigen and LPS stimulation associated with the chronic infection rather than primary defects that predispose to it. Mechanistic explanations for differences in immunologic function between CF and normal cells that relate to ion transport abnormalities associated with CFTR mutations are lacking. Thus, it currently is impossible to associate any immunologic abnormality with basic defects in CFTR.

Anti-Pseudomonas Antibodies in Patients with Cystic Fibrosis

Antibody responses to most standard antigens are normal in CF (1,48,49). Although 22% of patients with CF who are younger than 10 years of age were reported to have decreased immunoglobulin G (IgG) levels in a 1980 report (48), other studies have reported normal IgG levels in this age group (1,49), and even in the 1980 study, older patients had normal or elevated IgG levels (48). The lower IgG levels may have been due to decreased antigen exposure from the gut secondary to chronic oral antibiotic usage. In general, adult patients with CF tend to be hyperglobulinemic, and their IgG levels increase progressively with age and severity of lung disease (21,50). This hyperglobulinemia likely represents the cumulative effects of prolonged antigen exposure in the respiratory tract and increased local IL-6 production in the lung.

In most patients with CF, IgG, IgA, and IgM antibodies develop against a broad array of Pseudomonas antigens, including exoenzymes, pili, LPS, mucoid exopolysaccharide (MEP), and outer membrane proteins. The titers of many of these antibodies increase after pulmonary exacerbations and may be used to help determine when increases in the burden of organisms occur (50–52). Reports of decreased levels of antibodies against the polysaccharides of microorganisms other than Pseudomonas (49) may represent decreased exposure to

other antigens because of frequent use of oral antibiotics because in contrast, most patients have increased levels of IgG2 and IgG4 antibodies to Pseudomonas antigens (49).

Among the most intriguing aspects of the immunology of CF are the observations that anti-Pseudomonas antibodies from CF fail to support, or actually block, phagocytosis of these organisms by macrophages in vitro (29–33,53). Studies in a model of chronic Pseudomonas infection in cats showed that initially antibodies were produced that facilitated phagocytosis (54). As the chronic infection continued, however, the same animals produced antibodies with inhibitory activity similar to that seen with the sera of patients with CF (54). This strongly suggests that the inhibitory activity is a secondary effect of the prolonged antigenic stimulation from the chronic infection rather than a primary defect that predisposes to it. Interestingly, almost all reports of this inhibitory activity use macrophages rather than neutrophils as the phagocytes. Because phagocytosis by alveolar macrophages depends primarily on high-affinity Fcγ receptors that preferentially bind IgG1 and IgG3 (55), a shift to IgG2 and IgG4 production may contribute to this inhibitory activity (53, 56). This phenomenon also may contribute to the apparent lack of phagocytosis by CF alveolar macrophages in vivo, as assessed by BAL (57). Antibodies that block phagocytosis also may be formed as a result of proteolytic cleavage of normal IgG molecules (see below).

The role of various Pseudomonas products in virulence and the corresponding protective or permissive effects of antibodies against any given Pseudomonas antigen is difficult to assess, particularly because the organisms persist in the presence of these antibodies, although their production of different surface antigens and exoproducts fluctuates from time to time. It is not known whether antibodies have a role in inducing the specific phenotypic adaptations typical of P. aeruginosa in the CF lung, such as the loss of type-specific LPS O-side chains (58) and elaboration of copious amounts of MEP. Pier et al. (59) reported that a subset of older patients who apparently were not infected chronically with Pseudomonas made anti-MEP antibodies that facilitated opsonophagocytic killing by neutrophils. Chronically infected patients with CF and controls also made antibodies to MEP, but these anti-MEP antibodies did not promote killing in this assay and the antibodies they had that did promote killing were directed against other antigens (59). Further studies from the same group have shown that animals immunized with low doses of MEP made protective opsonic antibodies, whereas animals immunized with higher doses of MEP made nonopsonic antibodies and had much more intense inflammatory responses (60). Recently, protein conjugation has been used to improve the response to experimental MEP vaccines (61). High molecular-weight forms of antigen and/or conjugation to proteins may facilitate T-cell cooperation in antibody production to polysaccharides and result in qualitatively and quantitatively better antibody responses. In contrast, it seems likely that low molecular-weight forms of MEP, which induce poorly opsonic antibodies, predominate in natural exposure of controls and in the massive exposure of chronically infected patients with CF. Thus, Tosi et al. (62) reported that both chronically infected and apparently uninfected patients with CF made opsonic as well as nonopsonic antibodies, but the opsonic antibodies were not protective. These results suggest that chronic infection occurs stochastically and after it becomes established, the titers of the nonopsonic antibodies increase dramatically (62). The MEP may act like the capsule of gram-positive cocci, restricting access of phagocyte receptors to the bacterial cell wall itself (63). Thus, the ability of certain antibodies to fix complement to the surface of the MEP may explain their increased opsonic efficacy (63) in comparison with the effects of anticapsular antibody in protection against pneumococcal infection.

Thus, it seems likely that patients with CF are intrinsically able to produce protective antibodies and that their immune systems basically are normal, but that as a result of persistent infection and chronic antigenic stimulus, shifts in the subclass and/or antigen specificity of their anti-Pseudomonas responses result in production of opsonically ineffective antibodies. These conclusions raise the hopes that manipulation of the immune system might allow better control or eradication of the chronic Pseudomonas infection that plagues patients with CF.

Susceptibility to Infection in Cystic Fibrosis: Why *P. aeruginosa?*

The link between mutations in the CF gene, its biochemical consequences, and the increased susceptibility to lung infection, particularly with the unique, mucoid forms of *P. aeruginosa* that nearly are pathognomonic of CF, remains an enigma. Except for mild dilatation of the acini of tracheal submucosal glands, the airways usually are histologically normal in early infancy (64). Plugging of small airways by abnormal mucus is the most prominent early manifestation, but it is not clear whether this is caused by infection (65). The abnormalities in mucous secretions, which probably relate directly to the basic defect, must play a role. The underhydration of secretions and/or specific chemical alterations in the mucins lead to inspissation of secretions in the ducts of multiple exocrine glands in CF and probably account for obstruction and obliteration in the vas deferens, pancreas, biliary tree, and, in some cases, even the intestine. A similar process begins in the lung, but because this organ is a blind pouch that is open to the outside environment, airway obstruction and impaired mucus clearance lead to infection. The increased mucus secretion and airway obstruction cannot, by themselves, explain the increased susceptibility to infection or the selection of the unique flora particular to CF. Mucus hypersecretion and airway obstruction also occur in asthma, but infection usually is absent in that condition. Impaired mucociliary clearance in primary ciliary dyskinesis syndromes results in chronic infection of the airways, but *P. aeruginosa* does not predominate. Similarly, primary antibody deficiency syndromes are associated with chronic and recurrent sinopulmonary infection, but *P. aerugi-*

nosa is involved only rarely and mucoid forms are even rarer; *Haemophilus influenzae, Streptococcus pneumoniae*, and other encapsulated organisms are much more common. Furthermore, the course and pathology of *P. aeruginosa* infection in CF differ from that in most other underlying conditions. In CF, the *P. aeruginosa* acts as a low-grade pathogen and the infection remains primarily endobronchial, whereas in conditions such as neutropenia and cancer, this organism is rapidly invasive. In view of the lack of increased susceptibility to infection outside of the respiratory tract or any characteristic immune defect, these observations all suggest that unique features of the CF lung must contribute to the increased susceptibility to a restricted spectrum of pathogens.

Although *Staphylococcus aureus* and *H. influenzae* commonly are cultured from patients with CF, there is nothing unique about CF isolates of these organisms. Both organisms are readily recoverable from the upper airway and pharynx of many healthy individuals, and their presence at these sites likely leads to lower airway infection when obstruction and/or epithelial damage occurs from other causes. Thus, lung infection with these organisms, which dominates the picture early in CF, probably does not reflect any specifically increased susceptibility in CF.

The most distinctive finding in CF, and the one that is most clearly associated with the progressive deteriorating course, is the chronic endobronchial infection with mucoid strains of *P. aeruginosa*. Although nonmucoid *P. aeruginosa* may colonize the oropharynx of non-CF patients and are widely prevalent in the environment, lower airways infection with this organism is unusual in immunocompetent hosts who do not have CF. *P. aeruginosa* also is present frequently in the sinuses of patients with CF, yet it is not a characteristic pathogen in sinusitis in patients who do not have CF, and when it does occur, it rarely is mucoid. An increased burden of this organism in the sinuses of patients with CF may serve as a reservoir for descending infection into the lower airways. Descending infections with *P. aeruginosa* and

Staph. aureus are seen in patients with CF after lung transplantation, but they frequently can be eradicated from the posttransplant lungs with appropriate antibiotic therapy (66).

Hypotheses for Association of *P. aeruginosa* with Cystic Fibrosis

Host Factors

Three major hypotheses have been advanced to account for the specific predilection of patients with CF to infection with mucoid Pseudomonas (Table 6–1). First, this organism may be selected by the chronic and/or recurrent treatment of Staphylococcus and Hemophilus infections with antibiotics to which Pseudomonas is resistant. Second, there may be a specific increase in the affinity of CF epithelial cells or airway mucins for Pseudomonas adhesion. Third, a unique but as yet undefined characteristic of the CF airway microenvironment might induce the Pseudomonas to shift to the mucoid phenotype which then protects it from eradication.

The source from which patients with CF acquire Pseudomonas remains controversial. Pseudomonas species are ubiquitous in the environment and most likely are acquired randomly, although some investigators have suggested cross-infection as a major route of initial acquisition (50,67,68). Several observations argue against either cross-infection or selection by antibiotics. Most importantly, many patients, even infants, already harbor Pseudomonas at the time of their initial diagnosis (69–71). By the use of sensitive methods, such as bronchoscopy, to obtain cultures from

TABLE 6–1. *Hypotheses that could account for specific association of* P. aeruginosa *with cystic fibrosis*

1. Selection by antibiotics used to treat other organisms
2. Increased expression of altered (asialo-) epithelial cell surface glycoconjugates that provide increased adherence for *P. aeruginosa*
3. Altered composition of airway surface fluid induces mucoid phenotype of *P. aeruginosa*

young infants and children who do not expectorate, it is becoming clear that the prevalence of *P. aeruginosa* even in asymptomatic young patients is much higher than previously suspected (2–6,71). These patients have not had prolonged courses of antibiotics, thus arguing against selective pressure because of antibiotic therapy. Conversely, many patients with other causes of chronic lung infection and/or bronchiectasis may be on antibiotics almost continuously for decades before they acquire Pseudomonas, if they ever do; even then, mucoid types are extremely rare. In contrast to *P. aeruginosa*, there is more universal agreement that *Burkholderia cepacia* is in fact spread by cross-infection between patients with CF and that the incidence of infection with the latter organism can be decreased by cohorting (72–74).

The second hypothesis considers the importance of adherence of Pseudomonas to the epithelial surface. Increased affinity of binding of Pseudomonas to CF airway epithelial cells and/or mucins (75,76) could facilitate retention of these specific organisms and lead to their persistence and overgrowth. Despite careful analyses *in vitro*, no enhanced specific binding of *P. aeruginosa* to CF mucins has been demonstrated (77). It also has been proposed that Pseudomonas might bind preferentially to airway cells that had been damaged by viruses or prior infection with staphylococcus or Hemophilus, or to cells migrating into the epithelium to repair damage (78). In particular, removal of fibronectin from epithelial cell surfaces by neutrophil elastase and/or other proteases increases binding of Pseudomonas (79–81). These phenomena also would occur in other diseases, particularly hypogammaglobulinemia, but *P. aeruginosa* is not a major problem in those patients, so it seems unlikely to account for the incidence of Pseudomonas infection in CF.

An intriguing possibility is suggested by the observations of Krivan et al. (82) that asialogangliosides may provide high affinity binding sites for *P. aeruginosa*. CF mucins are undersialylated (83); other glycoconjugates, including cell surface glycolipids, might be undersialylated as well. Such specific alterations in the chemical structure of complex carbohydrates could serve well as the basis for selection of one particular type of organism by increasing its adherence. The hypothesis that decreased activity of CFTR could alter the pH of intracellular organelles such as the Golgi apparatus (84) provides a theoretical link between the basic defect and alterations in the chemical structure of cell surface or mucin carbohydrates because different enzymes involved in posttranslational modification of proteins and other glycosylated structures have different pH optima. This might explain why mucins and cell-surface glycolipids may be undersialylated and oversulfated in CF (83,85). Prince and colleagues (86–89) have reported increased binding of Pseudomonas to nasal epithelial cells from patients with CF compared with cells from controls and to CF versus normal cell lines. However, the differences were modest, and there was much overlap. At least some of the increased binding was attributed to increased expression on the CF cells of asialoGM1, which can bind to Pseudomonas pili (87,89). The increased adherence of Pseudomonas to CF epithelial cells has been associated with increased IL-8 production by CF versus normal epithelial cell lines on addition of the bacteria *in vitro* (90). It also has been suggested that *P. aeruginosa* might increase its own adherence by producing neuraminidase, which could expose additional asialogangliosides (86).

The third hypothesis centers on the most unique feature of the Pseudomonas infection in CF, the peculiar mucoid phenotype, and proposes that alterations in CF airway lining fluids or other changes in the CF microenvironment induce this phenotype (91). This particular adaptation likely confers a selective advantage to the organism because it favors its persistence in a number of ways. Recent studies suggest that mucoid *P. aeruginosa* grows as a biofilm that physically obstructs phagocytosis (92,93). Earlier electron microscopic studies showed that the individual organisms in mucoid colonies are dispersed extensively in copious amounts of amorphous mucoid exopolysaccharide "slime," which is chemically similar to seaweed alginate (94). It is easy to visualize this material physically interfering with phagocytosis by keeping the cells at "arm's length" and also stabilizing the organisms as a microcolony on the airway wall. In addition, the MEP is highly anionic and may serve to bind aminoglycosides and other antibiotics (95,96), as well as antibodies and/or complement components, again restricting their access to organisms deep within the mucoid microcolony. Furthermore, MEP can scavenge bactericidal products of host phagocytes' oxidative respiratory burst, conferring resistance to killing by hypochlorite *in vitro*. Thus, this extracellular MEP "slime," which gives mucoid strains of *P. aeruginosa* their characteristic phenotype, most likely makes a major contribution to the pathogenicity of this organism in CF.

Patients with CF are infected initially with classical, nonmucoid strains of *P. aeruginosa* (50,58). Animal studies have shown that the shift to mucoidy can occur during prolonged persistent infection, even in otherwise healthy hosts (98). This shift is accompanied by characteristic changes in the restriction fragment length polymorphism (RFLP) patterns of the Pseudomonas chromosome (98), which may correlate with mutations in genes that normally suppress MEP production (99). The shift to mucoidy can be induced *in vitro* under dehydrating conditions (91,100), suggesting that abnormalities in the fluid and/or ion content of CF airway secretions could have the same effect *in vivo*. This suggestion is consistent with the observation that mucoid strains are rarely recovered from individuals who do not have CF. Conversely, mucoid phenotypes occasionally have been reported in other gram-negative bacteria recovered from patients with CF. Mucoid *P. aeruginosa* isolates from patients with CF rapidly revert to the nonmucoid phenotype in the laboratory, although spontaneous shifts in the opposite direction are rare. It thus seems likely that the specific milieu in the CF lung

accelerates, stabilizes, and/or induces the shift to the mucoid phenotype of *P. aeruginosa* and that this plays a major role in the persistence of this particular organism. However, the actual features of the CF airway that cause this shift remain unidentified.

Other investigators have focused on determining whether the altered ionic milieu of CF airway epithelial cells could impair local epithelial defense mechanisms, allowing persistent infection to stimulate inflammation. These also would tie CFTR dysfunction to the abnormal inflammation in the lung. It has been suggested that phagocytosis and bactericidal activity of neutrophils are impaired by a *hypo*tonic milieu in CF (101); conversely, other investigators have proposed that the *increased* Na and Cl concentrations in this milieu interfere with the function of bactericidal peptides that can kill Pseudomonas (102). Clearly, additional data on the actual milieu *in vivo* is necessary before the importance of these *in vitro* observations can be understood fully. Another recent report suggests that normal airway epithelial cells can ingest and kill *P. aeruginosa* and that cell lines expressing mutant forms of the CFTR are defective in cellular uptake of this organism (103).

Although presented here as competing hypotheses, all the aforementioned mechanisms could operate together and contribute to the overall predilection of patients with CF to infection with mucoid Pseudomonas. Cross-infection could result in larger inocula than would be obtained randomly, and the use of oral antibiotics that are ineffective against *P. aeruginosa* could provide an early advantage to these organisms. In that context, even a minor degree of increased adherence could promote persistence, and continued growth of the organism in the CF milieu could rapidly induce or select mucoid organisms. The *P. aeruginosa* infection in CF is not rapidly invasive as it is in patients with neutropenia or neutrophil defects, but the shift to mucoidy leads to a state in which the patient with CF no longer can eradicate the organism from the lung (see below). Dysregulated cytokine production by CF airway epithelial cells (see Role of Macrophages and Cytokines section) could contribute to the excessive nature of the local inflammatory response, which exacerbates the lung damage.

Bacterial Factors

Although animal models and the rapidly invasive nature of Pseudomonas infections in non-CF hosts suggest that extracellular virulence factors secreted by the organisms play important roles in Pseudomonas infections in those settings, they may be less important in CF. Pseudomonads are highly adaptable species, as evidenced by their survival in a broad range of environments in nature. *P. aeruginosa* is capable of secreting exotoxin A, alkaline protease, and elastase, as well as low molecular-weight siderophores and phenazine pigments. The enzymes and toxins may be important early in the establishment of Pseudomonas in the airway by directly inhibiting phagocytosis, but they are unlikely to play much of a role in the chronic, progressive lung damage that ensues because extensive necrosis is not a prominent feature of CF lung disease. Furthermore, these secreted proteins induce neutralizing antibodies that are found at high titer in most patients with CF (49–52,104). Nevertheless, increasing titers of antibodies to these antigens after exacerbations suggest that they may play a role under some circumstances (50–52). The pigments and siderophores may avoid immunologic neutralization because of their low molecular weights. Phenazines may contribute to persistence of Pseudomonas by inhibiting lymphocyte responses (105), thus depriving macrophages of cytokines such as γ-interferon that enhance their phagocytic and bactericidal activity. These pigments also can inhibit ciliary activity (106). The siderophores may enable the bacteria to obtain the iron they need to grow despite the presence of host iron-binding proteins (107). In addition, these compounds may increase the toxicity of reactive oxygen species formed by macrophages and neutrophils (108). Because there is not yet an animal model that mimics the initial colonization with *P. aerugi-nosa* and the conversion to chronic infection, the importance of any of these factors *in vivo* remains difficult to evaluate.

When classical strains of *P. aeruginosa* shift to the mucoid phenotype, they generally decrease production of extracellular toxins and of the long O-polysaccharide side chains on their LPS (58). This shift from smooth to rough types of LPS is associated with a marked increase in the susceptibility to the bactericidal activity of serum *in vitro*, but despite the presence of antibodies and active complement in the lung, the CF host still is unable to eradicate these organisms. In addition to protecting the organisms, MEP may play an important role in the elaboration of lung damage in CF because it is highly antigenic. Although the anti-MEP antibodies may have poor opsonic activity (59,62), they likely still contribute to the formation of immune complexes *in situ*. These, in turn, stimulate the inflammatory response and intensify the local tissue damage.

Regardless of how bacterial factors and the host–bacteria interactions lead to the establishment of chronic Pseudomonas infection (reviewed in 91), conversion to the mucoid phenotype clearly is a critical event (109). Establishment of chronic infection with mucoid organisms is responsible for turning the inflammatory response into a self-perpetuating process that escapes from homeostatic control. This unchecked inflammatory response leads to a vicious cycle in which the products of the continued neutrophil influx actually impair clearance of the bacteria and eventually destroy the lung.

THE INFLAMMATORY RESPONSE IN THE CYSTIC FIBROSIS LUNG AND ITS RELATION TO INFECTION

Both clinically and pathologically, CF is characterized by an inflammatory response focused on the airways rather than the interstitium or the alveoli. As noted below, BAL fluids even from stable patients with mild disease generally culture positive for *P. aeruginosa* and, as compared with controls, demonstrate marked increases in inflammatory cells, immunoglobulins, and mediators such as active elastase, which are capable of tissue damage (5,110). These findings suggest that even in relatively asymptomatic patients, the presence of Pseudomonas and/or other organisms reflects local "infection" rather than harmless commensal "colonization," even though there may be no systemic signs (5,111). This pathologic process is confined initially to the lumen but then spreads across the epithelium into the submucosa and attacks the airway wall and supporting structures. Signs of early epithelial damage include denudation, loss of cilia, and squamous metaplasia. There also is hyperplasia of goblet cells and hypertrophy of mucous glands, even in infants (112). These changes are compatible with the effects of elastase (see below), and because recent results suggest that both infection and neutrophil influx begin in infancy, it seems likely that even these early changes are secondary to infection. With time, mucopurulent plugging of the airways occurs in nearly all patients and is accompanied by inflammatory infiltrates in the mucosa and submucosa. These cause ulceration and formation of microabscesses in the airway wall, and finally, progressive bronchiectasis. Breaching of the epithelial barrier is accompanied by infiltration into the parenchyma, which occurs to some extent in almost all patients older than 2 years of age (65,112). As with the exudate in the lumen, the lesions in the bronchial wall and the organized infiltrates consist largely of neutrophils, with a relative paucity of mononuclear cells. Similarly, with time and progression of clinical lung disease, the numbers of neutrophils in BAL increase tremendously and they become the predominant cell type recovered. Although there may be focal areas of lymphocytic infiltrates and even the local formation of germinal centers, these are relatively rare, and granulomas are not common.

The predominance of the inflammation in and around the airways suggests that the inflammatory reaction is related intimately to intraluminal infection. Immunohistologic studies have shown *P. aeruginosa* antigens primarily in an endobronchiolar distribution, in associa-

tion with intense inflammation and obliteration of small airways less than 1 mm in diameter (113). Although organisms also were found to a lesser extent in alveolar spaces, they were not often identified in interstitial areas. Thus, the primary pathologic process seems to be an intense inflammatory response to a relatively noninvasive pathogen. This is in marked contrast to the deeply necrotizing infection *P. aeruginosa* often causes in patients with cancer and neutropenia, in which severe tissue damage is produced by invasive organisms secreting enzymes and other extracellular toxins as they cross tissue planes. Similarly, the formation of granulomas containing small numbers of organisms that are resistant to killing by host phagocytes, as might be found in tuberculosis or histoplasmosis, is not a major component of CF lung disease. This peculiar pattern of inflammatory disease in CF is most likely related to the unique characteristics of the mucoid *P. aeruginosa* and the interplay of the host inflammatory response with this infection.

Most clinicians agree that the establishment of mucoid Pseudomonas in the CF lung is a critical turning point that marks the beginning of an inexorably accelerating downhill course (109). This association likely reflects the role of this infection and the elaboration of large amounts of MEP and other antigens as stimuli for the chronic inflammatory response. This inflammatory response itself becomes the major cause of the functional abnormalities and the structural damage that destroys the lung. In particular, recent studies have emphasized the role of neutrophil-derived DNA in increasing the viscosity of the secretions and the likely role of neutrophil elastase in inducing secretory hyperplasia and in stimulating additional chemoattractant formation. Elastase also causes impairments of local phagocytic defense mechanisms that interfere with eradication of the infection. Thus, a vicious cycle of infection and inflammation is established (Fig. 6–1). With the continued elaboration of bacterial antigens and LPS and the continued release of neutrophil products, the normal homeostatic mechanisms are overwhelmed and this vicious cycle escapes from control. Addi-

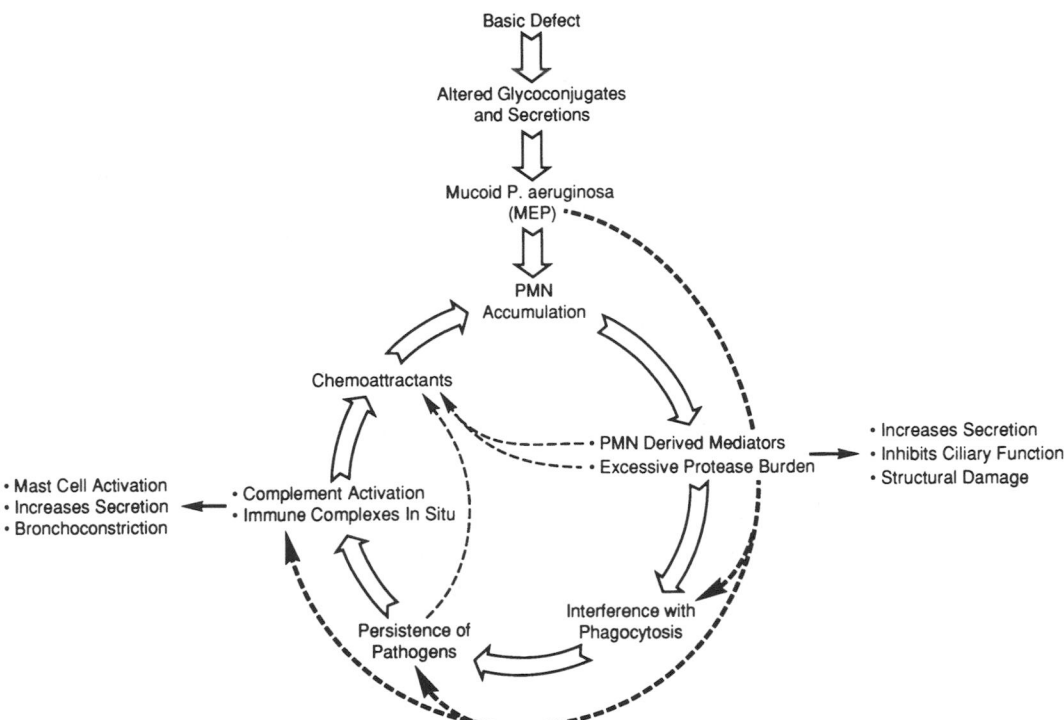

FIG. 6–1. The inflammatory response in the CF lung as a vicious cycle initiated by Pseudomonas infection. Conversion to the mucoid phenotype with production of mucoid exopolysaccharide (MEP) by *P. aeruginosa* is critical because it physically impedes access of phagocytes to the bacteria. Persistence of bacteria leads to chronic neutrophil (PMN) influx by contributing bacterial chemoattractants per se as well as antigens that activate, complement, and generate C5a. In addition, leukotriene B_4 (LTB$_4$) produced by the PMNs themselves and interleukin-8 (IL-8), which is induced by PMN elastase, also contribute to the PMN influx. The PMNs bring an excess protease burden to the lung, which causes structural damage and impairs phagocytic killing of the organisms, exacerbating the vicious cycle. (Reprinted from Konstan MW, Berger M. Infection and inflammation in the lung in cystic fibrosis. In: Davis PB, ed. *Cystic Fibrosis.* New York: Marcel Dekker Inc, 1993:219–276.)

tional inflammatory mediators cause bronchoconstriction, increased secretions, and other functional changes that exacerbate the underlying pulmonary abnormalities, as well as recruitment of additional inflammatory cells that perpetuate the cycle. The combination of these effects leads to the destruction of the lung and the death of the patient.

Role of Macrophages and Cytokines

Early in the course of CF, there are increased numbers of macrophages as well as neutrophils recovered by BAL (2,3,5,110, 114). Electron microscopy studies suggest that these macrophages are not involved actively in phagocytosis (57). This may be at least partly due to the presence of "blocking" and/or proteolytically cleaved antibodies that interfere with the opsonic activity of IgG (29–33), because recent studies suggest that both CF and normal alveolar macrophages rely primary on Fcγ receptors for phagocytosis (55). Nevertheless, immunofluorescence studies of BAL cells fixed immediately on removal from the lung shows abundant staining of the macrophages for intracellular cytokines, suggesting that these cells may be important sources of chemoattractants and other proinflammatory mediators *in vivo* (15).

Despite their quiescent appearance, the airway macrophages in CF are important sources of TNF, IL-1, and IL-8, (15,115). This is not unexpected because the chronic Pseudomonas infection provides a continuous source of LPS, which induces their synthesis. Indeed, many of the manifestations of CF, including the massive neutrophil influx into the lung, hyperglobulinemia, and cachexia resemble known effects of cytokines. Studies of IL-1 and TNF concentrations and their production by circulating cells in peripheral blood of patients with CF have yielded conflicting results (116–119), but it is important to remember that many cytokines are produced and act locally (120). In addition to the chemokine IL-8 (15,121–123), other cytokines, including IL-1, TNF/cachectin (TNF-α) and IL-6, all have been found at elevated concentrations in CF BAL (15,124–126), although the concentration of the antiinflammatory cytokine IL-10 is reduced (127). TNF enhances neutrophil oxidative and secretory responses (128,129), and both TNF and IL-1 can induce fever and other systemic effects as well as induce production of IL-6 and IL-8 by macrophages and epithelial cells. TNF also causes alterations in lipoprotein metabolism and may be responsible for the cachexia that accompanies many chronic diseases (130). IL-1 stimulates acute phase responses and muscle protein catabolism. Thus, it is speculated widely that in addition to stimulating the local inflammatory response in the lung, IL-1 and TNF may contribute to the poor weight gain and other systemic manifestations of CF. Because IL-6, in addition to other activities, stimulates antibody production by B-cells, it may be important in the hyperglobulinemia found in most patients with CF.

It seems likely that IL-8 and TNF are major contributors to the overall chemotactic and neutrophil-activating activity in the CF lung. Cytokines have short half-lives, and circulating concentrations or activities may not be representative of local effects. Many binding factors and receptor antagonists are produced at the same time as the cytokines themselves and may be induced by the same stimuli. For example, we have found high levels of IL-1 receptor antagonist and soluble TNF receptor fragments in CF BAL (15). These may reduce the systemic response to the cytokines, accounting for the lack of fever; the cytokines' effects may predominate in the local microenvironment. Recent work focusing on IL-8 production by bronchial epithelial cell lines in vitro (131,132) and the observations of elevated IL-8 concentrations in the BAL of infants diagnosed by neonatal screening (2) have emphasized the importance of this particular chemotactic cytokine even in the earliest stages of CF lung disease. Several studies have shown that the concentration of IL-8 in BAL correlates strongly with the concentration of neutrophils, DNA, and active elastase (2,6,133,134). IL-8 is of additional interest because it can be produced by pulmonary epithelial cells as well as macrophages. We have shown that fresh airway epithelial cells from patients with CF stain markedly positive for IL-8 by immunofluorescence and spontaneously secrete this chemoattractant on culture in vitro (135). Neutrophil elastase, soluble products of P. aeruginosa, and adherence of intact Pseudomonas all have been shown to induce IL-8 production from bronchial epithelial cell lines in vitro (90,131,132). Richman-Eisenstat et al. (123) demonstrated that most of the in vitro chemotactic activity of CF sputum can be inhibited by an anti–IL-8 monoclonal antibody, confirming the overall importance of this chemokine in vivo. Even in the BAL of infants younger than 1 year of age who were diagnosed with CF by neonatal genetic screening, the concentration of IL-8 correlated well with the amount of DNA (from decomposing neutrophils) in the same samples (134), suggesting a role for this chemoattractant very early in the development of CF lung disease. Recent reports that expression of viral proteins in human lung cell lines also induces IL-8 production (136) suggests one mechanism by which viral infection may lead to exacerbation of CF lung disease.

In addition to dramatically increased concentrations of the proinflammatory cytokines, CF airways are relatively deficient in the antiinflammatory cytokine IL-10 (15,127). This may be particularly important because IL-10 inhibits the production of IL-1, IL-8, and TNF by inflammatory cells, including LPS-activated macrophages (137). In our laboratory, we have shown that normal bronchial epithelial cells constitutively produce IL-10 in the healthy lung (127), but that production of IL-10 by CF bronchial epithelial cells is decreased *in vivo* and *in vitro* (127). Decreased IL-10 production by CF epithelial cells may allow excessive and/or persistent inflammatory responses to transient infection, helping to fuel the vicious cycle of inflammatory damage at early stages of CF lung disease, when infection still can be cleared. We have speculated that the decreased IL-10 production may be related directly to defective CFTR function, perhaps through autocrine mechanisms, but this has not yet been tested conclusively.

The multiple inflammatory mediators present in the milieu of the CF lung act in concert to exert their overall effects. This may be beneficial in the normal host because pretreatment with TNF increases the bactericidal activity of neutrophils (128,129) and can prime cells for secretion, which would not be induced by IL-8 itself (138). In the chronic infection in CF, however, the combined effects of these cytokines may be particularly deleterious in the local microenvironment. For example, TNF and IL-1 may increase the local inflammatory damage by causing increased release of toxic oxygen radicals from phagocytes and by inducing increased expression of adhesion molecules such as intracellular adhesion molecule 1 (ICAM-1). Increased ICAM expression on endothelial cells is important in stopping neutrophils in the circulation and allowing them to begin following the gradient of chemoattractants to the tissue site of inflammation, but it also promotes endothelial cell damage (139–141). In addition, both TNF and IL-1 can induce ICAM-1 on human tracheal epithelial cells *in vitro*, and this molecule is expressed prominently in CF lung tissue *in vivo*—on the epithelial as well as the endothelial cells (142,143). This increased expression of adhesion molecules on the epithelium may intensify the functional and toxic effects of PMN on the epithelial cells and cause their retention on the epithelium, retarding their clearance in the respiratory secretions.

Significance of Neutrophils as the Primary Inflammatory Cell in the Lung

Normally, alveolar macrophages are the predominant phagocytes recovered by BAL, but even in patients with mild CF, neutrophils predominate (Table 6–2). Recent studies show similar changes in infants diagnosed by neonatal screening who have little or no clinical evidence of lung problems (2,3). As the lung dis-

TABLE 6–2. *Bronchoalveolar lavage (BAL) findings in stable patients with CF with mild lung disease (FEV$_1$ = 79 ± 4% of predicted, n = 18) vs. non-CF controls (n = 23)[a]*

	CF	Non-CF	CF/Non-CF ratio
Neutrophils (× 10^6/mL ELF)	38 ± 14 (1–222)	0.10 ± 0.04 (0–0.6)	380
Neutrophils/total cells (%)	57 ± 5 (13–95)	3.0 ± 0.5 (0–9)	19
Active elastase (μmol/L ELF)	2.3 ± 0.9 (0–14.1)	0 —	∞
Total α$_1$-PI (μmol/L ELF)	2.7 ± 0.6 (0.3–8.0)	0.9 ± 0.2 (0.1–3.1)	3

[a]Values expressed as mean ± SEM (range). Epithelial lining fluid (ELF) in recovered BAL fluid was calculated from simultaneous determination of urea concentration in BAL and serum. Elastase was assayed by hydrolysis of MeO-Suc-Ala-Ala-Pro-Val-pNa, which measures active elastase, above and beyond that which may be present in an inactive, complexed form. Patients with CF were 12 to 36 years of age, and non-CF controls were healthy adults 18 to 38 years of age.
Adapted from reference 5.

ease progresses, the number of neutrophils increases progressively and the sputum becomes markedly purulent and increasingly tenacious. Barton et al. (144) showed that leukocytes were the major source of the greatly increased amount of DNA in CF sputum. Improvements in pulmonary function after intensive inpatient antibiotic and pulmonary toilet "cleanouts" are associated with decreased density of *P. aeruginosa* and decreased content of DNA and other neutrophil products in the sputum and/or BAL, implying decreased neutrophil infiltration (17–20,114,145–147). These correlations strengthen the etiologic relationship between the Pseudomonas infection, the neutrophilic response, and decreased pulmonary function.

In addition to furthering the inflammatory response by both direct and indirect contributions to the total chemoattractant activity (see Fig. 6–1 and Table 6–3), neutrophils may directly injure the lung by releasing highly reactive oxygen metabolites, as well as lysosomal enzymes and proteases (148). After stimulation, neutrophils and macrophages assemble a multienzyme complex that reduces molecular oxygen to produce several highly reactive and toxic species, including singlet oxygen, superoxide, hydroxyl radical, and hydrogen peroxide (H_2O_2) (149,150). Together with the neutrophil enzyme myeloperoxidase, H_2O_2 can react with halides such as Cl^- to produce hypochlorous acid (bleach), which has potent microbicidal activity but may be less toxic to normal tissues than the oxygen radicals (148). These oxidative products generally are considered important in killing bacteria intracellularly, and the proteases and lysosomal enzymes are believed to be necessary to break down and digest the bacterial remnants. However, these

same oxidative products and enzymes may act extracellularly at inflammatory sites, damaging the surrounding tissues and altering the inflammatory milieu (140,148).

Many stimuli, including C5a and TNF, which are chemotactic for neutrophils, also cause secretion of granular contents (149,150). Enzymes such as collagenase and gelatinase that are released during neutrophil activation normally may facilitate movement of the neutrophil through basement membranes and tissue planes, whereas proteins such as lactoferrin, lysozyme, and low molecular-weight defensins may exert direct bactericidal effects. Thus, the neutrophil has been described as a "secretory organ of inflammation" (149,150). It is obvious, however, that excess enzymes and/or oxidative products can digest connective tissue and damage normal tissues (148). When the target of phagocytosis is too large to be ingested and/or if the neutrophils' receptors are engaged by antibody and/or complement fragments bound to surfaces, phagocytosis may be "frustrated," and the toxic oxidative and granular enzymes are released onto the surface rather than into a phagocytic vacuole (151,152). This may occur on a microcolony or biofilm of *P. aeruginosa*, the surface of which is coated with antibodies to the MEP. Obviously, this could be an important mechanism of tissue damage, although organisms deep in the colony might remain unaffected. Once a neutrophil has left the vascular space and migrates into the tissues, it does not return to the circulation. Reports that respiratory epithelial cells express ICAM-1 and other adhesion molecules *in vivo* in CF (143) suggest that adhesion molecules on the epithelial cells may hold the neutrophils in place and retard their removal as in-

TABLE 6–3. *Chemoattractants for neutrophils in the cystic fibrosis lung*

Attractant	Likely sources
Formylated oligopeptides (f-MLP, etc.)	Bacteria, including *P. aeruginosa*
C5a and C5a des Arg	Plasma, following complement activation or nonspecific proteolysis
IL-8	Macrophages, PMN, epithelial cells
LTB$_4$	Macrophages, PMN

IL-8, interleukin-8; LTB$_4$, leukotriene B$_4$; PMN, neutrophils

tact cells by mucociliary clearance. Thus, many neutrophils probably die and decay *in situ*, releasing their entire content of proteases, digestive enzymes, and nuclear DNA to contribute to tissue damage and dysfunction at the inflammatory site.

Because macrophages are larger than neutrophils and can survive for extended periods of time in the tissue, it is tempting to speculate that a given amount of phagocytosis by macrophages might cause less tissue damage than the equivalent amount of ingestion by neutrophils. However, studies from several laboratories, including our own, show that the overall phagocytic activity of lung macrophages is less than that of neutrophils, even given optimal opsonization (55), and suggest that these cells are present primarily as scavengers and to exert immunomodulatory effects.

Neutrophil Chemoattractants in the Cystic Fibrosis Lung

Several potent neutrophil attractants are present in CF lung fluids (see Table 6–3), including those produced by the host as well as bacterial oligopeptides that resemble the prototypic synthetic chemoattractant N-formyl-Met-Leu-Phe (153). Bacterial LPS and/or other products also are important inducers of chemotactic cytokine production from alveolar macrophages and epithelial cells.

Reports showing that *P. aeruginosa* in CF sputum are coated with immunoglobulin and complement (37) and that soluble C3c in sputum correlates with *P. aeruginosa* infection (38) strongly suggest that complement is activated *in situ*. This leads to local generation of C5a and C5a des-Arg, the most important chemoattractant/neutrophil activators of the complement system. Fick et al. (154) have shown that C5a is present in CF BAL fluid and that the overall chemotactic activity of these fluids can be reduced by antibodies that neutralize C5a. Furthermore, CF sputum contains noncomplement proteases that can liberate chemotactic fragments from C5 *in vitro*. In addition to important chemoattractant activities, complement-derived anaphylatoxins can induce histamine release, bronchospasm, and mucous secretion (155), all of which contribute to the functional abnormalities in the CF airways.

In addition, leukotriene B$_4$ (LTB$_4$), which can be produced by both macrophages and neutrophils (156,157), has been shown to be the major eicosanoid present in CF BAL and sputum (158–161). The observation that the LTB$_4$ content of CF sputum samples increases on incubation *in vitro* suggests that neutrophils in the airways may be major sources of this chemoattractant *in vivo*. This is another example of how the neutrophils themselves can establish and perpetuate a positive feedback cycle. It has been difficult to single out any one chemoattractant as "the most important," and, similarly, it seems unlikely that any single type of antagonist will be effective at significantly reducing the neutrophil influx into the lung.

Effects of Neutrophil Products

DNA

One of the consequences of the massive recruitment of neutrophils into the CF airways is that they decompose in place, releasing large amounts of their granular enzymes and their nuclear DNA. This release may be exacerbated by the adherence of neutrophils, which are maximally expressing their CD11b/CD18 adherence molecules (162), to epithelial cells, which are expressing large amounts of ICAM-1, the major ligand for this adherence molecule (139). The resulting interaction may tether the neutrophil in place until it decomposes rather than allowing it to be swept away while it still is relatively intact. The physicochemical properties of solutions of free DNA are very different than the properties of suspensions of cells containing equal amounts of DNA because the long strands of DNA that impart high viscosity to the solutions are kept condensed and coiled up inside intact cells. Recombinant human DNase decreases the molecular weight of the DNA strands in CF sputum and the sputum viscosity in parallel (163), and it currently is in widespread clinical use (see Chapter 7).

The highly anionic nature of the DNA leads to many ionic interactions with other constituents in CF sputum. For example, much of the elastase in sputum is bound to DNA because elastase is highly cationic. Because of this, adding DNase to sputum *in vitro* increases the free elastase in the supernatant (164). Although similar effects are seen acutely *in vivo*, with longer term use of DNase *in vivo*, the elastase content of the sputum decreases (164,165), presumably because of better clearance of airway neutrophils. Intact DNA also may bind aminoglycosides, which are very basic as well, and decrease their efficacy. Thus, the use of DNase may allow reductions in the dosages of aerosolized tobramycin or other antibiotics. It also has been reported that DNA copurifies with mucous glycoproteins when sputum is fractionated (166), and treatment of isolated mucus fractions with DNase *in vitro* reduces their viscosity just as it does for unfractionated sputum (166). Thus, DNA can impair mucociliary clearance and eradication of infection in several ways. Thus, it is hoped that in addition to short-term effects of DNase in facilitating clearance of viscous secretions, this agent also will allow more rapid removal of effete neutrophils and will contribute in other ways to the eradication of the chronic intraluminal infection.

Oxidase Products

In contrast to the effects of DNA and proteases, whose roles in CF lung disease have been clearly documented, the effects of oxidative mechanisms have received less attention. It is difficult to document oxidation of structural proteins or membrane lipids *in situ*, and increased plasma concentrations of oxidized products such as malonaldehyde or dioenoic acid may be secondary to decreases in dietary antioxidants (167). However, the large amounts of free myeloperoxidase in CF lung fluids (114,146,168,169) suggest that the neutrophils express their full oxidative capacity *in situ*. Furthermore, the demonstration that on the addition of H_2O_2, CF sputum is cytotoxic for respiratory epithelial cells in culture (170) strongly suggests that similar activity occurs *in vivo*.

H_2O_2 itself has potent bactericidal activity, but this is increased markedly by reaction with halide ions, which is catalyzed by myeloperoxidase. The product of this reaction is the hypohalous acid or anion—in the case of Cl^-, hypochlorous acid or hypochlorite (bleach). Hypochlorite has potent antibacterial effects but is fairly noninjurious to normal cells and tissues (148). In contrast, the hydroxyl radical, $\cdot OH$, is a much more reactive and toxic product that can be formed from H_2O_2 in the presence of Fe^{++}. In the so-called Haber-Weiss reaction, the Fe^{++} then is regenerated by an electron from O_2^-. Currently, it is believed that $\cdot OH$ is the major toxic oxidative species formed by activated phagocytes. Unlike H_2O_2, it can rapidly oxidize a number of different cell and tissue constituents and can cause DNA strand breaks (148,171,172).

Thus, the availability of Fe^{++} is believed to be a critical determinant of the amount of tissue injury that accompanies neutrophil activation. The release of large amounts of the iron-binding protein lactoferrin at inflammatory sites serves as a homeostatic mechanism that limits local oxidative damage by removing Fe^{++}. At the same time, this protein enhances local defenses by depriving bacteria of the iron that is essential to their growth. In the chronic Pseudomonas infection in CF, there are several ways in which the production of $\cdot OH$ might be enhanced (171–173). First, *P. aeruginosa* can secrete important low molecular compounds, including the siderophores pyochelin and pyoverdin and the redox dye pyocyanin. The siderophores are secreted by Pseudomonas and other bacteria to facilitate their own iron uptake and growth. Iron bound to pyochelin is an effective catalyst of Haber-Weiss reactions, and ferripyochelin increases the amount of cellular toxicity when target cells are incubated with activated PMN or their products (171, 172). In addition, pyocyanin can participate in cell-mediated redox cycling, which can generate O_2^- and H_2O_2. This by itself does not cause cytotoxicity *in vitro*, but if ferripyochelin also is present, cell injury and death occur because ·OH is produced (172). Finally, the active proteases present in the milieu of the chronically infected CF lung can cleave lactoferrin and other iron-binding proteins and change their protective functions into injurious ones. For example, the combination of Pseudomonas elastase and neutrophil elastase can cleave ferric transferrin much more efficiently than either enzyme acting alone. The resulting fragments continue to bind iron and can catalyze ·OH production (171,173).

In addition to the well-recognized effects of oxidants in inactivating α_1-protease inhibitor (174,175), inflammatory proteases may increase oxidative tissue injury by altering functions of cellular enzymes. In the presence of activated neutrophils, intracellular xanthine dehydrogenase is converted into an oxidase, the reactions of which generate H_2O_2 and O_2^- in addition to the end product, uric acid (140, 141). This conversion requires active neutrophil elastase and tight adhesion of neutrophils to cultured endothelial cells because it is blocked by antibodies to the adhesion molecule CD11b (141). This additional oxidizing system is believed to be of major importance in neutrophil-mediated injury to endothelial cells. The observations by Tosi et al. that CF airway cells express large amounts of ICAM-1, to which PMN can adhere through CD11b/CD18 (142, 143), suggest that a similar mechanism could operate in the CF airway, injuring the epithelial cells. Although it is difficult to identify end products of oxidative tissue damage or to quantitate the *in vivo* effects of these systems, there is a great deal of circumstantial evidence suggesting that these mechanisms do in fact operate *in vivo* in the chronically infected CF lung.

Proteases

Mechanisms of Protease/ Antiprotease Imbalance

Although host protease inhibitors should limit the injury caused by proteolytic enzymes, once the inhibitory capacity of these inhibitors has been exceeded, additional enzyme activity is unimpeded and tissue damage may become extensive. This occurs in CF because of the continuous, massive neutrophil influx. BAL studies show that the concentration of α_1-protease inhibitor in the BAL of patients with mild CF is several-fold higher than in healthy subjects (see Table 6–2), but that the numbers of neutrophils in the same specimens are elevated several hundred-fold. Thus, there is a corresponding several hundred-fold excess of elastase and other neutrophil proteases, which clearly exceeds the inhibitory capacity of the inhibitors.

The lung normally is protected against proteolytic damage by α_1-protease inhibitor (α_1-PI, α_1-antitrypsin), secretory leukocyte protease inhibitor (SLPI, formerly termed bronchial mucus protease inhibitor), and, to a lesser extent, α_2-macroglobulin. The latter may play some role at tissue sites, particularly if there is increased vascular permeability, but its high molecular weight (725,000 daltons) limits its penetration into tissues and its efficacy at inflammatory sites. Local synthesis of α_2-macroglobulin by alveolar macrophages is difficult to assess. SLPI is produced and secreted by airway mucosal cells and is the predominant inhibitor in the conducting airways (176,177). α_1-PI (molecular weight = 45,000 daltons) diffuses from the blood and predominates in smaller airways and alveoli. Both SLPI and α_1-PI can be inactivated by Pseudomonas proteases (178,179), which may limit their efficacy in CF, although the extent to which this occurs *in vivo* is difficult to assess (180). α_1-PI also can be inactivated by the reactive oxygen species released during neutrophil activation (174) because its active site contains a critical methionine residue whose oxidation reduces the affinity of α_1-PI for neutrophil elastase by three orders of magnitude (174,175). This type of inactivation also can be produced by cell-free systems containing myeloperoxidase, H_2O_2, and Cl^- (174), which takes on particular significance because free myeloperoxidase is readily demonstrable in CF sputum (114,146,168,169).

Inactivated α_1-PI then can be cleaved by a variety of proteases, as can α_1-PI complexed to serine proteases it has inhibited. Several studies suggest that proteolytic cleavage by excess elastase is the major cause of fragmentation of α_1-PI in CF sputum (181,182). Because there is a tremendous excess of proteases over inhibitors in the CF lung, it is not surprising that most of the α_1-PI in CF BAL or sputum is in the form of low molecular-weight cleavage fragments rather than high molecular-weight complexes (146,181,182).

In most studies of free proteases in CF BAL and/or sputum, the majority of the activity—regardless of the substrate—is inhibitable by inactivators of serine proteases, such as phenylmethyl sulfonyl fluoride (PMSF), soybean trypsin inhibitor, and exogenous α_1-PI; rather than by chelators, such as edetic acid (EDTA) or phenanthrolene; or by phosphoamidon, a relatively specific inhibitor of Pseudomonas elastase (162). This strongly suggests that neutrophil elastase and cathepsin G are the major enzymes present because macrophage and Pseudomonas elastases are metalloenzymes (183,184). Several studies have shown correlations between protease activity in CF sputum or BAL, or serum concentrations of elastase– α_1-PI complexes, with the clinical condition of the patient and/or the occurrence of exacerbations (18–20). Even in the first 6 months of life, there are significant increases in the amount of elastase bound to α_1-PI and excess free elastase that are readily detectable in BAL of infants with CF identified by neonatal screening (2). In addition to direct structural damage, neutrophil elastase and other proteases that are present chronically in CF cause functional changes that exacerbate the abnormalities in secretion, contribute to the excessive inflammatory response, and interfere with local host defense mechanisms, as explained below.

Role in Tissue Damage

Considerable evidence suggests that neutrophil-derived proteases play major roles in damaging lung tissue in CF. It is well estab-lished that unchecked neutrophil elastase is the major cause of emphysema in patients with α_1-protease inhibitor deficiency. An analogous mechanism may account for the emphysema occasionally seen in CF. However, because the airways are the primary locus of neutrophil accumulation in CF, the effect of the uninhibited proteases primarily is on the airway wall rather than the interstitium or the alveoli, which are the sites most exposed to neutrophils normally emigrating from the bloodstream. Thus, proteolytic destruction of structural proteins leads to bronchiectasis in CF rather than alveolar destruction, as in α_1-PI deficiency. Incubation of human bronchial epithelial cell monolayers with concentrations of elastase found in CF BAL leads to loss of tight junctions (185), which also has been found in biopsy specimens. This in turn could lead to increased access of neutrophil products and inflammatory mediators to the submucosa, increasing their ability to damage the structural framework of the airway and to further stimulate the inflammatory response.

Many studies have documented active proteases in CF sputum and BAL (see Tables 6–2 and 6–4). Bruce et al. (186) provided direct evidence for proteolytic destruction of lung tissue *in vivo* in CF by demonstrating disruption and exfoliation of elastin fibers in areas of inflammation *in situ*. They also demonstrated increased urinary excretion of desmosines, cross-linked amino acid degradation products of elastin, with higher concentrations correlating with increased severity of lung disease (186). Stone et al. (187) recently confirmed that patients with CF excrete larger amounts of desmosines in their urine than controls or patients with other lung diseases, providing further evidence that proteases released as part of the inflammatory response cause substantial lung injury in CF.

Role in Hypersecretory State

Although administration of high doses of human neutrophil extracts or purified elastase to animals causes pulmonary hemorrhage,

TABLE 6–4. *Adverse effects of proteases in the cystic fibrosis lung*

On epithelium	
Structural damage	Bruce et al., 1985 (186)
	Stone et al., 1995 (187)
Increased secretion and induction	Snider et al., 1984 (188)
of secretory metaplasia	Sommerhoff et al., 1990 (190)
Inhibit ciliary beating	Tegner et al., 1979 (193)
Induction of IL-8	Nakamura et al., 1992 (131)
On opsonophagocytic defense	
Cleavage of IgG	
Production of inhibitory fragments	Fick et al., 1984 (199)
Inhibition of cell activation by	Döring et al., 1986 (224)
immune complexes	
Inactivation of C3	Suter et al., 1984 (225)
Cleavage of C5 and generation	Fick et al., 1986 (154)
of chemoattractants	
Cleavage and inactivation	Suter et al., 1988 (80)
of fibronectin	
Cleavage of C3b receptor (CR1)	Berger et al., 1989 (162)
from neutrophils	
Cleavage of iC3b on Pseudomonas	Tosi et al., 1990 (197)

IL-8, interleukin-8; IgG, immunoglobulin G.

lower doses cause less acute damage but can cause dramatic secretory metaplasia (188). Elastase inhibitors such as SLPI block these effects, confirming that they are the result of enzymatic activity per se (189). Sommerhoff et al. (190) have shown that human neutrophil elastase and cathepsin G are extremely potent secretagogues for cultured bovine tracheal serous gland cells, releasing almost 50-fold more high molecular weight mucin glycoproteins than optimal doses of histamine. These results extend to human cells as well (191), and Pseudomonas enzymes also have similar effects (192). Although the mechanisms by which the proteases induce secretion and/or secretory metaplasia are unknown, the results suggest that uninhibited neutrophil elastase may cause similar effects in CF, both acutely and chronically. In light of the abnormalities in CF secretions, it seems likely that any increased secretory stimulus would increase the amount of mucus plugging and airway obstruction. It also has been shown that purulent sputum and purified elastase inhibit the beating of respiratory cilia *in vitro* and that these effects can be inhibited by α_1-PI (193,194). Together, these effects of elastase may compound and se-

riously exacerbate the problems of abnormal secretions and decreased mucociliary clearance in CF.

Role in Generating Chemoattractants

Another important functional change caused by elastase is the induction of IL-8 synthesis by respiratory epithelial cells (131,133). Both the isolated enzyme and CF BAL induce IL-8 production by bronchial epithelial cell lines *in vitro* (131), and we have shown that CF bronchial epithelial cells produce IL-8 *in vivo* (135). McElvaney et al. (133) have shown that aerosol administration of recombinant SLPI caused proportional decreases in the concentration of active elastase and number of PMN in CF BAL, suggesting a causal relationship between elastase and IL-8 secretion *in vivo* as well.

Neutrophil elastase also is capable of releasing a C5a-like chemotactic peptide from C5, which is not surprising because many complement components can be activated by other serine proteases, and Fick et al. (154) have demonstrated such activity in CF sputum. These activities of elastase provide further examples of how the inflammatory process may become a vicious cycle that feeds on itself and escapes from control.

Interference with Phagocytic Host Defenses

As noted previously, no primary systemic immunologic or phagocytic defect has ever been documented in CF, leading to the conclusion that local factors in the lung must interfere with eradication of the infection. Uninhibited proteases in the inflammatory milieu seem likely candidates for causing such local interference because in the lung, their activity greatly exceeds the activities of their inhibitors; elsewhere in the body, the normal excess inhibitory capacity is maintained (18–20,146). Studies from several laboratories have documented that soluble proteins important in host defense against bacteria can be cleaved and inactivated by proteases in CF BAL or sputum, as summarized in Table 6–4. In most cases, the proteolytic activity is inhibitable by serine protease inhibitors such as PMSF, suggesting that elastase and, to a lesser extent, cathepsins are responsible.

Optimal phagocytosis requires deposition of opsonins on the bacteria that can interact with specific surface receptors on the phagocytes and that the latter, neutrophils and macrophages, must be activated to ingest and kill the bound bacteria. The opsonins include fibronectin, antibodies, and complement fragments derived from C3. Surfactant protein A, which binds to a receptor on macrophages, also may play an important role in opsonization in the lung (195). All these can be inactivated by proteases in CF sputum or BAL, reducing their efficacy *in vivo* or even producing inhibitory fragments that may block antigenic sites on the bacteria or occupy receptors on phagocytes. The effects of cleavage of fibronectin may further complicate the situation in CF because removal of epithelial cell surface fibronectin has been shown to increase the adherence of gram-negative bacteria (79–81,196). Our work has focused on the effects of proteases on cell surfaces, but in the context of opsonophagocytosis. These studies have shown that neutrophils in CF BAL are lacking C3b receptors and that a serine protease in the BAL, most likely elastase, can efficiently remove this receptor from the cell surface, disabling one of the two major complement receptors and markedly decreasing the phagocytic and bactericidal activity of the cells (162). Studies by Tosi et al. (197) showed that elastase also has effects on the opsonized bacteria, removing iC3b, the ligand for the other major complement receptor, further decreasing the bactericidal activity by creating an "opsonin-receptor mismatch" (197).

Because the concentration of elastase necessary for the latter effect is less than one tenth of the amount necessary to remove C3b receptors from neutrophils (197), the observation that the neutrophils in fresh BAL already are lacking C3b receptors (5,162) suggests that concentrations of elastase commonly present in the lung fluid of patients with CF virtually eliminate the activity of the complement system *in vivo*. Administration of α_1-PI *in vitro* or *in vivo* can reverse these effects and eliminate the inhibitory effects of CF BAL on neutrophil killing of Pseudomonas *in vitro* (198). Comparisons of the roles of IgG and complement in enhancing the phagocytic activity of alveolar macrophages and neutrophils for Pseudomonas show that by far, the greatest enhancement of activity occurs when complement is included with neutrophils (52). Thus, elimination of complement's opsonic function *in vivo* is likely to reduce greatly the overall local phagocytic activity. Furthermore, because the macrophages rely primarily on IgG, proteolysis of this antibody reduces their phagocytic activity as well (199,200). This may contribute to their quiescent appearance on electron microscopy of BAL (57).

Macrophage function may be further compromised by proteases because optimal intracellular killing by macrophages depends on activation of these cells by γ-interferon produced by activated T-cells. Pseudomonas proteases have been shown to be capable of cleaving lymphocyte surface molecules, including CD4 (201), and can inhibit lymphocyte activation and natural killer-cell activity (202). It is likely that excess host proteases also can mediate similar effects in the local environment. Inhibition of lymphocyte activation would consequently decrease γ-interferon production and alter production of other immunoregulatory cytokines as well. In addition, Pseudomonas alkaline protease and elastase degrade and inactivate γ-interferon (203,204), suggesting that human elastase also may have similar effects. Thus, neutrophil elastase is likely to exert a number of effects in the CF lung that specifically exacerbate the major morbidity of this disease by increasing secretions, attracting more neutrophils, and interfering with eradication of the chronic infection. These effects of the neutrophil's own products create a vicious cycle that leads to the severe inflammatory damage to the lung that is ultimately responsible for the death of the patient.

IMPLICATIONS FOR THERAPY

To summarize the current thinking, inflammation in the CF lung occurs primarily in response to infection, most notably with mucoid types of *P. aeruginosa,* which essentially are impossible for the CF patient to eradicate. This inflammatory response is dominated by neutrophils and leads to a vicious cycle that actually exacerbates the infection, has deleterious functional effects, and eventually destroys the airways. The excessive and counterproductive nature of this inflammatory response is well illustrated by our study in which ibuprofen was administered to rats with the agar bead model of chronic *P. aeruginosa* infection (205). Most importantly, the drug caused a significant reduction in the percentage of lung area that was inflamed without increasing the burden of bacteria recovered (205). There are several steps in the inflammatory process at which intervention could be imagined, and because the overall inflammatory process can be viewed as a vicious cycle, significant improvement at any stage might result in overall improvement. However, the severity of the inflammatory response and the overlap of multiple effector mechanisms in eliciting the neutrophil infiltrate and damaging the tissues suggests that no single intervention is likely to be a panacea. Therefore, simultaneous attack at multiple points will be necessary.

Many therapies that primarily target other aspects of CF lung disease have some efficacy in interrupting the vicious cycle of inflammation as well [see Chapter 7, and (206,207)]. Thus, efforts to prevent or control infection, particularly with *P. aeruginosa*, are likely to reduce inflammation in the long run. Immunologic approaches, including vaccines (208) and/or passive immunotherapy (209–211), may prove promising as adjuncts to antibiotics, but their efficacy has yet to be demonstrated. Perhaps more aggressive use of antibiotics on a chronic basis might be effective in reducing the burden of bacteria in the airways, with the expectation that less inflammation would follow. Strategies that help clear the airways also indirectly reduce inflammation. DNase, by hydrolyzing the DNA released from neutrophils, decreases the viscoelasticity of purulent secretions and currently is in clinical use (163,212). Other agents with similar effects, such as gelsolin (213) and thymosin β4 (214), also are being considered. Ion transport regulators such as amiloride and uridine triphosphate (UTP) also are under investigation (215–217), in the hope that normalizing the hydration and ion composition of airway secretions not only would improve their clearance, but also may allow for improved function of local defense mechanisms in eradicating the infection. One must not minimize the beneficial effect of physically relieving obstruction and removing injurious products of inflammation. Thus, airway clearance techniques remain an important mainstay of treatment, and new techniques and devices are being developed.

Specifically attempting to decrease the persistent neutrophil influx is a relatively new strategy for treating CF lung disease. Efforts thus far have focused primarily on the therapeutic potential of corticosteroids and nonsteroidal antiinflammatory drugs (NSAIDs). Alternate-day prednisone may be beneficial (218,219), and trials have not been associated with exacerbation of infection (218,219), but unacceptable systemic effects of corticosteroids limit their long-term use (219). Inhaled corticosteroids are under investigation as a safer alternative. High-dose ibuprofen, taken twice daily for 4 years, was shown to decrease the progression of CF lung disease and currently is being used clinically in patients with mild lung disease (220). This particular drug has the advantage of interfering with neutrophil migration and degranulation, as well as inhibiting LTB_4 production at concentrations achievable *in vivo* (205). Clinical investigations of other NSAIDs (piroxicam), as well as pentoxifylline and fish oil, which may directly interfere with neutrophil function and decrease chemoattractant production, also are in progress [reviewed in (206, 207)]. The rationale for the use of all of these agents ultimately lies in their potential to decrease neutrophil influx into the lung. Preclinical work also is being done on other potential therapies intended to decrease the neutrophil influx. Although LTB_4 receptor antagonists and other agents specifically targeted against individual chemoattractants and cytokines in the lung are under development, their usefulness in CF may be limited by their specificity because many different chemoattractants and proinflammatory cytokines act synergistically in the CF airway. Therapies targeted at preventing neutrophils from migrating into the lung, such as antibodies to adhesion molecules on the neutrophil and/or endothelium, may prove to be more useful. Because of the large burden of uninhibited neutrophil elastase in the CF airway, and its many deleterious effects, attention also has focused on administering exogenous antiprotease to the airways of patients with CF (133,198,221). Antioxidant therapy also is under consideration (222,223). These and other antiinflammatory approaches are discussed in further detail in Chapter 11 and in references 206 and 207.

Experience to date suggests that therapies directed against the intense inflammatory response should be added to existing strategies aimed at decreasing the progression of CF lung disease. To counteract the adverse effects of the excessive inflammatory response that destroys the lungs of CF patients, more studies are required to better understand the mechanisms of action of antiinflammatory agents in the CF lung, to determine which agents would provide the most benefit to patients with CF and to determine which therapies are most appropriate at each age and/or stage of lung disease. The availability of noninvasive measures of local inflammatory activity would facilitate greatly studies aimed at optimizing the use of antiinflammatory agents to combat CF lung disease. Increasing use of antiinflammatory therapies in addition to already comprehensive therapeutic programs hopefully will decrease morbidity and improve the quality of life for patients with CF.

SUMMARY

Pulmonary infection and inflammation begin very early in the infancy of patients with CF and continue in an unabated vicious cycle throughout their lives. Inflammation plays key roles in the early pathogenesis of CF lung disease and is the major cause of the chronic destructive changes that eventually claim the life of most patients with CF. Although no primary immune defect has been recognized, poorly defined local mechanisms clearly lead to increased susceptibility to lower airway infection with *Staph. aureus, H. influenzae,* and *P. aeruginosa,* and to the subsequent transformation of the latter to the mucoid phenotype that is pathognomonic of CF. This shift in the phenotype of the predominant organism is associated with an inability of the host to eradicate the infection and a marked increase in the rate of progression of the lung disease. Although there is no animal model for the initial infection with Pseudomonas and its shift to mucoidy, several testable hypotheses have been advanced that may account for the predilection of patients with CF to this unusual infection. Hopefully, further investigation will allow a clearer understanding of the pathogenic links between the molecular defect and the organ-level disease. Evolving insights already have provided novel approaches to treatment, including antiinflammatory therapy and agents such as DNase, which can reverse pernicious effects of the excessive inflammatory response. Ongoing research into the etiology of lung infection and the dysregulated inflammatory response hold promise for additional therapies that should impact positively the quality and length of the lives of patients with CF.

REFERENCES

1. Abman SH, Ogle JW, Harbeck RJ, et al. Early bacteriologic, immunologic, and clinical courses of young infants with cystic fibrosis. *J Pediatr* 1991;119(2): 211–217.
2. Kahn TZ, Wagener JS, Bost T, et al. Early pulmonary inflammation in infants with cystic fibrosis. *Am J Respir Crit Care Med* 1995;151:1075–1082.
3. Armstrong DS, Grimwood K, Carzino R, et al. Lower respiratory infection and inflammation in infants with newly diagnosed cystic fibrosis. *Br Med J* 1995;310:1571–1572.
4. Armstrong DS, Grimwood K, Carlin JB, et al. Bronchoalveolar lavage or oropharyngeal cultures to identify lower respiratory pathogens in infants with CF. *Pediatr Pulmonol* 1996;21:267–275.
5. Konstan MW, Hilliard KA, Norvell TM, et al. Bronchoalveolar lavage findings in cystic fibrosis patients with stable, clinically mild lung disease suggest ongoing infection and inflammation. *Am J Respir Crit Care Med* 1994;150(2):448–454.
6. Balough K, McCubbin M, Weinberger M, et al. The relationship between infection and inflammation in the early stages of lung disease from cystic fibrosis. *Pediatr Pulmonol* 1995;20:63–70.
7. Harper TB, Gaumer HR, Waring W, et al. Cell mediated immunity and suppressor T cell function in children with cystic fibrosis. *Lung* 1980;157(4):219–228.
8. Knutsen AP, Slavin RG, Roodman ST, et al. Decreased T helper cell function in patients with cystic fibrosis. *Int Arch Allergy Appl Immunol* 1988;85(2): 208–212.
9. Lahat N, Rivlin J, Iancu TC. Functional immunoregulatory T-cell abnormalities in cystic fibrosis patients. *J Clin Immunol* 1989;9(4):287–295.
10. Sorensen RU, Waller RL, Klinger JD. Cystic fibrosis. Infection and immunity to pseudomonas. *Clin Rev Allergy* 1990;9:47–74.
11. Fauci A. Immunoregulation in autoimmunity. *J Allergy Clin Immunol* 1980;66(1):5–17.
12. Markham RB, Pier GB, Goellner JJ, et al. *In vitro* T cell-mediated killing of *Pseudomonas aeruginosa*: the role of macrophages and T cell subsets in T cell killing. *J Immunol* 1985;134(6):4112–4117.
13. Powderly WG, Pier GB, Markham RB. T lymphocyte-mediated protection against *Pseudomonas aeruginosa* infection in granulocytopenic mice. *J Clin Invest* 1986;78:375–380.
14. Krogh Johansen H, Espersen F, Stenvang Pedersen S, et al. Chronic *Pseudomonas aeruginosa* lung infection in normal and athymic rats. *APMIS* 1993;101: 207–225.
15. Bonfield TL, Panuska JR, Konstan MW, et al. Inflammatory cytokines in cystic fibrosis lungs. *Am J Respir Crit Care Med* 1995;152:2111–2118.
16. Glass S, Hayward C, Govan JRW. Serum C-reactive protein in assessment of pulmonary exacerbations and antimicrobial therapy in cystic fibrosis. *J Pediatr* 1988;113(1 pt 1):76–79.

17. Rayner RJ, Wiseman MS, Cordon SM, et al. Inflammatory markers in cystic fibrosis. *Respir Med* 1991;85(2):139–145.
18. Suter S, Schaad UB, Roux-Lombard P, et al. Relation between tumor necrosis factor α and granulocyte elastase-α 1-proteinase inhibitor complexes in the plasma of patients with cystic fibrosis. *Am Rev Respir Dis* 1989;140(6):1640–1644.
19. Meyer KC, Lewandoski JR, Zimmerman JJ, et al. Human neutrophil elastase and elastase/alpha$_1$-antiprotease complex in cystic fibrosis. *Am Rev Respir Dis* 1991;144(3 pt 1):580–585.
20. O'Connor CM, Gaffney K, Keane J, et al. α$_1$-Proteinase inhibitor, elastase activity, and lung disease severity in cystic fibrosis. *Am Rev Respir Dis* 1993; 148:1665–1670.
21. Wheeler WB, Williams M, Matthews M, et al. Progression of cystic fibrosis lung disease as a function of serum immunoglobulin G levels: a 5-year longitudinal study. *J Pediatr* 1984;104(5):695–699.
22. McCarthy MM, Rourk MH, Spock A. Bacteremia in patients with cystic fibrosis. *Clin Pediatr* 1980;19 (10):746–748.
23. Fahy JV, Keoghan MT, Crummy EJ, et al. Bacteremia and fungaemia in adults with cystic fibrosis. *J Infect* 1991;22(3):241–245.
24. Mantzouranis EC, Rosen FS, Colten HR. Reticuloendothelial clearance in cystic fibrosis and other inflammatory lung diseases. *N Engl J Med* 1988;319 (6):338–343.
25. McFarlane H, Holzel A, Brenchley P, et al. Immune complexes in cystic fibrosis. *Br Med J* 1975;1(5755): 423–428.
26. Moss RB, Lewiston NJ. Immune complexes and humoral response to *Pseudomonas aeruginosa* in cystic fibrosis. *Am Rev Respir Dis* 1980;121(1):23–29.
27. Wisnieski JJ, Todd EW, Fuller RK, et al. Immune complexes and complement abnormalities in patients with cystic fibrosis: increased mortality associated with circulating immune complexes and decreased function of the alternative complement pathway. *Am Rev Respir Dis* 1985;132(4):770–776.
28. Santos JI, Hill HR. Neutrophil function in cystic fibrosis. In: Shapira E, Wilson GB, eds. *Immunological aspects of cystic fibrosis*. Boca Raton, FL: CRC Press, 1984:29–37.
29. Biggar WD, Holmes B, Good RA. Opsonic defect in patients with cystic fibrosis of the pancreas. *Proc Natl Acad Sci U S A* 1971;68(8):1716–1719.
30. Boxerbaum B, Kagumba M, Matthews LW. Selective inhibition of phagocytic activity of rabbit alveolar macrophages by cystic fibrosis serum. *Am Rev Respir Dis* 1973;108(4):777–783.
31. Cassino RJJ, Sordelli DO, Macri CN, et al. Pulmonary nonspecific defense mechanisms in cystic fibrosis: I, phagocytic capacity of alveolar macrophages and neutrophils. *Pediatr Res* 1980;14(11):1212–1215.
32. Fick RB Jr, Naegel GP, Matthany RA, et al. Cystic fibrosis pseudomonas opsonins-inhibitory nature in an *in vitro* phagocytic assay. *J Clin Invest* 1981;68(4): 899–914.
33. Thomassen MJ, Boxerbaum B, Demko CA, et al. Inhibitory effect of cystic fibrosis serum on pseudomonas phagocytosis by rabbit and human alveolar macrophages. *Pediatr Res* 1979;13(9):1085–1088.

34. Gotz M, Lubec G. Complement in cystic fibrosis. *Eur J Pediatr* 1978;127(2):133–139.

35. Reynolds HY, Newball HH. Analysis of proteins and respiratory cells obtained from human lungs by bronchial lavage. *J Lab Clin Med* 1974;84(4):559–573.

36. Robertson J, Caldwell JR, Castle JR, et al. Evidence for the presence of components of the alternative (properdin) pathway of complement activation in respiratory secretions. *J Immunol* 1976;117(3):900–903.

37. Hann S, Holsclaw DS. Interactions of *Pseudomonas aeruginosa* with immunoglobulins and complement in sputum. *Infect Immunol* 1976;14(1):114–117.

38. Schiotz PO, Sorensen H, Hoiby N. Activated complement in the sputum from patients with cystic fibrosis. *Acta Pathol Microbiol Scand (C)* 1979;87C(1):1–5.

39. Yoshimura K, Nakamura H, Trapnell BC, et al. Expression of the cystic fibrosis transmembrane conductance regulator gene in cells of non-epithelial origin. *Nucleic Acids Res* 1991;19(19):5417–5423.

40. McDonald TV, Nghiem PT, Gardner P, et al. Human lymphocytes transcribe the cystic fibrosis transmembrane conductance regulator gene and exhibit CF-defective cAMP-regulated chloride current. *J Biol Chem* 1992;267(5):3242–3248.

41. Chen JH, Schulman H, Gardner P. A cAMP-regulated chloride channel in lymphocytes that is affected in cystic fibrosis. *Science* 1989;243:(4891)657–660.

42. Bubien JK, Kirk KL, Rado TA, et al. Cell cycle dependence of chloride permeability in normal and cystic fibrosis lymphocytes. *Science* 1990;248(4961):1416–1419.

43. Krauss RD, Bubien JK, Drumm ML, et al. Transfection of wild-type CFTR into cystic fibrosis lymphocytes restores chloride conductance at G_1 of the cell cycle. *EMBO J* 1992;11(3):875–883.

44. Krauss RD, Berta G, Rado TA, et al. Antisense oligonucleotides to CFTR confer a cystic fibrosis phenotype on B lymphocytes. *Am J Physiol* 1992;263 (6 pt 1):C1147–1151.

45. Monaco JJ, Cho S, Attaya M. Transport protein genes in the murine MHC: possible implications for antigen processing. *Science* 1990;250(4988):1723–1726.

46. Regelmann WE, Skubitz KM, Herron, JM. Increased monocyte oxidase activity in cystic fibrosis heterozygotes and homozygotes. *Am J Respir Cell Mol Biol* 1991;5(1):27–33.

47. Pfeffer KD, Huecksteadt TP, Hoidal JR. Expression and regulation of tumor necrosis factor in macrophages from cystic fibrosis patients. *Am J Respir Cell Mol Biol* 1993;9(5):511–519.

48. Matthews WJ Jr, Williams M, Oliphint B, et al. Hypogammaglobulinemia in patients with cystic fibrosis. *N Engl J Med* 1980;302(5):245–249.

49. Moss RB, Hsu YP, Van Eede PH, et al. Altered antibody isotype in cystic fibrosis: impaired natural antibody response to polysaccharide antigens. *Pediatr Res* 1987;22(6):708–713.

50. Pedersen SS. Lung infection with alginate-producing, mucoid *Pseudomonas aeruginosa* in cystic fibrosis. *APMIS Suppl* 1992;28:1–79.

51. Hoiby N. *Pseudomonas aeruginosa* infection in cystic fibrosis: diagnostic and prognostic significance of *Pseudomonas aeruginosa* precipitins determined by means of crossed immunoelectrophoresis, a survey. *Acta Pathol Microbiol Scand Suppl (C)* 1977;262: 1–96.

52. Hollsing AE, Granstrom M, Vasil ML, et al. Prospective study of serum antibodies to *Pseudomonas aeruginosa* exoproteins in cystic fibrosis. *J Clin Microbiol* 1987;25(10):1868–1874.

53. Eichler I, Joris L, Hsu YP, et al. Nonopsonic antibodies in cystic fibrosis. *Pseudomonas aeruginosa* lipopolysaccharide-specific immunoglobulin G antibodies from infected patient sera inhibit neutrophil oxidative responses. *J Clin Invest* 1989;84(6):1794–1804.

54. Winnie GB, Klinger JD, Sherman JM, et al. Induction of phagocytic inhibitory activity in cats with chronic *Pseudomonas aeruginosa* pulmonary infection. *Infect Immunol* 1982;38(3):1088–1093.

55. Berger M, Norvell TM, Tosi MF, et al. Tissue-specific Fcγ and complement receptor expression by alveolar macrophages determines relative importance of IgG and complement in promoting phagocytosis of *Pseudomonas aeruginosa*. *Pediatr Res* 1994; 35(1):68–77.

56. Hornick DB, Fick RB Jr. The immunoglobulin G subclass composition of immune complexes in cystic fibrosis. Implications for the pathogenesis of the *Pseudomonas* lung lesion. *J Clin Invest* 1990;86(4): 1285–1292.

57. Thomassen MJ, Demko CA, Wood RE, et al. Ultrastructure and function of alveolar macrophages from cystic fibrosis patients. *Pediatr Res* 1980;14(5): 715–721.

58. Hancock REW, Mutharia LM, Chan L, et al. *Pseudomonas aeruginosa* isolates from patients with cystic fibrosis: a class of serum-sensitive, nontypable strains deficient in lipopolysaccharide O side chains. *Infect Immunol* 1983;42(1):170–177.

59. Pier GB, Saunders JM, Ames P, et al. Opsonophagocytic killing antibody to *Pseudomonas aeruginosa* mucoid exopolysaccharide in older noncolonized patients with cystic fibrosis. *N Engl J Med* 1987;317 (3):793–798.

60. Pier GB, Small GJ, Warrens HB. Protection against mucoid *Pseudomonas aeruginosa* in rodent models of endobronchial infections. *Science* 1990;249(4968): 537–540.

61. Thornton MO, Fuller SA, Pekoe GM, et al. Progress of clinical trials with a mucoid *Pseudomonas aeruginosa* (MEP) vaccine and an opsonic anti-MEP hyperimmune immunoglobulin for use in cystic fibrosis patients. *Pediatr Pulmonol Suppl* 1993;9:161–162 (abstract).

62. Tosi MF, Zakem-Cloud H, Demko CA, et al. Cross-sectional and longitudinal studies of naturally-occurring antibodies to *Pseudomonas aeruginosa* in cystic fibrosis indicate absence of antibody mediated protection and decline in opsonic quality after infection. *J Infect Dis* 1995;172:453–461.

63. Pier GB, Grout M, Desjardins D. Complement deposition by antibodies to *Pseudomonas aeruginosa* mucoid exopolysaccharide (MEP) and by non-MEP specific opsonins. *J Immunol* 1991;147(6):1869–1876.

64. Sturgess J, Imrie J. Quantitative evaluation of the development of tracheal submucosal glands in infants with cystic fibrosis and control infants. *Am J Pathol* 1982;106(3):303–311.

65. Tomashefski JF Jr, Vawter GF, Reid L. Pulmonary pathology. In: Hodson ME, Norman AP, Batten JC, eds. *Cystic fibrosis.* London: Bailliere Tindall, 1983: 31–51.

66. Smyth RL, Higenbottam T, Scott J, et al. Cystic fibrosis: 5, the current state of lung transplantation for cystic fibrosis. *Thorax* 1991;46(3):213–216.

67. Hoiby N, Pedersen SS. Estimated risk of cross-infection with *Pseudomonas aeruginosa* in Danish cystic fibrosis patients. *Acta Pediatr Scand* 1989;78(3): 395–404.

68. Pedersen SS, Jensen T, Pressler T, et al. Does centralized treatment of cystic fibrosis increase the risk of *Pseudomonas aeruginosa* infection? *Acta Pediatr Scand* 1986;75(5):840–845.

69. Stern RC, Boat TF, Doershuk CF, et al. Cystic fibrosis diagnosed after age 13: twenty-five teenage and adult patients including three asymptomatic men. *Ann Intern Med* 1977;87(12):188–191.

70. May JR, Herrick NC, Thompson D. Bacterial infection in cystic fibrosis. *Arch Dis Child* 1972;47(256): 908–913.

71. Ramsey BW, Wentz KR, Smith AL, et al. Predictive value of oropharyngeal cultures for identifying lower airway bacteria in cystic fibrosis patients. *Am Rev Respir Dis* 1991;44:331–337.

72. LiPuma JJ, Dasen SE, Nielson DW, et al. Person-to-person transmission of *Pseudomonas cepacia* between patients with cystic fibrosis. *Lancet* 1990;336 (8723):1094–1096.

73. Tablan OC, Martone WJ, Doershuk CF, et al. Colonization of the respiratory tract with *Pseudomonas cepacia* in cystic fibrosis: risk factors and outcomes. *Chest* 1987;91(4):527–532.

74. Thomassen MJ, Demko CA, Doershuk CF, et al. *Pseudomonas cepacia*: decrease in colonization in patients with cystic fibrosis. *Am Rev Respir Dis* 1986;134(4):669–671.

75. Vishwanath S, Ramphal R. Adherence of *Pseudomonas aeruginosa* to human tracheobronchial mucin. *Infect Immunol* 1984;45(1):197–202.

76. Vishwanath S. Ramphal R. Tracheobronchial mucin receptor for *Pseudomonas aeruginosa*: predominance of amino sugars in binding sites. *Infect Immunol* 1985;48(2)331–335.

77. Sajjan U, Reisman J, Doig P, et al. Binding of nonmucoid *Pseudomonas aeruginosa* to normal human intestinal mucin and respiratory mucin from patients with cystic fibrosis. *J Clin Invest* 1992;89(2):657–665.

78. Plotkowski MC, Chevillard M, Pierrot D, et al. Differential adhesion of *Pseudomonas aeruginosa* to human respiratory epithelial cells in primary culture. *J Clin Invest* 1991;87(6):2018–2028.

79. Woods DE, Straus DC, Johanson WG, Jr et al. Role of fibronectin in the prevention of adherence of *Pseudomonas aeruginosa* to buccal cells. *J Infect Dis* 1981;143(6):784–790.

80. Suter S, Schaad UB, Morgenthaler JJ, et al. Fibronectin-cleaving activity in bronchial secretions of patients with cystic fibrosis. *J Infect Dis* 1988;158 (1):89–100.

81. Plotkowski MC, Beck G, Tournier JM, et al. Adherence of *Pseudomonas aeruginosa* to respiratory epithelium and the effect of leucocyte elastase. *J Med Microbiol* 1989;30(4):285–293.

82. Krivan HC, Ginsburg V, Roberts DD. *Pseudomonas aeruginosa* and *Pseudomonas cepacia* isolated from cystic fibrosis patients bind specifically to gangliotetraosylceramide (asialo-GM1) and gangliotriaosylceramide (asialo-GM2). *Arch Biochem Biophys* 1988; 260(1):493–496.

83. Cheng PW, Boat TF, Cranfill K, et al. Increased sulfation of glycoconjugates by cultured nasal epithelial cells from patients with cystic fibrosis. *J Clin Invest* 1989;84(1):68–72.

84. Barasch J, Kiss B, Prince A, et al. Defective acidification of intracellular organelles in cystic fibrosis. *Nature* 1991;352(6330):70–73.

85. Wesley A, Forstner J, Qureshi R, et al. Human intestinal mucin in cystic fibrosis. *Pediatr Res* 1983;17: 65–69.

86. Saiman L, Cacalano G, Gruenert D, et al. Comparison of adherence of *Pseudomonas aeruginosa* to respiratory epithelial cells from cystic fibrosis patients and healthy subjects. *Infect Immunol* 1992;60(7): 2808–2814.

87. Saiman L, Prince A. *Pseudomonas aeruginosa* pili bind to asialoGM1 which is increased on the surface of cystic fibrosis epithelial cells. *J Clin Invest* 1993; 92(4):1875–1880.

88. Zar H, Saiman L, Quittell L, et al. Correlation between CF genotype and *P. aeruginosa* adherence to respiratory epithelial cells. *Pediatr Res* 1993;33(4 pt 2):389A (abstract).

89. Imundo L, Barasch J, Prince A, et al. Cystic fibrosis epithelial cells have a receptor for pathogenic bacteria on their apical surface. *Proc Natl Acad Sci U S A* 1995;92:3019–3023.

90. DiMango E, Zar HJ, Bryan R, et al. Diverse *Pseudomonas aeruginosa* gene products stimulate respiratory epithelial cells to produce interleukin-8. *J Clin Invest* 1995;96:2204–2210.

91. May TB, Shinabarger D, Maharaj R, et al. Alginate synthesis by *Pseudomonas aeruginosa*: a key pathogenic factor in chronic pulmonary infections of cystic fibrosis patients. *Clin Microbiol Rev* 1991;4(2):191–206.

92. Anwar H, Strap JL, Costerton JW. Susceptibility of biofilm cells of *Pseudomonas aeruginosa* to bactericidal actions of whole blood and serum. *FEMS Microbiol Lett* 1992;71(3):235–241.

93. Meluleni GJ, Grout M, Evans DJ, et al. Mucoid *Pseudomonas aeruginosa* growing in a biofilm *in vitro* are killed by opsonic antibodies to the mucoid exopolysaccharide capsule but not by antibodies produced during chronic lung infection in cystic fibrosis patients. *J Immunol* 1995;155:2029–2038.

94. Lam J, Chan R, Lam K, et al. Production of mucoid microcolonies by *Pseudomonas aeruginosa* within infected lungs in cystic fibrosis. *Infect Immunol* 1980;28(2):546–556.

95. Slack MPE, Nichols WW. The penetration of antibiotics through sodium alginate and through the exopolysaccharide of a mucoid strain of *Pseudomonas aeruginosa*. *Lancet* 1981;11(8245):502–503.

96. Bayer AS, Speert DP, Park S, et al. Functional role of mucoid exopolysaccharide (alginate) in antibiotic-induced and polymorphonuclear leukocyte-mediated killing of *Pseudomonas aeruginosa*. *Infect Immunol* 1991; 59(1):302–308.

97. Learn DB, Brestel EP, Seetharama S. Hypochlorite scavenging by *Pseudomonas aeruginosa* alginate. *Infect Immunol* 1987;55(8):1813–1818.

98. Woods DE, Sokol PA, Bryan LE et al. *In vivo* regulation of virulence in *Pseudomonas aeruginosa* associated with genetic rearrangement. *J Infect Dis* 1991; 163(1):143–149.

99. Martin DW, Schurr MJ, Mudd MH, et al. Mechanism of conversion to mucoidy in *Pseudomonas aeruginosa* infecting cystic fibrosis patients. *Proc Natl Acad Sci U S A* 1993;90(18):8377–8381.

100. Roychoudhury S, Zielinski NA, Devault JD, et al. *Pseudomonas aeruginosa* infection in cystic fibrosis: biosynthesis of alginate as a virulence factor. *Antibiot Chemother* 1991;44(1):63–67.

101. Mizgerd JP, Kobzik L, Warner AE, et al. Effects of sodium concentration on human neutrophil bactericidal functions. *Am J Physiol* 1995;269 (*Lung Cell Mol Physiol* 13):L388–L393.

102. Smith JJ, Travis SM, Greenberg EP, et al. Cystic fibrosis airway epithelia fail to kill bacteria because of abnormal airway surface fluid. *Cell* 1996;85:229–236.

103. Pier GB, Grout M, Zaidi TS, et al. Role of mutant CFTR in hypersusceptibility of cystic fibrosis patients to lung infections. *Science* 1996;271:64–67.

104. Klinger JD, Straus DC, Hilton CB, et al. Antibodies to proteases and exotoxin A of *Pseudomonas aeruginosa* in patients with cystic fibrosis: demonstration by radioimmunoassay. *J Infect Dis* 1978;138(1): 49–58.

105. Nutman J, Berger M, Chase PA, et al. Studies on the mechanism of T cell inhibition by the *Pseudomonas aeruginosa* phenazine pigment pyocyanine. *J Immunol* 1987;138(10):3481–3487.

106. Wilson R, Pitt T, Taylor G, et al. Pycocyanin and 1-hydroxyphenazine produced by *Pseudomonas aeruginosa* inhibit the beating of human respiratory cilia *in vitro*. *J Clin Invest* 1987;79(1):221–229.

107. Sokol PA, Woods DE. Relationship of iron and extracellular factors to *Pseudomonas aeruginosa* lung infections. *J Med Microbiol* 1984;18(1):125–133.

108. Coffman TJ, Cox CD, Edeker BL, et al. Possible role of bacterial siderophores in inflammation. *J Clin Invest* 1990;86(4):1030–1037.

109. Demko CA, Byard PJ, Davis PB. Gender differences in cystic fibrosis: *Pseudomonas aeruginosa* infection. *J Clin Epidemiol* 1995;48:1041–1049.

110. Birrer P, McElvaney NG, Rüdeberg A, et al. Protease-antiprotease imbalance in the lungs of children with cystic fibrosis. *Am J Respir Crit Care Med* 1994;150:207–213.

111. Cantin A. Cystic fibrosis lung inflammation: early, sustained, and severe. *Am J Respir Crit Care Med* 1995;151:939–941.

112. Bedrossian CWM, Greenberg SD, Singer DB, et al. The lung in cystic fibrosis: a quantitative study including prevalence of pathologic findings among different age groups. *Hum Pathol* 1976;7(2):195–204.

113. Baltimore RS, Christie CDC, Smith GJ. Immunohistopathologic localization of *Pseudomonas aeruginosa* in lungs from patients with cystic fibrosis: implications for the pathogenesis of progressive lung deterioration. *Am Rev Respir Dis* 1989;140(6): 1650–1661.

114. Meyer KC, Zimmerman J. Neutrophil mediators, Pseudomonas, and pulmonary dysfunction in cystic fibrosis. *J Lab Clin Med* 1993;121(5):654–661.

115. Shute JK. IL-8 in cystic fibrosis and its regulation by complexation with macromolecules. *Pediatr Pulmonol Suppl* 1996;13:187–188.

116. Tichatschek E, Sanz C, Gotz M. IL-1, IL-6 and TNF alpha in peripheral mononuclear cells secreted after stimulation with LPS in patients with cystic fibrosis. *Pediatr Pulmonol Suppl* 1991;6:303 (abstract).

117. Pfeffer K, Huecksteadt T, Hoidal J. Tumor necrosis factor: *in vitro* production and expression in macrophages from CF patients. *Pediatr Pulmonol Suppl* 1991;6:303 (abstract).

118. Allen ED, Allen JN, McCoy KS. Comparison of interleukin-1β production in normals vs. CF patients. *Pediatr Pulmonol Suppl* 1991;6:304 (abstract).

119. Wilmott RW, Kociela V, Frenzke M. Relationship of peripheral blood cytokine concentrations and cytokine production to clinical status in cystic fibrosis (CF). *Pediatr Pulmonol Suppl* 1991;6:304 (abstract).

120. Tracey KJ, Cerami A. TNF and regulation of metabolism in infection: role of systemic vs. tissue levels. *Proc Soc Exp Biol Med* 1992;200:233–239.

121. Fick RB, Standiford TJ, Kunkel SL, et al. Interleukin-8 (IL-8) and neutrophil accumulation in the inflammatory airways disease of cystic fibrosis (CF). *Clin Res* 1991;39(2):292A (abstract).

122. Dean TP, Dai Y, Shute JK, et al. Interleukin-8 concentrations are elevated in bronchoalveolar lavage, sputum, and sera of children with cystic fibrosis. *Pediatr Res* 1993;34:159–161.

123. Richman-Eisenstat JB, Jorens PG, Heberg CA, et al. Interleukin-8: an important chemoattractant in sputum of patients with chronic inflammatory airway diseases. *Am J Physiol* 1993;264(4 pt 1):L413–L418.

124. Wilmott RW, Kassab JT, Kilian PL, et al. Increased levels of interleukin-1 in bronchoalveolar washings from children with bacterial pulmonary infections. *Am Rev Respir Dis* 1990;142(2):365–368.

125. Balcom DF, Kushmericks PS, Casey SC, et al. Cytokines and clinical status in CF patients. *Pediatr Pulmonol Suppl* 1991;6:302 (abstract).

126. Brown MA, Scuderi P, McIntosh JC, et al. Relation between tumor necrosis factor-α and granulocyte elastase-α1-proteinase inhibitor complexes in the plasma of patients with cystic fibrosis. *Am Rev Respir Dis* 1990;142(4):984–985.

127. Bonfield TL, Konstan MW, Burfeind P, et al. Normal bronchial epithelial cells constitutively produce the anti-inflammatory cytokine IL-10 which is downregulated in cystic fibrosis. *Am J Respir Cell Mol Biol* 1995;13:257–261.

128. Hostoffer RW, Krukovets I, Berger M. Enhancement by tumor necrosis factor-α of Fca receptor expression and IgA mediated superoxide generation and killing of *P. aeruginosa* by polymorphonuclear leukocytes. *J Infect Dis* 1994;170(1):82–87.

129. Klebanoff SJ, Vadas MA, Harlan JM, Gamble JR, Agosti JM, Waltersdorph M. Stimulation of neutrophils by tumor necrosis factor. *J Immunol* 1986; 136:4220–4225.

130. Cerami A, Beutler B. The role of cachectin/TNF in endotoxic shock and cachexia. *Immunol Today* 1988;9(1):28–31.

131. Nakamura, H, Yoshimura K, McElvaney NG, et al. Neutrophil elastase in respiratory epithelial lining fluid of individuals with cystic fibrosis induces interleukin-8 gene expression in a human bronchial epithelial cell line. *J Clin Invest* 1992;89(5):1478–1484.

132. Massion PP, Inoue H, Richman-Eisentat J, et al. Novel Pseudomonas product stimulates interleukin-8 production in airway epithelial cells *in vitro. J Clin Invest* 1994;93(1):T26–T32.

133. McElvaney NG, Nakamura H, Birrer P, et al. Modulation of airway inflammation in cystic fibrosis: *in vivo* suppression of interleukin-8 levels on the respiratory epithelial surface by aerosolization of recombinant secretory leukoprotease inhibitor. *J Clin Invest* 1992;90(4):1296–1301.

134. Kirchner KK, Khan TZ, Wagener JS, et al. Increased DNA levels in bronchoalveolar lavage fluid obtained from infants with cystic fibrosis. *Am J Respir Crit Care Med* 1996;154:1426–1429.

135. Bonfield TL, Konstan MW, Panuska JR, et al. Normal bronchial epithelial cells produce the anti-inflammatory cytokine IL-10 which is down regulated in CF, while IL-8 is upregulated. *Pediatr Pulmonol* 1995; 19:73 (abstract).

136. Garofalo R, Manganaro M, Mei F, et al. Respiratory syncytial virus (RSV) glycoproteins induce interleukin-8 (IL-8) production by airway epithelial cells. *Clin Res* 1993;41(4):764A.

137. Moore KW, O'Garra A, de Waal Malefyt R, et al. Interleuken-10. *Annu Rev Immunol* 1993;11:165–190.

138. Jorens PG, Richman-Eisenstat JBY, Housset BP, et al. Interleukin-8 induces neutrophil accumulation but not protease secretion in the canine trachea. *Am J Physiol* 1992;263(G pt 1):L708–L713.

139. Albelda SM, Smith CW, Ward PA. Adhesion molecules and inflammatory injury. *FASEB J* 1994;8:504–512.

140. Jesaitis AJ, Quinn MT, Mukherjee G, et al. Death by oxygen: radical views, the molecular basis of oxidative damage by leukocytes. A Montana State University/Keystone Symposium, Big Sky, January 28–February 3, 1991. *New Biol* 1991;3(7):651–655.

141. Phan SH, Gannon DE, Ward PA, et al. Mechanism of neutrophil-induced xanthine dehydrogenase to xanthine oxidase conversion in endothelial cells: evidence of a role for elastase. *Am J Respir Cell Mol Biol* 1992;6(3):270–278.

142. Tosi MF, Stark JM, Smith CW, et al. Induction of ICAM-1 expression on human airway epithelial cells by inflammatory cytokines: effects on neutrophil-epithelial cell adhesion. *Am J Respir Cell Mol Biol* 1992;7:(2)214–221.

143. Tosi M, Hamedani A, Zakem H, et al. Induction of intercellular adhesion molecule-1 (ICAM-1) on cultured primary human airway epithelial cells by supernatants of bronchoalveolar lavage fluid (BAL) from patients with CF. *Pediatr Pulmonol Suppl* 1994; 10:284 (abstract).

144. Barton AD, Ryder K, Lourenco RV, et al. Inflammatory reaction and airway damage in cystic fibrosis. *J Lab Clin Med* 1976;88(3):423–426.

145. Smith AL, Redding G, Doershuk C, et al. Sputum changes associated with therapy for endobronchial exacerbation in cystic fibrosis. *J Pediatr* 1988;112 (4):547–554.

146. Goldstein W, Doring G. Lysosomal enzymes from polymorphonuclear leukocytes and proteinase inhibitors in patients with cystic fibrosis. *Am Rev Respir Dis* 1986;134(1):46–56.

147. Regelmann WE, Elliott GR, Warwick WJ et al. Reduction of sputum *Pseudomonas aeruginosa* density by antibiotics improves lung function in cystic fibrosis more than do bronchodilators and chest physiotherapy alone. *Am Rev Respir Dis* 1990;141:914–921.

148. Weiss SJ. Tissue destruction by neutrophils. *N Engl J Med* 1989;320(6):365–376.

149. Weissmann G, Smolen JE, Korchak, HM. Release of inflammatory mediators from stimulated neutrophils. *N Engl J Med* 1980;303(1):27–34.

150. Gallin JI. Neutrophil specific granules: a fuse that ignites the inflammatory response. *Clin Res* 1984;32 (3):320–328.

151. Wright SD, Silverstein SC. Phagocytosing macrophages exclude proteins from the zones of contact with opsonized targets. *Nature* 1984;309(5966): 359–361.

152. Rice WG, Weiss SJ. Regulation of proteolysis at the neutrophil-substrate interface by secretory leukoprotease inhibitor. *Science* 1990;249(4965):178–181.

153. Fontan PA, Amura CR, Garcia VE, et al. Preliminary characterization of *Pseudomonas aeruginosa* peptide chemotactins for polymorphonuclear leukocytes. *Infect Immunol* 1992;60(6):2465–2469.

154. Fick RB, Jr, Robbins RA, Squier SU, et al. Complement activation in cystic fibrosis respiratory fluids: *in vivo* and *in vitro* generation of C5a and chemotactic activity. *Pediatr Res* 1986;20(21):1258–1268.

155. Marom Z, Shelhamer J, Berger M, et al. Anaphylatoxin C3a enhances mucous glycoprotein release from human airways *in vitro. J Exp Med* 1985;161 (4):657–668.

156. Martin TR, Altman LC, Albert RK, et al. Leukotriene B4 production by the human alveolar macrophage: a potential mechanism for amplifying inflammation in the lung. *Am Rev Respir Dis* 1984;129(1):106–111.

157. Martin TR, Pistorese BP, Chi Ey, et al. Effects of leukotriene B4 in the human lung: recruitment of neutrophils into the alveolar spaces without a change in protein permeability. *J Clin Invest* 1989;84(5):1609–1619.

158. Cromwell O, Walport MJ, Morris HR, et al. Identification of leukotrienes D and B in sputum from cystic fibrosis patients. *Lancet* 1981;ii(8239):164–165.

159. Zakrzewski JT, Barnes NC, Costello JF, et al. Lipid mediators in cystic fibrosis and chronic obstructive pulmonary disease. *Am Rev Respir Dis* 1987;136 (3):779–782.

160. Konstan MW, Walenga RW, Hilliard KA, et al. Leukotriene B$_4$ markedly elevated in the epithelial lining fluid of patients with cystic fibrosis. *Am Rev Respir Dis* 1993;148(4 pt 1):896–901.

161. Lawrence R, Sorrell T. Eicosapentaenoic acid in cystic fibrosis: evidence of a pathogenetic role for leukotriene B4. *Lancet* 1993;342(8869), 465–469.

162. Berger M, Sorensen RU, Tosi MF, et al. Complement receptor expression on neutrophils at an inflammatory site, the Pseudomonas-infected lung in cystic fibrosis. *J Clin Invest* 1989;84(4):1302–1313.

163. Shak S, Capon DJ, Hellmiss R, et al. Recombinant human DNase I reduces the viscosity of cystic fibro-

sis sputum. *Proc Natl Acad Sci U S A* 1990;87 (23):9188–9192.

164. Shah PL, Scott SF, Knight RA, et al. The effects of recombinant human DNase on neutrophil elastase activity and interleukin-8 levels in the sputum of patients with cystic fibrosis. *Eur Respir J* 1996;9:531–534.

165. Costello CM, O'Connor CM, Finlay GA, et al. Effect of nebulised recombinant DNase on neutrophil elastase load in cystic fibrosis. *Thorax* 1996;51:619–623.

166. Boat TF, Cheng PW, Iyer RN, et al. Human respiratory tract secretions: mucous glycoproteins of nonpurulent tracheobronchial secretions, and sputum of patients with bronchitis and cystic fibrosis. *Arch Biochem Biophys* 1976;177(1):95–104.

167. Cross CE, Halliwell B. Considerations of free radical injury in CF. *Pediatr Pulmonol Suppl* 1993;9:112 (abstract).

168. Witko-Sarsat V, Delacourt C, Rabier D, et al. Neutrophil-derived long-lived oxidants in cystic fibrosis sputum. *Am J Respir Crit Care Med* 1995;152: 1910–1916.

169. Regelmann WE, Siefferman CM, Herron JM, et al. Sputum peroxidase activity correlates with the severity of lung disease in cystic fibrosis. *Pediatr Pulmonol* 1995;19:1–9.

170. Cantin A, Woods DE. Protection by antibiotics against myeloperoxidase-dependent cytotoxicity to lung epithelial cells *in vitro*. *J Clin Invest* 1993;91(1): 38–45.

171. Britigan BE, Edeker BL. Pseudomonas and neutrophil products modify transferrin and lactoferrin to create conditions that favor hydroxyl radical formation. *J Clin Invest* 1991;88(4):1092–1102.

172. Britigan BE. Pseudomonas secretory products, hydroxyl radical production, and lung injury in CF. *Pediatr Pulmonol Suppl* 1993;9:110 (abstract).

173. Britigan BE, Hayek MB, Doebbeling BN, et al. Transferrin and lactoferrin undergo proteolytic cleavage in the Pseudomonas-infected lungs of patients with cystic fibrosis. *Infect Immunol* 1993;61(12): 5049–5055.

174. Carp H, Janoff A. Potential mediator of inflammation: Phagocyte-derived oxidants suppress the elastase-inhibitory capacity of α_1-proteinase inhibitor *in vitro*. *J Clin Invest* 1980;66(5):987–995.

175. Janoff A. Emphysema: proteinase-antiproteinase imbalance. In: Goldstein IM, Snyderman R, eds. *Inflammation: basic principles and clinical correlates.* New York: Raven Press, 1988:803–814.

176. Tegner H. Quantitation of human granulocyte protease inhibitors in non-purulent bronchial lavage fluids. *Acta Otolaryngol* 1978;85(3–4):282–289.

177. Ohlsson K. Interactions between granulocyte proteases and protease inhibitors in the lung. *Clin Respir Physiol* 1980;16(suppl):209–222.

178. Johnson DA, Carter-Hamm B, Dralle WM. Inactivation of human bronchial mucosal proteinase inhibitor by *Pseudomonas aeruginosa* elastase. *Am Rev Respir Dis* 1982;126(6):1070–1073.

179. Morihara K, Tsuzuki H, Oda K. Protease and elastase of *Pseudomonas aeruginosa*: inactivation of human plasma α_1-proteinase inhibitor. *Infect Immunol* 1979; 24(1):188–193.

180. Tournier JM, Jacquot J, Puchelle E, et al. Evidence that *Pseudomonas aeruginosa* elastase does not inactivate the bronchial inhibitor in the presence of leukocyte elastase: studies with cystic fibrosis sputum and with pure proteins. *Am Rev Respir Dis* 1985;132(3):524–528.

181. Suter S, Chevallier I. Proteolytic inactivation of α_1-proteinase inhibitor in infected bronchial secretions from patients with cystic fibrosis. *Eur Respir J* 1991;4(1):40–49.

182. Cantin A, Bilodeau G, Begin, R. Granulocyte elastase-mediated proteolysis of alpha₁-antitrypsin in cystic fibrosis bronchopulmonary secretions. *Pediatr Pulmonol* 1989;7:12–17.

183. Mandl I, Keller S, Cohen B. Microbial elastases: a comparative study. *Proc Soc Exp Biol Med* 1962;109 (4):923–925.

184. Banda MJ, Werb Z. Mouse macrophage elastase: purification and characterization as a metalloproteinase. *Biochem J* 1981;193(2):589–605.

185. Chung Y, Kercsmar CM, Davis PB. Ferret tracheal epithelial cells grown *in vitro* are resistant to lethal injury by activated neutrophils. *Am J Respir Cell Mol Biol* 1991;5(2):125–132.

186. Bruce MC, Poncz L, Klinger JD, et al. Biochemical and pathologic evidence for proteolytic destruction of lung connective tissue in cystic fibrosis. *Am Rev Respir Dis* 1985;132(3):529–535.

187. Stone PJ, Konstan M, Berger M, et al. Elastin and collagen degradation products in urine of patients with cystic fibrosis. *Am J Respir Crit Care Med* 1995;152:157–162.

188. Snider GL, Lucey EC, Christensen TG, et al. Emphysema and bronchial secretory cell metaplasia induced in hamsters by human neutrophil products. *Am Rev Respir Dis* 1984;129(1):155–160.

189. Lucey EC, Stone PJ, Ciccolella DE, et al. Recombinant human secretory leukocyte-protease inhibitor: *in vitro* properties, and amelioration of human neutrophil elastase-induced emphysema and secretory cell metaplasia in the hamster. *J Lab Clin Med* 1990;115(2):224–232.

190. Sommerhoff CP, Nadel JA, Basbaum CB, et al. Neutrophil elastase and cathepsin G stimulate secretion from cultured bovine airway gland serous cells. *J Clin Invest* 1990;85(3):682–699.

191. Schuster A, Ueki I, Nadel JA. Neutrophil elastase stimulates tracheal submucosal gland secretion that is inhibited by ICI 200,355. *Am J Physiol* 1992;262(1 pt 1):L86–L91.

192. Klinger JD, Tandler B, Liedtke CM, et al. Proteinases of *Pseudomonas aeruginosa* evoke mucin release by tracheal epithelium. *J Clin Invest* 1984;74(5): 1669–1678.

193. Tegner H, Ohlsson K, Toremalm NG, et al. Effect of human leukocyte enzymes on tracheal mucosa and its mucociliary activity. *Rhinology* 1979;17(3):199–206.

194. Smallman LA, Hill SL, Stockley RA. Reduction of ciliary beat frequency *in vitro* by sputum from patients with bronchiectasis: a serine proteinase effect. *Thorax* 1984;39(9):663–667.

195. LeVine AM, Bruno MD, Whitset JA, et al. Group B streptococcal infection in SP-AA deficient mice. *Pediatr Pulmonol Suppl* 1996;13:332.

196. Abraham SN, Beachey EH, Simpson WA. Adherence of *Streptococcus pyogenes*, *Escherichia coli*, and *Pseudomonas aeruginosa* to fibronectin-coated and

uncoated epithelial cells. *Infect Immunol* 1983;41(3): 1261–1268.

197. Tosi MF, Zakem H, Berger M. Neutrophil elastase cleaves C3bi on opsonized pseudomonas as well as CR1 on neutrophils to create a functionally important opsonin receptor mismatch. *J Clin Invest* 1990;86(1): 300–308.

198. McElvaney NG, Hubbard RC, Birrer P, et al. Aerosol α₁-antitrypsin treatment for cystic fibrosis. *Lancet* 1991;337(8738):392–394.

199. Fick RB Jr, Naegel GP, Squier SU, et al. Proteins of the cystic fibrosis respiratory tract: fragmented immunoglobulin G opsonic antibody causing defective opsonophagocytosis. *J Clin Invest* 1984;74(1):236–248.

200. Fick RB Jr, Baltimore RS, Squier SU, et al. IgG proteolytic activity of *Pseudomonas aeruginosa* in cystic fibrosis. *J Infect Dis* 1985;151(4):589–598.

201. Pedersen BK, Kharazmi A, Theander TG, et al. Selective modulation of the CD4 molecular complex by *Pseudomonas aeruginosa* alkaline protease and elastase. *Scand J Immunol* 1987;26(1):91–94.

202. Pedersen, BK, Kharazmi, A. Inhibition of human natural killer cell activity by *Pseudomonas aeruginosa* alkaline protease and elastase. *Infect Immunol* 1987; 55(4):986–989.

203. Horvat RT, Parmely MJ. *Pseudomonas aeruginosa* alkaline protease degrades human gamma interferon and inhibits its bioactivity. *Infect Immunol* 1988;56 (1):2925–2932.

204. Horvat RT, Clabaugh M, Duval-Jobe C, et al. Inactivation of human gamma interferon by *Pseudomonas aeruginosa* proteases: elastase augments the effects of alkaline protease despite the presence of α2-macroglobulin. *Infect Immunol* 1989;57(6):1668–1674.

205. Konstan MW, Vargo KM, Davis PB. Ibuprofen attenuates the inflammatory response to *Pseudomonas aeruginosa* in a rat model of chronic pulmonary infection: implications for anti-inflammatory therapy in cystic fibrosis. *Am Rev Respir Dis* 1990;141: 186–192.

206. Konstan MW. Evolving anti-inflammatory therapy in cystic fibrosis. In: Ramsey BW, Hodson ME, eds. *New insights into cystic fibrosis.* Califon, NJ: Gardiner-Caldwell SynerMed, 1995:3(2):7–11.

207. Ramsey BW. Management of pulmonary disease in patients with cystic fibrosis. *N Engl J Med* 1996;335: 179–188.

208. Cryz SJ Jr, Wedgwood J, Lang AB, et al. Immunization of noncolonized cystic fibrosis patients against *Pseudomonas aeruginosa*. *J Infect Dis* 1994;169: 1159–1162.

209. Winnie GB, Cowan RG, and Wade NA. Intravenous immune globulin treatment of pulmonary exacerbations in cystic fibrosis. *J Pediatr* 1989;114:309–314.

210. Van Wye JE, Collins MS, Baylor M, et al. Pseudomonas hyperimmune globulin passive immunotherapy for pulmonary exacerbations in cystic fibrosis. *Pediatr Pulmonol* 1990;9:7–18.

211. Moss R, Fink R, Schroeder S, et al. Safety and pharmacokinetics of a mucoid Pseudomonas aeruginosa immune globulin, intravenous (human) in patients with cystic fibrosis: preliminary results of a phase I/II trial. *Pediatr Pulmonol* 1995;19:85 (abstract).

212. Fuchs HJ, Borowitz DS, Christiansen DH, et al. Effect of aerosolized recombinant human DNase on exacerbations of respiratory symptoms and on pulmonary function in patients with cystic fibrosis. *N Engl J Med* 1994;331:637–642.

213. Vasconnelles CA, Allen PG, Wohl ME, et al. Reduction in viscosity of cystic fibrosis sputum *in vitro* by gelsolin. *Science* 1994;263:969–971.

214. Rubin BK, Kater AP, Dian T, et al. Effects of thymosin b4 on cystic fibrosis sputum. *Pediatr Pulmonol Suppl* 1995;12:234.

215. Knowles MR, Church NL, Waltner WE, et al. A pilot study of aerosolized amiloride for the treatment of lung disease in cystic fibrosis. *N Engl J Med* 1990; 322:1189–1194.

216. Tomkiewicz RP, App EM, Zayas JG, et al. Amiloride inhalation therapy in cystic fibrosis: influence on ion content, hydration, and rheology of sputum. *Am Rev Respir Dis* 1993;148:1002–1007.

217. Knowles MR, Clarke LL, Boucher RC. Activation by extracellular nucleotides of chloride secretion in the airway epithelia of patients with cystic fibrosis. *N Engl J Med* 1991;325:533–538.

218. Auerbach HS, Williams M, Kirkpatrick JA, et al. Alternate-day prednisone reduces morbidity and improves pulmonary function in cystic fibrosis. *Lancet* 1985;2(8457):686–688.

219. Eigen H, Rosenstein BJ, FitzSimmons S, et al. A multicenter study of alternate-day prednisone therapy in patients with cystic fibrosis. *J Pediatr* 1995;126: 515–523.

220. Konstan MW, Byard PJ, Hoppel CL, et al. Effect of high-dose ibuprofen in patients with cystic fibrosis. *N Engl J Med* 1995;332:848–854.

221. Berger M, Konstan M, Hilliard J, et al. Aerosolized Prolastin (α1-protease inhibitor) in CF. *Pediatr Pulmonol* 1995;20:421 (abstract).

222. Rouhm JH, Buhl R, McElvaney NG, et al. Systemic deficiency of glutathione in cystic fibrosis. *J Appl Physiol* 1993;75:2419–2424.

223. Winklhofer-Roob BM, Schlegel-Haueter SE, Khoschsorur G, et al. Neutrophil elastase/α1-proteinase inhibitor complex levels decrease in plasma of cystic fibrosis patients during long-term oral beta-carotene supplementation. *Pediatr Res* 1996;40: 130–134.

224. Döring G, Goldstein W, Botzenhart K, et al. Elastase from polymorphonuclear leucocytes: a regulatory enzyme in immune complex disease. *Clin Exp Immunol* 1986;64(3):597–605.

225. Suter S, Schaad UB, Roux L, et al. Granulocyte neutral proteases and pseudomonas elastase as possible causes of airway damage in patients with cystic fibrosis. *J Infect Dis* 1984;149(4):523–531.

Cystic Fibrosis in Adults,
edited by J. R. Yankaskas and M. R. Knowles,
Lippincott-Raven Publishers, Philadelphia, 1999.

7

Standard Therapy of Cystic Fibrosis Lung Disease

Peadar G. Noone and Michael R. Knowles

Cystic Fibrosis/Pulmonary Research and Treatment Center, Division of Pulmonary and Critical Care Medicine, University of North Carolina School of Medicine, Chapel Hill, North Carolina

Cystic fibrosis (CF) is a multisystem disorder, but pulmonary disease is the predominant cause of morbidity and mortality (1,2). Although the airways of neonates with CF are not infected, chronic bacterial infection with *Staphylococcus aureus*, *Hemophilus influenzae*, and *Pseudomonas aeruginosa* occurs early in life. This is followed by chronic inflammation, ultimately leading to bronchiectasis. Despite aggressive therapy with airway clearance maneuvers and intravenous antibiotics, the clinical course is notable for slow but progressive deterioration in lung function and ultimately respiratory failure. Careful attention to detail with a therapeutic regimen can retard the progression of pulmonary disease in patients with CF. This chapter outlines a systematic approach for achieving that goal. Table 7–1 outlines an approach to the monitoring of CF in adults, as recommended by the Cystic Fibrosis Foundation guidelines committee (3).

Although our understanding of the pathogenesis of CF lung disease remains incomplete, a knowledge of the organ-level pathobiology is important to develop a rational approach to the management of patients with CF. In addition, a team, including specialized nurses, physical therapists, nutritionists and social workers is important to address the multifaceted aspects of the disease (Fig. 7–1). Patient compliance is an integral part of a successful therapeutic approach, and the patient must be involved in the contract of therapy. As patients grow older, partners and spouses can become involved.

In this chapter, established or recently published therapeutic modalities (4–10) are discussed. Better understanding of pathophysiologic events at molecular and cellular levels will give rise to newer, more specific approaches to treatment. For example, pharmacotherapy of ion transport mechanisms, antiinflammatory therapy, and gene transfer techniques are dealt with in other chapters. The treatment of significant pulmonary complications, such as respiratory failure, massive hemoptysis, pneumothorax, and lung transplantation, are addressed in Chapters 8 and 9.

THERAPIES

Airway Clearance

The airway secretions of patients with CF are thick, tenacious, and difficult to clear from the tracheobronchial tree. The pathophysiology underlying the abnormality in airway secretions in CF is complex, and a variety of mechanisms contribute to defective airway clearance. These mechanisms include abnormal ion transport, mucus hypersecretion involving abnormal mucin macromolecules, chronic inflammation, and high concentrations of DNA (see Chapter 3 for a full review of the pathophysiology of CF airways disease).

TABLE 7–1. *Outline of surveillance approach to adult patients with cystic fibrosis*

Three monthly clinic visits (more if required in individual cases), with a complete physical examination, including nasal examination for polyps

Spirograms on each visit (at least every 6 months)

Sputum culture on each visit (at least annually)

Chest radiograph at least annually, and when clinically indicated

Influenza vaccine annually

Arterial blood gases at least annually on patients with an FEV_1 less than 40% predicted value, including assessment of the need for nocturnal oxygen, or oxygen on exercise

Complete pulmonary function (lung volumes) annually

Review of chest physical therapy techniques and adherence to exercise on each visit (at least annually)

Psychosocial assessment, including vocational aspects, annually

Nutritional assessment annually, including serum albumin and liver function tests, and with assessment for diabetes mellitus

Fertility, pregnancy, and sexuality issues should be discussed, when appropriate

These recommendations are based on the minimum guidelines as recommended by the Cystic Fibrosis Foundation Guidelines Committee (some of the guidelines may not be absolute in individual patients, e.g., annual lung volumes or sputum cultures at each visit).

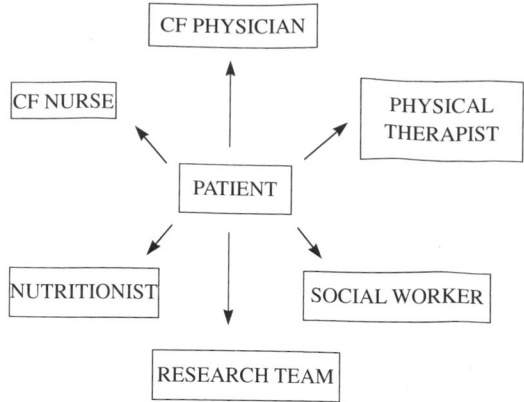

FIG. 7–1. Diagram illustrating the multidisciplinary team approach to the care of a patient with cystic fibrosis.

Defective cystic fibrosis transmembrane conductance regulator (CFTR)-mediated Cl⁻ secretion, coupled to Na⁺ hyperabsorption, contributes to the abnormality of airway secretions by limiting the ability of airway epithelium to regulate the consistency and depth of the periciliary fluid layer such that mucociliary clearance is impaired (11–13). To compound this problem, abnormal quantity and quality of mucin secretion further impairs the ability of cilia to clear the airways effectively (6). Whether this is a result of the basic defect in CF or whether it is a result of chronic inflammation is unclear as yet, but regardless, inflammation appears early in the course of the disease. Inflammatory mediators from both infectious agents and host defense cells are significant factors in damaging airway surfaces and further reducing effective mucociliary clearance (14,15). Human neutrophil elastase, in particular, is a major factor in damaging air-

way epithelial surfaces, disrupting ion transport and mucociliary clearance, and interfering with immune-mediated defenses (15). After chronic infection and inflammation is established, high concentrations of DNA are released from dead inflammatory cells, which adds to the viscosity of airway secretions. The end result of these factors is reduced airway clearance, with a cycle of infection and inflammation following. Ultimately airways damage ensues, leading to floppy, collapsing airways (ectasia) and significant lung damage (1).

The goal of airway clearance techniques is to aid in mechanical removal of these highly viscid airway secretions, which contain high concentrations of bacteria (10^8/mL purulent secretions), elastases, cytokines, and bacterial products. Reducing the burden of these agents limits this ongoing cycle of events. This can be achieved by several methods, ranging from traditional chest physiotherapy and physical exercise to the use of mechanical devices and specific breathing or coughing techniques (16). Although an extensive and controversial literature exists as to the benefits of the various forms of treatment in relation to each other, CF physicians agree that regular adherence to a planned regimen to clear airway secretions is beneficial (17). A recent meta-analysis of 35 studies using various combinations of chest physical therapy modalities concluded that standard chest physical therapy enhances sputum production and produces an improvement in forced expiratory volume in 1 second (FEV_1) (18).

Early aggressive therapy to clear airway secretions is warranted as early in the course of the disease as possible, even in patients with only mild lung dysfunction. Tests of mucociliary clearance indicate a reduction in small airways clearance in these patients with mild disease (19) and support the notion that efforts to clear the airways in such patients is important. In addition, inflammatory mediators and significant amounts of bacteria also are present very early in the course of the disease, even in very young children, which also suggests that early intervention to clear airway secretions would be beneficial (14,20).

Chest Physical Therapy

For decades, traditional chest physical therapy (CPT) has been a mainstay of clearance of airway secretions from patients with CF and comprises postural drainage, percussion/vibration techniques, breathing exercises, and directed cough. Newer techniques and devices strive to optimize the efficiency of airway clearance techniques and are dealt with in the following sections. Examples of such measures include use of the flutter valve, autogenic drainage (AD), the forced expiration technique (FET), positive expiratory pressure (PEP) mask, and high-frequency chest compression (vest). No specific form of chest physiotherapy has been demonstrated to be superior, and various combinations of all of the aforementioned are in general usage (16,17,21).

Postural drainage involves the use of gravity-assisted positions to assist clearance, either alone or with another individual performing physical percussion (postural drainage and percussion). This method can be used as the primary method of airway clearance, and many patients find this the optimal way to ensure adequate airway clearance. However, some patients prefer to employ other methods in addition to postural drainage. For example, postural drainage with the FET or percussive techniques can prove more efficient than postural drainage alone. Data showing increased tracheal mucus clearance and improved pulmonary function tests in stable patients in the short term support this notion (22,23). Postural drainage can be used with other techniques. The addition of phasic energies through percussion or vibration techniques through the chest wall enhances removal of secretions in stable patients with CF with moderate functional impairment, but without changes in tracheobronchial clearance rates (24). The overall aim of all of these techniques is to loosen secretions and facilitate mucociliary clearance. Cough also can be used as an adjunct to CPT (25). Cough alone can be as effective as other techniques at assisting removal of secretions in certain patients (26). However, conventional CPT is more effective than cough in patients with more severe disease, possibly because central airways collapse and increased obstruction occurs with cough alone (27,28).

Physical Exercise

Physical exercise has a central role in the management of patients with CF and physical conditioning is a strong predictor of survival. It augments airway clearance, improves cardiovascular physiologic parameters, and provides psychological benefits. The beauty of exercise also lies in its ease of use at home. The form of exercise need not be limited to any particular type but can be tailored to the individual's personal situation and preferences (29).

Several studies have addressed the role and benefits of exercise in CF, with documented objective physiologic improvements (see Chapter 17). The bronchodilator effects of exercise have been demonstrated (30). Sputum production can be increased with regular exercise (31), although there is no demonstrable increase in mucociliary clearance (32). Lung function can be improved, as can exercise endurance and cardiorespiratory fitness, even during an exacerbation (33–35). In a 10-week study of children with CF, a 30-minutes-a-day period of training improved many physiologic parameters, including vital capacity, total lung capacity, exercise tolerance, and inspiratory muscle strength (36). Most authors agree that exercise should be part of the maintenance therapy of patients with CF (17).

Patients with milder disease will usually have better exercise tolerance than those with more severe disease. Those with significant impairment of lung function should be assessed carefully for the risks of oxyhemoglobin desaturation when exercise is recommended as an adjunctive method of augmenting airway clearance. This assessment can be relatively easily done. The FEV_1/forced vital capacity (FVC) ratio correlates well with the risk of oxyhemoglobin desaturation—the lower the ratio, the more likely the patient will have a significant (5% to 10%) decrease in oxyhemoglobin saturation (37). Generally, most patients with CF are limited in their exercise by ventilatory capacity rather than cardiovascular factors. Thus, appropriate cardiovascular and lung function assessment during the setting up of an exercise program, with the help of experienced physical therapists, should make some form of exercise possible even for those with severe disease. Supplemental oxygen should be used if necessary to prevent arterial oxygen percent saturation (SaO_2) less than 90% (33).

Newer Breathing Techniques for Airway Clearance

Specific breathing techniques, such as the FET and autogenic drainage, appeal to certain groups of patients, particularly those who cannot tolerate postural drainage because of gastroesophageal reflux, or in those who have no one to assist them with percussion at home. However, these techniques do require intensive teaching and follow-up evaluation by a knowledgeable therapist.

The FET consists of huffs (forced expirations) through an open glottis followed by relaxation and controlled breathing, commencing from the midlung region and progressing to total lung capacity. As secretions reach upper airways, coughing completes clearance. The idea behind huffing is to produce less airway com-

pression than during coughing. Percussion or vibration by an assistant can enhance the technique, as can use of a PEP mask, which helps stent airways open during expiration (38, 39–41). Studies of the FET—with and without additional modalities as aforementioned—yield mixed results, with short-term studies demonstrating a benefit in those patients with mild to moderate disease; however, in the longer term, conventional CPT seems to be superior (23,42).

Autogenic drainage (self-drainage) is an airway clearance method used extensively in Europe, where it was first developed. The technique uses controlled breathing techniques to optimize airflow in different generations of bronchi, particularly in those prone to collapse, and it has been shown to be beneficial in terms of improved pulmonary function and enhanced clearance of secretions (43). By controlling breathing at various lung volumes from expiratory reserve volume through to inspiratory reserve volume, optimal airflow in different generations of bronchi can mobilize secretions without causing collapse. The technique requires education by an experienced therapist, a sensing on the part of the patient as to the area of lung that requires clearance, and training to control rate and depth of breathing. A disadvantage of this technique is the time it takes to clear airways adequately, that is, twice daily (approximately 30 minutes). It also requires a clear understanding on the part of the patient of the technique. However, it is attractive to some patients because it is relaxing and can be performed without assistance. It can be taught to younger patients and can be practiced anywhere, without special equipment. Like the active cycle of breathing technique, it is less likely to cause oxyhemoglobin desaturation, is better tolerated by patients, and is very effective at sputum clearance (44,45).

The active cycle of breathing technique is used very commonly in Britain and encompasses several techniques in combination—starting with breathing control, alternating with thoracic expansion exercises, and finishes with FET maneuvers—huffs and expectoration. Thoracic expansion exercises couple deep inspiration with relaxed expiration, allowing mobilization of secretions because of distal air flow (17). The technique often is used in conjunction with postural drainage positions and an assistant (unlike autogenic drainage), but it is possible to use the technique independently in the seated position (16).

Devices

The flutter valve recently was developed as a simple device to aid in clearance of airway secretions. It is approximately the same size as a metered dose inhaler, and one of the main advantages of this device is its portability. When the patient exhales through the device, a small metal ball oscillates inside the device, thus delivering a combination of positive end-expiratory pressure (PEEP) and oscillating wave forms. In the short term, it enhances sputum expectoration. A study of 18 patients with mild to moderate CF lung disease showed a threefold increase in sputum production with use of the flutter valve device compared with cough alone or a 15-minute postural drainage and percussion session (9). The evidence for its advantages over the long term remains to be seen (21,46). In the meantime, pending such data, patients appreciate its benefits and its ease of usage.

Another device to aid sputum clearance is the PEP mask, which is designed to deliver pressures from 10 to 20 cm H_2O. The patient uses it for approximately 2 minutes before other clearance maneuvers, such as the FET, if airway collapse during such maneuvers is perceived to be a problem. A system can be set up to use the device in conjunction with aerosolized bronchodilators to save time for patients. The patient uses a slightly forced expiratory technique, to prevent airways from collapsing. Studies to support usage of the PEP mask are few, but some do show that it is equivalent to conventional CPT alone (39). Most data, however, indicate that other methods clearly are superior, particularly in those patients with large (> 20 g daily) amounts of sputum (38). Therefore, data supporting the PEP mask is mixed, but some therapists and patients like it (39).

External thoracic devices, such as high-frequency chest compression (HFCC) performed via an inflatable vest, and ultrasonic percussors have been demonstrated to facilitate mucociliary clearance in animals, but their efficacy in CF is less certain. The oscillating compression of the thorax is conducted during exhalation and presumably produces intermittent increases in gas flow and increases removal of secretions. Some patients like the fact that these devices can be used without any assistance, in a passive manner, but this may lull the patients into a false sense of security that they themselves do not need to do anything else because the machine does it for them. Generally, data on the efficacy of these devices are scarce, although some evidence does perhaps support their usage, primarily through secondary advantages like increased independence in younger patients (47,48). Given the convenience and efficacy of the flutter valve and the expense of the vest system, it seems reasonable to initiate therapy with the more simple device with most patients who appear to require help with regular CPT.

In summary, regular airway clearance is undoubtedly beneficial for patients with CF, although the optimal modality has not been defined. Such clearance maneuvers should be a mainstay of any regimen, with physical exercise being a desired component and the flutter valve providing a simple extra support technique. Tailoring the regime to the individual patient's lifestyle and preferences is the best approach, to maximize compliance.

Antibiotic Therapy

Antibiotic therapy for patients with CF has remained a cornerstone of treatment since its first usage (49). Indeed, the development of potent broad-spectrum antibiotics, particularly antipseudomonal antibiotics, has had a major impact on the increasing survival of patients with CF in the past several decades (50). The rationale for antibiotic usage is clear. The host response to chronic bacterial infection induces inflammation of the airways, obstructive airways disease, and ectasia (bronchiectasis). The main offending organisms in adults are *P. aeruginosa* and *Staph. aureus*, whereas other, more drug resistant or multidrug-resistant strains of these and other organisms—for example, *Burkholderia cepacia*—can appear later in the course of the disease.

P. aeruginosa cannot be eradicated despite aggressive therapy. However, the burden of infection usually can be reduced by antibiotic therapy (in conjunction with other measures such as airway clearance), with improvement in symptoms and lung function (51). Monitoring the sputum culture is important because pathogens develop variable antibiotic sensitivities. Other pathogens may emerge, for example, nontuberculous mycobacteria (NTM), *Aspergillus fumigatus*, and *Stenotrophomonas maltophilia* (formerly *Xanthomonas maltophilia*), that can impact on the clinical status of the patient (52) (see Chapter 5).

Antibiotics can be delivered via three routes—intravenous, oral, and aerosolized. The mode of delivery depends on the clinical situation for individual patients. The medications can be used to intervene during an exacerbation to reverse the decline in clinical status and lung function or as maintenance therapy to prevent a decrease in pulmonary status. Definition of an exacerbation has been relatively imprecise, but a decline in lung function, increasing volumes of sputum, a decrease in exercise tolerance, and weight loss are among the most common markers (Table 7–2) (51,53). Recent data suggest that a decrease in exercise tolerance and fatigue correlates well with an exacerbation (53). Standard markers of infection such as fever and an increase in leukocyte count over baseline are atypical, although a low-grade fever may be present (~38°C). A chest radiograph is not a

TABLE 7–2. *Findings that suggest the need for antibiotic therapy in pulmonary exacerbations*

Increase in daily volume of sputum
Increase in cough, dyspnea
Decreased exercise tolerance
Deterioration in lung function or oxyhemoglobin saturation
Decreased appetite or weight
New chest auscultatory findings
New bacterial pathogen
Fever (uncommon)

useful marker of an exacerbation, except to rule out major complications, such as pneumothorax (54). To further complicate matters, particularly in relation to intravenous versus oral antibiotics as the treatment of choice for a given situation, there is no good definition of mild versus moderate versus severe exacerbation.

The ultimate aim of therapy is to return the patient to baseline (preexacerbation) status, including symptoms, volume of daily sputum production, and lung function. A point that cannot be overemphasized regarding antibiotic therapy is that doses of most antibiotics need to be higher than in the non-CF population because of altered pharmacokinetics in patients with CF (see Chapter 16). Figure 7–2 provides a treatment algorithm for planning therapy in a patient with CF experiencing an exacerbation.

Exacerbations

Acute/Subacute Exacerbation: Intravenous Antibiotics

The cornerstone of treatment for moderate to severe acute exacerbations is intravenous antibiotics. Intravenous antibiotics also can be given for subacute deterioration, in which a decline in clinical status and lung function (particularly the FEV_1) occurs over a longer time period. This mode of therapy is clinically efficacious, and several excellent reviews and studies are available (55–60). The targets are the specific bacterial pathogens in CF, such as *P. aeruginosa*, *Staph. aureus*, or *B. cepacia*. Because of the predilection of *P. aeruginosa* for CF airways, intravenous therapy usually includes medications active against that organism. One recent study clearly demonstrated the superiority of antipseudomonal antibiotics over placebo with intensive physiotherapy. This effect of antibiotics correlated with a reduction in *P. aeruginosa* colony-forming units (60).

The most important aspect of intravenous antibiotic therapy for CF is using the appropriate combination of drugs, at adequate dosage, for a sufficient length of time. Failure to adhere to these basic principles is the most frequent reason for lack of clinical response. Sputum bacte-

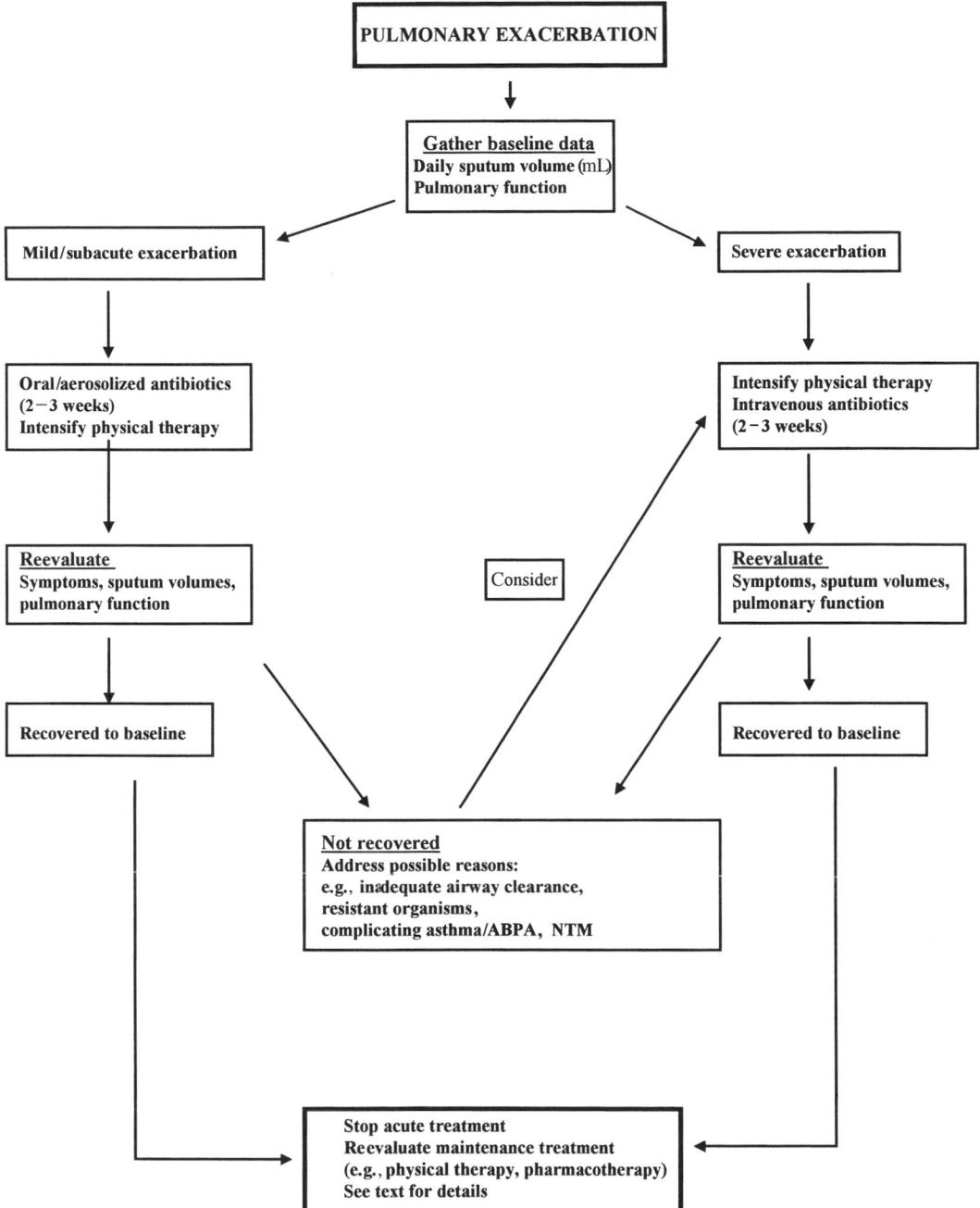

FIG. 7–2. Algorithm illustrating the treatment of a pulmonary exacerbation in cystic fibrosis.

riology can guide the choice of drugs. A combination of an aminoglycoside, such as gentamicin (or tobramycin, depending on drug sensitivity testing), with ceftazidime is optimal because of drug synergy against *Pseudomonas* species, and because a combination of drugs limits the emergence of drug-resistant bacteria (see Chapter 5) (55,56). Ceftazidime is the best third-generation cephalosporin because of its antipseudomonal activity and advantageous dosing frequency (twice or three times daily). If ceftazidime cannot be used, a semisynthetic penicillin, such as piperacillin, can be used, but a disadvantage of this combination is the frequency of dosage of the penicillins (every 4 to 6 hours). This latter point is particularly important for home therapy. Even if sensitivity results suggest resistance to one of the aforementioned drugs, *in vivo* clinical responses often are seen because of synergism between the antibiotics (61). This can be tested, as discussed in the section addressing the issue of resistance.

The doses of both the aminoglycosides and beta-lactam antibiotics (including the semisynthetic penicillins and cephalosporins) need to be considerably higher than in patients who do not have CF, for several reasons (62,63) (see Chapter 16). Patients with CF have a higher volume of distribution and whole-body clearance and, as a result, have reduced concentrations and activity of both classes of drugs in sputum (55,64). To add to this problem, tobramycin may be inactivated by binding to free DNA in infected CF airway secretions (64). Because optimal efficiency of antibiotics in CF airways depends on achieving bactericidal levels of drugs in airway secretions, lesser concentrations will be ineffective at killing bacteria (64). In addition, certain properties of *P. aeruginosa* render the organism more difficult to treat, that is, there are usually coexistent populations of varying drug sensitivities and mucoid strains produce alginate. The target peak serum level (30 minutes after completion of a 30-minute infusion) of tobramycin or gentamicin should be 10 to 12 µg/mL, with a trough level less than 2 µg/mL. The problem with aminoglycosides lies in the narrow therapeutic/toxic window at those higher levels and the unfamiliarity of most non-CF clinicians with such high levels. However, monitoring of drug levels and renal function usually results in safe administration of such large doses, without renal or overt ototoxicity. Despite this, some patients do get ototoxicity in the form of hearing loss or vestibular toxicity. Obviously, the risk of further damage in these patients needs to be balanced against the risks of ongoing lung disease.

If *Staph. aureus* is isolated in the sputum of patients with CF, the antipseudomonal aforementioned antibiotics provide limited coverage, although treatment may not be judged necessary when the culture results suggest a light burden of organisms. Overall therapy may include oral dicloxacillin, a penicillin/sulbactam combination, or a first-generation cephalosporin, again at a higher-than-standard dose. Methicillin-resistant *Staph. aureus* is becoming a problem, and vancomycin occasionally is necessary (65). Vancomycin pharmacokinetics do not appear to be altered in patients with CF, but reactions to the drug ("Red Man syndrome") are common (66). Therapy against *H. influenzae* also can be guided by sputum sensitivities and the perceived significance of the organism in sputum as indicated by the density of the culture growth and previous sputum culture results.

Occasionally, a patient will demonstrate allergy to the parenteral antibiotics, with the penicillins being the biggest culprits (67). Given that *P. aeruginosa* can be multidrug-resistant, desensitization to the semisynthetic penicillins may be necessary. This usually can be accomplished safely with attention to detail (68). Other side effects of broad-spectrum antibiotics include vulvovaginal candidiasis in females with CF. Care must be taken to ask females having antibiotic therapy about such symptoms because treatment with local antifungal therapy may be required—for example, nystatin or miconazole.

The aim of therapy is a return to pre-exacerbation status, that is, symptoms, sputum production, and lung function, particularly the FEV_1 and FVC. Two weeks usually suffice for patients who have not received recurrent courses of treatment, but return to pre-exacerbation status can take up to 3 weeks in patients with more severe disease (69). *P. aeruginosa* cannot be eradicated from the airways of adults with CF; therefore, this should not be one of the goals. Table 7–3 lists the commonly used antibiotics and dose regimens for therapy in CF exacerbations, with target serum concentrations for aminoglycosides.

Intravenous antibiotics need not necessarily be administered exclusively in the hospital,

TABLE 7–3. *Intravenous antibiotic regimens for treatment of CF lung infections*

Antibiotic	Dose	Doses/day	Max dose g/24hr	Pathogens
Aminoglycosides				
Gentamicin and			(Peak 10–12)[a]	P. aer., H. flu.
Tobramycin	6–15 (mg/kg/24 hr)	2–3	(Trough <1–2 µg/mL)[a]	
Amikacin	20–30 (mg/kg/24 hr)	2–3	(Peak 25–30)[a]	
			(Trough <5 µg/mL)[a]	
Cephalosporins				
Ceftazidime	2 g	3	12	P. aer., B. cep., H. flu.
Cefuroxime	0.75–1.5 g	3	5	H. flu.
Penicillins				
Piperacillin, (±tazobactam)	3–4 g	4–6	20	P. aer., H. flu.
Ticarcillin + clavulanic acid	3 g	4–6	24	P. aer., H. flu.
Ampicillin/sulbactam	1.5–2 g	4	8	S. aur., H. flu.
Oxacillin	1–2 g	4	8	S. aur.
Other				
Imipenem/cilastin	0.5–0.75 g	3–4	4	P. aer., S. aur., H. flu.
Ciprofloxacin	0.4 g	2	0.8	P. aer., H. flu.
Aztreonam	1–2 g	4	8	P. aer., H. flu.
Chloramphenicol	50 (mg/kg/24 hr)	4	4	B. cep., H. flu.
Trimethoprim-sulfamethoxazole	12–20 (mg/kg/24 hr)	2–4	1.5	B. cep., S. aur., H. flu.
Vancomycin	1 g	2	2	S. aur.
Clindamycin	0.15–0.9 g	3	4	S. aur.

P. aer., *Pseudomonas aeruginosa;* H. flu., *Hemophilus influenzae;* B. cep., *Burkholderia cepacia;* S. aur., *Staphylococcus aureus.*

[a]Doses guided by peak and trough serum levels, as indicated.

and many physicians and patients now opt for in-home therapy. This approach is attractive from many standpoints. Patients undergo less disruption to their lives, they can continue with work and education, and the cost is less than that of a hospital admission (70). However, there are several important considerations related to home intravenous therapy. For example, if the patient does not have indwelling intravenous access, a decision must be made as to whether an intravenous line can be placed at home by appropriately experienced personnel or whether the patient needs to attend the hospital for such placement. Delivery of adequate supplies of medication, with appropriate monitoring of serum drug levels, is required. Home intravenous therapy also depends on the ability of the patient to understand medication administration, particularly timing and doses, and care of a central or peripheral line. Most studies show that these aspects of home care are manageable, particularly as professional home care companies become established in most parts of the United States (71–74).

In considering home versus hospital intravenous treatment, medical considerations need to be addressed. For example, the patient may be so ill that the traditional benefits of hospital care are required (e.g., oxygen therapy, professional physical therapy, rest, nursing care), at least until the patient shows a response. Parenteral antibiotics for hemoptysis beyond mere blood streaking of the sputum associated with infection need to be initiated in hospital, should additional intervention such as embolization become necessary. Similarly, failure to clear secretions or excessive amounts of sputum production in association with an exacerbation need intensive CPT, and this may be optimally provided in hospital. Bearing these considerations in mind, there is evidence that home care compares well with hospital care. For example, there are data from retrospective studies on the efficacy of home antibiotics as compared with in-hospital management of exacerbations (70,71,74). In these studies, there was a return to baseline of initially measure parameters, for example, lung function, arterial blood gases, leukocyte count, and chest radiograph score, and the results were similar between those patients treated in the hospital and those treated at home (72,74).

Long-term indwelling intravenous catheters facilitate repeated courses of intravenous antibiotics, both in and out of hospital. There are several choices available, ranging from the removable midline catheter to the permanent indwelling catheter. The choice of an indwelling line depends very much on the individual patient's requirements for intravenous antibiotics and the expertise available for placement of such devices. For example, a patient who has mild pulmonary disease, who practices good airway clearance, who has minimal requirement for intravenous antibiotics on an annual basis, does not need a long-term indwelling subcutaneous catheter, but could easily have a temporary catheter placed when the need arises. These devices are relatively easy to place, have few complications, and provide access for a 2- to 3-week course of antibiotics (75). In a patient who has a frequent requirement for intravenous access, a long-term indwelling line should be considered. With experienced personnel and care over the long term, such devices offer advantages such as ready access for blood samples and rapid commencement of antibiotics. Patients themselves express a favorable opinion of these catheters and their advantages (76). However, there are disadvantages, such as thrombosis and sepsis (77,78). With good care, including an aseptic technique by personnel and the patient when accessing the catheter, and monthly flushing, these catheters can provide years of trouble-free venous access (79). Indwelling catheters should be considered in patients with CF who require frequent intravenous antibiotics, particularly those with poor peripheral venous access, and should be considered in those patients who have very severe lung disease.

Thus, home intravenous therapy is a very useful, proven, and cost-saving option for some patients who require intravenous antibiotics for an exacerbation of pulmonary disease, but consideration needs to be given to the more

extensive issues involved, and some patients continue to require in-hospital treatment. Midline catheters and long-term indwelling venous catheters provide useful alternatives in those patients who require frequent venous access.

Acute/Subacute Exacerbation: Oral Antibiotics

Oral therapy (Table 7–4) is best limited to those exacerbations that are mild to moderate in severity. One challenge, however, is in differentiating between mild to moderate and more severe flare-ups (53). Increase in cough and volumes of sputum, without a change in lung function, significant weight loss, or fever would qualify in most clinicians' opinion as a mild exacerbation. Patients with a mild exacerbation often report increased daytime cough, whereas nocturnal cough and difficulty sleeping usually are associated with more severe exacerbations. Patients often will be able to judge the severity of a flare-up themselves from previous experience. From the physician's point of view, a history of the patient's previous requirement for oral versus intravenous antibiotics, and their responses, also is very useful, and clinical judgment must suffice in the absence of precise definitions of mild/moderate/severe exacerbations.

A limitation of oral therapy is the narrow choice of effective antipseudomonal drugs, that is, the quinolones (ciprofloxacin, norfloxacin, ofloxacin). Broad-spectrum antibiotics may provide clinical benefit, for example, amoxicillin, first-generation cephalosporins, or macrolide antibiotics, even if they are not active against *Pseudomonas* species. These broad-spectrum antibiotics are effective because other nonpseudomonal bacteria (i.e., normal respiratory flora) are present in significant quantities in the lower respiratory tract (80,81). Broad-spectrum antibiotics also may reduce the release of bacterial toxins, limiting inflammation (82). Oral chloramphenicol has been used in this context in the past and is available from the Cystic Fibrosis Pharmacy on a compassionate basis for patients with CF. Patients in whom chloramphenicol is being considered should have bacteria sen-

TABLE 7–4. Oral antibiotics and regimens for treatment of CF lung infections in adults

Antibiotic	Dose (mg)	Frequency per day	Pathogen
Penicillins			
Amoxicillin	500	3	S. aur., H. flu.
Amoxicillin/clavulanic acid	500	3	S. aur., H. flu.
Dicloxacillin	500	4	S. aur.
Cephalosporins			
Cefuroxime	500	2	S. aur., H. flu.
Cephalexin	500	4	S. aur.
Cefaclor	500	3	S. aur., H. flu.
Others			
Trimethoprim/ sulfamethoxazole	2 DS	2	S. aur., H. flu.
Erythromycin	500	4	S. aur.
Azithromycin		500 mg day 1 250 mg daily days 2–5	S. aur., H. flu.
Clindamycin	450	3	S. aur.
Tetracycline	500	4	H. flu.
Doxycycline	100	2	H. flu.
Quinolones			
Ciprofloxacin	500–750	2–3	P. aer., S. aur., H. flu.
Ofloxacin	400	2–3	P. aer., S. aur., H. flu.

S. aur., *Staphylococcus aureus;* H. flu., *Hemophilus influenzae;* DS, double-strength tablets; P. aer., *Pseudomonas aeruginosa.*

sitive to the drug and resistant to other oral drugs. For specific antipseudomonal therapy, ciprofloxacin compares well with intravenous antibiotics in patients with CF with mild to moderate acute exacerbations, with excellent bioavailability in airway secretions (83,84), and offers the obvious advantage of convenience and lower cost. This efficacy of ciprofloxacin often is observed in those patients who have not had repeated courses of ciprofloxacin previously. It generally is well tolerated, although arthropathy is among the sporadically reported side effects, which must be differentiated from the other arthropathies associated with CF (85) (see Chapter 20). Drug resistance is common after 3 to 4 weeks of monotherapy with ciprofloxacin (86). Therefore it should be reserved for intermittent courses of treatment, for example, 2 to 3 weeks in duration, no more than every 3 to 4 months. Long-term use of ciprofloxacin should be discouraged vigorously. In this manner, it is an adjunct in the management of CF lung inflections, saving on hospital admissions and usage of intravenous antibiotic courses. Follow-up is mandatory to define return to baseline of symptoms, sputum produc-

tion, and FEV_1. If oral antibiotics do not result in full recovery, more aggressive parenteral therapy may be required.

Acute/Subacute Exacerbation: Inhaled Antibiotics

It generally is acknowledged that aerosolized antibiotics may have some role in the management of mild acute or subacute exacerbations, although definitive data are lacking. Minimal additional benefit is seen when aerosolized antibiotics are used as adjunctive treatment to standard therapy with intravenous antibiotics (55). However, occasionally, patients will demonstrate a benefit in response to various forms and doses of aerosolized antibiotics when experiencing acute exacerbation. Aerosolized antibiotics do have a role in maintenance therapy, as discussed below.

Maintenance Therapy

Oral Antibiotics

One approach to try to prevent a decrease in symptoms and lung function in CF is to use regular oral antibiotics, and various antibiotic schedules still are used empirically in individual patients (87,88). The rationale is similar to that employed in an acute/subacute exacerbation, that is, that suppression of nonpseudomonal organisms and limiting the release of bacterial toxins proves useful over the long term. A concerning problem in relation to the liberal use of broad-spectrum antibiotics and antistaphylococcal antibiotics is the recent increase of methicillin-resistant *Staph. aureus* (MRSA) in general and in CF (65). In addition, *P. aeruginosa* may perhaps increase in pathogen density in patients treated in this manner (87). Some CF physicians recommend continuous use of dicloxacillin or trimethoprim/sulfamethoxazole to suppress *Staph. aureus*, on the basis that therapy directed against this organism is useful over the long term. This needs to be scrutinized carefully in light of the increasing numbers of patients with drug-resistant organisms. In addition, a study to address the role of prophylactic antistaphylococcal therapy in children failed to demonstrate a benefit (89).

A recent study using 10 days of ciprofloxacin every 3 months to reduce the need for intravenous antibiotics and improve lung function yielded mixed results. Although the drug was well tolerated and there was a decrease in cough and sputum production, with improvement in peak flow measurements, there were no changes in FEV_1, FVC, or need for hospitalizations, as compared with placebo. In addition, the minimum inhibitory concentration (MIC) for *P. aeruginosa* increased after 1 year of the study in the ciprofloxacin group (90).

Inhaled Antibiotics

From a theoretical perspective, inhaled antibiotics would appear to offer advantages over intravenous therapy in terms of higher concentration of drug in airways while avoiding toxicity (91,92). Chronic bacterial suppression via this method might limit the ongoing proliferation of bacteria and resultant inflammation that is present even when patients appear clinically well (14).

Initially unblinded, uncontrolled studies of inhaled antibiotics were carried out in the early 1980s, and most suggested modest beneficial effects on pulmonary function or hospitalization rates (93). Side effects were not uncommon, particularly wheezing or chest tightness with colistin (94). The use of different nebulizers and doses and volumes of drug made definitive comparisons and conclusions difficult, although clinical use of inhaled antibiotics became common practice (95,96). A multicenter, double-blind crossover study administering high-dose tobramycin (600 mg three times daily) via a cumbersome ultrasonic nebulizer was carried out over two 28-day periods (97). This showed an improvement in FEV_1 of 9% over placebo, with a decrease in *P. aeruginosa* density during the tobramycin treatment period. No toxicity from tobramycin was observed. In addition, there was no difference in *P. aeruginosa* resistance in either group, although longer-term usage may yield more data in this regard. Although expensive and not logistically easy, this prevention of lung function decline, with the potential for reducing hospital admissions, may offer advantages over the long term. A more practical approach involves a recent study using a jet nebulizer and a smaller dose (300 mg) of preservative-free tobramycin (TOBI) taken twice daily. This treatment, taken on alternate months for three cycles, improved lung funtion, decreased bacterial burden, and decreased relative risk for hospitalization and use of other anti-Pseudomonal antibiotics as compared with placebo (165). It is also logistically easier for patients to use. For clinicians, the condundrum is whether smaller doses of drugs administered via aerosol also may be useful. For example, gentamicin or tobramycin can be used at a dose of 80 mg two to four times a day, or colistin at a dose of 50 to 75 mg two to three times a day. Colistin should be diluted in 3.5 to 4 mL of sterile water initially, then further diluted in normal saline, to ensure dissolution of the drug and to avoid bubbling during nebulization and irritative cough.

In general, the decision regarding whether to place individual patients on aerosolized antibiotics should be made on a case-by-case basis.

A test dose should be carried out in the clinic or hospital setting, to educate the patient in the correct use of the nebulizer and to monitor for side effects, to optimize the outcome. To achieve best delivery, slow inhalation to total lung capacity, with a breath hold for 3 to 4 seconds, followed by slow exhalation to functional residual capacity maximizes the deposition of drug on airway surfaces. Using jet nebulizers, optimizing the air flow and volume of fill in the medication cup increases the amount of respirable drug (98). Other, smaller ultrasonic devices may offer advantages over jet nebulizers from the point of view of efficiency and portability (99).

Intravenous Antibiotics

Regular "scheduled" usage of intravenous antibiotics has been employed in some centers, notably the Danish Cystic Fibrosis Center, on a prophylactic basis (50,56). This approach has not become accepted in the United States because of the risk of drug resistance, and because it has not been studied in a larger, less homogeneous population than exists in Denmark (58). This method employs routine usage of intravenous antipseudomonal antibiotics (tobramycin plus a beta-lactam) approximately four times a year, with standard treatment of exacerbations when required also. The annual mortality after institution of this regimen was compared with that of historical controls, with improved survival. However, an increased resistance in *P. aeruginosa* was apparent (58,100), with increased cross-infection, side effects, and cost. Although still used in Denmark, this method has not received widespread acceptance elsewhere.

In summary, antibiotic therapy remains one of the most important aspects of the long-term management of patients with CF. There is no question as to the benefit of antibiotics for acute exacerbations if therapy is administered appropriately. The choice of drug and mode of administration are directed by the nature and severity of the episode. Home therapy is an alternative to prolonged hospitalizations for many patients. From a preventive point of view, oral antibiotics directed against *Staph. aureus* have been regarded as useful in the past, but because of emerging resistance of *Staph. aureus*, this approach needs to be reassessed. Inhaled antipseudomonal therapy for selected patients also is a useful option. As emphasized previously, all these measures should be in the context of regular mechanical airway clearance, exercise, and good nutrition.

Special Situations

Multidrug Resistant Bacteria

An increasing concern in the management of adult patients with CF has been the increase in antibiotic resistance in the bacterial pathogens that infect the airways of these patients. *P. aeruginosa*, *B. cepacia*, and *Staph. aureus* are the organisms of most concern (100–102).

Resistance to *P. aeruginosa* is problematic but usually only later in the course of the disease. In contrast to *B. cepacia* (see below), *P. aeruginosa* initially is sensitive to a host of antibiotics, including the aminoglycosides, beta-lactam antibiotics, imipenem, and the quinolones. However, after repeated courses of intravenous antibiotics for exacerbations of lung disease, resistance often emerges to most classes of drugs. Resistance can emerge for a variety of reasons, including mutation and selective advantage, plasmid acquisition of penicillinases, or modification of binding proteins (103) (see also Chapter 5). To try to circumvent the emergence of resistance in *P. aeruginosa*, the strategies outlined in the preceding sections for treatment should be employed. These include avoidance of monotherapy, use of antibiotics with complementary actions on the bacteria, and usage in high dosage. As indicated previously, overuse of oral ciprofloxacin as monotherapy generally results in resistance, which often wanes with time; for this reason, ciprofloxacin should be used sparingly as a single agent. When *P. aeruginosa* becomes multiresistant, successful treatment becomes difficult. However, there are strategies that can be employed. Avoidance of overuse of antibiotics, unless necessary, may allow nonresistant strains to repopulate the airways. Combinations of drugs still can prove efficacious clinically, despite the laboratory evidence of resistance, presumably because of *in vivo* synergy (104). *In vitro* laboratory synergy testing can provide guidelines in regard to useful combinations of drugs. Doses of some antibiotics can be increased to overcome apparent resistance, for example, ceftazidime (up to 4 g tid). Concentrations of tobramycin higher than the MIC for *Pseudomonas* can be achieved in the airway secretions of patients with CF via high-dose aerosolized tobramycin (up to 600 mg tid), which may be useful when few alternatives are apparent (93,97). Measures to treat multidrug-resistant *P. aeruginosa* ideally should be undertaken in conjunction with experienced CF center physicians.

B. *cepacia* is particularly problematic. The Toronto Cystic Fibrosis Center and centers in the United Kingdom reported an increase in isolation and mortality in patients with this organism in the late 1980s. Person-to-person transmission is the mode of transmission, usually among patients indulging in close social contact. As evidence for this became apparent, steps were taken to reduce the possibility (105,106). Transmission of *B. cepacia* to the United Kingdom may have occurred as a result of patients traveling from Cardiff to CF camps in Canada in 1987, and contacting patients with *B. cepacia* from the Toronto center. To reduce possible transmission of *B. cepacia*, measures to reduce the likely person-to-person transmission of this organism have been instituted, including the closure of the CF summer camps in 1993 by the Cystic Fibrosis Foundation (107). Since then, molecular techniques have elucidated the epidemiology of *B. cepacia*. Ribotyping, pulse field gel electrophoresis analysis of the organism, and comparison of the isolates at various centers have proved helpful in tracing the contact sources of *B. cepacia* (108). Differences in the adherent properties of strains of *B. cepacia* may explain differences in how the organism is transmitted and the clinical course of disease once acquired (see Chapter 5). The pili are structures that allow the organism to stick to respiratory epithelium and other adjacent organisms to form microcolonies, and it has been shown that the cable pilus on the surface of the epidemic strain of *B. cepacia* allows enhanced binding (108). To reduce transmission, general precautionary measures in and out of the hospital are advisable. Patients who carry *B. cepacia* in their sputum are best isolated from other patients not infected with *B. cepacia*. This means single rooms and separate physical therapy sessions for all patients infected with *B. cepacia* when hospitalized. In the outpatient setting, there should be some effort made to separate these patients from noninfected patients also. These patients should not indulge in close social contact with other noninfected patients, both in hospital (e.g., at the same physical therapy session) and out of hospital (e.g., handshaking, shared utensils, towels). Obviously, these measures have significant psychological and social implications for patients.

An important property of *B. cepacia* is its inherent resistance to antibiotics. This makes the organism difficult to treat once it is established in the airways. It may be sensitive initially to the lactam antibiotics, including piperacillin, ceftazidime, and imipenem, but not to aminoglycosides or the quinolones. After exposure to antibiotics, however, the organism quickly develops resistance even to those drugs to which it initially was sensitive. The mechanism likely reflects failure of the drugs to penetrate the outer-cell envelope. With no alternative therapeutic strategies, use of a combination of aminoglycosides and lactam antibiotics may effect a beneficial response, despite the fact that synergy studies may show no effect of the combination *in vitro* (109). As outlined previously for *P. aeruginosa*, other measures may be useful, including higher doses of intravenous or aerosolized antibiotics.

Three clinical patterns with *B. cepacia* have been described—chronic asymptomatic carriage, progressive deterioration over many months, and a more rapid, usually fatal deterioration (110). Patients with more severe disease are particularly prone to deterioration once *B. cepacia* is isolated (111). The problem becomes even more difficult when patients are being evaluated for lung transplantation because most centers have been reluctant to consider such patients for surgery because of the risks of resistant infection in an immunocompromised host postoperatively. The data are somewhat conflicting, with some centers having less problems with patients infected with *B. cepacia* posttransplant (112). This difference may be related to differing virulence between strains of the bacteria, perhaps related to the differences in adherence alluded to previously (108).

Drug-resistant *Staph. aureus* also is becoming more of a problem. Data from our institution, and others, suggest that the incidence in patients with CF is on the rise (~10% of *Staph. aureus* isolates in 1994–1995, compared with ~3% to 4% in 1993), with resistance to the beta-lactam antibiotics a particular problem (65) (see Chapter 5). The mechanism usually is via penicillin-binding proteins. These methicillin- and oxacillin-resistant organisms (MRSA/ORSA) have reduced sensitivity to the macrolides and tetracyclines, although they may retain sensitivity to ciprofloxacin and trimethoprim-sulfamethoxazole. The strategy to reduce the infectious effects of *Staph. aureus*, including continuous maintenance use of oral dicloxacillin or trimethoprim-sulfamethoxazole, may need to be reconsidered in light of these observations. Fortunately, most (~90%) of *Staph. aureus* recovered from adult patients with CF remain sensitive to most antistaphylococcal antibiotics. When MRSA/ORSA are isolated in the sputum, a decision must be made regarding the need for treatment. If the gram-stain and culture results suggest a significant burden of organisms, or if *Staph. aureus* is judged to be contributing to complications such as hemoptysis, intravenous vancomycin can be used. Vigilant follow-up with lung function and sputum bacteriology to see whether the organism is eradicated is mandatory. There are no data with respect to the likelihood of eradication of *Staph. aureus*, and a more likely outcome in most situations is one similar to that of *P. aeruginosa*, with exacerbation followed by treatment and remission, but without complete eradication.

Stenotrophomonas maltophilia (formerly *Xanthomonas maltophilia*) and *Alcaligenes xylosoxi-* dans are being seen increasingly in patients with CF. *S. maltophilia* is seen in patients after many courses of intravenous antibiotics, particularly imipenem, which it degrades via beta-lactamase. *S. maltophilia* is resistant to many antibiotics, although it may retain sensitivity to minocycline, trimethoprim-sulfamethoxazole, and ticarcillin/clavulanic acid, which may be used in combination. There are no firm data on either the pathogenicity or the successful treatment of either of these organisms in CF.

Nontuberculous Mycobacteria (NTM)

Recent data suggest a relatively high prevalence of NTM in the lower airway secretions of patients with CF. Organisms include *Mycobacterium avium* complex (MAC), *M. abscessus* (formerly *M. chelonei*), *M. fortuitium*, *M. gordonae*, *M. kansasii*, and various untyped organisms. Collectively, data from studies at eight North American and European CF centers using prospectively screened patients suggests a prevalence of approximately 13%, with some regional variation (101,102,113,114). Older patients tend to be affected, and a lower clinical score correlates to some extent with the presence of NTM in the sputum of these patients (113). Currently, there is a multicenter study to rigorously define the incidence and significance of NTM in CF.

There are several potential reasons why there should be an apparent increase in the prevalence of NTM in CF. The data may be influenced to some extent by an increasing awareness of NTM in CF, and subsequently, an increased search for such organisms on a routine basis (114). Additionally, modified culture techniques may improve the yield of NTM—for example, prevention of *P. aeruginosa* overgrowth (115). Alternatively, the increased longevity of adult patients with CF may increase the variety of pathogens, including NTM, to which patients with CF are predisposed. Another interesting theory has been put forth that patients with CF may represent a sentinel population, heralding a general increase in pulmonary infections by these organisms in the

United States. The reason for increasing NTM in the general population may reflect changes in habit, for example, showering as a method of personal hygiene, thus facilitating transmission of the organism by aerosolization (114).

It is difficult to define the precise pathogenic role of these organisms in CF airways disease. The concept that NTM may be colonizing the airways, as opposed to causing overt infection, arose because of observations that there appears to be some correlation between clinical manifestations and burden of organisms. For example, cavitary disease in patients who do not have CF appears to correlate with a repeatedly positive acid-fast bacillus smear, or a heavy growth of organisms. The converse also appears true, that is, that absence of cavitary changes correlates with a light growth. Supporting data include a small study in which 65% of (non-CF) patients without cavitary infiltrates cleared NTM from their sputum after a course of intense bronchial hygiene (116). However, difficulties arise in patients with CF because of the variability in the sampling of lower airway secretions in this population such that sputum may not yield a growth of organisms, despite a heavy presence in distal airways. In addition, bacterial overgrowth, as aforementioned, may confound the results of sputum culture, unless steps are taken to safeguard against such an occurrence. Finally, antibacterial drugs such as ciprofloxacin and the aminoglycosides used against *P. aeruginosa* have some activity against some NTM, and thus interfere with the sputum culture results.

The clinical evaluation of patients with CF whose sputum show a growth of NTM is not straightforward. The overlap between symptoms due to NTM and bacterial exacerbations in CF is considerable, including increase in cough, sputum production, dyspnea, chest pain, anorexia, and weight loss. Night sweats and fevers perhaps are more common in NTM-related disease. Radiographic changes of NTM-related infection are difficult to separate from those of CF lung disease, although radiologic assessment may be improving. Recent studies in patients without CF suggest that middle and lower lobe predominance, peripheral nodules, and patchy air space disease—as imaged by high-resolution computed tomography (HRCT)—correlates well with NTM infection, as opposed to bacterial infection (117,118). Multiple sputum specimens should be obtained over a period of time for repeated stain and culture for NTM, and other diagnostic methods may need to be employed, including bronchoscopic acquisition of secretions for stain and culture and biopsies of endobronchial mucosa looking for granulomatous disease. Skin testing shows promise as a screening tool, showing a good degree of sensitivity and specificity for MAC infection in adults with CF (118,119).

There currently are no firm guidelines for identifying those patients who require treatment. Pending better information, the best approach is to consider carefully those patients who seem more likely to have active infection. For example, those patients who are repeatedly smear positive, with a heavy growth of organisms, may be at greater risk of the NTM contributing to the progression of lung disease. A temporal decline in lung function that does not respond to conventional airway clearance and antibacterial antibiotics further supports the notion that NTMs are contributing to disease pathogenesis. An HRCT scan showing peripheral nodularity also may be useful. Ultimately, a response to treatment for NTM in clinical and radiologic terms is very supportive (114).

Once a decision to treat has been reached, one must consider choice of antimicrobials and the potential for side effects, given the prolonged courses needed to control infection. Dosage is critical, given the abnormal gastrointestinal absorption and pharmacokinetics in patients with CF as described previously, and serum levels are mandatory to guide the correct dosage (Table 7–5). Although no specific consensus with regard to treatment existed among CF physicians, a recent pamphlet has been issued from the coordinators of a multicenter study addressing the incidence and pathogenic significance of NTM in patients with CF. The emphasis is on vigorous pursuit of evidence of

TABLE 7–5. *Guidelines for treatment of nontuberculosis mycobacterium in patients with cystic fibrosis with well-defined pathogenic infection*

General

Start with a single drug, adding sequentially every 3–4 days, observing for side effects with each new drug.
Dose at bedtime to improve absorption and to mask gastrointestinal side effects
Because of altered metabolism and absorption in patients with CF,
    Monitor serum levels two weeks after all medications started
    Draw peak serum levels 2 hours postdosing
Follow up cultures monthly
Consider adding or changing drugs at 6 mos if adequate levels obtained and
    No clinical response
    No microbiologic response (no reduction in colony counts, positive smear)
In vitro drug susceptibility testing may be useful in selecting alternate drugs

Specific

Organism	Agent	Dose[a]	Comments
MAC	Clarithromycin	30 mg/kg/day (max 1,000 mg) po	Levels decreased by rifampicin, rifabutin, increased by azoles
	Rifabutin	5 mg/kg/day (max 300 mg) po	Discontinue if leukocytes <2,000 or granulocytes <1,000
	Ethambutol	25 mg/kg/day po	Baseline eye examination/ monitor acuity and color monthly

Duration: Not established, probably 1 yr after negative culture
Drugs to consider adding include: clofazamine, streptomycin, amikacin three times weekly, (serum peaks 40 μg/mL), ciprofloxacin

Organism	Agent	Dose[a]	Comments
M. abscessus (formerly M. chelonei, subspecies abscessus)	Cefoxitin	200 mg/kg/day IV	Max 12 g/day
	Amikacin	15 mg/kg/day IV every 12 hrs audiogram, monitor renal function	Peak 18–24 μg/mL, baseline
M. fortuitum	Clarithromycin	30 mg/kg/day (max 1,000 mg)	As above

Duration: 6–12 mos
If resistance to clarithromycin noted on susceptibility testing, use ciprofloxacin

Organism	Agent	Dose[a]	Comments
M. kansasii	Isoniazid	10–20 mg/kg/day po qd, max 300 mg	LFTs at baseline, then monthly, D/C if > 3 ×normal
	Rifampin	10–20 mg/kg/day po qd, max 600 mg	LFTs at baseline, then monthly, D/C if > 3 ×normal
	Ethambutol	25 mg/kg/day po qd × 2 months, then decrease to 15 mg/kg/day po qd	Baseline eye examination/ monitor acuity and color monthly

Duration: 18 mos, monthly cultures until negative, then at completion of therapy

D/C, discontinue; IV, intravenous; LFT, liver function test; MAC, *Mycobacterium avium* complex; po, by mouth; qd, every day.
[a]Doses and maximums are for initial dosing only; subsequent doses guided by peak serum levels.

mycobacterial disease wherever possible, with bronchoscopic and biopsy techniques, if applicable. Additionally, an emphasis on a uniform approach to the management is contained in the document, including obtaining susceptibility testing, drug concentrations in blood, and specific regimens for particular NTM (see Table 7–5). Data from such a uniform approach will give the best chance of meaningful analyses in the future. If *M. tuberculosis* organisms

are recovered in the sputum of patients with CF, the management is no different than that of the non-CF population.

Viruses/Chlamydia

Although definitive data are lacking regarding the role of viruses in CF lung disease, there are suggestions that they play a role in the pathogenesis of acute infection (121–123). In a

small study in children, infection with respiratory syncytial virus (RSV) appeared to be associated with severe and prolonged deterioration in pulmonary status (123). In contrast, however, in a 2-year study of school-aged patients with CF, patients seemed to have no difference in the incidence of infection with RSV than controls, and RSV had no adverse effects on pulmonary function (124). Anecdotal evidence for viruses playing an important role in acute disease also exists for influenza A. In addition to the possibility for prevention with annual vaccination, there is some evidence that amantadine given early in the course of this infectious complication may modulate the course of the disease, at least in patients who do not have CF (121). Other viruses also may impact on the clinical course of CF. A small number (n = 5) of patients demonstrating serologic evidence of active Epstein-Barr virus (EBV) infection had a worse clinical course during and after exacerbation than controls (122).

Although a role for viruses in chronic airways disease in CF still is uncertain, animal model systems suggest a role for latent adenovirus 5 infection in the pathogenesis of non-CF chronic airway inflammation and obstructive lung disease (125,126). If latent adenoviral infection does play a role in chronic CF lung disease, such data may be important from a number of perspectives, including that of potential new therapies. Gene therapy using adenoviral vectors raises the possibility of interactions between host latent adenoviral infection and the vector. Ongoing studies are addressing this role of adenovirus in chronic CF airways disease.

Most physicians would elect to treat patients with exacerbations vigorously with antibacterial agents, regardless of whether a viral cause is possible or not, because of the hypothesis that viral exacerbations act in conjunction with bacterial exacerbations and because proof that a virus alone is causing exacerbation often is difficult to obtain rapidly. In addition, patients should receive the annual influenza vaccine as part of routine care.

Chlamydia pneumoniae recently has been studied in regard to a possible role in acute ex-acerbation in CF (127). In a prospective study of 32 patients admitted to the hospital because of worsening lung status, four patients (three adults and one child) had evidence of *C. pneumoniae* infection (positive nasopharyngeal culture) as compared with none of 24 stable CF control patients. Three of the patients had serologic evidence, that is, high immunoglobulin M (IgM) or IgG titers, suggestive of acute infection, and the other patient had an IgG titer suggestive of past infection. IgE specific for *C. pneumoniae* also was elevated in all four patients, three of whom had problematic wheezing, leading to speculation that infection with this organism may trigger airway reactivity. This may be an important organism to consider in the setting of acute exacerbation, where standard antipseudomonal therapy will not be active against *C. pneumoniae*, and addition of a tetracycline may be worth considering.

Aspergillus

Allergic bronchopulmonary aspergillosis (ABPA) has been reported to occur in 5% to 10% of patients with CF, although these were pediatric patients, and the incidence in adult patients with CF probably is lower (128,129). More recent data suggest an incidence of 2.3% in adults and 1.5% in children (Cystic Fibrosis Foundation, National CF Patient Registry). The other diseases caused by aspergillus, cavitary mycetomas, and invasive aspergillosis are very uncommon in CF. Although not common in adults, ABPA should be considered in any patient with CF who is not doing well despite other maximal therapy, and who exhibits any of the many criteria of ABPA (Table 7–6). Refractory wheezing and new unexplained infiltrates on the chest radiograph are particularly useful indications toward the diagnosis. The diagnosis can be difficult because of the overlap between the criteria for ABPA and common CF symptoms. For example, positive criteria for ABPA can be present in patients with CF who do not necessarily have clinically overt ABPA. Moreover, the criteria can be present in a variety of combinations, limiting their usefulness (130). The serum IgE and immediate as-

TABLE 7–6. *Allergic bronchopulmonary aspergillosis (ABPA)*

Major criteria
  Episodic reversible bronchoconstriction
  Peripheral blood eosinophilia
  Positive immediate skin test
  Precipitating antibodies to *Aspergillus fumigatus*
  Increased IgE
  Pulmonary infiltrates
  Central bronchiectasis
Minor criteria
  Aspergillus fumigatus in sputum
  Sputum plugs
  Late Arthus skin reaction

IgE, immunoglobulin E.

pergillus skin test are very good screening tools. A normal IgE or a negative skin test certainly help to exclude the diagnosis, but either test may be positive in the absence of ABPA, that is, a positive skin test occurs in up to 60% of patients with CF, and elevated IgE levels (> 150 international units/mL) occur in up to 15% to 20% of patients without ABPA. Those patients with a very high serum IgE levels (e.g., > 1,000 international units/mL) and higher specific IgE and IgG levels versus aspergillus are more likely to have active disease. Interestingly, ABPA subsequently may develop in those patients with very high IgE levels but previously lacking other diagnostic criteria (130). Aspergillus precipitins are nonspecific, occurring in up to 40% of patients with CF. A negative aspergillus precipitin is more helpful to exclude ABPA, although occasionally a patient may have ABPA with very high specific IgE and IgG levels but a negative precipitin test. Establishing a diagnosis often is a question of considering all the data in the clinical context. Excluding the diagnosis is easier than confirming it, and laboratory data alone—without the accompanying clinical syndrome—is insufficient evidence to warrant treatment.

Steroids remain the mainstay of treatment for ABPA, the dose being 0.5 to 1 mg/kg daily initially, with a gradual reduction as symptoms and markers of activity improve (131). The best monitors are the clinical improvement and the serum IgE level, although occasionally a patient may not show a decrease in the serum IgE level (128). Although duration of required treatment varies, therapy should be continued for at least several months, during which time the dose can be reduced gradually, while watching for either a return in symptoms, a decrease in FEV_1, or an increase in IgE levels (131). Also, inhaled steroids may have a complementary role (132). Vigorous removal of secretions from the airways via mechanical methods is advisable to reduce the antigenic burden during treatment.

Other agents may be useful in the treatment of ABPA, although the data are scarce. An oral antifungal agent, itraconazole, has been reported anecdotally to be of benefit in patents when used in addition to prednisone treatment; in two patients who showed no improvement with steroid alone, there was an improvement in IgE, specific IgG, lung function, and weight. In those patients, however, the duration of high-dose steroids may not have been of adequate duration to demonstrate a response in those parameters (133).

Supplemental Oxygen Therapy/Cor Pulmonale

Supplemental oxygen therapy is very useful to prevent hypoxemia (< 55 torr in room air) at rest, on a continuous basis (18 to 24 hours per day), in patients with chronic obstructive airways disease, including CF (see Chapter 8). It limits the development of pulmonary hypertension and cor pulmonale, and reduces mortality (134). The target partial pressure of oxygen in arterial blood (PaO_2) is more than 60 torr, without a substantial increase in partial pressure of carbon dioxide ($PaCO_2$) or a decrease in pH. Clearly, in those patients who manifest a drop in pH, caution should be exercised, and the administered oxygen level adjusted accordingly.

More oxygen may be required on exercise or at night, and this may require extra monitoring to determine the level required (see Chapter 17). A 6-minute walk with continuous monitoring of the oxyhemoglobin level may be useful for guidance regarding dosage of oxygen during exercise. In a study involving 22 patients with CF with severe lung disease (FEV_1 38%

predicted), the investigators found an improvement in exercise capacity, maximal volume of oxygen utilization (VO_2), and O_2 pulse when using supplemental oxygen as compared with room air (135). In a similar fashion, monitoring of oxyhemoglobin during sleep can help assess the need for nocturnal oxygen. The risk of nocturnal hypoxemia can be assessed to some extent from lung function and resting levels of oxyhemoglobin saturation. An oxyhemoglobin level of less than 94% saturation during the day predicted nocturnal hypoxemia fairly well (136).

Although supplemental oxygen limits the development of pulmonary hypertension, severe end-stage CF lung disease can be accompanied by cor pulmonale. Physical examination reveals evidence of pulmonary hypertension, with an accentuated pulmonic second sound, and possibly a right ventricular heave. If right ventricular failure occurs, an enlarged heart should be detectable either on physical examination or on a chest radiograph, with an enlarged liver and edema. Treatment of the underlying disease determines the intermediate and long-term outcome, and clearly, with very severe irreversible disease, this goal may not be achievable without lung transplantation. Supplemental oxygen reduces pulmonary vascular resistance and should be used as the primary therapy. There is little place for diuretics, digitalis, or vasodilators in CF because disadvantages such as intravascular volume depletion, reduction in systemic pressure, and arrhythmias outweigh the few potential advantages (134). In general, the prognosis becomes worse if cor pulmonale develops, thus emphasizing the need for early aggressive prophylaxis and treatment in regard to the underlying lung disease.

Resectional Surgery

Surgery on focally affected areas of lung occasionally is considered for those patients refractory to aggressive standard therapy (see Chapter 8). The hypothesis is that if chest physiotherapy, bronchodilators, and antibiotics have not controlled the problem adequately,

the affected areas act as a reservoir for ongoing infection, resulting ultimately in damage to the remaining areas of lung. Resectional surgery yields best results in those patients with localized disease. Patients with more generalized disease and poor lung function ($< \sim 30\%$ FEV_1) fare badly postoperatively (137,138). Critical evaluation of patients being considered for surgery includes ventilation perfusion scanning and thin-section computerized tomographic scanning. Adequate pre- and postoperative care is vital to optimize the results, including pre- and postoperative chest physiotherapy, antibiotics, and hydration (137). Overall, such surgery only should be contemplated in conjunction with an experienced CF clinician and surgeon.

Other Therapies

DNase

Although traditional mucolytic therapies, such as N-acetylcysteine and isotonic saline aerosol, have been used for many years, none have been demonstrated to confer any benefit in CF. Recent data suggest a benefit from more specific targeting of DNA in airway secretions of patients with CF using recombinant technology. DNA is present in very high concentrations in purulent CF airway secretions. Treatment directed at cleaving the DNA should reduce the viscosity of airway secretions and enhance airway clearance.

An enzyme to cleave DNA, recombinant human deoxyribonuclease (rhDNase), recently has been cloned via molecular techniques, tested in clinical trials, and approved by the U.S. Food and Drug Administration (139). Preliminary data from *in vitro* studies indicated that DNase reduced viscoelastic properties of CF sputum, as assayed by a viscometer and "pourability." Subsequent clinical studies supported these data. Phase I and II studies confirmed the safety and efficacy of the drug, with modest (10% to 15% above baseline) acute improvements in FEV_1 and FVC, and improvements in dyspnea and well-being (140–143). The improvement in FEV_1 usually is apparent within 3 days, with a reversion to previous levels once the drug is stopped. The largest trial of DNase involved 968 patients in 51 CF centers, in a randomized, double-blind, placebo-controlled study, conducted in conjunction with usual therapy for CF (7). Clinically stable patients with CF older than 5 years of age with a predicted FVC greater than 40% were studied. Two doses of DNase were used—2.5 mg daily or 2.5 mg twice daily, for 24 weeks, compared with placebo. Respiratory exacerbations (protocol defined before start) were reduced by 28% and 37% in the 2.5 mg daily and 2.5 mg twice daily groups, respectively, compared with placebo. FEV_1 was improved by approximately 5% to 6% above baseline in both dosage groups. Other advantages of DNase were marginal, for example, time spent in hospital (~1.2 fewer days over 6 months in the treatment groups) and treatment with parenteral antibiotics (~2.5 fewer days in the treatment groups). There were no differences in dyspnea or well-being scores between the groups. Hoarseness and chest pain were among the side effects seen at greater frequency in the treatment groups. There was no evidence of hypersensitivity to the drug.

A medium-term treatment study involving fewer patients also was conducted in the United Kingdom (144). This was an open-label study with follow-up for 6 months, using the same patients (n = 59) who had completed the phase II study in the same center, with 57 patients completing treatment. DNase, 2.5 mg, twice daily was administered, with an improvement in FEV_1 of 13% over baseline in the first month of treatment. The improvement in FEV_1 stabilized at 6% over the next 5 months, and there was an improvement in FVC of 7% for most of the study period. These improvements reverted to baseline after medication was discontinued. Ongoing studies in patients with predicted FVC of less than 40% are in progress.

Thus, DNase confers modest benefits and may be useful in slowing the decline in lung function over time, although definitive data are lacking. Its risk/benefits ratio over the long

term remain to be seen, particularly because of the cost involved (approximately $30 daily for the single daily dose schedule) (145). Prescribing physicians should use a rigorous protocol for therapy with DNase; it probably is best used in a systematic fashion, that is with baseline objective data such as daily sputum quantities and FEV_1 recorded. These data should be collected again after a defined period, to ensure efficacy of the medication. If patients have a clear-cut improvement in lung function or symptoms, it is reasonable to continue the drug.

Antiinflammatory Therapy: Ibuprofen

Prevention of the decrease in lung function remains the real goal in the management of CF lung disease. Antiinflammatory therapy would seem a logical approach, particularly because evidence of inflammation early in life has been demonstrated, which contributes to the damage inflicted on airway mucosa over time. A previous study using systemic corticosteroids for this purpose was limited by a high incidence of side effects (146). A more recent study using the nonsteroidal antiinflammatory agent ibuprofen also examined the potential benefit on lung function and other clinical parameters by inhibiting the inflammatory response (8,147).

In vitro studies previously demonstrated that ibuprofen inhibited the ability of neutrophils to migrate and release damaging enzymes. Because these and other studies indicated that at low plasma concentrations (< 50 µg/mL), neutrophil influx into alveolar crevices of the oral mucosa in patients with CF was increased rather than inhibited, low-dose ibuprofen actually might be detrimental. Therefore, a high-dose regimen was chosen for the study to achieve peak plasma concentrations of 50 to 100 µg/mL of ibuprofen. A randomized, double-blind, placebo-controlled protocol was performed in which 85 patients, stratified by age, with mild disease (predicted FEV_1 > 60%), were studied. The study was carried out over 4 years, with the rate of change of FEV_1 as the primary outcome measure. The secondary outcome measures were the annual rate of change of FVC, FEF_{25-75}, residual volume/total lung capacity (RV/TLC), percentage change in ideal body weight, change in chest radiograph scores at 4 years, and number of hospitalizations and days of intravenous antibiotics. A profile of adverse effects also was compiled.

Of the 85 patients enrolled in the study, 84 were included in the intent-to-treat analyses and 57 patients were included in the completed treatment analysis. Compliance was similar in both the ibuprofen and the placebo groups. The number of younger (< 13 years of age) patients enrolled was 49. For the primary outcome measure, lung function, there was a significant difference in favor of ibuprofen, particularly in the younger patients and in those who completed treatment. Overall, the FEV_1 decreased more slowly in those who completed ibuprofen treatment (-1.48% of predicted value per year) than in the placebo group (-3.57% predicted per year) a 59% relative improvement. This effect was most noticeable in the younger patients, where ibuprofen slowed the annual decrease in FEV_1 by 65% in the intention-to-treat group and by 88% in the completed treatment group. In those patients older than 13 years of age, there was no significant difference in lung function between ibuprofen and placebo. In short, the benefits of ibuprofen in subset analyses were seen only in those patients younger than 13 years of age.

Of the secondary outcome measures, there was less decrease in ideal body weight in the younger patients treated with ibuprofen, with greater effect in those who completed treatment. Changes in chest radiograph scoring were slowed in all age groups by ibuprofen. There were small, nonsignificant differences in favor of ibuprofen in terms of hospitalizations and days of care. Surprisingly, considering the high dose of ibuprofen used, adverse effects—particularly those usually seen in conjunction with nonsteroidal antiinflammatory agents—were surprisingly few. It should be noted that at baseline, approximately 50% of all patients enrolled were on antacids or histamine receptor blockers, with a similar increase in usage over

the study period between the two groups. Epistaxis and conjunctivitis clearly were related to ibuprofen in two cases, but gastrointestinal problems such as abdominal pain and esophagitis were no more common in the ibuprofen group than in the placebo group.

Ibuprofen holds promise as an agent to be used in patients with mild disease, particularly younger patients. If FEV_1 and ideal body weight are preserved over longer periods of time, then this probably will significantly impact survival. The reasons for the lack of effect of the medication on older patients are unclear. They may be related to small numbers or a different rate of loss of lung function in older patients that make it difficult to demonstrate a difference, even over 4 years. In addition, over a longer time period, it remains to be seen whether more significant adverse effects will emerge as a significant problem. Nonetheless, the concept of an antiinflammatory agent as a prophylactic intervention early in the course of CF is exciting and heralds a new era in the management of the disease.

Bronchodilators

Certain agents that are in common use for other airway diseases may benefit patients with CF because of accompanying airway hyperresponsiveness (e.g., bronchodilators, anticholinergic agents).

Some patients with CF clearly also have asthma, so a careful history for symptoms suggestive of asthma and a search for evidence of atopy is warranted in all patients with CF because these patients will benefit from bronchodilator therapy directed against this component of their lung disease. β-adrenergic agents (with the newer more selective $β_2$ agonists preferred) and anticholinergic agents play a significant role in therapy of these patients with CF, particularly in those patients who demonstrate significant beneficial postbronchodilator effects on spirometric testing (148,149). In this context, ipratropium bromide recently has emerged as a potentially useful agent in CF (148–150). Ipratropium is at least as useful, and in some cases marginally better than, some β_2 agonists, for example, metaproterenol (although this agent currently is not used much) (151). Therefore, this agent is worth bearing in mind as potentially useful in some patients with CF for reducing airway obstruction and augmenting airway clearance. Side effects have been described, for example, meconium ileus equivalent (152). It should be noted that although a proportion of patients exhibit hyperresponsiveness on simple pre- and postbronchodilator spirometry testing, some patients demonstrate worsening of flow rates after inhalation of such agents. In addition, long-term, β-adrenergic stimulation may increase the already accelerated Na^+ absorption across CF airway epithelia via cyclic adenosine monophosphate (cAMP) stimulation (153). This may lead to worsening of airway surface liquid rheology and mucociliary clearance, with further deleterious effects on airway obstruction.

Thus, all patients with CF should be screened for symptoms and other evidence of reactive airways disease, and a trial of bronchodilator and/or anticholinergic therapy should be instituted. It should be kept in mind that a proportion of patients will not receive benefit from such therapy, and their condition may even worsen.

Future Therapies

An intense research effort currently is underway to develop more specific therapies for CF, targeting the underlying pathophysiology of the disease (see Chapters 3 and 11 for a detailed discussion) These new approaches address the underlying pathophysiologic defects that result from the mutated CFTR at several levels. Gene therapy for CF has been studied in initial trials, and others currently are under way (154–158). Therapies directed at the inflammatory process are under investigation, including pentoxifylline (inhibits cytokines that attract neutrophils) and antiproteases [e.g., α-1–antiprotease inhibitor and recombinant secretory leukoprotease inhibitor (rSLPI)] (6).

Another route of research is directed at the ion transport defects in CF, including amiloride and

uridine-5'-triphosphate (UTP). Amiloride blocks the excessive sodium transport on CF airway epithelia, and UTP stimulates chloride secretion via the alternative (i.e., not the CFTR) chloride channel. Pilot studies demonstrated an improvement in the biorheology of airway secretions and a slowing in the decline in lung function over time after aerosolization with amiloride (159,160). Subsequent studies, however, have been less promising in older patients with established disease (161,162). More recent studies have shown an improvement in mucociliary clearance in healthy subjects and patients with CF after acute administration of aerosolized UTP (163,164). UTP has multiple actions, including stimulation of Cl^- secretion, goblet cell degranulation, and ciliary beat frequency, so it is particularly attractive as a potential therapy for CF. Drugs targeting abnormal ion transport, such as amiloride and UTP, probably would be used optimally in patients with mild disease, possibly in combination, because of their complementary actions.

Hypertonic saline represents another approach to the hydration of airway secretions. Recent studies from Australia suggest a benefit in the short term from inhalation of hypertonic saline, with improvements in lung function and measures of mucociliary clearance (165,166). The first study addressed the effects of hypertonic saline on lung function, with an improvement in FEV_1 of 15% after inhalation of 6% saline, which was significantly better than after isotonic (0.9%) saline. There were surprisingly few side effects, but patients were premedicated with inhaled albuterol (165). In the second study, measures of mucociliary and cough clearance were significantly better after treatment with 7% saline (with and without amiloride) compared with isotonic saline (166). These patients also did not report any undue side effects such as wheezing or cough. Hypertonic saline may represent a new, relatively inexpensive treatment for improving airway clearance and reducing airway obstruction in CF. Long-term studies will be necessary to confirm efficacy and address safety considerations.

Other approaches include the use of antipseudomonal vaccines and intravenous immunoglobulin therapy, with the aim of reducing the effects of chronic infection with *P. aeruginosa*. New antibiotics that decrease the adherence of *P. aeruginosa* also are being studied.

SUMMARY

As indicated in the introduction, patients with CF currently have a significantly better prognosis than in previous decades, which reflects the institution of a broad approach to the treatment of the disease, including airway clearance techniques, intravenous antibiotics, and newer adjunctive therapies. The general approach to monitoring of patients with CF should include frequent (3 to 4 monthly) visits to a physician versed in the special needs of such individuals, with regular measurement of lung function and studies of sputum microbiology, and vigilance for additional problems that can cause a deterioration in symptoms, such as asthma and ABPA. Although other newer therapies hold promise and appear exciting, physicians and patients should not lose sight of what currently is the best available standard care, which is a careful, methodical approach, as outlined in this chapter.

Note: M.R. Knowles is a founding scientist of Inspire Pharmaceuticals, which licensed the patent for aerosolized UTP from the University of North Carolina on March 10, 1995. M.R. Knowles and the University of North Carolina hold equity in Inspire Pharmaceuticals.

REFERENCES

1. Davis PB. Pathophysiology of the lung disease in cystic fibrosis. In: Davis PB, ed. *Cystic fibrosis.* New York: Marcel Dekker Inc, 1993:193–218.
2. Welsh MJ, Tsui L, Boat TF, et al. Cystic fibrosis. In: Scriver CR, Beaudet AL, Sly WS, Valle D, eds. The metabolic and molecular bases of inherited diseases. 7th ed. New York: McGraw-Hill, 1996;3799–3876.
3. The Cystic Fibrosis Foundation Center Committee and Guidelines Subcommittee. Cystic Fibrosis Foundation guidelines for patient services, evaluation and monitoring in cystic fibrosis centers. *Am J Dis Children* 1990;144:1311–1312.
4. Turpin SV, Knowles MR. Treatment of pulmonary disease in patients with cystic fibrosis. In: Davis PB, ed. *Cystic fibrosis.* New York: Marcel Dekker, 1993:277–344.
5. Rolfe MW, Schnapf BM. Management of the adult patient with cystic fibrosis. *Clin Pulm Med* 1995;2:75–87.
6. Davis PB, Drumm M, Konstan MW. Cystic fibrosis—state of the art. *Am J Respir Crit Care Med* 1996;154:1229–1256.
7. Fuchs HJ, Borowitz DS, Christiansen DH, et al. Effect of aerosolized recombinant human DNase on exacerbations on respiratory symptoms and on pulmonary function in patients with cystic fibrosis. *N Engl J Med* 1994;331:637–642.
8. Konstan MW, Byard PJ, Hoppel CL, Davis PB. Effects of high-dose ibuprofen in patients with cystic fibrosis. *N Engl J Med* 1995;332:848–854.
9. Konstan MW, Stern RC, Doershuk CF. Efficacy of the Flutter device for airway mucus clearance in patients with cystic fibrosis. *J Pediatr* 1994;124:689–693.
10. Ramsey BW. Management of pulmonary disease in patients with cystic fibrosis. *N Engl J Med* 1996;335:179–188.
11. Boucher RC. Human airway ion transport: part 1. *Am J Respir Crit Care Med* 1994;150:271–281.
12. Boucher RC. Human airway ion transport: part 2. *Am J Respir Crit Care Med* 1995;150:581–593.
13. Noone PG, Olivier KN, Knowles MR. Modulation of the ionic milieu of the airway in health and disease. In: Coggins CH, Hancock EW, eds. *Annual Review of Medicine.* Palo Alto, CA: Annual Reviews Inc, 1994:421–434.
14. Konstan MW, Hilliard KA, Norvell TM, Berger M. Bronchoalveolar lavage findings in cystic fibrosis patients with stable, clinically mild lung disease suggests ongoing infection and inflammation. *Am J Respir Crit Care Med* 1994;150:448–454.
15. Moss RB. Inflammatory response in cystic fibrosis lung disease. *New Insights Cystic Fibrosis* 1995;3:1–6.
16. Davidson AGF, McIlwaine M. Airway clearance techniques in cystic fibrosis. *New Insights Cystic Fibrosis* 1995;3:6–11.
17. Williams MT. Chest physiotherapy and cystic fibrosis: why is the most effective form of treatment still unclear? *Chest* 1994;106:1872–1882.
18. Thomas J, Cook DJ, Brooks D. Chest physical therapy management of patients with cystic fibrosis: a meta-analysis. *Am J Respir Crit Care Med* 1995;151:846–850.
19. Regnis JA, Robinson M, Bailey DL, et al. Mucociliary clearance in patients with cystic fibrosis and normal subjects. *Am J Respir Crit Care Med* 1994;150:66–71.
20. Khan TZ, Wagener JS, Bost T, Martinez J, Accurso FJ. Early pulmonary inflammation in infants with cystic fibrosis. *Am J Respir Crit Care Med* 1995;151:1075–1082.
21. Pryor JA, Webber BA. Physiotherapy for cystic fibrosis—which technique? *Physiotherapy* 1992;78:105–108.
22. Webber BA, Hofmeyr JL, Morgan MDL, Hodson ME. Effects of postural drainage, incorporating the forced expiratory technique, on pulmonary function in cystic fibrosis. *Br J Dis Chest* 1986;80:353–359.
23. Pryor JA, Webber BA. An evaluation of the forced expiration technique as an adjunct to postural drainage. *Physiotherapy* 1979;65:304–307.

24. Sutton PP, Lopez-Vidriero MT, Pavia D, et al. Assessment of percussion, vibratory-shaking and breathing exercises in chest physiotherapy. *Eur J Respir Dis* 1985;66:147–152.

25. Rossman CM, Waldes R, Samspon D, Newhouse MT. Effect of chest physiotherapy on the removal of mucus in patients with cystic fibrosis. *Am Rev Respir Dis* 1982;126:131–135.

26. de Boeck C, Zinman R. Cough versus chest physiotherapy: a comparison of the acute effects on pulmonary function in patients with cystic fibrosis. *Am Rev Respir Dis* 1984;129:182–184.

27. Bateman JRM, Newman SP, Daunt KM, Sheahan NF, Pavia D, Clarke SW. Is cough as effective as chest physiotherapy in the removal of excessive tracheobronchial secretions? *Thorax* 1981;36:683–687.

28. Zapletal A, Stefanova J, Horak J, Vavrova V, Samanek M. Chest physiotherapy and airway obstruction in patients with cystic fibrosis: a negative report. *Eur J Respir Dis* 1983;64:426–433.

29. de Jong W, Grevink RG, Roorda RJ, Kaptein KA, Van Der Schans CP. Effect of a home exercise training program in patients with cystic fibrosis. *Chest* 1994;105:463–468.

30. Van Haren EH, Lammers JW, Festen J, Van Herwaarden CL. Bronchial vagal tone and responsiveness to histamine, exercise and bronchodilators in adult patients with cystic fibrosis. *Eur Respir J* 1992;5:1083–1088.

31. Baldwin DR, Hill AL, Peckham DG, Knox AJ. Effect of addition of exercise to chest physiotherapy on sputum expectoration and lung function in adults with cystic fibrosis. *Respir Med* 1994;88:49–53.

32. Olseni L, Midgren B, Wollmer P. Mucus clearance at rest and during exercise in patients with bronchial hypersecretion. *Scand J Rehab Med* 1992;24:61–64.

33. Freeman W, Stableforth DE, Cayton RM, Morgan MD. Endurance exercise in adults with cystic fibrosis. Respir Med 1993;87:541–549.

34. Alison JA, Donnelly PM, Lennon M, et al. The effect of a comprehensive, intensive inpatient treatment program on lung function and exercise capacity in patients with cystic fibrosis. *Phys Ther* 1994;74:591–593.

35. Orenstein DM, Franklin BA, Doershuk CF, et al. Exercise conditioning and cardiopulmonary fitness in cystic fibrosis. *Chest* 1981;80:392–398.

36. Sawyer EH, Clanton TL. Improved pulmonary function and exercise tolerance with inspiratory muscle conditioning in children with cystic fibrosis. *Chest* 1993;104:1490–1497.

37. Orenstein DM, Nixon PA. Patients with cystic fibrosis. In: Franklin BA, Gordon S, Timmis GS, eds. *Exercise in modern medicine.* Baltimore: Williams and Wilkins, 1989; 204–214.

38. Hofmeyr JL, Webber BA, Hodson ME. Evaluation of positive expiratory pressure as an adjunct to chest physiotherapy in the treatment of cystic fibrosis. *Thorax* 1986;41:951–954.

39. McIlwaine PM, Wong LT, Peacock D, Davidson AG. Long-term comparative trial of conventional postural drainage and percussion versus positive expiratory pressure physiotherapy in the treatment of cystic fibrosis. *J Pediatr* 1997;131(4):570–574.

40. Coates AL. Chest physiotherapy in cystic fibrosis: spare the hand and spoil the cough? *J Pediatr* 1997 Oct;131(4):506–508.

41. Ramsey B, Burns J, Smith A. Safety and efficacy of tobramycin solution for inhalation in patients with cystic fibrosis: the results of two phase III placebo controlled clinical trials. *Pediatr Pulmonol* 1997; Suppl 14, 137–138.

42. Reisman JJ, Rivington-Law B, Corey M, et al. Role of conventional chest physiotherapy in cystic fibrosis. *J Pediatr* 1988;113:632–636.

43. Pfleger A, Theissl B, Oberwaldner B, Zach MS. Self administered chest physiotherapy in cystic fibrosis: a comparative study of high pressure PEP and autogenic drainage. *Lung* 1992;170:323–330.

44. Giles DR, Wagener JS, Accurso FJ, Butler-Simon N. Short term effects of postural drainage with clapping vs autogenic drainage on oxygen saturation and sputum recovery in patients with cystic fibrosis. *Chest* 1995;108:952–954.

45. Miller S, Hall DO, Clayton CB, Nelson N. Chest physiotherapy in cystic fibrosis: a comparative study of autogenic drainage and the active cycle of breathing techniques with postural drainage. *Thorax* 1995; 50:165–169.

46. Pryor JA, Webber BA, Hodson ME, Warner JO. The flutter VRP1 as an adjunct to chest physiotherapy in cystic fibrosis. *Respir Med* 1994;88:677–681.

47. Warwick WJ, Hansen LG. The long term effect of high frequency chest compression therapy on pulmonary complications of cystic fibrosis. *Pediatr Pulmonol* 1991;11:265–271.

48. Arens R, Gozal D, Omlin KJ, et al. Comparison of high frequency chest compression and conventional chest physiotherapy in hospitalized patients with cystic fibrosis. *Am J Respir Crit Care Med* 1994;150: 1154–1157.

49. di Sant 'Agnese PA, Andersen DH. Celiac syndrome: IV, chemotherapy in infections of the respiratory tract associated with cystic fibrosis of the pancreas: observations with penicillins and drugs of the sulfonamide group, with special reference to the penicillin aerosol. *Am J Dis Children* 1946;72:17–65.

50. Pedersen SS, Jensen T, Hoiby N, Koch C, Flensborg EW. Management of *Pseudomonas aeruginosa* lung infection in Danish cystic fibrosis patients. *Acta Paediatr Scand* 1987;76:955–961.

51. Smith AL, Redding G, Doershuk C, et al. Sputum changes associated with therapy for endobronchial exacerbation in cystic fibrosis. *J Pediatr* 1988;112: 547–554.

52. Gilligan PH. Microbiology of airway disease in patients with cystic fibrosis. *Clin Microbiol Rev* 1991;4:35–51.

53. Ramsey BW, Pepe M, Williams Warren J. Pulmonary exacerbation (PE): How do we define it? (abstract) *Pediatr Pulmonol* 1994 (suppl. 9):77–78.

54. Greene KE, Takasugi JE, Godwin JD, Richardson ML, Burke W, Aitken ML. Radiographic changes in acute exacerbations of cystic fibrosis in adults: a pilot study. *Am J Roentgenol* 1994;163:557–562.

55. Mouton JW, Kerrebijn KF. Antibacterial therapy in cystic fibrosis. *Med Clin North Am* 1990;74:837–850.

56. Hoiby N. Antibiotic therapy for chronic infection of pseudomonas in the lung. In: Coggins CH, Hancock EW, eds. *Annual Review of Medicine.* Palo Alto, CA: Annual Reviews Inc, 1993:1–10.

57. Marks MI. Antibiotic therapy for bronchopulmonary infections in cystic fibrosis: the American approach. *Antibiotic Chemother* 1989;42:229–236.

58. Jensen T, Pedersen SS, Hoiby N, Koch C, Flensborg EW. Use of antibiotics in cystic fibrosis: the Danish approach. *Antibiotic Chemother* 1989;42:237–246.

59. Szaff M, Hoiby N, Flensborg EW. Frequent antibiotic therapy improves survival of cystic fibrosis patients with chronic *Pseudomonas aeruginosa* infection. *Acta Paediatr Scand* 1983;72:651–657.

60. Regelmann WE, Elliot GR, Warwick WJ, Clawson CC. Reduction of sputum *Pseudomonas aeruginosa* density by antibiotics improves lung function in cystic fibrosis more than do bronchodilators and chest physiotherapy alone. *Am Rev Respir Dis* 1990;141:914–921.

61. Govan JRW, Doherty C, Glass S. Rational parameters for antibiotic therapy in patients with cystic fibrosis. *Infection* 1987;15:300–306.

62. Horrevorts AM, Driessen OMJ, Michel MF, Kerrebijn KF. Pharmacokinetics of antimicrobial drugs in cystic fibrosis. Aminoglycoside antibiotics. *Chest* 1988;94:S120–S125.

63. Lindsay CA, Bosso JA. Optimisation of antibiotic therapy in cystic fibrosis patients: pharmacokinetic considerations. *Clin Pharmacokinet* 1993;24:496–506.

64. de Groot R, Smith AL. Antibiotic pharmacokinetics in cystic fibrosis: differences and clinical significance. *Clin Pharmacokinet* 1987;13:228–253.

65. Branger C, Fournier JM, Loulergue J, et al. Epidemiology of *Stapylococcus aureus* in patients with cystic fibrosis. *Epidemiol Infection* 1994;112:489–500.

66. Pleasants RA, Michalets EL, Williams DM, Samuelson WM, Rehm JR, Knowles MR. Pharmacokinetics of vancomycin in adult cystic fibrosis patients. *Antimicrob Agents Chemother* 1996;40:186–190.

67. Pleasants RA, Walker TR, Samuelson WM. Allergic reactions to parenteral beta-lactam antibiotics in patients with cystic fibrosis. *Chest* 1994;106:1124–1128.

68. Earl HS, Sullivan TJ. Acute desensitization of a patient with cystic fibrosis allergic to both beta-lactam and aminoglycoside antibiotics. *Clin Immunol* 1987;79:477–483.

69. Rosenberg SM, Schramm CM. Predictive value of pulmonary function testing during pulmonary exacerbations in cystic fibrosis. *Pediatr Pulmonol* 1993;16:227–235.

70. Kane RE, Jennison K, Wood C, Black PG, Herbst JJ. Cost saving and economic considerations using home intravenous antibiotic therapy for cystic fibrosis patients. *Pediatr Pulmonol* 1988;4:84–89.

71. Winter RJD, George RJD, Deacock SJ, Shee CD, Geddes DM. Self administered home intravenous antibiotic therapy in bronchiectasis and adult cystic fibrosis. *Lancet* 1984;i:1338–1339.

72. Pond MN, Newport M, Joanes D, Conway SP. Home versus hospital intravenous antibiotic therapy in the treatment of young adults with cystic fibrosis. *Eur Respir J* 1994;7:1640–4.

73. Hammond LJ, Caldwell S, Campell PW. Cystic fibrosis, intravenous antibiotics, and home therapy. *J Pediatr Health Care* 1991;5:24–30.

74. Strandvik B, Hjelte L, Malmorg AS, Widen B. Home intravenous antibiotic treatment of patients with cystic fibrosis. *Acta Paediatr Scand* 1992;81:340–342.

75. Harwood IR, Greene LM, Kozakowski-Koch JA, Rasor JS. New peripherally inserted midline catheter: a better alternative for intravenous therapy for patients with cystic fibrosis. *Pediatr Pulmonol* 1992;12:233–239.

76. Davies MJ, Wilson RG, Nixon SJ. Implantable venous access catheters: what the patients say. *J R Coll Surg Edinb* 1992;2:125–126.

77. Sola JE, Stone MM, Wise B, Colombani PM. Atypical thrombotic and septic complications of totally implantable venous access devices in patients with cystic fibrosis. *Pediatr Pulmonol* 1992;14:239–242.

78. Peckham D, Hill J, Manshire AR, Knox AJ. Resolution of superior vena cava obstruction following thrombolytic therapy in a patient with cystic fibrosis and a long term in-dwelling catheter. *Respir Med* 1994;88:627–629.

79. Yung B, Campbell IA, Elborn JS, Harvey JS, Shale DJ. Totally implantable venous access devices in adult patients with cystic fibrosis. *Respir Med* 1996;90:353–356.

80. Myers MG, Koontz FP, Weinberger M. Lower respiratory infections in patients with cystic fibrosis. In: Lloyd-Still JD, ed. *Textbook of cystic fibrosis.* Boston: John Wright, 1983:91–107.

81. Jewes LA, Spencer RC. The incidence of anaerobes in the sputum of patients with cystic fibrosis. *J Med Microbiol* 1990;31:271–274.

82. Morris G, Brown MRW. Novel modes of action of aminoglycoside antibiotics against *Pseudomonas* infection. *Lancet* 1988;2:1359–1360.

83. Baldwin DR, Wise R, Andrews JM, Gill M, Honeybourne D. Comparative bronchoalveolar concentrations of ciprofloxacin and lomefloxacin following oral administration. *Respir Med* 1993;87:595–601.

84. Bosso JA, Black PG, Matsen JM. Ciprofloxacin versus tobramycin plus azlocillin in pulmonary exacerbations in adult patients with cystic fibrosis. *Am J Med* 1987;82:180–184.

85. Samuelson WM, Pleasants RA, Whitaker MS. Arthropathy secondary to ciprofloxacin in an adult cystic fibrosis patient. *Ann Pharmacother* 1993;27:302–303.

86. Scully BE, Nakatomi M, Ores C, Davidson S, Neu HC. Ciprofloxacin therapy in cystic fibrosis. *Am J Med* 1987;82:196–200.

87. Loening-Baucke VA, Mischler E, Myers MG. A placebo-controlled trial of cephalexin therapy in the ambulatory management of patients with cystic fibrosis. *J Pediatr* 1979;95:630–637.

88. Nolan G, McIvor P, Levinson H, Fleming PC, Corey M, Gold R. Antibiotic prophylaxis in cystic fibrosis: inhaled cephaloridine as an adjunct to oral cloxacillin. *J Pediatr* 1982;101:626–630.

89. Accurso FJ. Lung disease in infants with cystic fibrosis. *New Insights Cystic Fibrosis* 1996;4:1–7.

90. Sheldon CD, Assoufi BK, Hodson ME. Regular three monthly ciprofloxacin in adult cystic fibrosis patients infected with *Pseudomonas aeruginosa*. *Respir Med* 1993;87:587–593.

91. Littlewood JM, Smye SW, Cunliffe H. Aerosol antibiotic treatment in cystic fibrosis. *Arch Dis Child* 1993;68:788–792.

92. Toso C, Williams D, Noone PG. Inhaled antibiotics in cystic fibrosis: a review. *Ann Pharmacother* 1996;30:840–850.

93. Fiel SB. Aerosol delivery of antibiotics to the lower airways of patients with cystic fibrosis. *Chest* 1995;107:61s–64s.

94. Maddison J, Dodd M, Webb AK. Nebulized colistin causes chest tightness in adults with cystic fibrosis. *Respir Med* 1994;88:145–147.

95. Weber A, Smith A, Williams-Warren J, Ramsey B, Covert DS. Nebulizer delivery of tobramycin to the lower respiratory tract. *Pediatr Pulmonol* 1994;17: 331–339.

96. Hodson ME. Antibiotic treatment: aerosol therapy. *Chest* 1988;94:157S–160S.

97. Ramsey BW, Dorkin HL, Eisenberg JD, et al. Efficacy of aerosolized tobramycin in patients with cystic fibrosis. *N Engl J Med* 1993;328:1740–1746.

98. O'Doherty MJ, Thomas S, Page C, Bradbeer C, Nunan TO, Bateman NT. Pulmonary deposition of nebulised pentamidine isethionate: effect of nebuliser type, dose and volume of fill. *Thorax* 1990;45: 460–464.

99. Noone PG, Regnis JA, Robinson J, et al. Airway deposition and clearance, and systemic pharmacokinetics of amiloride following aerosolization with an ultrasonic nebulizer. *Chest* 1997;112:1283–1290.

100. Ciofu O, Giwercman B, Pedersen SS, Hoiby N. Development of antibiotic resistance in *Pseudomonas aeruginosa* during two decades of antipseudomonal treatment at the Danish CF center. *APMIS* 1994;102: 674–680.

101. Kilby JM, Gilligan PH, Yankaskas JR, Highsmith WE, Edwards LJ, Knowles MR. Nontuberculous mycobacteria in adult patients with cystic fibrosis. *Chest* 1992;102:70–75.

102. Simpson IN, Finlay J, Winstanley DJ, et al. Multi resistant isolates possessing characteristics of both *Burkholderia (Pseudomonas) cepacia* and *Burkholderia gladioli* from patients with cystic fibrosis. *J Antimicrob Chemother* 1994;34:353–361.

103. Zabner R, Quinn JP. Antimicrobials in cystic fibrosis: emergence of resistance and implications for treatment. *Semin Respir Infect* 1992;7:210–217.

104. Saiman L, Mehar F, Niu WW. Antibiotic susceptibility testing of multiply resistant *Pseudomonas aeruginosa* from patients with cystic fibrosis, including candidates for transplantation. *Clin Infect Dis* 1996; 23: 532–537.

105. Millar-Jones L, Paull A, Saunders Z, Goodchild M. Transmission of *Pseudomonas cepacia* among cystic fibrosis patients. *Lancet* 1992;340:491.

106. Smith DL, Smith EG, Gumery LB, Stableforth DE. *Pseudomonas cepacia* infection in cystic fibrosis patients. *Lancet* 1992;339:252.

107. Hoogkamp-Korstanje JAA, Meis JFGM, Kissing J, van der Laag J, Melcehers WJG. Risk of cross colonization and infection by *Pseudomonas aeruginosa* in a holiday camp for cystic fibrosis. *J Clin Microbiol* 1995;33:572–575.

108. Goldstein R, Sun L, Jiang R, Sajjan U, Forstner JF, Campanelli C. Structurally variant classes of pilus appendage fibers coexpressed from *Burkholderia (Pseudomonas) cepacia*. *J Bacteriol* 1995;177:1039–1052.

109. Peckham D, Crouch S, Humphreys H, Lobo B, Tse A, Knox AJ. Effect of antibiotic treatment on inflammatory markers and lung function in cystic fibrosis patients with *Pseudomonas cepacia*. *Thorax* 1994;49: 803–807.

110. Lewin LO, Byard PJ, Davis PB. Effect of *Pseudomonas cepacia* colonization on survival and pulmonary function of cystic fibrosis patients. *J Clin Epidemiol* 1990;43:125–131.

111. Taylor RF, Gaya H, Hodson ME. *Pseudomonas cepacia*: pulmonary infection in patients with cystic fibrosis. Respir Med 1993;87:187–192.

112. Egan TM, Detterbeck FC, Mill MR, et al. Improved results of lung transplantation for patients with cystic fibrosis. *J Thor Cardiovasc Surg* 1995;109:224–235.

113. Aitken ML, Burke W, McDonald G, Wallis C, Ramsey B, Nolan C. Nontuberculous mycobacterial disease in adult cystic fibrosis patients. *Chest* 1993;103: 1096–1099.

114. Olivier KN, Yankaskas JR, Knowles MR. Nontuberculous mycobacterial pulmonary disease in cystic fibrosis. *Semin Respir Infect* 1996;11:272–284.

115. Whittier S, Hopfer RL, Knowles MR, et al. Improved recovery of mycobacteria from respiratory secretions of patients with cystic fibrosis. *J Clin Microbiol* 1993;31:861–864.

116. Ahn CH, McLarty CW, Ahn SS. Diagnostic criteria for pulmonary diseases caused by *Mycobacterium kansasii* and *Mycobacterium avium intracellulare*. *Am Rev Respir Dis* 1982;125:388–391.

117. Moore EH. Atypical mycobacterial infection in the lung; CT appearance. *Radiology* 1993;187:777–782.

118. Swensen SJ, Hartman TE, Williams DE. Computed tomographic diagnosis of mycobacterium avium-intracellulare complex in patients with bronchiectasis. *Chest* 1994;105:49–52.

119. Olivier KN, Thiede SG. Non tuberculous mycobacteria in the adult CF patient: colonizers or pathogens. *Pediatr Pulmonol* 1994;S10:176–177.

120. Pinto-Powell R, Olivier KN, Marsh BJ, et al. Skin testing with *Mycobacterium avium* sensitin to identify with *M. avium* complex in patients with cystic fibrosis. *Clin Infect Dis* 1996;22:560–562.

121. Conway SP, Simmonds EJ, Littlewood JM. Acute severe deterioration in cystic fibrosis associated with influenza A virus infection. Thorax 1992;47:112–114.

122. Winnie BG, Cowan RG. Association of Epstein-Barr virus infection and pulmonary exacerbations in patients with cystic fibrosis. *Pediatr Infect Dis* 1992; 11:722–726.

123. Abman SJ, Ogle JW, Butler-Simon N, Rumack CM, Accurso FJ. Role of respiratory syncitial virus in early hospitalizations for respiratory distress of young infants with cystic fibrosis. *J Pediatr* 1988; 113:826–830.

124. Ramsey BW, Gore E, Smith AL, Cooney MK, Redding GJ, Foy H. The effect of respiratory viral infections on patients with cystic fibrosis. *Am J Dis Children* 1989;143:662–668.

125. Matsuse T, Hayashi S, Kuwano K, Keunecke H, Jefferies WA, Hogg JC. Latent adenoviral infection in the pathogenesis of chronic airways obstruction. *Am Rev Respir Dis* 1992;146:177–184.

126. Vitalis TZ, Keicho N, Itabashi S, Hayashi S, Hogg JC. A model of latent adenovirus 5 infection in the guinea pig (*Cavia porcellus*). *Am J Respir Cell Mol Biol* 1996;14:225–231.

127. Emre U, Bernius M, Roblin PM, et al. *Chlamydia pneumonia* infection in patients with cystic fibrosis. *Clin Infect Dis* 1996;22:819–23.

128. Mroueh S, Spock A. Allergic bronchopulmonary aspergillosis in patients with cystic fibrosis. *Chest* 1994;105:32–36.

129. Becker JW, Burke W, McDonald G, Greenberger PA, Henderson WR, Aitken ML. Prevalence of allergic bronchopulmonary aspergillosis and atopy in adult patients with cystic fibrosis. *Chest* 1996;109:1536–1540.

130. Hutcheson PS, Rejent RJ, Slavin RG. Variability in parameters of allergic bronchopulmonary aspergillosis in patients with cystic fibrosis. *J Allergy Clin Immunol* 1991;88:390–394.

131. Knutsen AP, Slavin RG. Allergic bronchopulmonary mycosis complication cystic fibrosis. *Semin Respir Infect* 1992;7:179–192.

132. Imbeault B, Cormier Y. Usefulness of high dose inhaled steroids in allergic bronchopulmonary aspergillosis. *Chest* 1993;103:1614–1617.

133. Mannes GPM, Van der Heide S, Alderen WMC, Gerritsen J. Itraconazole and allergic bronchopulmonary aspergillosis in twin brothers with cystic fibrosis. *Lancet* 1993;341:492.

134. Schidlow DV, Taussig LM, Knowles MR. Cystic Fibrosis Foundation consensus conference report on pulmonary complications of cystic fibrosis. *Pediatr Pulmonol* 1993;15:187–198.

135. Marcus CL, Bader D, Stabile MW, Wang C, Osher AB, Keens TG. Supplemental oxygen and exercise performance in patients with cystic fibrosis with severe pulmonary disease. *Chest* 1992;101:52–57.

136. Versteegh FGH, Bogaard JM, Raatgever JW, Stam H, Neijens HJ, Kerrebijn KF. Relationship between airway obstruction, desaturation during exercise and nocturnal hypoxaemia in cystic fibrosis patients. *Eur Respir J* 1990;3:68–73.

137. Steinkamp G, von der Hardt H, Zimmerman HJ. Pulmonary resection for localized bronchiectasis in cystic fibrosis. *Acta Paediatr Scand* 1988;77:569–575.

138. Smith MB, Hardin WD, Dressel DA, Beckerman RC, Moynihan PC. Predicting outcome following pulmonary resection in cystic fibrosis patients. *J Pediatr Surg* 1991;26:655–659.

139. Shak S. Aerosolized recombinant human DNase 1 for the treatment of cystic fibrosis. *Chest* 1995;107:65S–70S.

140. Hubbard RC, McElvaney NG, Birrer P, et al. A preliminary study of aerosolized recombinant human deoxyribonuclease in the treatment of cystic fibrosis. *N Engl J Med* 1992;326:812–815.

141. Aitken ML, Burke W, McDonald G, Shak S, Montogemery AB, Smith A. Recombinant human DNase inhalation in normal subjects and patients with cystic fibrosis: a phase 1 study. *JAMA* 1992;267:1947–1951.

142. Ramsey BW, Astley SJ, Aitken ML, et al. Efficacy and safety of short term administration of aerosolized recombinant human deoxyribonuclease 1 in patients with cystic fibrosis. *Am Rev Respir Dis* 1993;148:145–151.

143. Rashasinha C, Assoufi B, Shak S, et al. Efficacy and safety of short term administration of aerosolized recombinant human DNase 1 in adults with stable stage cystic fibrosis. *Lancet* 1993;342:199–202.

144. Shah PL, Scott SF, Fuchs HJ, Geddes DM, Hodson ME. Medium term treatment of stable stage cystic fibrosis with recombinant human DNase 1. *Thorax* 1995;50:333–338.

145. Davis PB. Evolution of therapy for cystic fibrosis. *N Engl J Med* 1994;331:672–673.

146. Rosenstein BJ, Eigen H. Risks of alternate day prednisone in patients with cystic fibrosis. *Pediatrics* 1991;87:245–246.

147. Colten HR. Airway inflammation in cystic fibrosis. *N Engl J Med* 1995;323:886–887.

148. Avital A, Sanchez I, Chernick V. Efficacy of salbutamol and ipratropium bromide in decreasing bronchial hyperreactivity in children with cystic fibrosis. *Pediatr Pulmonol* 1992;13:34–37.

149. Sanchez I, Holbrow J, Chernick V. Acute bronchodilator response to a combination of beta-adrenergic and anticholinergic agents in patients with cystic fibrosis. *J Pediatr* 1992;120:486–488.

150. Tobin MJ, Maguire O, Reen D, Tempany E, Fitzgerald MX. Atopy and bronchial reactivity in older patients with cystic fibrosis. *Thorax* 1980;35:807–813.

151. Weintraub SL, Eschenbacher WL. The inhaled bronchodilators ipratropium bromide and metaproterenol in adults with CF. *Chest* 1989;95:861–864.

152. Mulherin D, Fitzgerald MX. Meconium ileus equivalent in association with nebulized ipratropium bromide in cystic fibrosis. *Lancet* 1990;1:552.

153. Boucher RC, Stutts MJ, Knowles MR, Cantley L, Gatzy JT. Na$^+$ transport in cystic fibrosis epithelia: abnormal rate and response to adenyl cyclase activation. *J Clin Invest* 1986;78:1245–1252.

154. Johnson LG, Olsen JC, Sarkadi B, Moore KL, Swanstrom R, Boucher RC. Efficiency of gene transfer for restoration of normal airway epithelial function in cystic fibrosis. *Nat Genet* 1992;2:21–25.

155. Alton EWFW, Middleton PG, Caplen NJ, et al. Non invasive liposome mediated gene delivery can correct the ion transport defect in cystic fibrosis mutant mice. *Nat Genet* 1994;5:135–142.

156. Crystal RG, McElvaney NG, Rosenfield MA, et al. Administration of an adenovirus containing the human CFTR cDNA to the respiratory tract of individuals with cystic fibrosis. *Nat Genet* 1994;8:42–51.

157. Caplen NJ, Alton EWFW, Middleton PG, et al. Liposome mediated CFTR gene transfer to the nasal epithelium of patients with cystic fibrosis. *Nat Med* 1995;1:39–46.

158. Knowles MR, Hohneker KW, Zhou Z, et al. A controlled study of adenoviral-vector-mediated gene transfer in the nasal epithelium of patients with cystic fibrosis. *N Engl J Med* 1995;333:823–831.

159. Knowles MR, Church NL, Waltner WE, et al. A pilot study of aerosolized amiloride for the treatment of lung disease in cystic fibrosis. *N Engl J Med* 1990;322:1189–1194.

160. Tomkiewicz RP, App EM, Zayas JG, et al. Amiloride inhalation therapy in cystic fibrosis: influence on ion content, hydration, and rheology of sputum. *Am Rev Respir Dis* 1993;148:1002–1007.

161. Granham A, Hasani A, Alton EWFW, et al. No added benefit from nebulised amiloride in patients with cystic fibrosis. *Eur Respir J* 1993;6:1243–1248.

162. Bowler IM, Kelman B, Worthington D, et al. Nebulised amiloride in respiratory exacerbations of cystic fibrosis: a randomised controlled trial. *Arch Dis Child* 1995;73:427–430.

163. Olivier KN, Bennett WD, Hohneker KW, et al. Acute safety and effects on mucociliary clearance of aerosolized uridine 5-triphosphate +/− amiloride in normal adults. *Am J Respir Crit Care Med* 1996; 154: 217–223.

164. Bennett WD, Olivier KN, Zeman KL, Hohneker KW, Boucher RC, Knowles MR. Effect of uridine 5-triphosphate plus amiloride on mucociliary clearance in adult cystic fibrosis. *Am J Respir Crit Care Med* 1996;153:1796–1801.

165. Eng PA, Morton J, Douglass JA, Riedler J, Wilson J, Robertson CF. Short term efficacy of ultrasonically nebulized hypertonic saline in cystic fibrosis. *Pediatr Pulmonol* 1996;21:77–83.

166. Robinson M, Regnis JA, Bailey DL, King M, Bautovich GJ, Bye PTP. Effect of hypertonic saline, amiloride, and cough on mucociliary clearance in patients with cystic fibrosis. *Am J Respir Crit Care Med* 1996;153:1503–1509.

Cystic Fibrosis in Adults,
edited by J. R. Yankaskas and M. R. Knowles,
Lippincott-Raven Publishers, Philadelphia, 1999.

8

Major Complications

James R. Yankaskas, *Thomas M. Egan, and †Matthew A. Mauro

Cystic Fibrosis/Pulmonary Research and Treatment Center, Division of Pulmonary and Critical Care
Medicine, *Division of Cardiothoracic Surgery, and †Departments of Radiology and Surgery,
University of North Carolina School of Medicine, Chapel Hill, North Carolina

The major pulmonary complications—respiratory failure, pneumothorax, and massive hemoptysis—are very common and cause significant morbidity and mortality. Pneumothorax and massive hemoptysis occur, respectively, in 0.7% and 1% of patients with cystic fibrosis (CF) annually (1), and the incidence increases with age. Respiratory failure is nearly uniform, causing 94% of CF deaths. The pathophysiology of these disorders is better understood and has resulted in the development of improved treatments for all these problems. In 1993, a Cystic Fibrosis Consensus Conference summarized the published literature and clinical practices regarding these complications (2). Recent experience suggests that intensive treatment of reversible complications can improve significantly the length and the quality of life for many adults with CF. Available therapy probably will continue to be refined and improved. In this chapter, the pathophysiology, presentation, and current diagnostic and therapeutic approaches to these potentially life-threatening problems in adult patients with CF are summarized.

RESPIRATORY FAILURE

Cystic fibrosis lung disease leads to progressive respiratory impairment and causes hypoxemic and hypercapnic respiratory failure. This complication leads to death in more than 90% of patients (1). Improvements in understanding the pathophysiology of respiratory failure and development of new treatment options, including lung transplantation, have prompted CF clinicians to reevaluate the clinical approach to respiratory failure. In the past, supplemental oxygen did not seem to improve survival (3) and limited prescription was encouraged (4). The demonstration of significant exercise (5) and nocturnal (6) hemoglobin oxygen desaturation suggests that earlier therapy with O_2 may delay complications and improve the overall quality of life. Early reports emphasized the limited benefits of assisted ventilation in patients with CF (7), but improved treatments for massive hemoptysis and pneumothorax and the development of successful lung transplantation capabilities have improved outcomes significantly. In the following section, the pathophysiology of hypoxemic and hypercapnic respiratory failure are described, therapy guidelines are suggested, and modes of therapy are outlined that may be effective in adult patients with CF who experience respiratory failure.

Pathophysiology

Cystic fibrosis causes abnormal ion transport in airway epithelial cells that leads to alterations in the quantity, composition, and clearance of airway secretions (see Chapters 1 and 4). Secondary chronic infection with characteristic bacteria produces inflammation and progressive airway damage and bronchiectasis (see Chapter 3). These processes cause airway obstruction from inflammatory mucosal edema, thickened airway secretions, and bronchoconstriction. The adverse effects of airway obstruction on ventilation and oxygenation may be exacerbated by increased ventilatory requirements, air-trapping, and respiratory muscle weakness and fatigue. These mechanisms lead to the development of hypoxemic and hypercapnic respiratory failure. Figure 8–1 displays these pathophysiologic events graphically.

Hypoxemia in patients with CF is caused by multiple mechanisms related to chronic airway inflammation. Hypoventilation, caused by mechanisms described below, increases alveolar partial pressure of carbon dioxide (P_ACO_2) and decreases partial pressure of oxygen (P_AO_2). Loss of pulmonary capillaries decreases diffusing capacity and O_2 transfer (8). Ventilation/ perfusion (V/Q) mismatch causes hypoxemia that responds to supplemental O_2, through mechanisms similar to those of chronic obstructive pulmonary disease (COPD) (9). Decreased mixed venous oxygen saturation caused by increased metabolic rate and oxygen consumption can amplify the hypoxemic effects of V/Q mismatch (5). Intrapulmonary shunts, an extreme form of V/Q mismatch, cause supplementary O_2-resistant hypoxemia. Sleep may decrease oxygenation by decreasing ventilation and by further altering V/Q relationships (10,11).

Hypercapnic respiratory failure primarily is the result of alveolar hypoventilation caused by severe airway obstruction. The mechanisms include limited alveolar emptying due to airway closure and increased dead space (V_D) with increased dead space/tidal volume ratio (V_D/V_T). Hyperinflation secondary to airway obstruction results in a short inspiratory time and limits V_T (12). Increased metabolic rates and CO_2 production contribute to hypercapnia when alveolar ventilation is limited. Muscle weakness and fatigue may limit further the ability to maintain adequate minute ventilation and alveolar ventilation (13).

Hypoxemic and hypercapnic respiratory failure in CF usually are caused by slowly progres-

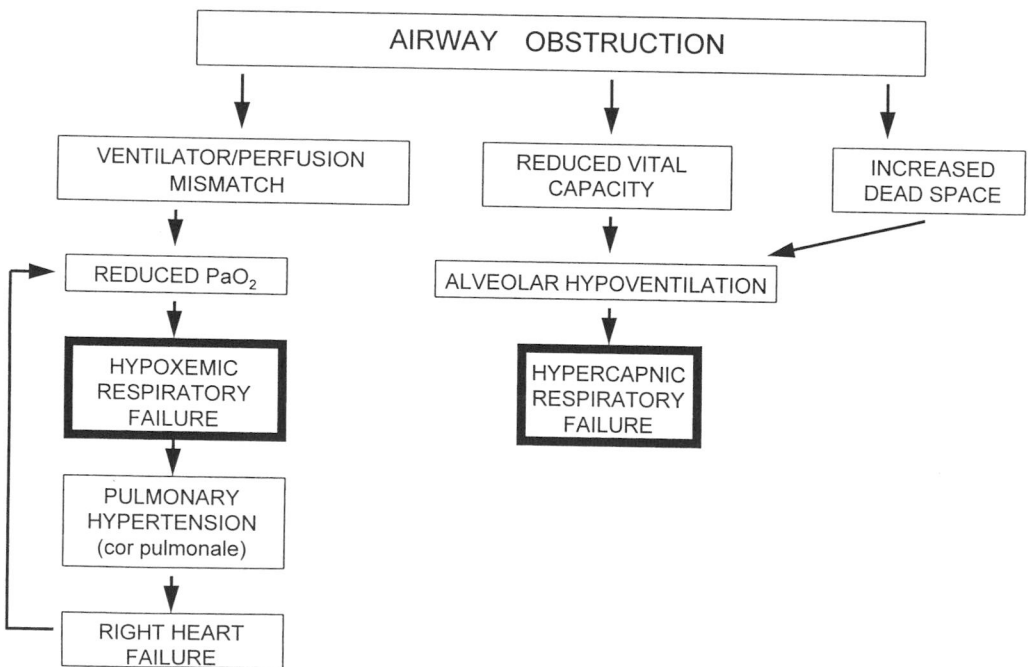

FIG. 8–1. Abnormalities contributing to hypoxemic and hypercapnic respiratory failure in cystic fibrosis.

sive airways disease. Such deterioration is most evident during exacerbations of bronchiectatic airways disease. Acute respiratory failure also may be precipitated by readily treatable complications, such as pneumothorax, hemoptysis, and bronchospastic airways diseases. All the contributing factors of respiratory failure should be identified to initiate the most appropriate therapies.

Treatment

General Measures

The goals of therapy are to correct hypoxemia and achieve alveolar ventilation adequate to permit normalization of arterial pH by respiratory and metabolic mechanisms. Specific treatments should focus on treating (a) reversible components of obstructive airways disease (infection, inflammation, retained airway secretions, and bronchoconstriction); (b) acute precipitating complications, such as pneumothorax or massive hemoptysis; and (c) the long-term complications of respiratory muscle weakness and fatigue. Diagnostic studies should include a search for new bacterial pathogens, including drug-resistant bacteria. Standard therapy (summarized in Chapter 7) should be intensified, including use of appropriate antibiotics and aggressive measures to clear airway secretions, including intensive care unit care, if required. Antibiotic selection should be based on recent sputum cultures and may include the use of synergistic antibiotic combinations identified by the Cystic Fibrosis Foundation-sponsored studies [14]. Concomitant bronchospastic disease or allergic bronchopulmonary aspergillosis may require treatment with inhaled bronchodilators and/or systemic steroids. Adequate nutrition is mandatory to maintain muscle mass, strength, and endurance. Enteral caloric supplements and adequate pancreatic enzyme replacement (described in Chapter 13) often are required. Exercise rehabilitation, which can improve cardiovascular and skeletal muscle conditioning (see Chapter 17) and assist in clearing of airway secretions,

usually is limited by the problems that precipitate respiratory failure. The high likelihood of disuse atrophy [15] suggests that early mobilization and exercise may be beneficial.

Hypoxemic Respiratory Failure

Effective treatment of hypoxemic respiratory failure will retard the development of pulmonary hypertension and cor pulmonale and prolong functional life. The use of supplemental oxygen to correct hypoxemia (Table 8–1) is considered standard therapy to limit the development of pulmonary hypertension and cor pulmonale [16,17]. Oxygen normally is delivered via nasal cannula, with flow titrated to maintain partial pressure of oxygen in arterial blood (PaO_2) greater than 60 torr (arterial saturation > 88% to 90%). Higher flows often are required during sleep [3,6,18] and during exercise [5,19,20]. Correction of hypoxemia may inhibit the hypoxemic respiratory drive mediated through the carotid chemoreceptors and induce a secondary increase in partial pressure of carbon dioxide in alveolar gas ($PACO_2$). This effect must be considered in selecting the O_2 flow rate, keeping correction of significant arterial oxygen desaturation as the primary goal, without significantly affecting $PaCO_2$ and pH. The benefits of continuous, nocturnal, or exercise supplemental oxygen therapy on quality of life and survival have not been established rigorously by controlled clinical trials in patients with CF. However, a nocturnal oxygen therapy trial in patients with COPD (due to causes other than CF) using continuous (18 to 24 hours per day) oxygen therapy showed a 50% decrease in mortality when compared with patients using

TABLE 8–1. *Indications for supplemental oxygen*

PaO_2 < 55 torr or SaO_2 < 88% breathing room air
Pulmonary hypertension
Cor pulmonale
Nocturnal SaO_2 < 88% for > 10% of sleep time
Exercise SaO_2 < 90%

Data from reference 2.

O_2 only 12 hours per day (21). Despite differences in age and etiology (5), most pulmonary physicians believe that these data should be extrapolated to adult patients with CF.

Sleep induces or worsens hypoxemia in patients with CF (6,11,18) as well as those who do not have CF (22,23,24). The mechanisms include decreased ventilation and alteration of V/Q relationships (10,25). Reactive polycythemia is not a good marker of nocturnal hypoxemia because it rarely is seen in patients with CF, even those with continuous hypoxemia. Consequently, nocturnal oximetry studies are required to document both nocturnal hypoxemia and appropriate response to therapy. Fortunately, recording pulse oximetry for outpatients is available in many regions. Patients with CF respond well to nocturnal supplemental oxygen (10,24). Home oxygen delivery is required for chronic therapy. An extensive variety of oxygen sources and delivery systems (Table 8–2) has been developed to meet this need (26). Concentrators are electricity dependent and provide continuous supplementation, but mobility is limited to the length of oxygen tubing. Compressed gas oxygen tanks are available in large and small sizes for home use and ambulation. Ambulatory use is limited by the size and weight of the tanks, and the duration is limited by the tank capacity. Portable liquid oxygen tanks generally are smaller and lighter than compressed gas tanks. Oxygen-conserving delivery devices add reservoirs or interrupted flow (only during inspiration), extending the effective capacity of tank and liquid oxygen systems. The system prescribed for an individual patient depends on availability of systems from local suppliers.

Patients with CF with predicted forced expiratory volume in 1 second (FEV_1) less than 30% (5,8,24) are prone to exercise hypoxemia and the potential complications of cor pulmonale and arrhythmia. Exercise capability (peak O_2 consumption) is an excellent predictor of survival (27). Aerobic exercise may improve clearance of airway secretions (28, 29,30) and skeletal muscle function (31) and thus may improve quality of life. The basic goals of an exercise program are to train to a level of activity commensurate to the maximum ventilatory capability while preventing significant oxygen desaturation of arterial hemoglobin. Supplemental O_2 flows should be titrated to maintain oxygen saturation in arterial blood (SaO_2) at a level greater than 88% to 90% (2). There is little evidence that staged exercise significantly increases PaCO2 (5,8). The regular pre- and postlung transplant physical rehabilitation program at the University of North Carolina (UNC) has improved airway clearance and improved exercise capability in many patients and provided prompt detection of clinical decrements (32).

Cor pulmonale and right-sided heart failure in CF are most commonly caused by hypoxemia, and treatment with supplemental oxygen is the most effective therapy. Although other drugs have been used for these complications, there is little role for diuretics, digitalis, or pulmonary vasodilators in treatment of hypoxemic respiratory failure in CF (33,34). Diuretics actually may have an adverse effect by decreasing systemic vascular volume and right heart filling without decreasing the pulmonary vascular pressures. This may lead to decreased cardiac output because the right ventricle

TABLE 8–2. *Home oxygen sources*

Type	Maximum flow	Duration at 2 L/min
O_2 concentrator	5 L/min	Indefinite
Compressed O_2 tanks		
D cylinder, 400 L	8 L/min	3.5 hrs
H cylinder, 6,700 L	"	5.5 hrs
Liquid		
Portable	15 L/min	4 hrs
Stationary	"	8 days

Data from reference 26.

serves primarily as a volume pump (35). Cardiac glycosides are of little use for right-sided failure (36) and increase the risk of cardiac dysrhythmia. Pulmonary vasodilators other than supplemental oxygen often reduce systemic vascular resistance as much as pulmonary vascular resistance. This effect may decrease cardiac output, leading to hypotension and possibly death (37). Theophylline may increase diaphragmatic muscle function (38), but it rarely is beneficial to overall function and may increase gastroesophageal reflux, a common problem in patients with CF.

Hypercapnic Respiratory Failure

Standard therapy for obstructive CF airways disease and treatment of acute complications form the basis of treating hypercapnic respiratory failure. Renal retention of bicarbonate partially compensates for the respiratory acidosis associated with CO_2 retention. Arterial pH levels greater than 7.3 generally are tolerated well, although consciousness often is impaired with PCO_2 greater than 100 torr, despite PaO_2 greater than 60 torr. Mechanical ventilation can acutely improve alveolar ventilation and respiratory acidosis, but its use may entail significant morbidity. Thus, when the decision is made to initiate ventilation through cuffed endotracheal tubes, the likelihood of improving the quality of life—as well as its duration—should be considered.

Experience with mechanical ventilation of patients with CF in the 1960s and 1970s achieved few long-term beneficial results. Few patients were weaned successfully from ventilators, and those who were extubated had short-term survival. A retrospective study (7) found poor outcome regardless of age at onset of respiratory failure. However, a more recent report of five infants with CF who required mechanical ventilation for acute respiratory failure (39) due to bronchiolitis or as an initial presentation of CF lung disease demonstrated 100% success at weaning and prolonged survival. The patients' Schwachmann scores and frequency of infectious exacerbations were comparable to those of 15 matched control patients with CF during 1 to 6 years of follow-up. Thus, infants and young children with CF should be afforded mechanical ventilation for acute and potentially reversible respiratory failure.

In contrast, in most adults with CF, largely irreversible respiratory insufficiency develops that limits the ability to wean from mechanical ventilation. Nevertheless, assisted ventilation is appropriate in several clinical circumstances (Table 8–3). Adults with respiratory failure due to an acute illness, such as bronchospasm, pneumothorax, massive hemoptysis, or a baseline suboptimal medical regimen, should be treated with standard medical therapy, including mechanical ventilation, as clinically indicated. The majority of these patients will survive short-term ventilatory support, as demonstrated by the cases summarized in Table 8–4. Their overall prognosis is determined primarily by the severity of the underlying irreversible lung disease, rather than by the episode of acute respiratory failure.

Individuals with extensive bronchiectatic disease in whom chronic and progressive hypercapnic respiratory failure develops that is unresponsive to aggressive standard therapy present difficult clinical and ethical challenges.

TABLE 8–3. *Hypercapnic respiratory failure in adult patients with CF: guidelines for assisted ventilation*

Indicated	Reversible or potentially reversible complications
	Pneumothorax
	Bronchospastic obstruction
	Central mucus plugging
	Suboptimal therapeutic regimen
Possible	Patients accepted as candidates for lung transplant
Not indicated	Progressive respiratory failure, unresponsive to intensive standard therapy

TABLE 8–4. *Adults with CF treated with mechanical ventilation for acutely reversible complications*

| Patient | Age (yrs) | Gender | Ventilator | | |
			Cause	Days	Survival
1	21	F	Initial presentation	45	12½ yrs
2	27	F	Bronchospasm	3	> 12 yrs
3	24	M	Massive hemoptysis	3	Died
4	31	M	Suboptimal regimen	8	> 6 yrs
5	24	M	Suboptimal regimen	4	> 6 yrs
6	16	F	Tension pneumothorax	1	2 yrs
7	26	F	Suboptimal regimen	38	1.1 yrs
8	22	M	Suboptimal regimen	3	> 4 yrs

Positive pressure ventilation through a cuffed endotracheal tube compromises the ability to clear secretions by cough and often results in worsening airway obstruction within days to weeks. Such therapy may be appropriate for listed lung transplantation candidates, provided that their waiting priority is high enough to make likely donor availability within several days or weeks. In the absence of a transplant option, few such patients would be weaned successfully from mechanical ventilation (7). A time-limited trial of intubation and mechanical ventilation occasionally is appropriate to assess responses to intensive therapy and to permit end-of-life tasks. The limitations of such therapy are best handled by careful education and planning before the end-stages of deteriorating health. Mask ventilation avoids some of the complications of standard mechanical ventilation via cuffed endotracheal tubes and may be a useful option for acute or chronic treatment of hypercapnic respiratory failure (see below).

Ventilatory Support Techniques

General Principles

Hypoxemic respiratory failure usually can be treated successfully with supplemental oxygen and treatment of the underlying disease. Assisted ventilation in patients with CF is appropriate therapy for hypercapnic respiratory failure due to acutely reversible causes and selected individuals with chronic hypercapnic failure, as described previously. The therapeutic goals are to increase alveolar ventilation

sufficiently to sustain life and to permit treatment of the underlying problems. Secretions cannot be cleared from small airways by endobronchial suctioning, and cough is less effective with an endotracheal tube in place. Intensive therapy must be instituted to correct acute and reversible components of respiratory failure and to limit the duration of tracheal intubation. Specific therapies for acute precipitating events (e.g., chest tube for pneumothorax) should be instituted, and an intensive regimen of intravenous antibiotics and effective chest physiotherapy to remove secretions is indicated. Inhaled or parenteral bronchodilators and/or corticosteroids should be considered for bronchospasm and mucosal edema unless contraindicated (e.g., some lung transplant centers limit the maximal doses and duration of steroid therapy before transplant). Adequate nutrition is essential and enteral feeding is preferred over total parenteral nutrition (TPN) to maintain gut epithelial integrity. Sedation use should be minimized, and a respiratory and skeletal muscle exercise program should be undertaken to minimize disuse atrophy.

Ventilation Through Endotracheal Tubes

Use of a large diameter orotracheal tube with a large-volume, low-pressure cuff is desirable to facilitate endotracheal suctioning of secretions and minimize mucosal damage. The optimal ventilatory mode has not been established by any controlled studies in patients with CF. Respiratory drive usually is excellent in patients with CF, and patient-initiated modes (e.g., pressure support) permit patient control of respiratory rate and synchronous use of respiratory muscles. Constant inspiratory pressure modes (e.g., pressure support and pressure control) provide lower peak airway pressures as compared with volume-limited (constant flow) modes. With pressure support ventilation, the inspiratory pressure should be titrated to permit a V_T adequate to maintain a respiratory rate less than 24 to 30 breaths/minute and a systemic arterial pH greater than 7.3. Tidal volumes for individuals with CF may be limited by hyperinflation and reduced respiratory system compliance and usually are less than 10 mL/kg. Positive end-expiratory pressure (PEEP) may be needed to compensate for auto-PEEP (40) and to improve ventilator triggering. PEEP increases functional residual capacity (FRC) and may improve ventilation by delaying airway closure, but it can significantly worsen air trapping and respiratory mechanics. Its utility to improve PO_2 is limited. As with asthma and COPD, respiratory rate, inspiratory flow, and V_T must be adjusted to provide a long and adequate expiratory time. High-frequency ventilation may be efficient at clearing airway secretions and maintaining arterial oxygenation but is less effective at CO_2 removal with bronchiectatic CF lungs. Hybrid high-frequency and low-frequency ventilators (e.g., the Volumetric Diffusive Respirator, Percussionaire Corp., Sandpoint, ID) may provide adequate oxygenation and ventilation while increasing clearance of secretions, but they may not support patient-initiated inspirations. At UNC, these principles have been used successfully to treat acute potentially reversible respiratory failure in seven of eight adults with CF (see Table 8–4) and in five CF transplant candidates (41). Over the same 3 years, one CF lung transplant candidate died before donor organs became available, after opting for time-limited mechanical ventilation.

Mask Ventilation

Positive pressure ventilation through nasal or face masks provides effective ventilatory assistance for some patients with hypercapnic respiratory failure due to neuromuscular weakness and some restrictive and obstructive lung diseases (42). Tracheal intubation is avoided; cough, verbal communication, and eating are possible; and intermittent use is feasible. Positive pressure ventilation is delivered via a tight-fitting nasal or face mask. Chin straps are available to minimize air loss through the mouth. Inspiratory flow may be generated at constant pressure (43) or with a constant-flow, volume-limited ventilator (15). The optimal V_T or pressure settings must be determined empirically because air leaks through the mask and mouth often are variable. The daily duration of treatment typically ranges from all night to continuous (except for meals and physiotherapy) and is based on clinical responses. Expiratory positive airway pressure can be added with either ventilator mode. Both methods achieve significant reductions in PCO_2 for several days to 6 months. The tight-fitting face masks often are uncomfortable, and high levels of patient motivation and cooperation are essential. Reports from Great Britain (43) and Australia (15) have demonstrated good results in individuals with CF. Benefits may be the result of increased tidal volumes, delayed airway closure secondary to expiratory positive airway pressure, and/or respiratory muscle rest. The Australian study demonstrated improved muscle strength within 1 month of starting nasal intermittent positive pressure ventilation.

Summary: Respiratory Failure

Patients with CF with respiratory failure should be treated with intensification of the standard therapy directed at intensive maneuvers to clear airway secretions, adequate antibacterial treatment, adequate nutrition, and reversal of mucosal edema and bronchoconstriction. Supplemental oxygen is the treatment of choice for hypoxemic respiratory failure. Therapy should be initiated when PO_2 is less than 55 torr or SaO_2 is less than 88%. Nocturnal pulse oximetry studies may be required to identify the indications for supplemental nocturnal O_2 and to determine adequacy of therapy. There is little role for diuretics, cardiac glycosides, or pulmonary vasodilators. Patients with CF with respiratory failure due to reversible causes such as acute illnesses or suboptimal standard therapy should be afforded mechanical ventilation by standard techniques using the principles outlined previously. Individuals with CF with progressive respiratory failure that has not responded to aggressive standard therapy and who are not transplant candidates should be advised that mechanical ventilation is unlikely to provide a long-term benefit. Occasionally, patients with CF on waiting lists for lung transplantation may be offered time-limited ventilatory support if donor lungs are likely to be available within a short time. New techniques, including mask ventilation, are establishing a useful role in the treatment of respiratory failure in some patients with CF.

PNEUMOTHORAX

Pneumothorax occurring in patients with CF can be either spontaneous or iatrogenic. Iatrogenic pneumothorax usually is due to puncture of the lung from placement of central venous lines. Spontaneous pneumothorax is caused by rupture of subpleural blebs. According to Cystic Fibrosis Registry data (44), the incidence of spontaneous pneumothorax in patients with CF is approximately 1% per year. The incidence increases with age and severity of disease such that up to 20% of adults with CF will experience a pneumothorax in their lifetime. Subpleural air cysts are common in patients with CF. In one autopsy study, they were present in 15 of 21 patients with CF. Six of these patients had pneumothorax at some point before their death (45). Although it has been suggested that degenerative pleural changes may predispose to pneumothorax in patients with CF (46), the frequency of subpleural air cysts is a more compelling reason for the high incidence. Because of the association of spontaneous pneumothorax with severity of disease, it has been considered an ominous complication (47).

Management of an Initial Pneumothorax

Members of a Cystic Fibrosis Consensus Conference have proposed a management strategy for patients with CF in whom pneu-

mothorax develops (2). Observation alone is a reasonable management strategy for asymptomatic patients with CF with a small pneumothorax (< 20% of the volume of the hemithorax). Conference members recommended hospital admission for any patients with newly diagnosed pneumothorax, even those who are asymptomatic. If the pneumothorax increases in size or the patient becomes symptomatic, then tube thoracostomy is indicated. The patient with CF who remains asymptomatic with evidence of resolution or no increase in size on a chest x-ray taken 24 hours after admission can be followed on an outpatient basis.

However, most pneumothoraces in patients with CF will cause symptoms of either chest discomfort or dyspnea. Additionally, a pneumothorax occupying a volume of the hemithorax in excess of 20% in a patient with CF should be drained with a tube thoracostomy. Chest tube placement is important to facilitate resolution of the pneumothorax. The tube should be inserted in a place that will not compromise a future incision for surgery for persistent pneumothorax. The tube should be inserted in an interspace where the lung has fallen away from the chest wall and should be advanced to the apex of the chest. Anteriorly placed chest tubes frequently are problematic because of increased local discomfort, the tendency of the tube to kink, and the difficulty in placing the tip of the chest tube in the apex of the chest. There also is a risk of injury to the internal thoracic artery if the tube is placed too medially. A chest tube placed in the mid or anterior axillary line in the sixth or seventh interspace, directed to the apex of the chest, minimizes these problems.

For evacuation of a large pneumothorax, the lung should be allowed to expand slowly by initially placing the chest tube to underwater seal only. When the air leak diminishes, then the tube can be placed to suction (-20 cm H_2O). There is no advantage to increasing the amount of suction applied to the chest tube; in fact, this may be detrimental. Although administration of 100% oxygen to facilitate resolution of a pneumothorax commonly is done, there is no evidence in humans that this is worthwhile.

The pneumothorax will resolve if the ruptured subpleural blebs seal. This is facilitated by apposition of the visceral and parietal pleura, which is the goal of tube thoracostomy therapy. Accordingly, if an air leak persists and the lung is not expanded fully on chest x-ray, consideration should be given to placement of additional chest tubes so that the lung can expand fully. Once the air leak ceases, the chest tube can be removed if the lung is expanded fully. In some asthenic patients with CF, placement of a purse-string suture around the chest tube site helps to prevent recurrence of pneumothorax caused by air leak through the tube tract.

For patients whose air leak persists beyond 5 days, the chest tube may be placed to underwater seal and removed if pneumothorax does not recur within 24 hours. For patients with recurrent pneumothorax or persisting pneumothorax, that is, those with a persistent air leak that results in lung collapse with the chest tube to underwater seal or clamped, some other intervention is warranted to resolve the pneumothorax.

Management of Persistent or Recurrent Pneumothorax

For patients whose pneumothorax persists beyond 5 days despite tube thoracostomy, or for patients in whom a second pneumothorax develops on the same side as a previously resolved pneumothorax, consideration should be given to a procedure to obliterate the pleural space.

Sclerosing agents have been used as a therapy for pneumothorax in patients with CF with varying results. McLaughlin et al. (48) reported a higher occurrence rate with tetracycline pleurodesis (6 of 7 patients) or silver nitrate pleurodesis (3 of 7 patients), although sclerosis with quinacrine was more effective. Quinacrine is no longer available for this purpose, and the only agent that has had moderate success at preventing recurrent pneumothorax is talc poudrage (49). Unfortunately, this requires a general anesthetic and insufflation of talc using the thoracoscope. Alternately, talc can be placed intrapleurally in a saline slurry.

This approach has been successful at resolving malignant pleural effusion 80% of the time (50). Talc causes an intense inflammatory reaction in the pleural space, with accompanying pleuritic pain and fever. It is a very effective agent in the management of malignant pleural effusion; however, the severity of adhesions produced makes subsequent explantation difficult and may increase the morbidity of lung transplantation. A theoretical concern is the calcification that can occur along pleural surfaces long after instillation of talc. Calcification of the diaphragm may occur and would be problematic in patients with CF. Another agent used as a sclerosant to manage malignant pleural effusions is bleomycin (51), but it is difficult to justify the use of such a potent antimetabolite in a patient with benign disease. Thus, the role of sclerosing agents in the management of CF pneumothorax is limited.

A surgical approach to recurrent or persistent pneumothorax is associated with a very low recurrence rate. Spector and Stern (47) reported a 95% success rate with thoracotomy and apical pleurectomy among 57 patients with pneumothorax. Schuster and colleagues (52) had a similar high success rate in a smaller series of 20 patients. Pleurectomy probably is not necessary because stapling across ruptured blebs and mechanical pleural abrasion produces similar satisfactory results in most non-CF patients with spontaneous pneumothorax. This approach can be performed through a small transaxillary thoracotomy (53), which provides excellent exposure of the apex of the lung and of the superior segment, sites of predilection for the formation of subpleural blebs.

There is growing interest in the use of the thoracoscope to approach problems in the pleural space, and thoracoscopy has been used to perform surgical bullectomy (54). Pleurodesis can be achieved through a thoracoscope, either mechanically or by insertion of an Nd:YAG or CO_2 laser (55). However, thoracoscopy may have limited application in patients with CF because of the tendency for CF lungs to deflate poorly because of airway obstruction and the fibrotic nature of the underlying lung. This may hinder visualization and

manipulation. There is no evidence that thoracoscopy is superior to transaxillary thoracotomy in the management of a pneumothorax.

Unfortunately, because pneumothorax is associated with advanced CF lung disease, instances occur where a pneumothorax fails to
resolve in patients with CF for whom even a
limited thoracotomy constitutes a significant
risk. In general, patients awaiting lung transplantation are poor candidates for any thoracic
surgical procedure except transplant because of
the requirement for a temporary period of intubation and mechanical ventilation and the impact of postoperative chest pain on ventilatory
mechanics. Attempts at chemical pleurodesis
may have some role in this group of very ill patients, in whom the risk of surgery may outweigh the benefits.

A surgical approach to pneumothorax does
not constitute a contraindication to future lung
transplantation. Previous surgery increases
blood transfusion requirements but is not associated with increased mortality after lung
transplantation (56). There is some consensus
at experienced CF lung transplant centers that
transplantation can proceed in patients with CF
who have had previous pleurodesis; these centers would prefer to offer transplants to patients
with CF who have had a surgical approach to
recurrent or persistent pneumothorax rather
than chemical pleurodesis (57,58).

Perioperative and Postoperative Considerations

Although transaxillary thoracotomy generally is tolerated well in young patients with recurrent spontaneous pneumothorax, it can be a
major hurdle in patients with CF, particularly
in those with significant compromise of lung
function. Postoperative analgesia is imperative
so that cough is preserved and clearance of airway secretions is facilitated. Chest physical
therapy should be initiated quickly after transplant. There is no evidence that properly performed chest physical therapy will interfere
with resolution of pneumothorax. In our experience, early ambulation also assists in mobi-
lizing airway secretions. Adequate nutrition
and sleep also are important for recovery. At-

tention must be paid perioperatively to gastrointestinal (GI) tract function of patients with
CF because narcotic analgesics may predispose
to the development of distal intestinal obstructive syndrome.

Pleural Effusions and Empyema

Despite the frequency of pulmonary infections in patients with CF, pleural effusions requiring drainage are unusual complications.
Although parapneumonic pleural effusions are
unusual in patients with CF, they should be
drained with thoracentesis or tube thoracostomy because these effusions can lead to
the development of an empyema. In the early
stages, tube thoracostomy usually is adequate
management of an empyema. Unfortunately,
drainage frequently is delayed, resulting in loc-
ulations and the formation of a thick pleural
peel that prevents the lung from expanding to
fill the space once it is drained. Thoracotomy
with decortication of underlying trapped lung
and evacuation of infected organized material
from the pleural space (59) is the preferred approach to a chronic empyema cavity (Fig. 8–2),
but it may not be a practical alternative in patients with CF with advanced lung disease (60).
In some circumstances, chronic drainage may
be necessary.

Summary: Pneumothorax

Management of pleural space problems in
patients with CF is based on general principles
of pleural space physiology in the context of
the needs of the individual patient, depending
on the severity of the patient's lung disease.
The prospect of future lung transplantation
should not interfere with good care for the patient. Because thoracic surgical procedures
generally are not considered absolute contraindications to future transplantation, the decision to treat a pleural space problem with surgery should be based on the patient's ability to
tolerate the surgery and the indications for surgery, rather than an overriding concern for
the impact of this intervention on future lung
transplantation. Surgical therapy of recurrent
or persistent pneumothorax is the preferred

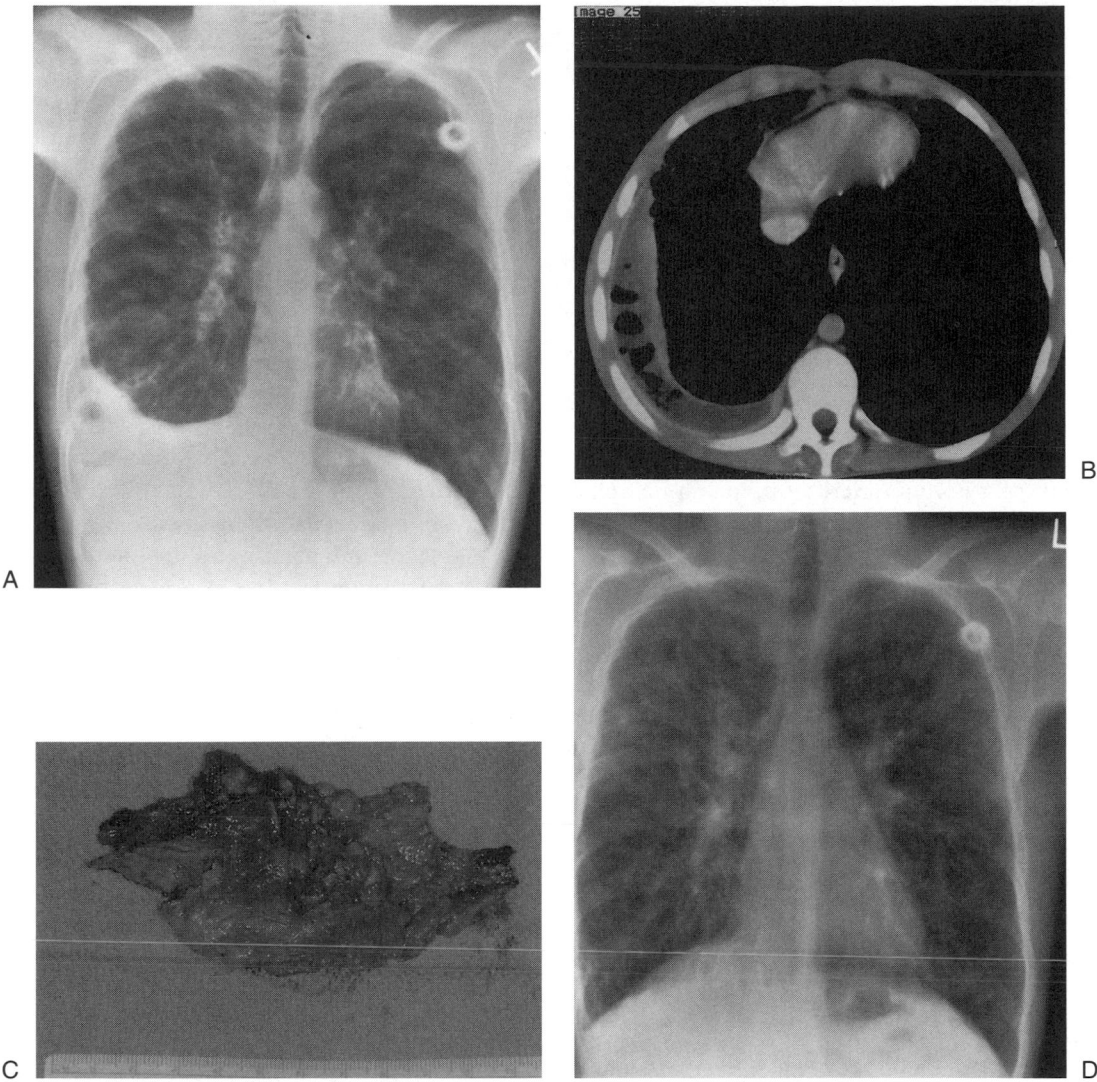

FIG. 8–2. (A) Chest x-ray of an 18-year-old male with CF and a complex empyema cavity growing *Pseudomonas aeruginosa*, which failed to resolve with chest tube drainage. **(B)** Computed tomography scan showing loculated collections and thick visceral pleura entrapping lung. **(C)** Portion of resected specimen retrieved at decortication through a posterolateral thoracotomy. **(D)** Convalescent chest x-ray 6 months later showing resolution. Two years postoperatively, the patient is listed for lung transplant. (Reproduced from reference 59.)

management alternative in the era of lung transplantation.

HEMOPTYSIS

Minor hemoptysis or simple "blood streaking" commonly is seen in patients with CF. Although it does not require treatment, minor hemoptysis may signal an acute pulmonary exacerbation that requires therapy. Massive hemoptysis, defined as bleeding greater than 240 to 300 mL of blood in a 24-hour period, carries a 50% to 85% mortality rate with conservative therapy alone (61). Death is due to asphyxiation from airway obstruction and, less commonly, exsanguination and acute hypotension. Recurrent episodes of moderate hemoptysis (3 or more bouts of 100 mL of blood per day within a week) also is considered a "major" bleeding event. These patients also require consideration for urgent therapy directed at hemorrhage control due to the threat of asphyxiation, airway obstruction, hypotension, anemia, chemical pneumonitis, and incitement of a pulmonary exacerbation (2,62−64). Recurrent hemoptysis is very debilitating and often precludes routine postural drainage of other lung regions. Approximately 1% of patients with CF will have at least one episode of major bleeding (> 240 mL/24 hours or requiring transfusion) each year. The majority of these patients will be 16 years of age or older.

Major bleeding in patients with CF is invariably of systemic arterial origin. The chronic airway inflammation leads to markedly enlarged and tortuous bronchial arteries, which are the source of bleeding. Effective means of therapy, including treatment of infections and embolization of hypertrophied bronchial arteries [bronchial artery embolization (BAE)] have been developed (61–64). Patients with CF often present with recurrent crescendo bleeds and are likely to have recurrent bleeds after successful management (62–64). A rich anastomosis exists between many of the mediastinal structures and the bronchial artery circulation. Even after successful BAE management, recurrent hemorrhages are likely to occur because of recanalization of previously embolized vessels or hypertrophy of collateral vessels from other systemic supplies. Therefore, patients who have undergone previously successful BAE therapy should not be excluded from subsequent attempts to arrest the hemorrhage by embolization.

Diagnosis

The source of bleeding must be defined and hemoptysis must be differentiated from bleeding from the upper airway or upper GI tract. The possibility of an aspirated foreign body always should be entertained. Patients with CF often will localize the bleeding to one side of the chest by noticing gurgling, fullness, or discomfort. Differentiating pulmonary and other sources may require a nasogastric tube aspiration or lavage or endoscopic examination of the pharynx, esophagus, and stomach. All medications that may contribute to bleeding [e.g., aspirin, nonsteroidal antiinflammatory drugs (NSAIDs), and high-dose penicillin derivatives] should be stopped. Coagulation profile (prothrombin time and partial thromboplastin time), platelet count, and blood type and crossmatch should be obtained. A sputum sample should be obtained for culture and sensitivity of microbiologic pathogens organisms, including bacteria, mycobacteria, and fungi (2).

A chest x-ray should be obtained to search for acute radiographic changes in the lung fields, localize site of bleeding, and discover other potential causes of bleeding, such as a foreign body or cavitary lung disease. If no localizing signs are present, recent or current chest computed tomograms may identify areas of severe bronchiectasis or new infiltrates that may help determine the probable site of bleeding. If embolotherapy is being considered, localization of the bleeding site will help direct treatment.

Bronchoscopy may help localize or a least lateralize the bleeding source. However, the bronchoscopic examination may be nondiagnostic in the setting of major bleeding because of limited visualization. Saumench et al. (65) found bronchoscopy of increased value when obtained early in the patient management. The site of hemorrhage was identified in 91% of patients when bronchoscopy was performed early compared with 50% when it was performed later in the clinical course (65). Bronchoscopy may be indicated when acute bleeding persists or recurs frequently or when local airway management will be used. Both flexible and rigid bronchoscopes should be available. When patients with CF are admitted with significant bleeding, a thoracic surgeon and interventional radiologist should be consulted to coordinate therapy. A multidisciplinary approach consisting of physicians who are experienced with managing this life-threatening complication is desirable. An experienced interventional radiologist familiar with BAE is an important member of this team.

Treatment: Noninvasive

Many patients with CF with hemoptysis will stop bleeding over several °days with medical management. All patients should be reassured and sedated if necessary. All drugs that interfere with coagulation should be discontinued, including aspirin, NSAIDs, and penicillin-derived antibiotics. Any coagulation defects should be corrected with vitamin K, fresh frozen plasma, or specific factors when indicated. Acute blood loss may require transfusion to provide adequate oxygen delivery. Inhaled irritants such as *N*-acetylcysteine and aerosolized antibiotics should be discontinued. The value of inhaled bronchodilators in this setting is controversial. Whereas many bleeding episodes are associated with pulmonary exacerbations, appropriate intravenous antibiotics should be instituted (2).

To avoid contamination of the nonbleeding pulmonary segments, placement of the offending lung in a dependent position may be of benefit with acute hemorrhage. Various positions may stimulate increased bleeding or breathing difficulty; therefore, the optimum position will need to be individualized. Exercise and chest physical therapy are discontinued temporarily and cough suppressants are administered for 24 to 48 hours to prevent dislodging immature blood clots. To maintain airway patency, cough and airway clearance measures are resumed gradually over several days, as permitted by reductions in bleeding. Intravenous conjugate estrogen and intravenous vasopressin have been reported to help control pulmonary bleeding by platelet, capillary, and cytokine effects (66) or by arteriolar smooth muscle contraction (67,68), respectively, but have been replaced largely by bronchial artery embolization.

Treatment: Invasive Endobronchial Therapy

When the bleeding appears immediately life-threatening, various local and topical treatments may be indicated. Positioning the patient with the bleeding lung dependent may reduce aspiration of blood into the contralateral lung.

Intubation with a large orotracheal tube provides access for suctioning of blood and providing mechanical ventilation. The tube may be advanced into the bronchus of the lung that is not bleeding to isolate the hemorrhagic lung and provide one lung ventilation. Double-lumen endotracheal tubes provide separate access to each lung, but the small lumen diameters significantly limit suction catheter effectiveness. Tamponade of the bleeding lobe or segment with an endobronchial balloon-tipped catheter has been reported (69), and the use of Gelfoam (absorbable gelatin sponge) pledgets, topical thrombin, α-adrenergic agonists, and iced saline lavage have been suggested (70). Rigid bronchoscopy typically is required for these procedures. These emergency measures are intended to forestall asphyxiation and excessive blood loss, whereas more definitive therapy (see below) is arranged. Fortunately, the use of these endobronchial treatments is not required frequently.

Bronchial Artery Embolization

Bronchial artery embolization (BAE) has been shown to play the key role in the management of hemorrhage in patients with CF with major and moderate episodes of hemoptysis (62–64,70). It now is a well-established technique to control acute hemorrhage rapidly and safely. Even more chronic or slowly increasing episodes of hemoptysis are being referred for limited BAE. The availability of lung transplantation also has stimulated this more aggressive approach to hemorrhage control in the CF population. Patients should undergo urgent angiography, when indicated, and preferably during a quiescent phase that optimizes the technical success of the procedure.

Bronchial Artery Anatomy

Bronchial arteries most commonly originate from the thoracic aorta at the T3 to T8 level and supply the trachea, bronchi, vagus nerve, posterior mediastinum, and esophagus. Eighty percent of all bronchial arteries arise the T5 to T6 level. The more common bronchial artery combinations include a single right intercostobronchial trunk with single left artery, single right intercostobronchial trunk with right and left arteries arising from a common trunk, and a single right intercostobronchial trunk with two left bronchial arteries (71,72). The right-sided arteries typically arise from the right lateral or anterolateral surface of the descending aorta, whereas the left bronchial arteries originate from a more anterior location. As many as 20% of bronchial arteries have anomalous origins other than the aorta. Bronchial arteries also may originate from the convex or concave surface of the aortic arch itself. Aberrant origins include the subclavian, thyrocervical, internal mammary, innominate, pericardiophrenic, superior intercostal, abdominal aorta, and inferior phrenic arteries (73–75). Transpleural systemic collaterals from intercostal, internal mammary, phrenic, thyrocervical, and axillary artery branches frequently are encountered in patients with CF who have undergone multiple previous BAE procedures (76).

In approximately 5% of cases, the artery of Adamkiewicz (the major supply to the anterior spinal artery) arises from a right intercostobronchial trunk. The right superior intercostal artery and right bronchial artery also may share a common trunk with a branch to the anterior spinal artery. Therapeutic approaches that endanger the arterial supply to the spinal cord must be avoided (77).

BAE Technique

A concise neurologic examination should be performed to establish a baseline before the embolization procedure. Diagnostic angiography is performed initially and often will entail a descending thoracic aortogram before selective catheterization of the bronchial arteries. If the site of hemorrhage is known, the feeding arteries are catheterized and embolized selectively. However, if the site of bleeding cannot be localized, any tortuous and hypertrophic bronchial artery should be treated. The bronchial artery search is begun at the T5 to T6 level. Once catheterized, a selective injection is performed to document its appearances and course and to verify that there is no supply to the anterior

spinal artery. Nonionic contrast material should be used for the entire procedure because it is less painful, will not stimulate coughing, and will lower the risk of transverse myelitis. Abnormal angiographic findings supporting a site of bleeding include tortuous and hypertrophied bronchial arteries, hypervascularity, and systemic-to-pulmonary artery or venous shunting (Fig. 8–3). The need to search for a nonbronchial systemic supply is particularly important in cases of recurrent hemoptysis following prior BAE procedures and in patients with unusual sites of bleeding or extreme severity. Vessels responsible for recurrent bleeding include a recannulated bronchial artery that was embolized previously, a bronchial artery not previously embolized (aberrant or nonaberrant), or a nonbronchial systemic collateral artery (Fig. 8–4).

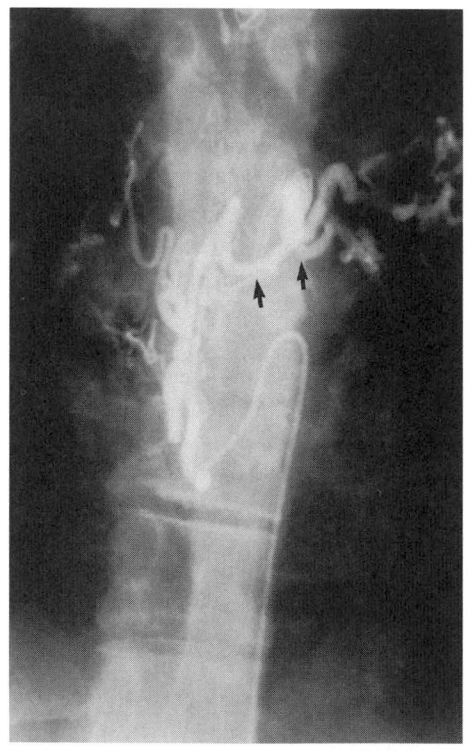

FIG. 8–3. Enlarged bronchial artery. Selective arteriogram shows a common trunk with an enlarged left (*arrows*) and smaller right bronchial artery in a patient referred for the first embolization procedure. The left bronchial artery was embolized successfully.

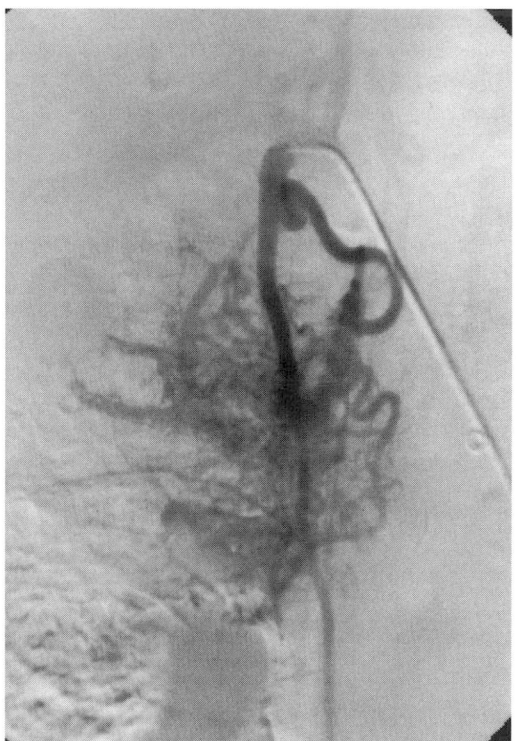 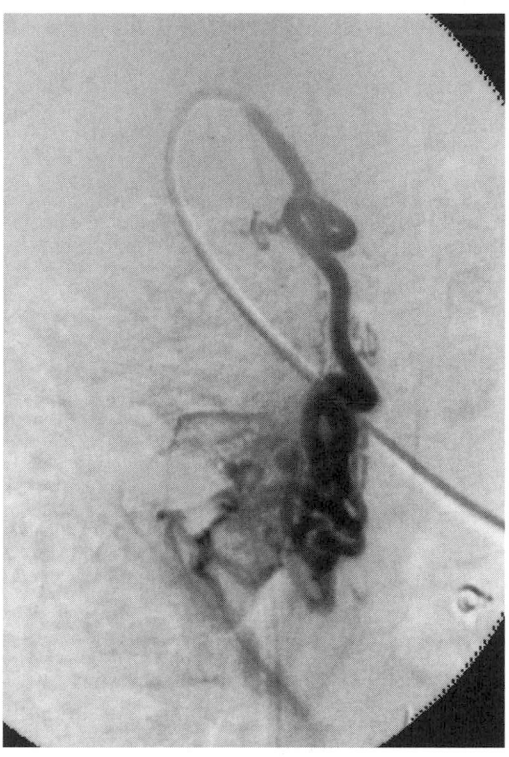

A B

FIG. 8–4. Nonbronchial systemic collaterals. Patient referred for fifth embolization procedure shows enlarged collaterals from **(A)** right internal mammary artery and **(B)** right thyrocervical trunk. Both were embolized successfully, and the patient was discharged 2 days later.

Any abnormal bronchial artery supplying the site(s) of bleeding should be embolized. A stable catheter position is mandatory for BAE to avoid nontarget embolization. If this is not possible with standard catheters, coaxial catheterization systems currently are available to complete the procedure in a safe manner. Distal embolization should be performed with particulate materials (polyvinyl alcohol or absorbable gelatin sponge) greater than 250 μm in size to avoid tissue ischemia and neurologic damage (63,72,78). Liquids such as ethanol or fine particles should be avoided because they produce very distal occlusion, leading to tissue infarction.

Results of BAE

Bronchial artery embolization has been shown to be a very effective technique in the immediate control of hemoptysis in patients with CF. In combining the series of patients with CF studied by Fellows et al. and Cohen et al., 94% of patients (31 of 33) treated by BAE for hemoptysis had immediate control of bleeding (63,64). At UNC, 13 patients have undergone 28 BAE procedures since 1990 (79). Nine patients required one embolotherapy session whereas four required multiple (2 to 3) sessions to control the hemorrhage during a single hospital admission. All patients ultimately had their hemorrhage controlled with BAE. Three of the 13 patients have returned for repeat BAE procedures for recurrent bouts of hemoptysis. Two patients had two recurrences, and one patient had three recurrences. All recurrent bouts of hemorrhage were controlled successfully with BAE. Intervals between recurrent bouts of hemorrhage following control with BAE averaged 20 months (range, 6 to 37 months).

The procedure should be performed urgently when indicated, and when good embolization techniques are employed, complications are quite infrequent. Early and effective palliative control of major and moderate bouts of hemoptysis in young patients with CF is particularly valuable as lung transplant programs become more prevalent. There currently are no data to indicate a change in long-term prognosis for any individual patient who has had a major bleeding episode.

Complications of BAE

Spinal cord ischemia and transverse myelitis are the most feared complications, which fortunately are extremely rare. The single case report of paralysis after embolization for hemoptysis was in a case of an embolized left seventh intercostal artery (80). The use of nonionic contrast has reduced significantly—if not eliminated—the risks of transverse myelitis (81,82).

Two cases of bronchial infarction have been reported following BAE. In both cases, a liquid sclerosing agent was used, which now is avoided (83,84). Bronchoesophageal fistulas have been reported in cases of combined bronchial and esophageal ischemia secondary to the use of very fine particulate materials (85,86). Chest pain and dysphagia commonly occur within the first week after BAE and are self-limiting.

Surgical Resection

Surgery may have a role in patients who fail to stop bleeding with BAE or whose bleeding recurs in the face of what is considered a complete embolization (87,88). Because BAE largely is ineffective at controlling hemoptysis from cavitary lung disease (72,78), patients with CF who are bleeding from known cavitary lung disease should undergo resection if they are suitable candidates for thoracotomy. In these circumstances, preoperative localization of the bleeding site is necessary. Computed tomography scan and bronchoscopy may be useful in this regard. Baseline pulmonary function studies are essential to assess surgical candidacy. If the lobe in question has been destroyed substan-

tially, then resection may have other benefits besides controlling hemoptysis. The high success rate of BAE lends some support to the notion that systemic devascularization on the side of bleeding may be adequate to control bleeding from massive hemoptysis without resection. This clinical approach has never been reported but may be reasonable, particularly in patients with minimal pulmonary reserve in whom BAE fails, and is based on the premise that hemoptysis from bronchiectasis always involves the systemic bronchial circulation. Presumably, failure of embolization to control hemoptysis is related to missing an aberrant bronchial artery or a collateral artery from the chest wall.

Summary: Hemoptysis

Hemoptysis is a common complication of CF in adults, and massive hemoptysis from hypertrophied bronchial arteries may be life-threatening. Many individual episodes of massive hemoptysis can be controlled with bed rest, temporary cough suppression, and intravenous antibiotics. The development of invasive BAE techniques has revolutionized the approach to this problem. Persistent hemoptysis usually can be controlled by embolization of the primary and collateral bronchial arteries to the bleeding area. In experienced hands, the procedure is safe, has a high success rate, and often prevents recurrent hemorrhage for at least 1 to 2 years. Local surgical resection for refractory bleeding is only rarely necessary. The frequency of massive hemoptysis increases with age, but there have been excellent improvements in its management and therapeutic options.

REFERENCES

1. FitzSimmons SC. *Cystic Fibrosis Foundation Patient Registry: 1995 Annual Report.* Bethesda, MD: 1996.
2. Schidlow DV, Taussig LM, Knowles MR. Cystic Fibrosis Foundation Consensus conference report on pulmonary complications of cystic fibrosis. *Pediatr Pulmonol* 1993;15:187–198.
3. Zinman R, Corey M, Coates AL, et al. Nocturnal home oxygen in the treatment of hypoxemic cystic fibrosis patients. *J Pediatr* 1989;114(3):368–377.

4. Coates AL. Oxygen therapy, exercise, and cystic fibrosis. *Chest* 1992;101(1):2–4.

5. Nixon PA, Orenstein DM, Curtis SE, et al. Oxygen supplementation during exercise in cystic fibrosis. *Am Rev Respir Dis* 1990;142(4):807–811.

6. Tepper RS, Skatrud JB, Dempsey JA. Ventilation and oxygenation changes during sleep in cystic fibrosis. *Chest* 1983;84(4):388–393.

7. Davis PB, di Sant'Agnese PA. Assisted ventilation for patients with cystic fibrosis. *JAMA* 1978;239(18): 1851–1854.

8. Lebecque P, Lapierre J, Lamarre A, et al. Diffusion capacity and oxygen desaturation effects on exercise in patients with cystic fibrosis. *Chest* 1987;91:693–698.

9. West JB. State of the art: ventilation–perfusion relationships. *Am Rev Respir Dis* 1977;116(5):919–943.

10. Coffey MJ, FitzGerald MX, McNicholas WT. Comparison of oxygen desaturation during sleep and exercise in patients with cystic fibrosis. *Chest* 1991;100 (3):659–662.

11. Ballard RD, Sutarik JM, Clover CW, et al. Effects of non-REM sleep on ventilation and respiratory mechanics in adults with cystic fibrosis. *Am J Respir Crit Care Med* 1996;153:266–271.

12. Coates AL, Canny G, Zinman R, et al. The effects of chronic airflow limitation, increased dead space, and the pattern of ventilation on gas exchange during maximal exercise in advanced cystic fibrosis. *Am Rev Respir Dis* 1988;138(6):1524–1531.

13. Regnis JA, Donnelly PM, Robinson M, et al. Ventilatory mechanics at rest and during exercise in patients with cystic fibrosis. *Am J Respir Crit Care Med* 1996; 154(5):1418–1425.

14. Saiman L, Mehar F, Niu WW, et al. Antibiotic susceptibility of multiply resistant *Pseudomonas aeruginosa* isolated from patients with cystic fibrosis, including candidates for transplantation. *Clin Infect Dis* 1996; 23:532–537.

15. Piper AJ, Parker S, Torzillo PJ, et al. Nocturnal nasal IPPV stabilizes patient with cystic fibrosis and hypercapnic respiratory failure. *Chest* 1992;102(3):846–850.

16. Stern RC, Borkat G, Hirschfeld SS, et al. Heart failure in cystic fibrosis. Treatment and prognosis of cor pulmonale with failure of the right side of the heart. *Am J Dis Child* 1980;134(3):267–272.

17. Goldring RM, Fishman AP, Turino GM, et al. Pulmonary hypertension and cor pulmonale in cystic fibrosis of the pancreas. *J Pediatr* 1964;65:501–524.

18. Stokes DC, McBride JT, Wall MA, et al. Sleep hypoxemia in young adults with cystic fibrosis. *Am J Dis Child* 1980;134(8):741–743.

19. Orenstein DM, Franklin BA, Doershuk CF, et al. Exercise conditioning and cardiopulmonary fitness in cystic fibrosis. *Chest* 1981;80:392–398.

20. Marcus CL, Bader D, Stabile MW, et al. Supplemental oxygen and exercise performance in patients with cystic fibrosis with severe pulmonary disease. *Chest* 1992;101:52–57.

21. Continuous or nocturnal oxygen therapy in hypoxemic chronic obstructive lung disease, a clinical trial: Nocturnal Oxygen Therapy Trial Group. *Ann Intern Med* 1980;93(3):391–398.

22. Boysen PG, Block AJ, Wynne JW, et al. Nocturnal pulmonary hypertension in patients with chronic obstructive pulmonary disease. *Chest* 1979;76(5): 536–542.

23. Wynne JW, Block AJ, Hemenway J, et al. Disordered breathing and oxygen desaturation during sleep in patients with chronic obstructive lung disease (COLD). *Am J Med* 1979;66(4):573–579.

24. Versteegh FGA, Bogaard JM, Raatgever JW, et al. Relationship between airway obstruction, desaturation during exercise and nocturnal hypoxaemia in cystic fibrosis patients. *Eur Respir J* 1990;3(1):68–73.

25. Regnis JA, Piper AJ, Henke KG, et al. Benefits of nocturnal nasal CPAP in patients with cystic fibrosis. *Chest* 1994;106(6):1717–1724.

26. Christopher KL. Long-term oxygen therapy. In: Pierson DJ, Kacmarek RM, ed. *Foundations of respiratory care.* New York: Churchill Livingstone, 1992:1155–1174.

27. Nixon PA, Orenstein DM, Kelsey SF, et al. The prognostic value of exercise testing in patients with cystic fibrosis. *N Engl J Med* 1992;327(25):1785–1788.

28. Salh W, Bilton D, Dodd M, et al. Effect of exercise and physiotherapy in aiding sputum expectoration in adults with cystic fibrosis. *Thorax* 1989;44:1006–1008.

29. de Jong W, Grenvink RG, Roorda RJ, et al. Effect of a home exercise training program in patients with cystic fibrosis. *Chest* 1994;105(2):463–468.

30. Baldwin DR, Hill AL, Peckham DG, et al. Effect of addition of exercise to chest physiotherapy on sputum expectoration and lung function in adults with cystic fibrosis. *Respir Med* 1994;88(1):49–53.

31. Strauss GD, Osher A, Wang CI, et al. Variable weight training in cystic fibrosis. *Chest* 1987;92(2):273–276.

32. Downs AM. Physical therapy in lung transplantation. *Phys Ther* 1996;76(6):626–642.

33. Geggel RL, Dozor AJ, Fyler DC, et al. Effect of vasodilators at rest and during exercise in young adults with cystic fibrosis and chronic cor pulmonale. *Am Rev Respir Dis* 1985;131(4):531–536.

34. Davidson A, Bossuyt A, Dab I. Acute effects of oxygen, nifedipine, and diltiazem in patients with cystic fibrosis and mild pulmonary hypertension. *Pediatr Pulmonol* 1989;6(1):53–59.

35. Matthay RA, Berger HJ. Cardiovascular function in cor pulmonale. *Clin Chest Med* 1983;4(2):269–295.

36. Mathur PN, Powles P, Pugsley SO, et al. Effect of digoxin on right ventricular function in severe chronic airflow obstruction: a controlled clinical trial. *Ann Intern Med* 1981;95(3):283–288.

37. Packer M. Vasodilator therapy for primary pulmonary hypertension: limitations and hazards. *Ann Intern Med* 1985;103(2):258–270.

38. Aubier M, de Troyer A, Sampson M, et al. Aminophylline improves diaphragmatic contractility. *N Engl J Med* 1981;305(5):249–252.

39. Garland JS, Chan YM, Kelly KJ, et al. Outcome of infants with cystic fibrosis requiring mechanical ventilation for respiratory failure. *Chest* 1989;96(1):136–138.

40. Marini JJ. Should PEEP be used in airflow obstruction? *Am Rev Respir Dis* 1989;140:1–3.

41. Flume PA, Egan TM, Westerman JH, et al. Lung transplantation for mechanically ventilated patients. *J Heart Lung Transplant* 1994;13(1 Pt 1):15–21.

42. Meyer TJ, Hill NS. Noninvasive positive pressure ventilation to treat respiratory failure. *Ann Intern Med* 1994;120(9):760–770.

43. Hodson ME, Madden BP, Steven MH, et al. Non-invasive mechanical ventilation for cystic fibrosis patients—a potential bridge to transplantation. *Eur Respir J* 1991;4(5):524–527.

44. FitzSimmons SC. The changing epidemiology of cystic fibrosis. J Pediatr 1993;122(1):1–9.

45. Tomashefski JF Jr, Bruce M, Stern RC, et al. Pulmonary air cysts in cystic fibrosis: relation of pathologic features to radiologic findings and history of pneumothorax. *Hum Pathol* 1985;16(3):253–261.

46. Tomashefski JF Jr, Dahms B, Bruce M. Pleura in pneumothorax: comparison of patients with cystic fibrosis and idiopathic spontaneous pneumothorax. *Arch Pathol Lab Med* 1985;109(10):910–916.

47. Spector ML, Stern RC. Pneumothorax in cystic fibrosis: a 26-year experience. *Ann Thorac Surg* 1989;47 (2):204–207.

48. McLaughlin FJ, Matthews WJ Jr, Strieder DJ, et al. Pneumothorax in cystic fibrosis: management and outcome. *J Pediatr* 1982;100(6):863–869.

49. Tribble CG, Selden RF, Rodgers BM. Talc poudrage in the treatment of spontaneous pneumothoraces in patients with cystic fibrosis. *Ann Surg* 1986;204(6):677–680.

50. Kennedy L, Rusch VW, Strange C, et al. Pleurodesis using talc slurry. *Chest* 1994;106(2):342–346.

51. Bitran JD, Brown C, Desser RK, et al. Intracavitary bleomycin for the control of malignant effusions. *J Surg Oncol* 1981;16(3):273–277.

52. Schuster SR, McLaughlin FJ, Matthews WJ Jr, et al. Management of pneumothorax in cystic fibrosis. *J Pediatr Surg* 1983;18(4):492–497.

53. Murray KD, Matheny RG, Howanitz EP, et al. A limited axillary thoracotomy as primary treatment for recurrent spontaneous pneumothorax. *Chest* 1993;103 (1):137–142.

54. Nathanson LK, Shimi SM, Wood RAB, et al. Videothoracoscopic ligation of bulla and pleurectomy for spontaneous pneumothorax. *Ann Thorac Surg* 1991;52(2):316–319.

55. Torre M, Belloni P. Nd:YAG laser pleurodesis through thoracoscopy: new curative therapy in spontaneous pneumothorax. *Ann Thorac Surg* 1989;47(6):887–889.

56. Detterbeck FC, Egan TM, Mill MR. Lung transplantation after previous thoracic surgical procedures. *Ann Thorac Surg* 1995;60(1):139–143.

57. Noyes BE, Orenstein DM. Treatment of pneumothorax in the era of lung transplantation (editorial). *Chest* 1992;101(5):1187–1188.

58. Egan TM, Detterbeck FC, Mill MR, et al. Improved results of lung transplantation for patients with cystic fibrosis. *J Thorac Cardiovasc Surg* 1995;109(2):224–235.

59. Egan TM. Thoracic surgery for patients with cystic fibrosis. In: Orenstein DM, Stern RC, eds. *Treatment of the hospitalized patient with cystic fibrosis.* New York: Marcel Dekker, 1998:231–247.

60. Miller JI Jr. Infections of the pleura. In: Shields TW, ed. *General Thoracic Surgery.* 3rd ed. Philadelphia: Lea & Febiger, 1989:633–649.

61. Wholey MH, Chamorro HA, Rao G, et al. Bronchial artery embolization for massive hemoptysis. *JAMA* 1976;236(22):2501–2504.

62. Tonkin ILD, Hanissian AS, Boulden TF, et al. Bronchial arteriography and embolotherapy for hemoptysis in patients with cystic fibrosis. *Cardiovasc Intervent Radiol* 1991;14(4):241–246.

63. Cohen AM, Doershuk CF, Stern RC. Bronchial artery embolization to control hemoptysis in cystic fibrosis. *Radiology* 1990;175:401–405.

64. Fellows KE, Taik Khaw K, Schuster S, et al. Bronchial artery embolization in cystic fibrosis: technique and long-term results. *J Pediatr* 1979;95:959–963.

65. Saumench J, Escarrabill J, Padro L, et al. Value of fiberoptic bronchoscopy and angiography for diagnosis of the bleeding site in hemoptysis. *Ann Thorac Surg* 1989;48(2):272–274.

66. Popper J. The use of Premarin IV in hemoptysis. *Dis Chest* 1960;37(6):659–660.

67. Magee G, Williams MH Jr. Treatment of massive hemoptysis with intravenous Pitressin. *Lung* 1982;160 (3):165–169.

68. Bilton D, Webb AK, Foster H, et al. Life threatening haemoptysis in cystic fibrosis: an alternative therapeutic approach. *Thorax* 1990;45(12):975–976.

69. Swersky RB, Chang JB, Wisoff BG, et al. Endobronchial balloon tamponade of hemoptysis in patients with cystic fibrosis. *Ann Thorac Surg* 1979;27 (3):262–264.

70. Schuster SR, Fellows KE. Management of major hemoptysis in patients with cystic fibrosis. *J Pediatr Surg* 1977;12:889–896.

71. Cauldwell EW, Siekert RG, Lininger RE, et al. The bronchial arteries: an anatomic study of 150 human cadavers. *Surg Gynecol Obstet* 1948;86(4):395–412.

72. Uflacker R, Kaemmerer A, Picon PD, et al. Bronchial artery embolization in the management of hemoptysis: technical aspects and long-term results. *Radiology* 1985;157(3):637–644.

73. Tan RT, McGahan JP, Link DP, et al. Bronchial artery embolization in management of haemoptysis. *J Intervent Radiol* 1991;6:67–74.

74. McPherson S, Routh WD, Nath H, et al. Anomalous origin of bronchial arteries: potential pitfall of embolotherapy for hemoptysis. *J Vasc Intervent Radiol* 1990;1(1):86–88.

75. Cohen AM, Antoun BW, Stern RC. Left thyrocervical trunk bronchial artery supplying right lung: source of recurrent hemoptysis in cystic fibrosis. *AJR Am J Roentgenol* 1992;158(5):1131–1133.

76. Keller FS, Rosch J, Loflin TG, et al. Nonbronchial systemic collateral arteries: significance in percutaneous embolotherapy for hemoptysis. *Radiology* 1987;164(3):687–692.

77. Stoll JF, Bettmann MA. Bronchial artery embolization to control hemoptysis: a review. *Cardiovasc Intervent Radiol* 1988;11(5):263–269.

78. Remy J, Arnaud A, Fardou H, et al. Treatment of hemoptysis by embolization of bronchial arteries. *Radiology* 1977;122(1):33–37.

79. Brinson GM, Noone PG, Mauro MA, Knowles MR, Yankaskas JR, Sandhu JS, Jacques PF. Bronchial artery embolization for the treatment of hemoptysis in cystic fibrosis patients. *Am J Respir Crit Care Med* 1998;158:1951–1958.

80. Vujic I, Pyle R, Parker E, et al. Control of massive hemoptysis by embolization of intercostal arteries. *Radiology* 1980;137(3):617–620.

81. Kardjiev V, Symeonov A, Chankov I. Etiology, pathogenesis, and prevention of spinal cord lesions in selective angiography of the bronchial and intercostal arteries. *Radiology* 1974;112(1):81–83.
82. Doppman JL, Girton M, Oldfield EH. Spinal WADA test. *Radiology* 1986;161(2):319–321.
83. Rabkin JE, Astafjev VI, Gothman LN, et al. Transcatheter embolization in the management of pulmonary hemorrhage. *Radiology* 1987;163(2):361–365.
84. Ivanick MJ, Thorwarth W, Donohue J, et al. Infarction of the left main-stem bronchus: a complication of bronchial artery embolization. *AJR Am J Roentgenol* 1983;141(3):535–537.
85. Helenon CH, Chatel A, Bigot JM, et al. Fistule oesophago-bronchique gauche apres embolisation bronchique. *Nouv Presse Med* 1977;6(45):4209.
86. Munk PL, Morris DC, Nelems B. Left main bronchial–esophageal fistula: a complication of bronchial artery embolization. *Cardiovasc Intervent Radiol* 1990;13(2):95–97.
87. Levitsky S, Lapey A, di Sant'Agnese PA. Pulmonary resection for life-threatening hemoptysis in cystic fibrosis. *JAMA* 1970;213(1):125–127.
88. Porter DK, Van Every MJ, Mack JW Jr. Emergency lobectomy for massive hemoptysis in cystic fibrosis. *J Thorac Cardiovasc Surg* 1983;86(3):409–411.

Cystic Fibrosis in Adults,
edited by J. R. Yankaskas and M. R. Knowles,
Lippincott–Raven Publishers, Philadelphia, 1999

9

Lung Transplantation for Cystic Fibrosis

Linda J. Paradowski and *Thomas M. Egan

*Division of Pulmonary and Critical Care Medicine, and *Division of Cardiothoracic Surgery,
University of North Carolina School of Medicine, Chapel Hill, North Carolina*

Progressive lung disease causes the greatest morbidity for patients with cystic fibrosis (CF) and continues to be the leading cause of death. In the face of incipient death due to respiratory failure, attention had been directed at ensuring comfort and minimizing distress. The development of successful lung transplant procedures brought new hope for patients with CF with severe respiratory disease. The clinical experience is significant, but many aspects of patient selection, pre- and intraoperative care, and long-term management remain controversial.

Lung transplantation for end-stage lung disease due to CF was approached initially with much trepidation. The patients, usually malnourished, would be at substantial risk for pleural contamination during the removal of their grossly purulent, abscessed lungs and would remain colonized in their upper airway with an assortment of pathogens. In this setting, the risks of infectious complications exacerbated by the required immunosuppression were substantial. Moreover, CF, as a multisystem disease, would continue to affect other organs. Although lung transplantation had been performed successfully in patients with end-stage respiratory disease due to chronic obstructive and interstitial lung diseases in the early 1980s, the first successful heart–lung transplants for CF were performed in the United Kingdom in 1985. Heart–lung transplantation lessened the risk of anastomotic airway complications due to the preservation of the donor bronchial–coronary collateral circulation (1). Bilateral sequential lung transplantation for CF was performed successfully in Toronto in 1988 (2). The bilateral sequential technique offered the advantages of avoiding cardiopulmonary bypass, with its attendant risk of bleeding, and eliminated the complications of heart transplantation. Bilateral lobar transplants from living donors is emerging as an alternative procedure in the appropriate setting (3).

As of April 1996, 761 patients with CF have undergone lung transplantation. This represents 14% of all transplanted patients listed with the St. Louis International Lung Transplant Registry. Their 5-year survival rate is 48% (Fig. 9–1) and is slightly higher than other transplant diagnoses (4,5). Causes of death rank in the same order as the overall lung transplant experience, but patients with CF tend to have an increased mortality in the early postoperative period from infectious complications, and a larger percentage of patients with CF die from chronic rejection or obliterative bronchiolitis in the later posttransplant period (4). In this chapter, patient selection, surgical approach, and postoperative care in this unique and challenging group of patients are discussed. Although a consensus exists about indications for lung transplantation in CF (5), many care issues have not been tested rigorously by controlled trials, and management is influenced by the experience at the local transplant teams.

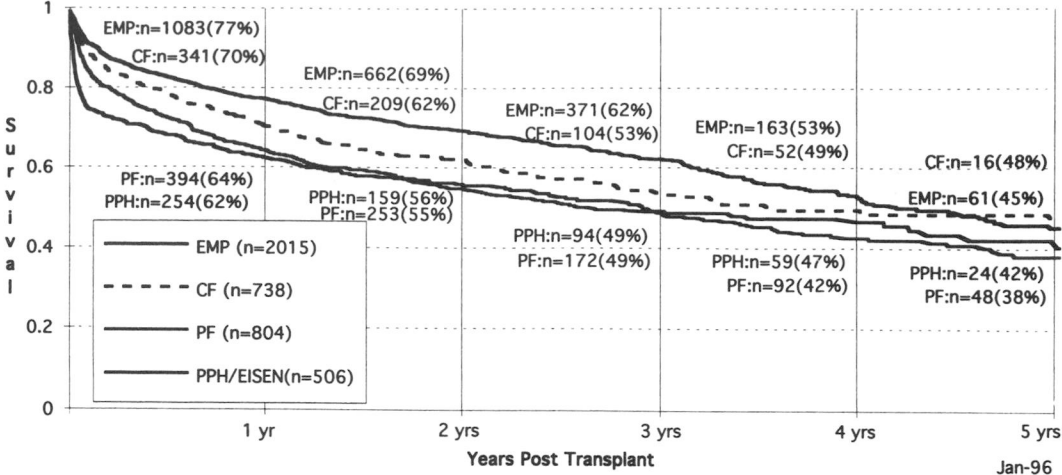

FIG. 9–1. From the St. Louis International Lung Transplant Registry, the actuarial survival for all reported lung transplant patients by diagnostic groups. EMP, emphysema; PPH, primary pulmonary hypertension; PF, pulmonary fibrosis

PRETRANSPLANTATION

Candidate Selection

Because of a static donor pool (6) and an ever-expanding transplant candidate list, the current waiting time for double lung transplant is approximately 18 to 24 months after patients are listed as transplant candidates. The clinical course of CF lung disease is highly variable, and 20% to 30% of all patients die waiting for transplant. Therefore, criteria for transplant candidacy must maximize the optimal use of scarce donor lungs, while simultaneously selecting the optimal "transplant window" for each potential recipient. For patients with CF, most pulmonary transplant centers have validated the criterion of a forced expiratory volume in 1 second (FEV_1) of less than 30% of predicted as an indicator of greater than 50% mortality rate within 2 years (7). Some individual considerations, for example, female gender and younger age, may suggest a lower threshold for listing. Patients with poor quality of life, high frequency of hospitalizations, and weight loss also may need to be considered earlier. Criteria for double lung transplant have been described previously (8) and are listed in Table 9–1. Patients awaiting lung transplant are assigned organs mainly by time accrued on

the transplant list and not by severity of illness, as with the transplantation of other organs.

Exclusion Criteria

Infections that would preclude perioperative and long-term survival contraindicate lung transplantation. These are human immunodeficiency virus (HIV), hepatitis B with surface antigen expression, and active tuberculosis. Significant psychological or social dysfunction (Table 9–2) preclude initial and continuing candidacy. Relative exclusions to lung transplant (Table 9–3) tend to be transplant center specific and are influenced by individual centers' experiences. Some centers will not accept patients who have undergone

TABLE 9–1. *Referral criteria*

Progressive pulmonary function impairment manifest by FEV_1 < 30% predicted, severe hypoxemia, and hypercarbia
Increased functional impairment, evidenced by increasing frequency and duration of hospital treatment for pulmonary exacerbations
Major life-threatening pulmonary complications, such as recurrent massive hemoptysis
Increasing antibiotic resistance of bacteria infecting the lungs

TABLE 9–2. *Psychological or social dysfunction contraindications*

Recent or current abuse of alcohol, tobacco, or other drugs (prescription or other)
Psychiatric illness that precludes adherence with the pre- and posttransplant regimen
Inability to adhere to a complex treatment plan
Lack of adequate social support systems

cardiothoracic surgery or pleurodesis (chemical or surgical) because of the difficulties encountered during the transplant surgery (9). Persistent isolation of multiresistant *Pseudomonas aeruginosa*, nontuberculous mycobacteria (NTM), or *Aspergillus* species also may be viewed as a relative contraindication (10). The presence of *Burkholderia cepacia*, especially multiresistant organisms, contraindicates lung transplantation in many centers (11–13).

Other relative contraindications to transplant include significant dysfunction of other organs. Kidney function is assessed by creatinine clearance and should be greater than 50 cc/minute. There should be no evidence of end-stage liver disease as assessed by the presence of portal hypertension with esophageal varices or hepatic encephalopathy. Cardiac function must be adequate—defined as a left ventricular ejection fraction greater than 50%. Patients with diabetes should have good control and no significant microvascular complications affecting the kidneys, eyes, or nervous system. Patients with severe osteopenia, as defined by the presence of vertebral fractures or poor mineralization as assessed by a bone density scan,

TABLE 9–3. *Noninfectious medical contraindications*

Significant left ventricular dysfunction
Significant hepatic dysfunction or portal hypertension
Renal insufficiency
Diabetes mellitus with significant end-organ damage
Malignancy within 5 years
Osteoporosis (i.e., below fracture threshold or with symptomatic vertebral fractures)
Inability to ambulate
Other systemic diseases that compromise long-term survival with or without lung transplantation

should not undergo lung transplantation since the immunosuppressive agents will contribute to further bone loss. Severe scoliosis would limit pulmonary function after lung transplantation and may be an absolute exclusion. History of cancer, unless at least 5 years have elapsed without any evidence of malignancy, is an absolute contraindication to transplantation because of the increased risk of neoplasm with immunosuppressives. Patients must be ambulatory and able to partake in an exercise rehabilitation program, although the value of the latter is not established rigorously (14). Lastly, but most importantly, patients must have the psychosocial skills and abilities to comply with a complex medical regimen.

Impact of Infections

Bacteria

Sepsis is the leading cause of death in the first few months posttransplant (15,16). Because the upper respiratory tract tends to remain colonized with bacteria that were present before transplant, the advisability of transplanting patients who are infected with antibiotic-resistant bacteria is of particular concern. *B. cepacia* is notoriously resistant to antibiotics (17,18). Patients with advanced CF lung disease and colonization with *B. cepacia* appear to have an increased risk of death when compared with noncolonized patients (17–19). *B. cepacia* may be acquired nosocomially through water or disinfectants (20), but strain identification through ribotyping has documented person-to-person transfer among patients with CF (2,11). This has led to segregation of colonized patients from noncolonized patients in hospital wards and in other activities (21) at some centers. The Toronto group (11) has reported that colonization with *B. cepacia* pretransplant is associated with excess morbidity and mortality postlung transplantation. Ramirez et al. (2) documented postoperative infections with *B. cepacia*, not only in previously colonized patients, but also in patients who did not have the organism preoperatively but who were in contact with other colonized patients after transplant. At the University of North Carolina (UNC), two of seven patients with CF colonized with *B. cepacia* preoperatively died within 6 weeks posttransplant as a direct result of *B. cepacia* infection. The other five patients experienced no excess morbidity attributable to *B. cepacia*. The different outcomes may be related to different *B. cepacia* strains (22), but uniform identification criteria and causality have not been established. Whether *B. cepacia* colonization should be considered a relative or absolute contraindication to transplantation remains controversial (12). The effects of other antibiotic species are of similar concern. One study reported that pretransplant infection with antibiotic-resistant *Pseudomonas* species had no effect on survival (13). At this time, the decision to list and to transplant patients infected with *B. cepacia* or other antibiotic-resistant bacteria is based largely on the experience of a given center. Microbiological and epidemiologic studies may provide additional guidance, especially in the setting of insufficient donor organs.

Fungi

Aspergillus species can be isolated from the respiratory tree of up to 60% of patients with CF (23). As many as 10% of all patients with CF fulfill some criteria of allergic bronchopulmonary aspergillosis. Posttransplant, the presence of *Aspergillus* species in the airway is associated with an increased risk of airway anastomotic stenosis, locally invasive disease, and dissemination (24,25). Patients with diabetes are believed to be at increased risk. Some centers treat all patients colonized preoperatively with *Aspergillus* species (12,24) with aerosolized or parental amphotericin B or oral itraconazole both before and after transplant. Conversely, some centers view any evidence of *Aspergillus* colonization as a possible contraindication to transplant (26). The Papworth Hospital lung transplant group (27) recently revised their criteria and currently list patients with *Aspergillus* "colonization" in the airways, but will not transplant patients with "active"

Aspergillus infection. Active infection is defined as evidence of an aspergilloma abutting the pleura (27), which could lead to significant pleural contamination with *Aspergillus* during surgery. At UNC, 52% of 71 patients with CF and none of 55 non-CF patients had *Aspergillus* isolated from their sputum pretransplant (28). After lung transplantation, *Aspergillus* was isolated from the respiratory secretions of 40% of the patients with CF (only 7% were positive both pre- and posttransplant) and 30% of the non-CF patients. Five patients died as a direct result of fungal infection, four non-CF patients and one patient with CF. None of these patients had evidence of preoperative colonization with fungus. All five patients either had severe bronchiolitis obliterans necessitating augmented immunosuppression, persisting cytomegalovirus (CMV) or bacterial infections, and/or major organ failure. These deaths occurred between 74 to 1,039 days posttransplantation. Therefore, measures to eradicate preoperative fungal sputum colonization may not impact significantly postoperative fungal mortality. Multicenter epidemiologic studies have not been reported, and policies for listing and treating *Aspergillus* isolates are center specific.

Nontuberculous Mycobacteria

The importance of NTM colonization or infection in airways of patients with CF undergoing transplant remains unclear. The prevalence of NTM may vary geographically because environmental exposure is the likeliest source (29). In patients with CF with NTM sputum isolates, it is difficult to distinguish airway colonization from active infection because of concomitant bacterial pathogens, abnormal chest radiographs, and the relatively high risks of bronchoscopic or open-lung biopsies. At UNC, six patients with CF were colonized with NTM [5 with *Mycobacterium avium* complex (MAC), 1 with *Mycobacterium abscessus*] preoperatively. In no case did the resected lungs reveal parenchymal granulomatous infection on pathologic examination. In one patient in this group, a soft tissue infection due to *M. abscessus* developed. She was treated successfully with a prolonged course of amikacin, cefoxitin, and azithromycin, but the disease recurred several months after cessation of her antibiotics. The prognosis for successful resolution of infections with rapidly growing *Mycobacterium* in the face of continued immunosuppression is quite poor (30). However, the actual risk of posttransplant NTM disease in those colonized preoperatively is unknown in the posttransplant group, and clinical management is center specific. One case of disseminated MAC infection led to death in a patient with CF after lung transplantation (R. Grad et al., personal communication, 1993).

Viruses

During their preoperative evaluation, patients are screened serologically for evidence of active or past infection with various viruses: HIV, hepatitis B and C, CMV, and Epstein-Barr virus (EBV). The presence of HIV antibodies precludes additional immunosuppression and, therefore, lung transplantation. Patients with the presence of hepatitis B surface antigen are at a high risk of recrudescence of hepatitis and fulminant liver disease (31). Seropositivity for antibodies to hepatitis C necessitates evaluation for the presence of hepatitis C nucleic acids by polymerase chain reaction to amplify hepatitis C virus (HCV) RNA in serum or liver samples (32). These patients testing positive would be at risk for severe liver disease development posttransplant (33,34). Overall, patients with CF tend to be a younger patient group and often are serologically negative for CMV and EBV. Transplantation of a CMV-positive organ into a CMV-negative recipient virtually guarantees posttransplant CMV disease, but in most cases it is manageable with perioperative antiviral prophylaxis and frequent screening for CMV disease activity. Apparently, EBV seronegativity pretransplant places a patient at increased risk for developing posttransplant lymphoproliferative disorder, but the mortality is low. This will be discussed in a later section.

Protozoa

Seronegativity to *Toxoplasma* places heart transplant patients at risk if they acquire primary infection when immunosuppressed (35). The risk to lung transplant patients is unknown because the risk of acquiring *Toxoplasma* from the graft is very low.

Sinus Disease

Because of their abnormal respiratory epithelium, patients with CF will remain colonized with microorganisms throughout the remaining upper respiratory tree despite the transplantation of "normal" lungs. Because sinus disease has been recognized not only as a reservoir of pathogenic bacteria but also as a potential cause of CF exacerbations (36), routine preoperative sinus drainage has been advocated (37). Several centers (26) perform maxillary sinus antrostomies in all CF candidates, with or without antibiotic irrigation of the sinuses, before lung transplantation. However, many institutions do not require sinus surgery before lung transplantation, particularly in the absence of sinus symptoms. In a comparison of the incidence of posttransplant lung infections in patients with CF (without prophylactic sinus surgery) and non-CF patients at UNC, there were no significant differences in the incidence of pneumonia or bronchitis requiring treatment (38). In a series of 27 patients with CF and 32 non-CF patients, after lung transplantation, 37% of patients with CF were treated for pneumonia versus 31% of non-CF patients (P = not significant). Similarly, 52% of the patients with CF and 69% of those who did not have CF were treated for bronchitis. Patients with CF with symptomatic sinus disease or nasal obstruction may require medical and/or surgical treatment. The need for prophylactic surgery, however, remains to be established by epidemiologic studies or controlled clinical trials.

Pretransplant Care

Nutrition

Patients with CF who present for lung transplantation often are extremely malnourished, with a mean percentage of ideal body weight (IBW) of 76 ± 11 percent predicted (39). Patients homozygous for the most common mutation (ΔF508) tend to have the most severe pulmonary disease, pancreatic insufficiency, and the lowest percentiles of weight (40). Malnutrition contributes to pulmonary mortality with decreased muscle function, impaired immunity, and recurrent infections. Conversely, the chronic catabolic stress of progressive pulmonary pathology leads to progressive malnutrition. Several studies support the use of nutritional rehabilitation with nocturnal feeding tubes to improve the quality of life and the length of survival in patients with end-stage CF lung disease (41,42). A trial of long-term aggressive nutritional rehabilitation in severely malnourished patients with CF (< 85% IBW) at Toronto did not measurably improve pulmonary function but was associated with less deterioration in spirometry when compared with control patients with CF (43). Although the patients were able to gain weight, they also increased their resting energy expenditure without increasing protein turnover. The authors suggested that despite refeeding, other confounding factors, either genetic or humoral, may limit the benefits of nutritional supplementation in patients with CF with end-stage lung disease. In summary, there are data that suggest that aggressive nutritional therapy may slow the decline in pulmonary status and increase respiratory and skeletal muscle strength (44).

The importance of nutritional support in CF lung transplantation has not been established rigorously. Experience from Papworth Hospital also suggests that malnourished patients with CF may have a poorer outcome from lung transplant (27). It is clear that adequate nutrition is essential for postoperative healing and physical rehabilitation. Enteral feeding is preferred for pretransplant patients with CF, to optimize gut function. Total parenteral nutrition as the main nutritional support mode risks gut atrophy and intravenous line infections but usually is necessary in the immediate postoperative period. Early return to enteral nutrition may improve gut barrier and absorptive functions and facilitate absorption of oral medications. Correction of detectable vitamin deficiencies (especially vitamin K) before transplant is essential.

Diabetes

Diabetes mellitus occurs in 5% to 15% of patients with CF (45) and increases in prevalence as patients grow older (46). Glucocorticoid treatment frequently unmasks or exacerbates glucose intolerance. Microvascular complications secondary to diabetes once were considered rare in patients with CF (46) primarily because of these patients' shortened life spans. Because patients with CF currently are living into adulthood, diabetic microangiopathy has been described in up to 20% of patients with CF with diabetes in one series (47). Because cyclosporine and high-dose corticosteroids will exacerbate diabetic symptoms after lung transplantation, diabetic control should be optimized before lung transplantation.

Osteoporosis

Patients with CF are at high risk for osteoporosis because of frequent malnutrition and exercise limitations (discussed in detail in Chapter 18). All candidates for lung transplantation are screened for osteoporosis with dual-energy photon absorptiometry. Bone mass densitometry of the radius, femoral neck, and spine has emerged as a reliable predictor of future spontaneous fractures in osteopenic patients (48). A decrease of more than one standard deviation in bone mass for age and gender by bone densitometry is associated with an increase of 50% to 100% in the incidence of spontaneous fractures in middle-aged women (49). Posttransplant patients are at an unavoidable increased risk of further bone loss because of the combination of high-dose and chronic glucocorticoid therapy, and possibly because of cyclosporine (50,51). Heart transplant patient data indicate that the greatest risk of bone loss is in the first 6 months after transplantation because of the highest incidence of acute rejection and subsequent use of high-dose steroids during that period (52). Patients with greater than one standard deviation below the norm in bone mass density should receive calcium and vitamin supplementation and additionally estrogen or testosterone if they are deficient. Those more than two standard deviations below the norm are encouraged to receive additionally biphosphonates (e.g., pamidronate) parenterally every 3 months and/or calcitonin. Posttransplant, these medications are continued indefinitely.

Exercise

The combined experience of several centers suggests that the most physically fit patients have the greatest likelihood of surviving lung transplant surgery and the postoperative period (9,27). Exercise in patients with CF also may enhance clearance of airway secretions and skeletal respiratory muscle function (53). Moreover, an individual patient's exercise tolerance may be a useful means of monitoring their clinical status both pre- and posttransplant. The requirements for formal supervised exercise rehabilitation before transplantation vary among different transplant centers (8,14). At UNC, patients are required to relocate to the center before transplant and to undergo a supervised exercise program. It is believed that aggressive exercise rehabilitation contributes to early postoperative extubation and ambulation (8). The Pittsburgh group does not require relocation or formal exercise rehabilitation before transplantation, and they have found a health maintenance education program to be as beneficial as education plus exercise (14).

Assisted Ventilation

Although patients dependent on mechanical ventilation are not evaluated routinely for transplant, intubation and mechanical ventilation may become issues for patients already listed, particularly if accrued waiting time on the list makes transplant within 1 to 2 weeks possible. As time on mechanical ventilation increases, the risk of nosocomial infections, respiratory muscle deconditioning, and line sepsis increases; this can make operative risk prohibitive (54). To avoid tracheal intubation, nasal intermittent positive pressure ventilation (NIPPV) may be useful to maintain deteriorating pulmonary patients before transplant (55,56). Nocturnal NIPPV also may prevent night-time oxygen desaturation and hypercapnea. Patients with CF frequently desaturate at night because of decreased functional reserve capacity secondary to airways closure and development of unventilated lung regions, and they show evidence of marked sleep disruption with occasional apneic episodes (57,58). Correction of nocturnal respiratory acidosis also may improve respiratory muscle function and prevent fatigue (59,60). Four patients with CF in Australia—some followed for 18 months—demonstrated improved daytime function, quality of sleep, and functional capacity with NIPPV (56). NIPPV could be an effective therapeutic approach for patients with end-stage lung disease secondary to CF (6) who have an extended waiting time. Controlled trials of NIPPV for CF have not been reported, but reports of its effectiveness in chronic alveolar hypoventilation (61) and for acute exacerbation of chronic obstructive pulmonary disease (COPD) (62) support its increasing use in CF lung transplant candidates.

Corticosteroids

It is common for patients with CF to be placed on systemic glucocorticoids for reversible airflow obstruction [which can occur in 40% of patients (46)], as treatment for allergic bronchopulmonary aspergillosis (ABPA) [10% of patients with CF may fulfill the criteria (63)], and to reduce airway inflammation (64). However, it has been demonstrated in animal models that administration of methylprednisolone at 2 mg/kg per day significantly compromises bronchial anastomosis strength (65). The adverse effects of corticosteroids on bone density and diabetes management are significant. Therefore, most centers minimize corticosteroid use in potential transplant recipients. No or minimal (i.e., < 0.2 mg/kg per day) prednisone or equivalent is permitted. Controlled studies in human transplant recipients are lacking, and maximal doses are established by individual centers.

Transfusions

Transplant candidates should avoid blood transfusion if at all possible because of the risk of generating preformed antibodies that could recognize donor lung epitopes and induce hyperacute graft rejection at the time of surgery. Hyperacute rejection occurs immediately and catastrophically and is the result of presensitization of class 1 major histocompatibility complex (MHC) antigens on leukocytes through blood transfusion. Preformed lymphocytotoxic antibodies directed against donor lymphocytes also have been associated with a significant decrement in long-term graft survival (54,66) in lung transplant recipients. The risk may be decreased by the use of washed, leukocyte-poor packed erythrocytes if blood transfusion is unavoidable.

Miscellaneous

There is no contraindication to the use of recombinant human DNase (rhDNase) during the preoperative period. Participation in other experimental protocols should not affect transplant status but should be reviewed with the transplant team.

In summary, all attempts to maximize the overall health and fitness of the lung transplant candidates are encouraged. Renal function must not be compromised, and care must be taken when treating with aminoglycosides and other potentially nephrotoxic drugs. Severe medical or psychosocial complications may compromise transplant candidacy. Well-coordinated comprehensive care programs developed at many transplant centers, combined with the care of the referring physicians, support the many and variable needs of the patient with CF.

SURGERY

Evolution of Surgical Technique

The first heart–lung transplant was performed at Stanford University in 1981 in a patient with Eisenmenger's syndrome (67). This operation was first performed for a patient with CF at the University of Pittsburgh in October 1983. The North American experience with heart–lung transplant for CF initially was very discouraging, with only 10 of 33 patients surviving through the first year (68). Better early results were reported from Harefield (69) and Papworth (70) Hospitals.

Early reports of isolated double lung transplantation for obstructive pulmonary disease were encouraging (71), but the *en bloc* double lung transplantation procedure was fraught with major complications, including a high incidence of airway necrosis. Necrosis of the entire donor airway was observed in 3 of the first 16 patients who underwent this procedure at the University of Toronto (72). In four other patients, airway strictures developed, necessitating dilatation and stent placement, for an airway complication rate of 44%. To address this issue, Noirclerc and colleagues (73) in Marseilles, France, introduced the technique of bilateral bronchial anastomosis, substantially reducing the amount of ischemic donor airway. Shortly afterward, Pasque and colleagues (74) from Washington University described a technique of bilateral lung transplantation through a transverse thoracosternotomy ("clamshell") incision, which has become the standard procedure for double lung transplantation in North America. This operative approach offers several advantages, particularly to patients with CF. Chronic infection predisposes to the formation of dense pleural adhesions and large tortuous bronchial arteries that supply the bronchiectatic airways and peribronchial lymph nodes. The need for cardiopulmonary bypass for *en bloc* double lung transplantation procedures made exsanguinating hemorrhage an all-too-frequent occurrence for patients with CF. The clamshell incision introduced by Pasque affords excellent exposure of the pleural spaces and hila, allowing for safer extraction of lungs

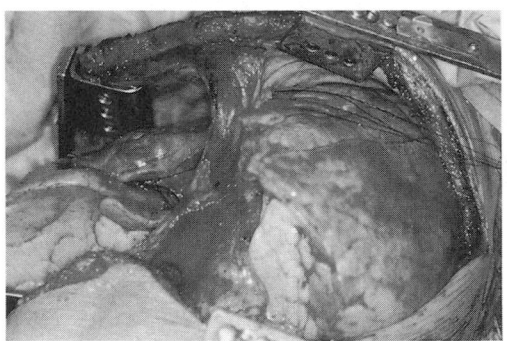

FIG. 9–2. Exposure of both pleural spaces is excellent through this approach. Ties are around branches of the pulmonary artery on each side. (From Egan TM, Detterbeck FC. Techniques and results of double lung transplantation. *Chest Surg Clin North Am* 1993;3:89–111.)

with severe pleural adhesions and control of the large bronchial vessels entering each hemithorax (Fig. 9–2). By implanting each lung sequentially, cardiopulmonary bypass frequently can be avoided, considerably reducing transfusion requirements.

The European experience with CF transplant operations supports the performance of heart–lung transplantation. de Leval et al. (75), from Papworth Hospital at Cambridge, reported a 67% actuarial 1-year survival rate of 32 patients with CF who underwent heart–lung transplantation. Yacoub's group at Harefield reported 79 patients with CF who underwent heart–lung transplantation; there were 18 deaths in the first 2 months and a 1-year actuarial survival rate of 69% (10). It is likely that the routine use of aprotinin (76) in the United Kingdom for these procedures reduced perioperative bleeding and improved survival.

Donor Lungs

Donor lungs are selected for transplant from brain-dead organ donors, after family consent, on the basis of adequate gas exchange characteristics [defined as a partial pressure of oxygen (PO_2) > 350 on 100% oxygen with 5 cm of positive end-expiratory pressure (PEEP)] (77). Bronchoscopy is an essential part of donor evaluation.

Evidence of purulent bronchitis may preclude a successful outcome (78). Unfortunately, aspiration frequently accompanies closed-head injuries (79). It has been estimated that only approximately 25% of cardiac donors will have lungs suitable for transplantation (80). The small number of organ donors severely limits the number of lung transplants that can be performed.

Donor and recipient ABO compatibility and some size matching are necessary, although the degree of allowable size mismatch is unclear. If implanted lungs are too small, there is a risk of graft injury because of overinflation and a likelihood of pleural fluid accumulation. The pleural space is contaminated unavoidably with lung microorganisms at the time of recipient pneumonectomy, and thus, pleural fluid is more susceptible to infection in patients with CF. Lungs that are too large may produce hemodynamic embarrassment when the chest is closed, or significant atelectasis may develop, which can predispose to postoperative pneumonia. Patients with CF frequently are of small stature, but lungs from larger donors can be used. UNC reported pneumoreduction procedures in nine CF bilateral lung transplant recipients (81). These procedures consisted of right middle lobectomies or nonanatomic lingular resection, or combinations of both. This pneumoreduction has not had an adverse effect on survival or posttransplant lung function and is an appropriate strategy for placing substantially larger donor lungs into smaller recipients.

Size discrepancy is likely to be a limiting factor in many living related donor lobe transplants for CF (3). Although this procedure may be suitable for children and small adults, many adults with CF—particularly men, who have larger lung volumes than women of similar age and height—may have thoracic volumes too large to allow performance of bilateral lobe transplant from parents or siblings.

Surgical Techniques

Anesthesia

Large-bore intravenous access is of paramount importance because of occasional exsanguinating hemorrhage from an injury to a pulmonary artery or vein. An oxymetric Swan-Ganz catheter is useful for monitoring cardiac function and pulmonary artery pressures, particularly during one-lung anesthesia. Meticulous management of intraoperative vascular volume is essential for a good outcome. Renal failure is a serious risk of extended hypovolemia. However, newly implanted lungs are prone to the development of pulmonary edema, so it is preferable to keep cardiac filling pressures as low as can be tolerated, subject to the limits of cardiac output and vital organ perfusion.

The maintenance of an adequate airway for ventilation is a vexing intraoperative problem. Large volumes of viscous airway secretions constantly threaten the integrity of the airway, particularly with surgical manipulation of the CF lung during explantation. It is useful to intubate recipients initially with a large-diameter endotracheal tube and aspirate airway secretions through a fiberoptic bronchoscope. Subsequently, a left-sided double lumen tube is placed. In children too small to accommodate a double lumen tube, bronchus blocking balloons have been used. The operation can be interrupted temporarily to change endotracheal tubes or perform bronchoscopy for aspiration of secretions. This approach may prevent instituting systemic anticoagulation and cardiopulmonary bypass. However, cardiopulmonary bypass is set up in the operating room and immediately available for all operations, with a perfusionist on standby.

Pneumonectomy

A preoperative radionuclide perfusion scan identifies the least perfused (presumably the worst functioning) lung. In general, this is the lung chosen for the first pneumonectomy. Both hemithoraces are entered through an anterior thoracotomy in the fourth or fifth interspace. The sternum is divided transversely. Adhesions are taken down in the pleural space with electrocautery. Adhesions at the apex can be particularly troublesome, especially in patients who have had previous pneumothoraces or who have undergone some type of pleural scleros-

ing procedure. However, the visibility afforded by this surgical approach allows for safe extraction of lungs, even when talc has been instilled in the pleural space or when surgical pleurectomy has been performed.

If there is any question about the patient's ability to tolerate one-lung anesthesia, the response to temporary occlusion of the pulmonary artery on the side of intended first pneumonectomy should be assessed. Preservation of cardiac output, mixed venous saturation, and oxygenation may confirm tolerance and allow pneumonectomy. If the patient cannot tolerate temporary occlusion of the chosen pulmonary artery, then the opposite side can be occluded. If the patient cannot be maintained on one lung, then cardiopulmonary bypass can be instituted easily by opening the pericardium vertically and cannulating the ascending aorta and right atrium.

Dissection of the hilum can be hazardous because of large, well-vascularized lymph nodes. There frequently are extensive adhesions of the lung to the hilum. It is preferable to divide the pulmonary artery distal to the upper lobe division on each side. Occasionally, there will be a considerable size discrepancy between the donor and recipient pulmonary arteries, particularly in patients who have had significant elevation of pulmonary artery pressures. In these instances, the pulmonary artery anastomosis to the recipient's pulmonary artery can be made distal to its first division.

The pulmonary veins are divided extrapericardially, using vascular stapling devices. Dividing the pulmonary ligament with electrocautery facilitates identification of the inferior pulmonary vein. Occlusive clamps are placed on the distal bronchial divisions in the lung parenchyma to minimize soiling of the pleural space with airway secretions. The bronchus proximal to the upper lobe takeoff then is divided using sharp dissection. After the lung is extracted from the chest, hemostasis is secured. There frequently are large bronchial arteries that bleed profusely, requiring clips or ligatures. The clamshell incision affords adequate exposure to see and control these vessels. The best retractor to expose the hilum, particularly if one encounters stubborn bleeding, is an assistant's hand. This minimizes the risk of phrenic nerve injury, which is more common when rigid metal retractors are used. After the native lung is explanted, the open airway and pleural space are irrigated with warm povidone–iodine solution. A considerable amount of purulent material that otherwise would end up in the newly transplanted organ usually is flushed from the airway by this maneuver.

Lung Implantation

The first donor lung to be implanted is prepared by trimming back the donor bronchus to within one or two rings of the upper lobe takeoff. The bronchial anastomosis is performed first because it is the most posterior. An end-to-end bronchial anastomosis is preferred by surgeons at UNC, although other groups have used a telescoping technique (82). Early in our experience, bronchial omentopexy was employed routinely (83). However, we have abandoned omentopexy, preferring instead to buttress the bronchial suture line with peribronchial tissue, as first described by Noirclerc et al. (73).

The pulmonary veins of the donor lung are attached as a cuff of left atrium. This is facilitated on the right side by development of the interatrial groove. Of necessity, an atrial cuff must be fashioned by incising the pericardium around the recipient pulmonary veins, including both of these in a Satinsky clamp. Amputation of the staple lines on the recipient pulmonary vein stumps allows for creation of a recipient atrial cuff, which is anastomosed to the donor atrial cuff using a running polypropylene suture. The pulmonary artery (PA) anastomosis then is performed. The donor PA must be aligned appropriately with the recipient PA to avoid torsion. This is most easily accomplished by noting the location of the upper lobe takeoff on the recipient PA and aligning this with the upper lobe takeoff on the donor PA.

On completion of the vascular anastomoses, de-airing of the lung blood vessels is important to prevent systemic air embolism. The newly inflated lung is back-bled to establish egress of air and blood through an open pulmonary

artery anastomosis. On completion of the first transplant, the opposite native lung is excised in the same fashion as described previously. The airway and pleural space once again is irrigated with povidone–iodine (Betadine), and the second transplant is performed. Cardiopulmonary bypass may be required if pulmonary edema should occur in the first implanted lung, which assumes all of the cardiac output during the second implantation.

After the second lung has been implanted, pressure gradients across the PA anastomoses are measured using a monitoring line and needle passed off to the anesthetist. In general, anastomoses with mean gradients greater than 5 mm Hg should be evaluated for stenosis or torsion, and revision should be considered.

Perioperative Complications

Early Graft Dysfunction

There are several factors that may contribute to early graft dysfunction, including the duration of ischemic time and the integrity of the endothelial/alveolar barriers in the donor lungs at the time of explantation. Unfortunately, organ donors may have sustained injuries that set the stage for a microvascular lung injury, and there are varying degrees of airway contamination and infection among intubated brain-dead individuals. Graft dysfunction is a substantial problem after lung transplantation, but it cannot be predicted from duration of ischemia alone. Significant pulmonary edema should raise the suspicion of a narrowed pulmonary venous anastomosis. Graft dysfunction is a major cause of morbidity and mortality in the early postoperative period after lung transplantation. At UNC, three CF lung transplant recipients have been retransplanted for life-threatening graft dysfunction, with two successful outcomes. Three other patients from a total of 67 recipients of double lung transplants for CF required ventilation for more than 7 days because of graft dysfunction.

Dysfunction of pulmonary lymphatic vessels contributes to interstitial fluid accumulation in the transplanted lung (84). Any pulmonary insult in the early posttransplant period may be manifest by an exaggerated degree of capillary leak.

Perioperative Blood Loss

Bleeding can be a significant problem for a variety of reasons. Vascular pleural adhesions frequently are present, and extrapleural dissection of the native lung for explantation often is necessary. Even without technical difficulties or significant pleural adhesions, an obligatory blood loss occurs consequent to removal of CF lungs, which do not collapse as readily as lungs of patients with other forms of end-stage disease. Thus, the CF lung is presumed to have a larger vascular capacitance at explantation. Each lung in turn is replaced with an organ that has been flushed empty of blood and that is atelectatic when implanted with a relatively empty vascular capacitance. This results in an obligatory blood volume loss at the time of reperfusion of the transplant.

A coagulopathy caused by blood loss is more likely to occur in CF transplant recipients, whose liver function usually is abnormal. The need for blood and coagulation factor replacement must be balanced against the risk of intravascular volume infusion, particularly in the presence of graft dysfunction. In addition, the necessity for cyclosporine therapy may predispose to renal failure, particularly in a hypovolemic patient.

Clot that accumulates in the pleural space must be evacuated to reduce the risk of infection with microbes spilled during lung explant. This occasionally necessitates a return to the operating room 1 or 2 days after successful transplantation if the pleural spaces have not been evacuated adequately with pleural drainage tubes. Similarly, postoperative pneumothoraces in patients with CF should be evacuated to obliterate the pleural space and reduce the risk of empyema.

Renal Failure

As alluded to previously, there frequently is a dilemma in perioperative fluid management because of ongoing fluid losses, the need to maintain an adequate intravascular volume for vital perfusion (especially renal perfusion), the effects of cyclosporine on glomerular blood flow, and the propensity for extravascular fluid to accumulate in newly transplanted lungs. Occasionally, serious intraoperative bleeding and hypotension have given rise to intraoperative oliguria or anuria. Postoperative hemodialysis is required occasionally. The use of α-adrenergic agents to maintain blood pressure should be tempered by their adverse effect on bronchial mucosal blood flow and the potential increased risk of bronchial anastomotic complications.

Anastomotic Complications

Vascular anastomotic complications should be suspect if there appears to be a significant pulmonary edema, or if significant asymmetry in vascular markings is apparent on the chest radiograph. Bronchial anastomotic complications become apparent only after the first or second week after transplantation. We have observed three instances of bronchial dehiscence in our CF recipients, two of which were contained and one of which was associated with a small air leak. All of these healed without further sequelae. In two other patients, strictures have developed in the bronchus intermedius distal to an apparently well-healed airway anastomosis. Both of these patients have required placement of a Dumon Silicone endobronchial stent (Bryan Corp., Woburn, MA) (85).

Infectious Complications

Despite the presence of multiple resistant organisms in the chest and pleural spaces of these patients, wound complications have been infrequent. One sternal dehiscence required reclosure. Three sternal wound infections have occurred. One patient succumbed from *B. cepacia* pneumonia, whereas another patient resolved his sternal wound infection as a small chronic draining sinus. One patient with *M. abscessus* required drainage, but this subsequently has healed. Infectious complications after lung transplantation in patients with CF have had a similar incidence and outcome to that of lung transplant recipients with other diseases (38).

Other Complications

Axillary vein thrombosis has been observed frequently. Patients with CF often have preexisting chronic central venous lines or have had lines in these veins. The contribution of axillary vein compression during surgery because of the clamshell approach may contribute to this complication. Patients in whom significant upper extremity edema develops are treated with anticoagulation which, unfortunately, complicates bronchoscopy and transbronchial lung biopsy.

POSTOPERATIVE CARE

Patients with CF who undergo lung transplantation have to deal with myriad complications inherent to transplantation plus all of the ramifications of their underlying systemic disease. This dual challenge is best exemplified by the unique—and at times unpredictable—pharmacodynamics of CF and immunosuppressive drugs.

Immunosuppression

Immunosuppression in the lung is based on a regimen of three nonspecific immune-modulators (Table 9–4). Cyclosporine and, more recently, tacrolimus act by blocking the production of and response to T-lymphocyte lymphokines. Neither drug is lymphotoxic nor indirectly inhibits monocyte function (86). Direct comparisons of cyclosporine versus tacrolimus have been few and so far have not conclusively shown significant difference in survival or in the incidence of acute rejection. However, the prevalence of obliterative bronchiolitis may be significantly lower with tacrolimus (87). Azathioprine and, more recently, mycophenolate are lymphocyte antimetabolites and decrease cell number. Corticosteroids are used for their wide range of antiinflammatory properties. All immunosuppressive agents have potent side effects (Table

TABLE 9–4. *Immunosuppression protocol, University of North Carolina*

Cyclosporine
  4 mg/hr IV (initiated at implantation)
  Daily cyclosporine levels in immediate
    postoperative period
  Dosage adjusted as follows using TDEX
    monoclonal antibody assay
    First 6 mos—400–450 ng/mL
    6 mos–1 year—350–400 ng/mL
    1 yr—300 ng/mL
    2 yrs—250 ng/mL
  Dosage may be adjusted according to renal
    function or patient pharmacokinetics
Azathioprine
  2 mg/kg/day (initiated on call to the OR)
  Given at 1600 hours once a day
  Monitor leukocyte count and hold if less than
    4,000/mL
Corticosteroids
  Started on day 1
  Dose: adults—125 mg IV every 8 hours for 24
    hours then 0.5 mg/kg twice a day
  Wean dose by 2.5-mg increments until patient is
    on maintenance dose of 15 mg every other day
    by 7 months posttransplant
  Rejection treated with prednisone boost and taper
    orally for 2–3 weeks after treatment with high-
    dose methylprednisolone 15 mg/kg/day IV for 1
    day and 7.5 mg/kg/day IV for 2 more days
Tacrolimus
  Substituted for cyclosporine in cases of acute or
    chronic rejection unresponsive to increased
    corticosteroids
  Cyclosporine is usually stopped for 3 days before
    tacrolimus is initiated
  Patients are placed on increased corticosteroids
    during that 3-day period
Mycophenolate
  Substituted for azathioprine because of unrelenting
    rejection or drug intolerance

IV, intravenous; TDEX, cyclosporine monoclonal antibody assay, Abbott Laboratories, Abbott Park, IL.

9–5) that must be monitored and considered when titrating dosage and serum levels.

Cyclosporine

Oral cyclosporine is the cornerstone of effective outpatient immunosuppression for solid-organ transplantation. For patients with CF, cyclosporine causes problems in terms of its absorption, metabolism, and biliary excretion (Table 9–4). Cyclosporine is absorbed variably and unpredictably throughout the gastrointestinal (GI) tract of individual patients

TABLE 9–5. *Immunosuppressive drug side effects*

Cyclosporine
  Nephrotoxicity
    Decreased renal perfusion
    Hyperkalemia
    Magnesium wasting
  Neurotoxicity
    Seizures
    Headaches
    Tremors
  Hepatotoxicity
    Cholestasis
  Photosensitivity
  Hypertension
  Hirsutism
  Increased risk of malignancy
  Gingival hyperplasia
Tacrolimus
  Similar to cyclosporine except for
    No hirsutism or gingival hyperplasia
    Increased risk of fungal infections
Azathioprine
  Bone marrow suppression
  Pancreatitis
  Hepatotoxicity
Mycophenolate
  Diarrhea
  Possible increased risk of cytomegalovirus
  Leukopenia
Corticosteroids
  Glucose intolerance
  Osteoporosis
  Peptic ulcers
  Cataracts
  Psychosis
  Peripheral edema
  Cushingoid features

blood by monoclonal antibody assay is targeted in the first 6 months, 350 to 400 ng/mL in the second 6 months, and 200 to 250 ng/mL thereafter. However, this method of monitoring blood levels neglects the actual peak level as well as the area under the curve for a given patient. This may lead to unexpected problems in terms of drug toxicity and efficacy. Because cyclosporine is metabolized in the liver via the cytochrome P450 system and excreted via the biliary tree, hepatotoxicity and cholestasis may be causes as well as effects of cyclosporine toxicity (90).

Any medication that affects the mixed-function oxidases of the liver will alter cyclosporine levels (Table 9–6). Medications that induce the P450 system, such as phenytoin (Dilantin, Parke-Davis, Morris Plains, NJ) and rifampin, can acutely lower the cyclo-sporine levels and thus precipitate acute rejection. Erythromycin, diltiazem, birth control pills, and ketoconazole (which may be used for this effect) may raise cyclosporine levels by inhibiting the liver enzymes (Table 9–6).

Common side effects of cyclosporine include neurotoxicity, nephrotoxicity, hepatic toxicity, and high blood pressure. Tremors and headaches are frequent but not totally specific for cyclosporine toxicity. In 14 of 68 patients with CF transplanted at UNC, focal seizures with grand mal extension both with and without EEG abnormalities (91) developed. These seizures occurred around the time of treatment

with CF (88); because cyclosporine is hydrophobic and lipid soluble, bioavailability may vary with diet and ability to absorb lipids (88). To achieve adequate blood levels with affordable oral doses, ketoconazole is used to inhibit cyclosporine liver metabolism and thus increase blood levels. The new cyclosporine preparation of Neoral (Novartis, East Hanover, NJ) is a microemulsion that appears to provide greater absorbability and does not necessitate the use of ketoconazole. Bioavailability with both preparations is enhanced by adequate pancreatic enzyme supplementation (89). It is routine to use a twice-a-day dosing schedule of cyclosporine and measure trough levels in the morning. A level of 400 to 450 ng/mL whole

TABLE 9–6. *Drug interactions with cyclosporine*

Will *decrease* blood cyclosporine levels
  Phenytoin
  Rifampin
  Phenobarbital
Will *increase* blood cyclosporine levels
  Erythromycin
  Clarithromycin
  Diltiazem
  Ketoconazole
  Birth control pills
Synergistic for cyclosporine nephrotoxicity
  Nonsteroidal antiinflammatory agents
  Diuretics
  Amphotericin B

of acute rejection with high-dose steroids, and these patients most frequently had serum cyclosporine levels within the range that is accepted as therapeutic for lung transplant patients. Seizures also have been reported to develop in other solid-organ transplant recipients who do not have CF, in the setting of administration of high-dose corticosteroids for organ rejection (92–94). Patients have had lumbar punctures that do not suggest infection by cell counts, chemistries, serologies, or cultures. Cerebrospinal fluid cyclosporine levels have been negligible. Magnetic resonance imaging (MRI) abnormalities in the brain have been noted at the time of seizures (Fig. 9–3), spontaneously regressed during a seizure-free period, and returned with a new bout of seizures. These lesions, which also have been

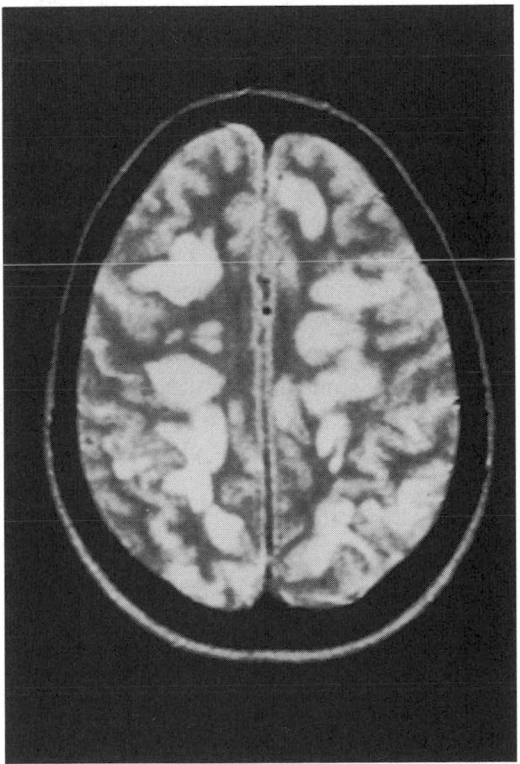

FIG. 9–3. Magnetic resonance imaging of the brain of a lung transplant patient with seizures consistent with cyclosporine neurotoxicity (1995). The scattered bright areas are seen on T2-weighted images.

described in other non-CF solid organ transplant patients, are hypodense nonenhancing white matter lesions with a prolonged T2 relaxation time indicative of increased water content (91,93). It is hypothesized that these lesions may represent focal breakdown of the blood–brain barrier related either to rejection, corticosteroids, or both (91). This may allow focally intense exposure of the brain to cyclosporine, which is highly lipophilic. Lorazepam is used both to treat the seizure episodes and as seizure prophylaxis for 1 week after corticosteroid treatment of acute rejection in those individuals susceptible to seizures in this context. The new antiepileptic gabapentin may be useful in these patients, especially in those individuals with a defined seizure focus. Gabapentin has been found to be useful in the management of refractory pain syndromes (95–97) and possibly may be used to treat severe cyclosporine-related headaches (98). Rare, idiosyncratic reactions to cyclosporine include encephalopathy, coma, and even brain death (88). Tacrolimus can be substituted successfully for cyclosporine even though the potential for neurotoxicity is similar to cyclosporine (99).

Nephrotoxicity from cyclosporine is almost universal. Decreased aminoglycoside clearance within the first postoperative week suggests a 25% to 50% reduction in renal function despite a serum creatinine level that is within the normal range. After 1 year, the average serum creatinine level is 2.4 mg/dL, having been normal preoperatively. Because cyclosporine reduces renal blood flow, dehydration, diuretic overuse, and nonsteroidal antiinflammatory agents may act synergistically to decrease renal function. Cyclosporine also causes magnesium wasting and hyperkalemia.

Cyclosporine has induced systemic high blood pressure in approximately one third to one half of lung transplant patients (100). Appropriate antihypertensives include calcium channel blockers (closely observing cyclosporine levels if using diltiazem), angiotensin-converting enzyme inhibitors, and clonidine alone or in combination. Angiotensin-converting enzyme inhibitors must be used with caution in patients who have cyclosporine-induced renal insufficiency and hyperkalemia.

Azathioprine

Most of the side effects of azathioprine center on marrow suppression (see Table 9–5). Occasionally, the dose may need to be decreased or the medication discontinued to maintain a leukocyte count greater than 4,000/µL. Patients may become chronically anemic and require transfusions. Interestingly, erythropoietin (EPO) levels are not elevated (101); therefore, EPO is "inappropriately" normal. Erythrocytes for transfusions either should be CMV negative or buffy coat poor to prevent infection with a new CMV strain.

Mycophenolate

Mycophenolate mofetil is an antimetabolite that perturbs the proliferation of T and B lymphocytes more selectively and may be somewhat more efficacious and less bone marrow toxic than azathioprine (102–104). Mycophenolate has been shown to be useful both in preventing and treating acute and chronic rejection in a variety of solid-organ transplants (105–107). It currently is being studied as an alternative to azathioprine.

Glucocorticoids

The side effects of glucocorticoids are well known (see Table 9–5). Glucocorticoids are the current standard treatment for acute rejection and obliterative bronchiolitis. Most patients are on chronic low-dose steroids as part of their immunosuppression regimen. After lung transplantation, patients are maintained on 0.5 mg/kg per day. After 3 months, this typically is reduced by 2.5 mg increments at weekly intervals if pulmonary function is maintained and there have been no episodes of acute rejection. The lowest chronic dose is 15 mg every other day. In the future, it may be possible to identify patients who tolerate glucocorticoid withdrawal. These patients would be identified by the absence of episodes of graft rejection, a favorable histocompatability match, and possibly by a negative mixed lymphocyte reaction (108).

Early Course:
The First 3 Months After Transplant

All lung transplant patients must monitor and record their temperature, systemic blood pressure, weight, and lung spirometry daily and are given parameters for notification of the transplant coordinator. When a post–lung transplant patient has a fever (defined as greater than 37.5°C) or a significant decrease in spirometry (defined as a greater than 10% decrease in FEV_1 over 48 hours), the main consideration is differentiating immunologic rejection from infection as a cause of graft dysfunction. For the first 3 months, both events are quite common and patients usually undergo bronchoscopy with transbronchial biopsy to establish the diagnosis.

Transbronchial biopsy is 90% sensitive for detecting CMV pneumonitis and 70% sensitive for detecting acute rejection (109). Therefore, nondiagnostic biopsies in the face of falling spirometry and fever usually will lead to treatment for rejection. However, CMV may follow the increased immunosuppression and may cause lack of improvement or relapse. Similarly, acute rejection may follow CMV pneumonitis because of the stimulation of the patient's native immune system. Therefore, a high index of suspicion must be maintained along with a low threshold for further diagnostic considerations and procedures when following these patients.

Acute Rejection

Acute rejection usually presents with a low-grade fever, malaise, and a persistent decrease in spirometry. Bilateral perihilar infiltrates with increases in pleural fluid often are evident on chest radiograph. The lung biopsy demonstrates perivascular lymphocytic cuffing without any evidence of a coexisting infectious etiology (Fig. 9–4). The clinical response to

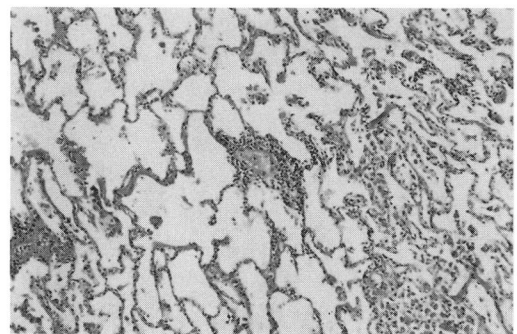

FIG. 9–4. Transbronchial lung biopsy specimen showing mild acute rejection under low power view. The blood vessel in the center has a lymphocytic cuff without extension into air spaces or interstitium.

high-dose intravenous methylprednisolone (1 g the first day, and 500 mg on days 2 and 3) supports the diagnosis. However, the longer the time away from transplant, the less classical the presentation for acute rejection, especially by chest radiograph (16). The sensitivity and specificity of computed tomography (CT) of the chest or high-resolution CT in differentiating acute rejection from other infectious etiologies of pneumonitis is not well documented (110). Therefore, a normal radiograph will not rule out rejection as a cause of declining pulmonary function.

Infection

Bacteria

Because the first 3 months also are the time of maximum immunosuppression, the lung allograft also is at risk for infection. Mucociliary clearance is diminished in denervated transplanted lungs (111) so that episodes of clinical bronchitis/pneumonitis are common. This is true for both patients with CF and non-CF patients (38), although the bacterial flora may differ. Because the upper airways of patients with CF remain colonized by *Pseudomonas*, these organisms frequently are isolated from expectorated sputum and from samples of the lower respiratory tree. Patients who do not

have CF are more likely to present with non-pseudomonal organisms. However, frequent bacterial infections, especially *Pseudomonas* later in the posttransplant course (i.e., > 6 months) may suggest the development of bronchiolitis obliterans in both patients with CF and non-CF patients.

Viruses

CMV disease is common, especially during the first 2 months after transplant (Fig. 9–5). The incidence of significant CMV disease varies according to the CMV status of donor (D) and recipient (R): with the D+,R− having the highest frequency, followed in order by the D+,R+, then D−,R+, and the D−,R− having the least (112). CMV prophylaxis after transplantation varies according to each center's experience. The group at Pittsburgh elects to give all D+ or R+ patients 90 days of parenteral gancyclovir and have published data showing less CMV disease and bronchiolitis obliterans in patients treated in this manner (113). However, based on data on management of CMV infection after bone marrow transplant, many centers prophylactically treat newly infected D+,R− patients with 4 weeks of gancyclovir and 6 weeks of intravenous CMV specific immunoglobulin because CMV disease is especially severe in this group. CMV disease has varied manifestations, from a systemic flu-like syndrome with neutropenia and appearance of

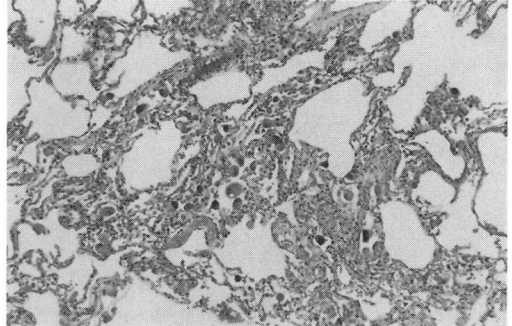

FIG. 9–5. Transbronchial lung biopsy specimen displaying the typical cytomegaloviral inclusions consistent with cytomegalovirus pneumonitis.

serum immunoglobulin M antibody to CMV, to multiple organ involvement reflected by gastritis, colitis, hepatitis, retinitis (rarely), and pneumonitis (15). An immune fluorescent monoclonal antibody test for CMV antigen using blood leukocytes may provide the earliest and most rapid detection of CMV disease (114,115). This test allows very sensitive detection of CMV viremia and may allow therapeutic intervention before a patient's symptoms develop. Treatment is with parenteral gancyclovir for 2 to 3 weeks, with renal adjusted dosing. The main side effects of gancyclovir "overdose" are bone marrow suppression with significant neutropenia or thrombocytopenia. Foscarnet is used for the rare occurrence of clinical gancyclovir resistance, as determined by lack of improvement, despite adequate doses of gancyclovir within 1 week (116). Foscarnet, however, has significant renal toxicity, affects serum electrolytes, and requires concurrent administration of saline. CMV disease refractory to either agent alone may respond to a combination of gancyclovir and foscarnet (116).

Herpes simplex 1 infections can be very painful. To prevent this complication, acyclovir (200 mg/day) may be given for the first year after transplantation. This practice varies among transplant centers.

Fungi

As stated in the pretransplant section, the correlation between recovery of *Aspergillus* organisms from preoperative sputum cultures and postoperative fungal complications is unclear. Serious *Aspergillus* infections in lung transplant patients has been reported to produce a mortality rate of 60% to 75% (117). These infections may be locally invasive *Aspergillus* at the anastomatic site of the large airways (118) or may involve parenchymal lung disease and dissemination (119). It has been suggested that persistent CMV disease (119) or augmented immunosuppression, especially with corticosteroids (120) in the setting of obliterative bronchiolitis (121), may increase the risk of serious *Aspergillus* disease.

There have been reports of patients developing ABPA after lung transplantation (122). These patients presented with progressive airflow obstruction and eosinophilic bronchitis on biopsy and have responded to systemic and inhaled steroid therapy. There may be an additional benefit in ABPA for administering antifungal agents, especially if moderate to heavy growth of *Aspergillus* is obtained from sputum or bronchoscopically obtained cultures.

Candidal organisms cause most of the fungal infections but not the most mortality in lung transplant recipients (123). Because oropharyngeal thrush frequently is troublesome, nystatin mouthwash is given indefinitely.

Pneumocystis carinii pneumonia, although once a common respiratory pathogen in immunosuppressed solid-organ transplant recipients, rarely has caused significant morbidity or mortality when effective prophylactic therapy is employed. Prophylactic treatment regimens are virtually identical to those used with HIV patients and may include trimethoprim/sulfamethoxazole (one double-strength tablet PO 3 times a week), dapsone (100 mg PO every day), or pentamidine (300 mg inhaled once a month) (124). Duration of prophylaxis varies, but lifelong treatment is prescribed at UNC.

Nontuberculous Mycobacteria

Infections with NTM are rare but potentially serious complications after lung transplantation. NTM are isolated from sputa of approximately 13% of patients with CF (125), but the prevalence of active infection, rather than colonization, probably is much lower. Active NTM infections that extend beyond the patient's native lungs may flourish when immunosuppression is initiated at the time of transplantation, but the incidence of disseminated NTM infection in the posttransplant CF population appears to be very low. Nevertheless, all lobes of CF lungs excised from individuals with NTM isolated from pretransplant sputum samples should be examined meticulously by the pathologist for granulomatous inflammation and other signs of active NTM infection after excision.

After transplantation, regular evaluation of symptoms, physical examinations, chest radiographs, and bronchoscopy specimens for evidence of NTM infection is warranted, particularly in recipients with preoperative NTM isolates. High-resolution CT may be useful (126), but its role in the diagnosis of NTM disease after lung transplantation has not been established. The isolation of NTM in sputum or bronchoalveolar lavage samples may necessitate transbronchial or open-lung biopsy to characterize disease activity. Diagnostic criteria for establishing NTM disease have been published (127,128), but treatment thresholds should be reduced because of the transplant-required immunosuppression. Optimal drug therapy has not been defined, but a number of multidrug regimens have been suggested (125). Caution must be exercised because of possible drug interference with cyclosporine or tacrolimus metabolism, especially with rifampin.

Late Course: After 3 Months

Obliterative Bronchiolitis

After a lung transplantation patient has survived 6 months, the leading cause of morbidity and mortality is obliterative bronchiolitis (OB) (16). OB is suggested by a progressive and consistent decrease (> 20%) of expiratory flows and the absence of other reversible causes. Frequently, an increase in the percentage of neutrophils in bronchoalveolar lavage (BAL) is seen, reflecting the development of bronchitis/bronchiectasis. Bronchoscopy with transbronchial biopsy is of low yield because of the patchy nature of OB and is used primarily to rule out other ongoing processes (16). Histopathologically, a lymphocytic bronchiolitis frequently precedes or accompanies OB, suggesting an "active immunologic" response (Fig. 9–6). This is believed to be analogous to coronary artery disease in heart transplant patients or to bile duct sclerosis in liver transplant patients and therefore is tantamount to chronic allograft rejection (16). Treatment is augmented immunosuppression, which may arrest or reverse the decline in pulmonary function.

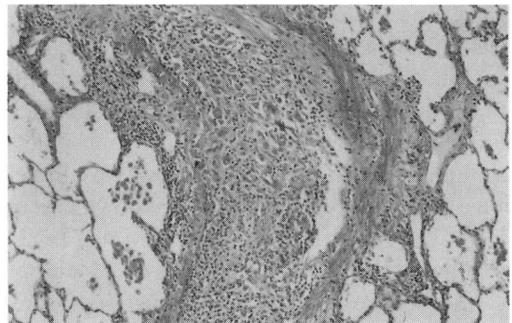

FIG. 9–6. Light microscopy of a transbronchial lung biopsy specimen that shows the histology consistent with obliterative bronchiolitis. The small airway in the center is denuded of epithelium and is filled with granulation tissue. The end result will be irreversible fibrosis and scarring of that airway.

Currently, standard therapy is high-dose corticosteroids (15 mg/kg intravenously for 3 days) followed by increased oral corticosteroids in a very slow taper (16). Antilymphocyte globulin, used both as induction immunosuppression posttransplant and as treatment for later episodes of acute and chronic rejection, has been reported to be variably efficacious (16,129–131) in controlling obliterative bronchiolitis. Tacrolimus (FK506) may be superior to cyclosporine in controlling episodes of acute rejection and may reduce subsequent development of OB (87). Methotrexate has been advocated as an adjunctive immunosuppressive agent in treating and preventing refractory allograft rejection (132–134). Other potential options to treat or prevent OB include aerosolized cyclosporine (135) and total lymphoid irradiation (136).

The etiology of OB is unclear, and its incidence has been reported to be between 20% and 50% (10,16). Many studies suggest that repeated and severe episodes of acute rejection are the most significant risk factors; hence, aggressive treatment of acute rejection is indicated (16). Others suggest that infection, particularly with CMV, may be etiologically important (137). Most likely, OB may be a final common pathway for any immunologic lung injury to denervated transplanted lungs

(138). The clinical and pathologic manifestations of OB are not unique to the transplanted lung and have been described in chronic graft versus host disease in bone marrow transplant patients and in individuals without transplants but with connective tissue diseases, viral infections, or some drugs, and from unknown causes (139). The clinical course of OB in lung transplant patients is variable; patients may stabilize at a lower level of pulmonary function or may experience progressive deterioration. For both patients with CF and non-CF patients with OB, airways become bronchiectatic and are colonized with *P. aeruginosa*. For patients with CF, this can cause a return to a life of regular antibiotics and chest physiotherapy, which may be quite disheartening. Given the youth of these patients, retransplantation may be considered.

OB is the leading indication for retransplantation (140), but the overall numbers of retransplants are quite small. Prolonged survival has been reported, but the 1-year actuarial survival after retransplantation is 40%, which is only approximately half that of first-time lung transplants (140). With the current shortage of donor organs, this presents extremely difficult ethical dilemmas. Short of prohibiting retransplant operations, one approach is to consider all these patients as presenting *de novo* for lung transplant candidacy. They then must meet the same listing criteria as first time candidates (i.e., creatinine clearance greater than 50 mL/minute, ambulatory, diabetes well controlled, etc.). These selection criteria may improve outcomes after retransplantation. Therapeutically, these patients are treated with antibiotics and antifungals as needed, and with increased chronic corticosteroids or other immunosuppressants as needed for exacerbations of their symptoms.

Posttransplant Lymphoproliferative Disorder

Potent immunosuppression that interferes with T-cell lymphocyte number and function also appears to allow tumor cell growth. The Pittsburgh group has described an 8% incidence of B-cell lymphoma in post–lung transplant patients, suggesting a role for T-cells in suppressing the growth of these neoplastic cells (141). Lymphomatous disease in these patients may be associated with primary EBV infection (142). Pediatric or adolescent patients, the majority of whom are patients with CF, are at the greatest risk because they are more likely to be EBV negative preoperatively.

At UNC, 14 patients who underwent lung transplantation were EBV seronegative at the time of their surgery. Twelve of those patients later seroconverted to EBV-seropositive status; of that group, posttransplant lymphoproliferative disorder (PTLD) developed in five. That experience suggests that the rate of PTLD in EBV-naive patients who seroconvert after transplant is approximately 42%. Conversely, the rate of PTLD in those who are seropositive for EBV before transplant is less than 2% (143). PTLD developed in one patient who was EBV seropositive before transplant. Two of the five patients in whom PTLD developed died as a result of their malignancy despite also receiving chemotherapy, and one died from progressive bronchiolitis obliterans. The rest of the patients attained PTLD remission by drastically reducing their immunosuppression. All the tumors in these patients were monoclonal polymorphic B-cell lymphomas (143), and the histopathology did not predict their clinical outcomes. Consequently, EBV-seronegative status may not be a contraindication to transplant, but these patients should receive close monitoring with EBV serologies and chest radiographs. Immunosuppression may need to be decreased at the first sign of EBV seroconversion.

General Medical Management

As to be expected, as overall pulmonary function improves posttransplant, so does nutrition. The average weight percentage improved from 76% of IBW before surgery to 89% at 1 year posttransplant (39). However, for individual patients, weight gain does not correlate strictly with improvement in pulmonary function (39). Therefore, correction of the pulmonary dysfunction does not necessarily correct the underlying malnutrition.

Immunosuppressants, especially cyclosporine, may exacerbate any underlying GI problems [i.e., esophageal reflux, distal intestinal obstruction syndrome (DIOS), or early satiety]. Because of the high incidence of delayed gastric emptying in all patients after lung transplantation, motility agents, such as metoclopramide or cisapride, commonly are administered (144). At times, bezoars may develop and require endoscopic mechanical removal. Osmotic laxatives (e.g., lactulose) are useful to prevent DIOS. Constipation always must be considered in a differential diagnosis of abdominal pain in these patients.

Glucose intolerance may be exacerbated and lead to initial insulin use or to increased insulin requirements. Increased glucose intolerance develops posttransplant because of CF pancreatic disease, steroid use, and cyclosporine inhibition of insulin release (145), as well as increased food intake. Dietary restrictions are avoided by frequent insulin injections (46,47) because the emphasis is on weight gain and avoidance of diabetic microvascular complications (46,47).

patients believe that they have a new life after transplant, and the majority will return to full-time work and school. They believe that they can participate in a whole new range of activities untethered by supplemental oxygen or parenteral medications. For many, this time may be abbreviated, but even those with posttransplantation OB state that they would undergo transplantation again if given the opportunity.

Although lung transplantation must be regarded as palliative therapy for end-stage pulmonary disease secondary to CF, a study from the Transplant Unit at Papworth Hospital compared patient survival and resource use for patients with CF between transplantation and conventional therapy. They found that not only did the transplanted group have a markedly lower risk of dying and a greatly improved health status, but also a measurably favorable cost profile when compared with the conventional therapy group (147). Therefore, we need to develop better approaches to organ donation because many of these courageous patients will die before a donor organ becomes available.

SUMMARY

After 10 years of experience in transplanting the lungs of patients with CF, this endeavor still is approached with much trepidation; however, knowledge and therapeutic options are increasing, and most complications are manageable. Although the infectious, pharmacologic, and nutritional issues inherent to CF add some complexity to the care of a given transplant patient, these patients demonstrate a lifelong commitment to compliance that makes for a successful transplant. Patients with CF usually are very good at coping with complex medical regimens, know how to self-monitor, and use their experience with the healthcare system to good avail.

Anyone who has dealt with end-stage patients with CF has experienced the frustration and sadness of losing these bright, highly motivated individuals in the prime of their lives (146). Lung transplantation offers an opportunity to prolong the duration and to significantly improve the quality of these patients' lives (27,146). Many

REFERENCES

1. Kotloff RM, Zuckerman JB. Lung transplantation for cystic fibrosis: special considerations. *Chest* 1996; 109(3):787–798.
2. Ramirez JC, Patterson GA, Winton TL, et al. Bilateral lung transplantation for cystic fibrosis: the Toronto Lung Transplant Group. *J Thorac Cardiovasc Surg* 1992;103(2):287–294.
3. Cohen RG, Barr ML, Schenkel FA, et al. Living-related donor lobectomy for bilateral lobar transplantation in patients with cystic fibrosis. *Ann Thorac Surg* 1994;57:1423–1428.
4. Cooper JD, Pohl MS, Patterson GA. An update on the current status of lung transplantation: report of the St. Louis International Lung Transplant Registry. *Clin Transplants* 1993:95–100.
5. Yankaskas JR, Mallory GB Jr. Lung transplantation in cystic fibrosis: Consensus Conference Statement. *Chest* 1998;113:217–226.
6. Hayden AM, Kriett JM, Kapelanski DP, et al. Survival awaiting lung transplantation. *J Heart Lung Transplant* 1994;13(1 Pt 2):S45 (abstract).
7. Kerem E, Reisman J, Corey M, et al. Prediction of mortality in patients with cystic fibrosis. *N Engl J Med* 1992;326(18):1187–1191.
8. Egan TM, Detterbeck FC, Mill MR, et al. Improved results of lung transplantation for patients with cystic fibrosis. *J Thorac Cardiovasc Surg* 1995;109(2): 224–235.

9. Marshall SE, Kramer MR, Lewiston NJ, et al. Selection and evaluation of recipients for heart–lung and lung transplantation. *Chest* 1990;98(6):1488–1494.

10. Madden BP, Hodson ME, Tsang V, et al. Intermediate-term results of heart–lung transplantation for cystic fibrosis. *Lancet* 1992;339(8809):1583–1587.

11. Snell GI, de Hoyos A, Krajden M, et al. *Pseudomonas cepacia* in lung transplant recipients with cystic fibrosis. *Chest* 1993;103(2):466–471.

12. Shennib H, Noirclerc M, Ernst P, et al. Double-lung transplantation for cystic fibrosis: the Cystic Fibrosis Transplant Study Group. *Ann Thorac Surg* 1992; 54(1):27–31.

13. Aris RM, Gilligan PH, Neuringer IP, et al. The effects of panresistant bacteria in cystic fibrosis patients on lung transplant outcome. *Am J Respir Crit Care Med* 1997;155:1699–1704.

14. Manzetti JD, Hoffman LA, Sereika SM, et al. Exercise, education, and quality of life in lung transplant candidates. *J Heart Lung Transplant* 1994;13(2):297–305.

15. Dauber JH, Paradis IL, Dummer JS. Infectious complications in pulmonary allograft recipients. *Clin Chest Med* 1990;11(2):291–308.

16. Trulock EP. Management of lung transplant rejection. *Chest* 1993;103(5):1566–1576.

17. Tablan OC, Martone WJ, Doershuk CF, et al. Colonization of the respiratory tract with *Pseudomonas cepacia* in cystic fibrosis. *Chest* 1987;91(4):527–532.

18. Thomassen MJ, Demko CA, Klinger JD, et al. *Pseudomonas cepacia* colonization among patients with cystic fibrosis. *Am Rev Respir Dis* 1985;131(5): 791–796.

19. Lewin LO, Byard PJ, Davis PB. Effect of *Pseudomonas cepacia* colonization on survival and pulmonary function of cystic fibrosis patients. *J Clin Epidemiol* 1990;43(2):125–131.

20. LiPuma JJ, Dasen SE, Nielson DW, et al. Person-to-person transmission of *Pseudomonas cepacia* between patients with cystic fibrosis. *Lancet* 1990;336 (8723):1094–1096.

21. Thomassen MJ, Demko CA, Doershuk CF, et al. *Pseudomonas cepacia*: decrease in colonization in patients with cystic fibrosis. *Am Rev Respir Dis* 1986;134(4):669–671.

22. Steinbach S, Sun L, Jiang RZ, et al. Transmissibility of *Pseudomonas cepacia* in clinic patients and lung-transplant recipients with cystic fibrosis. *N Engl J Med* 1994;331:981–987.

23. Gilligan PH. Microbiology of airway disease in patients with cystic fibrosis. *Clin Microbiol Rev* 1991; 4(1):35–51.

24. Westney G, Maurer JR, de Hoyos A, et al. Aspergillus infections in lung transplant recipients. *Am Rev Respir Dis* 1993;147(4 Pt 2):A600 (abstract).

25. Levine SM, Peters JI, Anzueto A, et al. Aspergillus infection in single lung transplant recipients. *Am Rev Respir Dis* 1993;147(4 Pt 2):A599 (abstract).

26. Starnes VA, Lewiston N, Theodore J, et al. Cystic fibrosis: target population for lung transplantation in North America in the 1990s. *J Thorac Cardiovasc Surg* 1992;103(5):1008–1014.

27. Dennis C, Caine N, Sharples L, et al. Heart–lung transplantation for end-stage respiratory disease in patients with cystic fibrosis at Papworth Hospital. *J Heart Lung Transplant* 1993;12(6 Pt 1):893–902.

28. Paradowski L. Saprophytic fungal infections and lung transplantation—revisited. *J Heart Lung Transplant* 1997;16:524–531.

29. Kilby JM, Gilligan PH, Yankaskas JR, et al. Nontuberculous mycobacteria in adult patients with cystic fibrosis. *Chest* 1992;102(1):70–75.

30. Ingram CW, Tanner DC, Durack DT, et al. Disseminated infection with rapidly growing *Mycobacteria*. *Clin Infect Dis* 1993;16(4):463–471.

31. Smedile A, Marzano A, Farci P, et al. Liver transplant for viral hepatitis: recurrence of reinfection. *J Hepatol* 1991;13(Suppl 4):S134–S137.

32. Wright TL, Donegan E, Hsu HH, et al. Recurrent and acquired hepatitis C viral infection in liver transplant recipients. *Gastroenterology* 1992;103(1):317–322.

33. Arnold JC, Kraus T, Otto G, et al. Recurrent hepatitis C virus infection after liver transplantation. *Transplant Proc* 1992;24(6):2646–2647.

34. Rohr MS, Lesniewski RR, Rubin CA, et al. Risk of liver disease in HCV-seropositive kidney transplant recipients. *Ann Surg* 1993;217(5):512–517.

35. Luft BJ, Naot Y, Araujo FG, et al. Primary and reactivated toxoplasma infection in patients with cardiac transplants: clinical spectrum and problems in diagnosis in a defined population. *Ann Intern Med* 1983;99(1):27–31.

36. Umetsu DT, Moss RB, King VV, et al. Sinus disease in patients with severe cystic fibrosis: relation to pulmonary exacerbation. *Lancet* 1990;335(8697):1077–1078.

37. Lewiston N, King V, Umetsu D, et al. Cystic fibrosis patients who have undergone heart–lung transplantation benefit from maxillary sinus antrostomy and repeated sinus lavage. *Transplant Proc* 1991;23(1 Pt 2):1207–1208.

38. Flume PA, Egan TM, Paradowski LJ, et al. Infectious complications of lung transplantation: impact of cystic fibrosis. *Am J Respir Crit Care Med* 1994;149 (6):1601–1607.

39. Robbins MK, Paradowski L, Thompson J. Nutritional status of cystic fibrosis patients before and after lung transplantation. *Pediatr Pulmonol Suppl* 1993;9:273–274 (abstract).

40. Kerem E, Corey M, Kerem B, et al. The relation between genotype and phenotype in cystic fibrosis—analysis of the most common mutation (DF_{508}). *N Engl J Med* 1990;323(22):1517–1522.

41. Levy LD, Durie PR, Pencharz PB, et al. Effects of long-term nutritional rehabilitation on body composition and clinical status in malnourished children and adolescents with cystic fibrosis. *J Pediatr* 1985; 107(2):225–230.

42. Shepherd RW, Holt TL, Thomas BJ, et al. Nutritional rehabilitation in cystic fibrosis: controlled studies of effects on nutritional growth retardation, body protein turnover, and course of pulmonary disease. *J Pediatr* 1986;109(5):788–794.

43. Vaisman N, Clarke R, Pencharz PB: Nutritional rehabilitation increases resting energy expenditure without affecting protein turnover in patients with cystic fibrosis. *J Pediatr Gastroenterol Nutr* 1991;13(4): 383–390.

44. Callow LJ, Ernst P, Shennib H. Is there a benefit of aggressive enteral feeding in cystic fibrosis patients

awaiting lung transplantation? *J Heart Lung Transplant* 1993;12(1 Pt 2):S92 (abstract).

45. Rosenecker J, Eichler I, Baermeier H, et al. Epidemiology of diabetes mellitus in patients with cystic fibrosis. *Pediatr Pulmonol Suppl* 1993;9:277 (abstract).

46. Penketh ARL, Wise A, Mearns MB, et al. Cystic fibrosis in adolescents and adults. *Thorax* 1987;42(7): 526–532.

47. Sullivan MM, Denning CR. Diabetic microangiopathy in patients with cystic fibrosis. *Pediatrics* 1989; 84(4):642–647.

48. Bachrach LK, Loutit CW, Moss RB. Osteopenia in adults with cystic fibrosis. *Am J Med* 1994;96(1):27–34.

49. Johnson CC Jr, Slemenda CW, Melton LJ III. Clinical use of bone densitometry. *N Engl J Med* 1991; 324(16):1105–1109.

50. Hollister JR. The untoward effects of steroid treatment on the musculoskeletal system and what to do about them. *J Asthma* 1992;29(6):363–368.

51. Julian BA, Benfield M, Quarles LD. Bone loss after organ transplantation. *Transplant Rev* 1993;7(2):82–95.

52. Sambrook PN, Kelly PJ, Keogh AM, et al. Bone loss after heart transplantation: a prospective study. *J Heart Lung Transplant* 1994;13(1 Pt 1):116–120.

53. Nixon PA, Orenstein DM, Kelsey SF, et al. The prognostic value of exercise testing in patients with cystic fibrosis. *N Engl J Med* 1992;327(25):1785–1788.

54. Dennis C, Wallwork J. Mechanical ventilation and lung transplantation. *J Heart Lung Transplant* 1993; 13(1 Pt 1):22–23.

55. Hodson ME, Madden BP, Steven MH, et al. Noninvasive mechanical ventilation for cystic fibrosis patients—a potential bridge to transplantation. *Eur Respir J* 1991;4(5):524–527.

56. Piper AJ, Parker S, Torzillo PJ, et al. Nocturnal nasal IPPV stabilizes patient with cystic fibrosis and hypercapnic respiratory failure. *Chest* 1992;102(3):846–850.

57. Tepper RS, Skatrud JB, Dempsey JA. Ventilation and oxygenation changes during sleep in cystic fibrosis. *Chest* 1983;84(4):388–393.

58. Braggion C, Pradal U, Mastella G. Hemoglobin desaturation during sleep and daytime in patients with cystic fibrosis and severe airway obstruction. *Acta Paediatr* 1992;81:1002–1006.

59. Juan G, Calverley P, Talamo C, et al. Effect of carbon dioxide on diaphragmatic function in human beings. *N Engl J Med* 1984;310(14):874–879.

60. Carrey Z, Gottfried SB, Levy RD. Ventilatory muscle support in respiratory failure with nasal positive pressure ventilation. *Chest* 1990;97(1):150–158.

61. Bach JR, Alba AS. Management of chronic alveolar hypoventilation by nasal ventilation. *Chest* 1990;97:52–57.

62. Brochard L, Mancebo J, Wysocki M, et al. Noninvasive ventilation for acute exacerbations of chronic obstructive pulmonary disease. *N Engl J Med* 1995; 333(13):817–822.

63. Feanny S, Forsyth S, Corey M, et al. Allergic bronchopulmonary aspergillosis in cystic fibrosis: a secretory immune response to a colonizing organism. *Ann Allergy* 1988;60(1):64–68.

64. Murphy S. Cystic fibrosis in adults: diagnosis and management. *Clin Chest Med* 1987;8(4):695–710.

65. Lima O, Cooper JD, Peters WJ, et al. Effects of methylprednisolone and azathioprine on bronchial

healing following lung autotransplantation. *J Thorac Cardiovasc Surg* 1981;82(2):211–215.

66. Smith JD, Rose ML, Pomerance A, et al. Reduction of cellular rejection and increase in longer-term survival after heart transplantation after HLA-DR matching. *Lancet* 1995;346(8986):1318–1322.

67. Reitz BA, Wallwork JL, Hunt SA, et al. Heart–lung transplantation: successful therapy for patients with pulmonary vascular disease. *N Engl J Med* 1982; 306(10):557–564.

68. Frist WH, Fox MD, Campbell PW, et al. Cystic fibrosis treated with heart–lung transplantation: North American results. *Transplant Proc* 1991;23:1205–1206.

69. Yacoub MH, Banner NR, Khagani A, et al. Heart–lung transplantation for cystic fibrosis and subsequent domino heart transplantation. *J Heart Transplant* 1990;9:459–467.

70. Scott J, Higenbottam T, Hutter J, et al. Heart–lung transplantation for cystic fibrosis. *Lancet* 1988;2: 192–194.

71. Cooper JD, Patterson GA, Grossman R, et al. Double-lung transplant for advanced chronic obstructive lung disease. *Am Rev Respir Dis* 1989;139:303–307.

72. Patterson GA, Todd TR, Cooper JD, et al. Airway complications after double lung transplantation: Toronto Lung Transplant Group. *J Thorac Cardiovasc Surg* 1990;99:14–21.

73. Noirclerc MJ, Metras D, Vaillant A, et al. Bilateral bronchial anastomosis in double lung and heart–lung transplantations. *Eur J Cardiothorac Surg* 1990;4(6): 314–317.

74. Pasque MK, Cooper JD, Kaiser LR, et al. Improved technique for bilateral lung transplantation: rationale and initial clinical experience. *Ann Thorac Surg* 1990;49:785–791.

75. de Leval MR, Smyth R, Whitehead B, et al. Heart and lung transplantation for terminal cystic fibrosis: a 4½-year experience. *J Thorac Cardiovasc Surg* 1991;101:633–642.

76. Royston D, Bidstrup BP, Taylor KM, et al. Effect of aprotinin on need for blood transfusion after repeat open-heart surgery. *Lancet* 1987;2(8571): 1289–1291.

77. Egan TM, Kaiser LR, Cooper JD. Lung transplantation. *Curr Probl Surg* 1989;26:673–751.

78. Egan TM: Selection and management of the lung donor. In: Kaye MP, O'Connell JB, eds. *Intrathoracic transplantation 2000*. Austin, TX: Landes Co, 1992:25–30.

79. Hsieh AHH, Bishop MJ, Kublis PS, et al. Pneumonia following closed head injury. *Am Rev Respir Dis* 1992;146(2):290–294.

80. Egan TM, Boychuk JE, Rosato K, et al. Whence the lungs? A study to assess suitability of donor lungs for transplantation. *Transplantation* 1992;53(2):420–422.

81. Egan TM, Thompson JT, Detterbeck FC, et al. Effect of size (mis)matching in clinical double-lung transplantation. *Transplantation* 1995;59(5):707–713.

82. Calhoon JH, Grover FL, Gibbons WJ, et al. Single lung transplantation: alternative indications and technique. *J Thorac Cardiovasc Surg* 1991;101(5):816–825.

83. Egan TM, Paradowski LJ, Detterbeck FC, et al. Is bronchial omentopexy helpful in human lung transplantation? *Chest* 1992;102 (Suppl):74S (abstract).

84. Eraslan S, Turner MD, Hardy JD. Lymphatic regeneration following lung reimplantation in dogs. *Surgery* 1964;56:970–973.

85. Dumon JF. A dedicated tracheobronchial stent. *Chest* 1990;97(2):328–332.

86. Bennett WM, Norman DJ. Action and toxicity of cyclosporine. *Annu Rev Med* 1986;37:215–224.

87. Keenan RJ, Konishi H, Kawai A, et al. Clinical trial of tacrolimus versus cyclosporine in lung transplantation. *Ann Thorac Surg* 1995;60(3):580–585.

88. Maurer JR. Therapeutic challenges following lung transplantation. *Clin Chest Med* 1990;11(2):279–290.

89. Mancel-Grosso V, Bertault-Peres P, Barthelemy A, et al. Pharmacokinetics of cyclosporine A in bilateral lung transplantation candidates with cystic fibrosis. *Transplant Proc* 1990;22(4):1706–1707.

90. Lorber MI, Van Buren CT, Flechner SM, et al. Hepatobiliary and pancreatic complications of cyclosporine therapy in 466 renal transplant recipients. *Transplantation* 1987;43(1):35–40.

91. Vaughn BV, Olivier KN, Paradowski LJ. Seizures in lung transplantation. *Epilepsia* 1996;37:1175–1179.

92. Durrant S, Chipping PM, Palmer S, et al. Cyclosporin A, methylprednisolone, and convulsions. *Lancet* 1982;ii(8302):829–830.

93. de Groen PC, Aksamit AJ, Rakela J, et al. Central nervous system toxicity after liver transplantation: the role of cyclosporine and cholesterol. *N Engl J Med* 1987;317(14):861–866.

94. Wilczek H, Ringden O, Tyden G. Cyclosporine-associated central nervous system toxicity after renal transplantation. *Transplantation* 1985;39(1):110.

95. Mellick GA, Seng ML. The use of gabapentin in the treatment of reflex sympathetic dystrophy and a phobic disorder. *Am J Pain Manage* 1995;5(1):7–9.

96. Mellick GA, Mellicy LB. Gabapentin in the management of reflex sympathetic dystrophy. *J Pain Symptom Manage* 1995;10(4):265–266.

97. Mellick LB, Mellick GA. Successful treatment of reflex sympathetic dystrophy with gabapentin. *Am J Emerg Med* 1995;13(1):96.

98. Mathew NT, Lucker C. Gabapentin in migraine prophylaxis: a preliminary open label study. *Neurology* 1996;46(2):A169 (abstract).

99. Maurer JR, Tewari S. Nonpulmonary medical complications in the intermediate and long-term survivor. *Clin Chest Med* 1997;18(2):367–382.

100. Morrison RJ, Short HD, Noon GP, et al. Hypertension after lung transplantation. *J Heart Lung Transplant* 1993;12(6 Pt 1):928–931.

101. Frost AE, Keller CA. Anemia and erythropoietin levels in recipients of solid organ transplants: the Multi-Organ Transplant Group. *Transplantation* 1993;56(4):1008–1011.

102. Mycophenolate mofetil—a new immunosuppressant for organ transplantation. *Med Lett* 1995;37(958):84–86.

103. Taylor DO, Ensley RD, Olsen SL, et al. Mycophenolate mofetil (RS-61443): preclinical, clinical, and three-year experience in heart transplantation. *J Heart Lung Transplant* 1994;13(4):571–582.

104. Ensley RD, Bristow MR, Olsen SL, et al. The use of mycophenolate mofetil (RS-61443) in human heart transplant recipients. *Transplantation* 1993;56(1):75–82.

105. Roberts JP, Lake JR, Hebert M, et al. Reversal of chronic rejection after treatment failure with FK506 and RS61443. *Transplantation* 1993;56(4):1021–1023.

106. Sollinger HW. Mycophenolate mofetil for the prevention of acute rejection in primary cadaveric renal allograft recipients: the U.S. Renal Transplant Mycophenolate Mofetil Study Group. *Transplantation* 1995;60(3):225–232.

107. Kirklin JK, Bourge RC, Naftel DC, et al. Treatment of recurrent heart rejection with mycophenolate mofetil (RS-61443): initial clinical experience. *J Heart Lung Transplant* 1994;13(3):444–450.

108. Hausen B, Morris RE. Review of immunosuppression for lung transplantation: novel drugs, new uses for conventional immunosuppressants, and alternative strategies. *Clin Chest Med* 1997;18(2):353–366.

109. Trulock EP, Ettinger NA, Brunt EM, et al. The role of transbronchial lung biopsy in the treatment of lung transplant recipients. An analysis of 200 consecutive procedures. *Chest* 1992;102(4):1049–1054.

110. Rota L, Callegari G, Fracchia C, et al. Infection and rejection in lung transplantation: no invasive diagnostic approach. *Am J Respir Crit Care Med* 1994;149(4 Pt 2):A740 (abstract).

111. Shankar S, Fulsham L, Read RC, et al. Mucociliary function after lung transplantation. *Transplant Proc* 1991;23(1 Pt 2):1222–1223.

112. Gould FK, Freeman R, Taylor CE, et al. Prophylaxis and management of cytomegalovirus pneumonitis after lung transplantation: a review of experience in one Center. *J Heart Lung Transplant* 1993;12(4):695–699.

113. Duncan SR, Grgurich WF, Iacono AT, et al. A comparison of ganciclovir and acyclovir to prevent cytomegalovirus after lung transplantation. *Am J Respir Crit Care Med* 1994;150(1):146–152.

114. Landry ML, Ferguson D. Comparison of quantitative cytomegalovirus antigenemia assay with culture methods and correlation with clinical disease. *J Clin Microbiol* 1993;31(11):2851–2856.

115. Grossi P, Minoli L, Percivalle E, et al. Clinical and virological monitoring of human cytomegalovirus infection in 294 heart transplant recipients. *Transplantation* 1995;59(6):847–851.

116. Lane HC, Laughon BE, Falloon J, et al. Recent advances in the management of AIDS-related opportunistic infections. *Ann Intern Med* 1994;120(11):945–963.

117. Guillemain R, Lavarde V, Amrein C, et al. Invasive aspergillosis after transplantation. *Transplant Proc* 1995;27(1):1307–1309.

118. Kramer MR, Denning DW, Marshall SE, et al. Ulcerative tracheobronchitis after lung transplantation: a new form of invasive aspergillosis. *Am Rev Respir Dis* 1991;144(3 Pt 1):552–556.

119. Yeldandi V, Laghi F, McCabe MA, et al. Aspergillus and lung transplantation. *J Heart Lung Transplant* 1995;14:883–890.

120. Berenguer J, Allende MC, Lee JW, et al. Pathogenesis of pulmonary aspergillosis: granulocytopenia versus cyclosporine and methylprednisolone-induced

immunosuppression. *Am J Respir Crit Care Med* 1995;152:1079–1086.

121. Bertocchi M, Thevenet F, Bastien O, et al. Fungal infections in lung transplant recipients. *Transplant Proc* 1995;27(2):1695.

122. Egan JJ, Yonan N, Carroll KB, et al. Allergic bronchopulmonary aspergillosis in lung allograft recipients. *Eur Respir J* 1996;9(1):169–171.

123. Chaparro C, Kesten S. Infections in lung transplant recipients. *Clin Chest Med* 1997;18(2):339–351.

124. Abramowicz M, ed. Drugs for AIDS and associated infections. *Med Lett* 1995;37(959):87–94.

125. Olivier KN, Yankaskas JR, Knowles MR. Nontuberculous mycobacterial pulmonary disease in cystic fibrosis. *Semin Respir Infect* 1996;11(4):272–284.

126. Tanaka E, Amitani R, Nimi A, et al. Yield of computed tomography and bronchoscopy for the diagnosis of *Mycobacterium avium* complex pulmonary disease. *Am J Respir Crit Care Med* 1997;155:2041–2046.

127. Wallace RJ Jr, O'Brien R, Glassroth J, et al. Diagnosis and treatment of disease caused by nontuberculous mycobacteria. *Am Rev Respir Dis* 1990;142(4):940–953.

128. Wallace RJ Jr, Cook J, Glassroth J, et al. Diagnosis and treatment of disease caused by nontuberculous *Mycobacteria. Am J Respir Crit Care Med* 1997 (in press).

129. Snell GI, Esmore DS, Williams TJ. Cytolytic therapy for the bronchiolitis obliterans syndrome complicating lung transplantation. *Chest* 1996;109(4):874–878.

130. Ross DJ, Jordan SC, Nathan SD, et al. Delayed development of obliterative bronchiolitis syndrome with OKT3 after unilateral lung transplantation: a plea for multicenter immunosuppressive trials. *Chest* 1996;109(4):870–873.

131. Rajagopalan N, Kesten S, Maurer J. Cytolytic treatment in chronic allograft rejection in lung transplantation. *Am J Respir Crit Care Med* 1994;149(2 Pt 2):A1093 (abstract).

132. Michael B, Francos GC, Burke JF Jr, et al. Methotrexate is effective in preventing acute and potentially chronic renal allograft rejection. *Transplant Proc* 1996;26(5):3046–3047.

133. Bouchart F, Gundry SR, Van Schaack-Gonzales J, et al. Methotrexate as rescue/adjunctive immunotherapy in infant and adult heart transplantation. *J Heart Lung Transplant* 1993;12(3):427–433.

134. Bourge RC, Kirklin JK, White-Williams C, et al. Methotrexate pulse therapy in the treatment of recurrent acute heart rejection. *J Heart Lung Transplant* 1992;11(6):1116–1124.

135. Iacono AT, Keenan RJ, Duncan SR, et al. Aerosolized cyclosporine in lung recipients with refractory chronic rejection. *Am J Respir Crit Care Med* 1996;153(4 Pt 1):1451–1455.

136. Valentine VG, Robbins RC, Wehner JH, et al. Total lymphoid irradiation for refractory acute rejection in heart–lung and lung allografts. *Chest* 1996;109(5):1184–1189.

137. Reinsmoen NL, Bolman RM, Savik K, et al. Are multiple immunopathogenetic events occurring during the development of obliterative bronchiolitis and acute rejection? *Transplantation* 1993;55(5):1040–1044.

138. Madden BP, Siddiqi AJ, Pomerance A, et al. Possible aetiological factors in obliterative bronchiolitis following lung transplantation. *Pediatr Pulmonol Suppl* 1993;9:273 (abstract).

139. Guerry-Force ML, Mueller NL, Wright JL, et al. A comparison of bronchiolitis obliterans with organizing pneumonia, usual interstitial pneumonia, and small airways disease. *Am Rev Respir Dis* 1987;135(3):705–712.

140. Novick RJ, Kaye MP, Patterson GA, et al. Redo lung transplantation: a North American-European experience. *J Heart Lung Transplant* 1993;12(1 Pt 1):5–16.

141. Armitage JM, Kormos RL, Stuart RS, et al. Post-transplant lymphoproliferative disease in thoracic organ transplant patients: ten years of cyclosporine-based immunosuppression. *J Heart Lung Transplant* 1991;10(6):877–887.

142. Randhawa PS, Jaffe R, Demetris AJ, et al. Expression of Epstein-Barr virus-encoded small RNA (by the EBER-1 gene) in liver specimens from transplant recipients with post-transplantation lymphoproliferative disease. *N Engl J Med* 1992;327(24):1710–1714.

143. Aris RM, Maia D, Neuringer IP, et al. Post-transplantation lymphoproliferative disorder (PTLD) in the EBV-naive lung transplant recipient. *Am J Respir Crit Care Med* 1996;154 (6 Part 1):1712–1717.

144. Berkowitz N, Schulman LL, McGregor C, et al. Gastroparesis after lung transplantation: potential role in postoperative respiratory complications. *Chest* 1995;108(6):1602–1607.

145. Draznin B, Metz SA, Sussman KE, et al. Cyclosporin-induced inhibition of insulin release: possible role of voltage-dependent calcium transport channels. *Biochem Pharmacol* 1988;37(20):3941–3945.

146. Gross CR, Savik SK, Edin C, et al. Long term health status and quality of life outcomes of lung allograft recipients. *J Heart Lung Transplant* 1994;13(1 Pt 2):S44 (abstract).

147. Caine N, Tait S, Sharples LD, et al. Cystic fibrosis patients survival and resource use: a comparative study of heart & lung transplantation and conventional treatment. *J Heart Lung Transplant* 1994;13(1 Pt 2):S69 (abstract).

Cystic Fibrosis in Adults,
edited by J. R. Yankaskas and M. R. Knowles,
Lippincott–Raven Publishers, Philadelphia, 1999.

10

Nasal and Sinus Disease

Robert C. Stern and *Kim Jones

*Department of Pediatrics, Rainbow Babies and Children's Hospital, Case Western Reserve
University School of Medicine, Cleveland, Ohio; and *Division of Otolaryngology, University of
North Carolina School of Medicine, Chapel Hill, North Carolina*

Distinguishing between nasal disease and sinus disease is difficult, even in uncomplicated patients. In patients with cystic fibrosis (CF), separating the two often is impossible. Symptoms of nasal obstruction, rhinorrhea, and postnasal drip may come from one or the other, or a combination of the two. Opacification seen on sinus radiographs or even computed tomography (CT) scans may represent simple nasal polyps or acutely infected mucosa. In this chapter, we attempt to differentiate between nasal disease (primarily polyposis) and sinus disease, although the two often coexist in patients with CF.

Treatment decisions can be even more difficult. There is no universally successful approach to either of the two primary CF problems (nasal polyposis and sinusitis). Deciding among surgical treatment, medical treatment, or no treatment at all requires substantial knowledge of the underlying pathophysiology, the natural history of the complication, and often the individual needs of the patient.

ANATOMY AND PATHOPHYSIOLOGIC MECHANISMS

The location of the paranasal sinuses is familiar, but the functional and surgical anatomy is complex. The frontal, maxillary, and anterior ethmoid sinuses all drain into the osteomeatal complex (Fig. 10–1), a region located lateral to the middle turbinate and surrounding the uncinate process, a thin bony plate. Secretions from

these sinuses pass out of the osteomeatal complex through the hiatus semilunaris, a thin slit in the lateral nasal wall, and then posteriorly down the lateral pharynx (Fig. 10–2). Secretions from the posterior ethmoids and the sphenoid sinuses drain into the sphenoethmoid recess, located superior and posterior to the osteomeatal complex.

In healthy infants, at birth only the maxillary and ethmoid sinuses are identifiable. The sphenoid sinus is very small at birth and does not begin to grow until approximately 4 years of age. The development of the frontal sinus is highly variable. It may appear as early as 4 years of age and is present radiographically in most children by 6 years of age. It does not reach adult proportions until after adolescence.

The sinuses of patients with CF may have abnormal development and final configuration. Mackay and Djazaeri (1) noted no discernible frontal sinus in 36% of patients with CF. The average size of the frontal sinus in the remaining patients with CF was smaller than that of age-matched controls. The maxillary sinus may be normal or somewhat attenuated, whereas the ethmoids usually are of normal size (see Figs. 10–1 and 10–2).

There are no published reviews of either the anatomic pathology or the radiologic findings of the sinuses in infants and young children with CF. Although cross-sectional data indicate that close to 100% of patients with CF have radiologic evidence of pansinusitis (2,3), the status of their sinuses shortly after they are

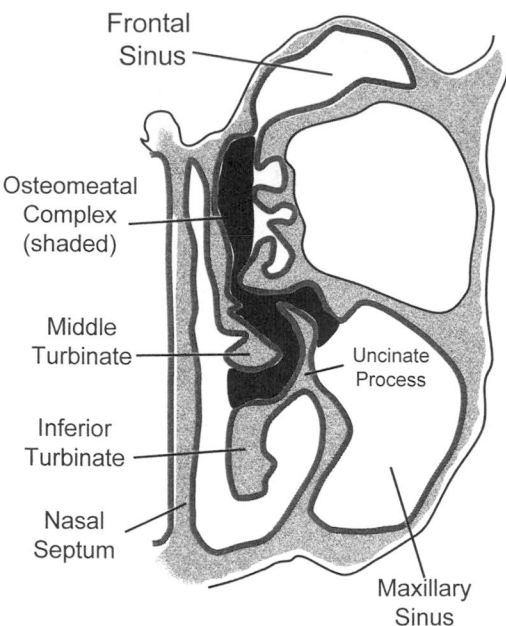

FIG. 10–1. The left osteomeatal complex (shaded). Blockage in this area can lead to secondary disease in the frontal and maxillary sinuses.

pneumatized during infancy is not known. Thus, there are no clinical data to help assess the role played by the fundamental cellular defect [abnormal cystic fibrosis transmembrane conductance regulator (CFTR) with resultant abnormal electrolyte and water transport] versus the role played by environmental/acquired factors (including infection) in generating sinus disease.

The bioelectrical manifestation of the CFTR-induced ion transport abnormalities in membrane function has been documented in nasal mucosa (4) and presumably is present in the sinuses as well. Using an argument similar to the one advanced to partially explain the pulmonary lesion, one could hypothesize that the mucus coating of the sinuses is abnormally thick/viscid because of abnormal electrolyte content and/or underhydration. These changes interfere with its drainage into the nasal cavity, where it normally would be swept back into the nasopharynx and eventually swallowed. Retained sinus secretions then could be further altered by water loss and become even more viscous (Fig. 10–3). If ab-

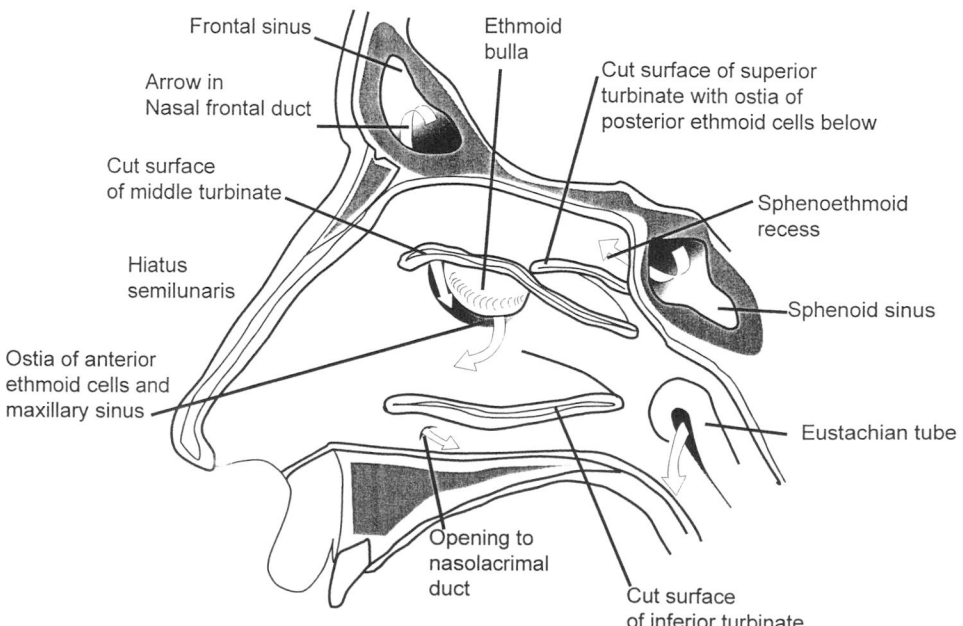

FIG. 10–2. The lateral nasal wall shown without the turbinates. The ostia of the paranasal sinuses open beneath the middle and superior turbinates and above the superior turbinate.

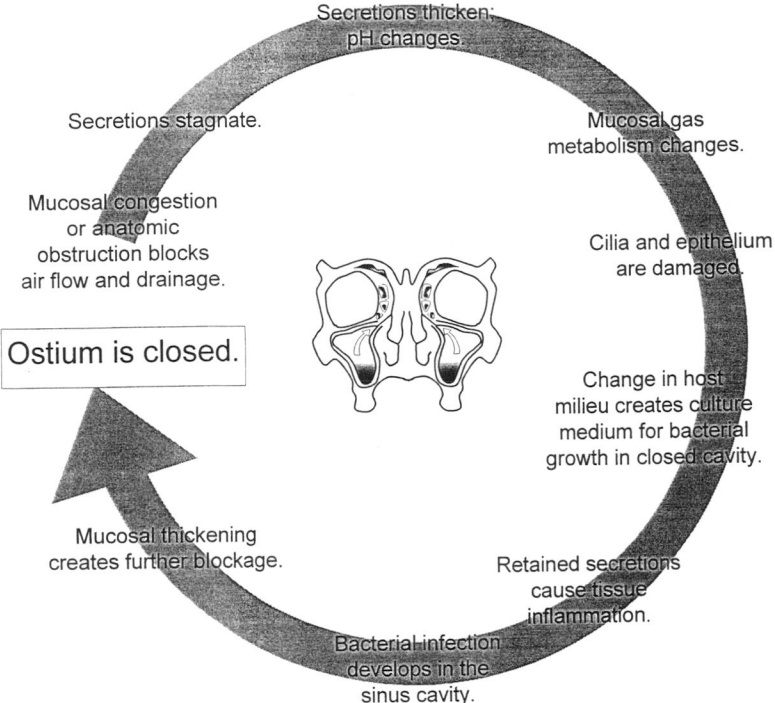

FIG. 10–3. Pathogenesis of sinus disease.

normalities of salt and water metabolism are the principal pathophysiology of sinus disease in CF, it is not surprising that all patients are affected early and that the radiologic abnormalities then are present for life.

Although stagnation of secretions also is believed to play an important part in the pathogenesis of the progressive lung infection in CF, the exact pathophysiology that leads to *Pseudomonas aeruginosa* emerging as the dominant pulmonary pathogen is not clear. There are few published studies concerning the microbiology of CF sinuses (see below), and it is not known whether infection plays a primary role in the genesis of the pansinusitis in every patient with CF. In fact, infection/inflammation may not be present in every patient. In one study (5), inflammatory cells were rare in material aspirated from CF sinuses, suggesting that bacterial colonization, rather than infection, occurred. Nonetheless, various pathogens have been recovered from CF sinuses, and it is reasonable to assume that infection contributes to sinus symptoms in some patients. Furthermore, the apparent success of aggressive antibiotic treatment of sinus disease in some patients with CF (see below) lends additional support to the argument that infection is involved in symptomatic CF sinus disease.

Chronic inflammation has been proposed as a major factor in the progression of CF pulmonary disease, and once established, it is believed to become self-perpetuating. A similar situation may be present in the sinuses of some patients; however, this certainly does not apply to all patients, and there are insufficient detailed biopsies/autopsy investigations available to reach a definitive conclusion.

Whether other factors [e.g., changes in pH and partial pressure of oxygen (PO_2) secondary to pulmonary disease] are involved is unknown. Low PO_2 does decrease respiratory ciliary activity (and presumably has the same effect on sinus mucosal cells). Thus, hypoxia could secondarily aggravate sinus problems in patients with CF with advanced pulmonary disease.

Nasal polyps (discussed in greater detail below) also can contribute to the progression of sinus disease by physically blocking the sinus ostia. This additional obstacle to sinus drainage could lead to increased infection and inflammation.

RADIOLOGIC ABNORMALITIES

Virtually all patients with classic CF (i.e., markedly elevated sweat chloride concentration, typical pulmonary and/or gastrointestinal manifestations, and/or a positive family history) have radiologic evidence of opacification of all the paranasal sinuses (2,6–8). Patients with variants of CF [e.g., those with normal (9,10) or intermediate (11) sweat chloride concentrations and/or sparing of the exocrine pancreas] have been reported sporadically for many years (but without specific genotype data); many of these patients have sinus opacification as well. However, it is not clear whether the greater than 90% prevalence in classic CF also occurs in patients with these and other mild genetic variants.

Some male patients with congenital bilateral absence of the vas deferens have two abnormal CFTR genes but no typical pulmonary or digestive symptoms (12). In the absence of a positive family history, CF cannot be diagnosed in these patients. Sinusitis also appears to be common in this group of patients (13), suggesting that the sinuses may be more susceptible to mild mutations than the lungs or pancreas.

Opacification of all the paranasal sinuses is extremely rare in healthy children and young adults, so any patient with this finding should be evaluated for CF (14). This evaluation should begin by sweat testing and/or CF genotyping, but may involve other tests as well [e.g., testing of pancreatic function and semen analysis (15)]. If CF can be excluded with reasonable certainty, additional immunologic work-up or endoscopy to look for otolaryngeal anatomic lesions may be justified. Uncomplicated allergy usually does not cause pansinusitis in children, teenagers, and young adults.

CLINICAL MANIFESTATIONS

Sinus Disease

The prevalence of daily symptoms suggestive of sinusitis in a large CF population is 10% or less in children (16,17) and approximately 24% in adults (18), despite the high prevalence of radiologic sinus abnormalities. However, suggestive symptoms and physical findings (headache, facial pain and tenderness, purulent nasal discharge, and pain in the upper jaw/teeth) would be attributed to sinusitis, based on the aforementioned radiologic findings. Although some radiologic findings clearly indicate clinically relevant disease (e.g., erosion of a sinus wall), the mere presence of opacification does not establish that CF-related sinus disease is causing the patient's acute symptoms. Thus, the true incidence and prevalence of symptoms caused by CF-related sinus disease (vs. symptoms unrelated to the sinuses or symptoms related to acute sinus disease, but unrelated to CF [e.g., an upper respiratory infection (URI) or allergic disease] is unknown.

The major manifestations of uncomplicated CF sinus disease (Table 10–1) are similar to those caused by chronic sinusitis in patients who do not have CF. Patients with CF also are subject to the same complications of sinusitis that occur in healthy persons. For example, mucopyocele, occasionally severe enough to be associated with erosion of one of the sinus walls, has been reported (19,20). These patients present with worrisome ophthalmologic

TABLE 10–1. *Clinical manifestations/presenting symptoms of sinus disease in patients with cystic fibrosis*

Headache
Nasal obstruction/mouth breathing/snoring
Facial pain/swelling/tenderness
Halitosis
Fever
Purulent nasal discharge
Ophthalmologic (visual) symptoms
Ophthalmologic signs (e.g., proptosis)
Postnasal drip/sore throat; "cobblestone" posterior
   pharynx
Worsening of pulmonary disease (?)

symptoms and signs (double vision, blurred vision, proptosis (19), and/or severe headache) (20). Surgical intervention is necessary (see below) in such patients.

Nasal Polyps

Approximately 25% of patients with CF have symptomatic nasal polyposis at some time in their lives. The incidence rate for the initial episode of nasal polyps varies with age, with the peak (8% to 12%) occurring between 5 and 19 years. The rate is much lower before 5 years of age and after 20 years of age (21). The incidence for asymptomatic nasal polyps presumably is much higher [43% in one series (3)]. Increases in the life expectancy for patients with CF should not appreciably increase the incidence of this complication. There is no gender difference in incidence.

No data on prevalence are available. However, as noted below, the recurrence rate after surgery is extremely high; thus, the prevalence probably approaches the total incidence by the mid to late teenage years. There seems to be some reduction in the recurrence rate after 20 years of age, and this, together with the dramatic decrease in initial episodes in this age group, should result in a reduction of the overall prevalence of this complication as the CF population continues to age. There are no published data on incidence and prevalence adjusted for genotype. However, nasal polyps have been reported in apparently mild CF variants (10,11). There is no clear concordance for the presence or absence of nasal polyps in families with two or more siblings with CF (21).

Nasal polyps can produce a variety of clinical manifestations (Table 10–2), any of which can be the presenting symptom. Surprisingly, however, CF-related nasal polyps and sinus abnormalities have not been associated with unusually serious or recurrent middle ear disease in patients with CF (22).

Nasal polyposis, like sinus opacification, is quite unusual in healthy persons younger than 20 years of age; therefore, a sweat test and, occasionally, genotyping and other tests are indicated to help rule out CF in these patients.

TABLE 10–2. *Clinical manifestations/presenting symptoms of nasal polyps in patients with cystic fibrosis*

Obstruction of nasal air flow[a]
Mouth breathing; snoring
Change in voice[b]
Rhinorrhea; purulent discharge[a]
Epistaxis
Nasal pain[b]
Polyp visible protruding from nose
Polyp or polyp tissue sneezed or blown from nose
Distortion of facial features/spreading of nasal bridge[a]
Halitosis
Decreased sense of smell (even before surgery)[b]
Worsening pulmonary status (?)[a,b]

[a]Most common indications for surgical intervention.
[b]Causation of symptom by nasal polyps not definitively established.

Nasal polyposis preceded respiratory symptoms in 1.6% of all patients in one large series (21) and often is the final symptom/sign that precipitates sweat testing in a large number of others.

Pathology

The polyp characteristically is lined by normal respiratory (pseudostratified columnar) epithelium, but scattered areas of squamous or transitional metaplasia can be seen. The basement membrane is normal or slightly thickened. However, although the lamina propria generally is thickened markedly and contains an edematous finely granular eosinophilic substance and varying numbers of inflammatory cells (plasma cells and lymphocytes), some polyps also contain many eosinophils. Blood vessels usually are normal (23,24).

The histopathology of CF nasal polyps generally has been thought to be indistinguishable from those of patients who do not have CF (25). However, one report (26) suggests that there are some differences that are detectable on routine staining with hematoxylin and eosin (H&E). In this study, unlike a previous claim (27), acid mucins did not predominate in the CF polyps. However, the absence of basement membrane thickening (< 10 μm) was characteristic of CF. Conversely, tissue eosinophilia

(> 100 eosinophils per 3 high-power fields) was more likely to be associated with allergic polyps.

RELATIONSHIP OF SINUSITIS TO PULMONARY DISEASE/EXACERBATIONS

Many patients report improvement in chronic (and unchanging) "sinus symptoms" after a course of intravenous antibiotics for a pulmonary exacerbation. However, pulmonary exacerbations have not been noted to be especially more common after exacerbation of chronic sinus symptoms, although URIs (7- to 10-day acute illnesses with coryza, sore throat, headache, etc.) can cause acute sinus symptoms and lead to pulmonary exacerbations (28). The pulmonary exacerbations may be the result of viral infection of the lung, rather than be related to sinus drainage. Furthermore, there is no clinically evident correlation between the presence of chronic sinus symptoms and frequent exacerbations or unusual rate of progression of pulmonary disease. Many adult patients with severe long-standing sinus symptoms, including some with severe complications of sinus disease, have relatively mild pulmonary disease.

As noted previously, the sequence of colonization of different parts of the respiratory tract with various pathogens, including *Staphylococcus aureus*, *Hemophilus influenzae*, and *P. aeruginosa* (and even *Burkholderia cepacia*, although that organism is almost always a latecomer), is not known. Sinus colonization may precede pulmonary colonization, at least in some patients; if so, sinus infection and postnasal drainage might be the source of the organism(s) that ultimately infect the lung. Serial sinus cultures (a problem to obtain at any age, let alone in infants and young children) would be needed to investigate this issue.

Sinus disease can result in nasal obstruction with conversion to mouth breathing, particularly during sleep. Bypassing the nasal mucosa could result in slightly dryer air entering the lung. Whether this, in and of itself, can precipitate or aggravate pulmonary exacerbations has

long been suspected, but it remains unproven. Similarly, although a relationship between sinusitis and asthma exacerbations has been proposed (29,30), relevant studies are not available (and may not be possible) in CF.

The upper airway, including the nose and sinuses, may act as a reservoir for pulmonary pathogens after bilateral pneumonectomy and single or double lung transplantation. This situation is analogous in some ways to the oncology concept of "sanctuaries" (e.g., the eye) in which tumor (e.g., leukemia) cells may escape destruction by chemotherapy. In CF, the transplanted lungs, although their epithelial cells do not have the abnormal genotype of CF, still occasionally become infected with typical CF pathogens, particularly *P. aeruginosa* and *B. cepacia*. It seems reasonable to assume that much of the "bacterial burden" present in the respiratory tract after transplant originates in the sinuses. This has led some transplant centers to treat sinus disease very aggressively pre- and postoperatively (see treatment sections).

INFECTIOUS PATHOGENS

In one study (22), the maxillary sinuses of 20 patients with CF were examined by radiographic techniques and cultured by transantral aspiration. Unlike childhood acute sinusitis, in which *Streptococcus pneumoniae, H. influenzae* (untypable) and *Branhamella catarrhalis* dominate (22), CF sinuses harbored mainly *P. aeruginosa* and *H. influenzae* (untypable)—in 13 and 10 patients, respectively—but streptococci and anaerobes also were encountered. In this study [and one other (31)], there was no association between the bacteria recovered from the sinus and those found in sputum/throat swabs.

MEDICAL TREATMENT

Sinus Disease

The demonstration of opacification of all the paranasal sinuses in a patient with CF is not itself an indication for specific treatment.

However, if the patient is symptomatic or if there is radiologic evidence of a clinically important complication of sinusitis, antibiotic and other treatment should be instituted. As with non-CF sinusitis, systemic and local antibiotics and local decongestants are the cornerstones of treatment. Antibiotic therapy should cover the organisms known to be present in the lungs, and if the patient does not respond, agents that cover the more classic sinus pathogens should be added. Doses should be the same as would be given for CF pulmonary disease. Local decongestants and nasal hygiene, as usually prescribed for chronic sinusitis, may be helpful.

Recombinant human deoxyribonuclease (rhDNase), a potent mucolytic agent, given by aerosol, recently has been approved for the treatment of CF-related pulmonary disease. Some clinicians have been concerned that sudden liquefaction of large amounts of pulmonary airway secretions could be dangerous if the patient is unable to clear them, and instead aspirates them further into the periphery. However, this theoretical concern does not apply to the sinuses. Liquefaction of sinus secretions, whether inadvertently as a side effect of pulmonary treatment or intentionally by nasal spray, intentional nasal inhalation, or direct intrasinus instillation, might be beneficial. The mucolytic effect of rhDNase depends on the presence of DNA in secretions; presumably, infected sinus secretions, with their high neutrophil content, would be more affected (and more in need of treatment) than uninfected sinus secretions. Regardless, however, the drug cannot yet be recommended specifically for sinus treatment.

Nasal Polyps

The possibility of coexisting allergic disease should be considered. Although CF-related nasal polyps are not caused clearly by allergies, polyps and nasal allergies can cause similar (and presumably) additive nasal symptoms. Control of the nasal allergy component may make the symptoms of nasal polyps tolerable. The effect of allergy treatment on polyp growth

and rate of recurrence after surgery is unknown, but it clearly is not totally effective.

Many other medical approaches have been tried. Conventional systematically administered decongestants are not effective. Nasal and systemic corticosteroids, nasal cromolyn, and various regimens for nasal hygiene all have individual patient and physician proponents, but no objective evidence of efficacy. A hyposensitization approach, using material extracted from the patient's own polyps, has been used, but again no consistent improvement from this or other innovative approaches has been reported (21).

Because chronic irritation of mucosa from sinusitis is one factor in the genesis of polyps, all measures noted for the medical treatment of sinusitis (see above) also may apply to some patients with recurrent nasal polyps.

SURGICAL TREATMENT

Preparation for Surgery

For "uncomplicated" nasal polyps and sinusitis, the patient should be advised that there is virtual certainty that immediate relief of nasal obstruction due to polyps will be possible (especially after the first procedure), but that recurrence of polyps is extremely common and may be very rapid. Synechiae may form and can cause recurrence of nasal obstruction even if polyps do not recur. Although patients with CF often undergo polypectomy many times, the procedure becomes more difficult and the risks of bleeding, penetration of cribriform plate, and injury to the optic nerve may increase. Simple sinus surgery (i.e., removal of sinus secretions and creation of drainage windows) is unlikely to result in long-lasting resolution.

A coronal CT scan of the sinuses should be obtained preoperatively to help the surgeon select the exact procedure. A coagulation screen (PT/APPT) should be performed before surgery, and the patient should receive an oral vitamin K analog the day before and/or the day of surgery to eliminate the most common treatable coagulopathy in patients with CF. Patients with CF with severe pulmonary disease, especially if they are to undergo general anesthesia, may benefit from aggressive antibiotic treatment of lung infection before surgery. One reasonable approach is to institute this treatment approximately 1 week before the procedure and then complete the course after surgery.

Nasal Polyps

It is generally recognized that simple polypectomy may be the most appropriate surgical treatment when the primary ailment is nasal obstruction secondary to polyps. However, the recurrence rate after simple polypectomy ranges from 58% to 89% (8,21,31,32). Performing more extensive sinus surgery in conjunction with a polypectomy reduces the rate of recurrence (32). The choice of such an aggressive approach requires evaluation of the individual's clinical course and risks and potential benefits of surgery.

Sinus Disease

Until the development of endoscopic sinus surgery (see below), surgical treatment of sinusitis alone (as opposed to nasal polyps and sinusitis) was rarely performed. Although multiple surgical techniques were used (intranasal ethmoidectomy, intranasal antrostomy, Caldwell-Luc procedure, etc.), the criteria for procedure selection were not clearly defined. Furthermore, results usually were reported as recurrence of polyps rather than recurrence of sinusitis or symptoms of sinusitis.

With the advent of endoscopic sinus surgery in the late 1980s, attention began to be focused on treating the symptoms of sinusitis alone in patients with CF (nasal discharge, postnasal drip, facial pain, etc.) versus those of nasal polyps (usually nasal obstruction). Almost all authors who report their results using this approach refer to it as functional endoscopic sinus surgery (FESS). However, this term should be reserved for the specific endoscopic techniques described by Stammberger and Posawetz (33), in which minimal surgical manipulation is employed to restore normal function

to the sinuses. Because no surgical techniques ever will restore normal function to the sinuses of patients with CF, this technique is best described simply as endoscopic sinus surgery.

Most results of endoscopic sinus surgery in patients with CF have been described in terms of subjective improvement of symptoms because radiographically almost all patients show rapid return of their sinus disease (34). Duplechain et al. (35) reported that nasal discharge was improved in 75% of their patients, whereas other symptoms, such as nasal congestion and headache, were improved in approximately 60%. Length of follow-up was not reported. Jones et al. (36) queried 17 patients with CF pre- and postoperatively (average follow-up, 29 months) and found significant improvement in nasal obstruction, nasal discharge, and postnasal drip. Improvements in halitosis, cough, and headache were minor, and the average number of hospitalizations per year for the group did not change. Nishioka et al. (37) reported improvement in a similar group of 21 pediatric patients with CF. No study has specifically reported surgical results in adult patients with CF.

A combined surgical/pharmacologic approach to the sinus problems of patients with CF has been reported (38). After endoscopic maxillary antrostomies, a flexible catheter is inserted into each maxillary sinus via the antrostomy and the other end is taped to the patient's cheek. Tobramycin (40 mg in 1 mL saline) then is instilled into each sinus three times a day with the head positioned so that the irrigated sinus is dependent. This procedure is continued for 7 to 10 days, after which the catheters are removed. The patient then returns once a month for repeat tobramycin instillations under local anesthesia. Compared with historical controls who had similar surgery but no tobramycin instillation, the frequency of repeat sinus surgery was decreased from 72% to 22% over 2 years (39).

Sinus surgery has been recommended for all patients with CF before lung transplantation (40,41) on the rationale that bacteria from the infected sinuses will be aspirated into the lungs and increase posttransplant morbidity and mortality. The goal of surgery is to improve aeration of the sinuses and to provide a surgically enlarged antrostomy so that the patients can instill tobramycin directly into the maxillary sinuses. The groups advocate tobramycin irrigations for 10 days postoperatively and for an additional 1 to 3 weeks whenever the patient becomes symptomatic (40), or indefinitely (41). Both groups reported a decrease in the incidence of *Pseudomonas* in posttransplant sputum cultures. Neither study, however, included nonsurgical controls, limiting the conclusions regarding morbidity and mortality. Another transplant center reported that subsequent sinus problems developed in only 11% of patients with CF who received lung transplants without prior sinus surgery. This low incidence suggests that a multicenter study would be required to test rigorously the impact of prophylactic sinus surgery on complications after lung transplantation.

Epistaxis

Minor episodes of epistaxis are common in healthy children and some young adults and usually respond to local pressure, but they occasionally require packing and/or cautery. Patients with CF are not immune to this problem, and bleeding may be prolonged if there is vitamin K deficiency. Nonetheless, these patients rarely require more than reassurance, instruction on first aid, and appropriate vitamin K replacement.

Epistaxis presents a more difficult problem when it complicates the use of supplemental oxygen by nasal cannulae. This problem is most troublesome in patients who have severe pulmonary disease and require high-flow oxygen (many patients with CF require as much as 6 L per min; in the absence of epistaxis, some can tolerate flow rates as high as 12 L per min). Such epistaxis can be addressed in several ways. Unilateral bleeding sometimes can be managed by temporarily using a single nasal cannula in the contralateral nares. This is likely to be successful only for patients who need low-flow oxygen, The drying effects of oxygen may be reduced by use of mask oxygen, either

exclusively for 1 or 2 days or intermittently every day or by light application of white petroleum jelly (Vaseline) to the distal nasal mucosa. Humidification of oxygen may be worth trying, but not much humidification is possible at room temperature, and systems that warm oxygen to body temperature are prone to condensation and accumulation of water in the tubing. Negative pressure activated ("demand") oxygen reduces delivery of oxygen to the nose by approximately 60%. A "nasal mask" with added humidification at the nose circumvents the aforementioned problems presented by warmed humidified oxygen. Transtracheal oxygen solves the nasal drying problem, but the transtracheal catheter may not be tolerated because of coughing.

Anosmia, Hyposmia, and Dysosmia

Anosmia/hyposmia has been reported in patients with CF before and after removal of nasal polyps, and in some patients who do not have visible polyps (42). Smell also could be impaired in CF because the thick viscous mucus characteristic of the disease blocks diffusion of odors to the olfactory receptors. In addition, inflammation of the nasal mucosa/sinusitis may impair olfaction. Anosmia also could be caused by an unrelated illness [e.g., it has been associated with hypogonadotropic hypogonadism (Kallman's syndrome)], including one patient who also had CF (43). In some patients, anosmia/hyposmia either is intermittent or temporary. Occasionally, normal olfaction returns, but not always immediately, after polypectomy. Otherwise, however, there is no effective treatment.

Dysosmia (disagreeable odor or altered perception of known scents) may be due to nasal pathology, but also could be caused partially by halitosis, raising the possibility of an anaerobic component to the patient's pulmonary problem. An empiric course of metronidazole or clindamycin may be worthwhile.

Although patients may implicate anosmia/ dysosmia as an explanation for anorexia and weight loss, there is no evidence that anosmia alone produces weight loss in otherwise healthy persons. Other causes of weight loss, notably increasing pulmonary disease, should be sought.

SUMMARY

Although radiologic examination usually shows sinus abnormalities in patients with CF, at any given time the majority of patients do not report overt sinus or nasal symptoms. Over the course of a lifetime, however, a substantial percentage of patients do note intermittent symptoms that could be caused by CF-related sinonasal disease. When nasal polyps are present on examination and are symptomatic, or when symptoms (e.g., headache and/or visual disturbance) are severe and are accompanied by CT demonstration of bone erosion, the need for clinical intervention is obvious. Nasal polypectomy, ethmoidectomy, creation of sinus drainage "windows," and sinus cavity obliteration may be necessary in these patients. In addition, some physicians believe that "prophylactic" surgical drainage and intensive local antibiotic treatment of sinus disease improves the results of lung transplantation.

The relationship of sinus disease to CF-related pulmonary disease is not clear. Pulmonary morbidity seems to decrease in some patients after aggressive drainage procedures and prolonged administration of local antibiotics. However, a properly controlled study has not been done, and the routine use of this approach to treat increasingly severe and/or frequent pulmonary exacerbations or inexorable slow progression of pulmonary disease cannot be recommended for all patients with CF on the basis of presently available information.

Other nasal problems, including recurrent epistaxis, allergic nasal symptoms, and anosmia and dysosmia, may be related to CF or its treatment and usually should be approached as they are for patients who do not have CF. Areas in which clinical research can be expected to reveal clinically relevant information in the near future include: (a) elucidation of which clinical problems deserve surgical intervention/local antibiotic treatment; and (b) determination whether there is any role for antiinflammatory agents with or without antibiotics as prophylaxis against the recurrence of nasal polyps. More definitive treatments, based on molecular pathophysiology (pharmacologic treatment), and/or gene therapy are being developed, but these have not been tested yet for clinical efficacy.

ACKNOWLEDGMENTS

This research was supported in part by Grant DK 27651 from the National Institutes of Health and by grants from the United Way Services of Greater Cleveland and the Cystic Fibrosis Foundation.

REFERENCES

1. Mackay IS, Djazaeri B. Chronic sinusitis in cystic fibrosis. *J R Soc Med* 1994;87(suppl 21):17–19.
2. Gharib R, Allen RP, Joos HA, et al. Paranasal sinuses in cystic fibrosis: incidence of Roentgen abnormalities. *Am J Dis Child* 1964;108(5):499–502.
3. Coste A, Gilain L, Roger G, et al. Endoscopic and CT-scan evaluation of rhinosinusitis in cystic fibrosis. *Rhinology* 1995;33:152–156.
4. Boucher RC. Human airway ion transport: part two. *Am J Respir Crit Care Med* 1994;150:581–593.
5. Shapiro ED, Milmoe GJ, Wald ER, et al. Bacteriology of the maxillary sinuses in patients with cystic fibrosis. *J Infect Dis* 1982;146(5):589–593.
6. Shwachman H, Kulczycki LL, Mueller HL, et al. Nasal polyposis in patients with cystic fibrosis. *Pediatrics* 1962;30(3):389–401.
7. di Sant'Agnese P, Davis PB. Cystic fibrosis in adults: 75 cases and a review of 232 cases in the literature. *Am J Med* 1979;66(1):121–132.
8. Reilly JS, Kenna MA, Stool SE, et al. Nasal surgery in children with cystic fibrosis: complications and risk management. *Laryngoscope* 1985;95(12):1491–1493.
9. Davis PB, Hubbard VS, di Sant'Agnese PA. Low sweat electrolytes in a patient with cystic fibrosis. *Am J Med* 1980;69(4):643–646.
10. Ludlow D, Lybass T, Knowles M, et al. A variant form of cystic fibrosis in two siblings with normal sweat tests and abnormal transmission potentials. *CF Club Abstracts* 1986;27:139 (abstract).
11. Stern RC, Boat TF, Abramowsky CR, et al. Intermediate range sweat chloride concentration and pseudomonas bronchitis: a cystic fibrosis variant with preservation of pancreatic function. *JAMA* 1978;239(25): 2676–2680.
12. Oates RD, Amos JA. The genetic basis of congenital bilateral absence of the vas deferens and cystic fibrosis. *J Androl* 1994;15(1):1–8.
13. Damur V, Gervais R, Rigot J-M, et al. Abnormal distribution of DF508 allele in azoospermic men with congenital aplasia of the epididymis and vas deferens (Letter to the Editor). *Lancet* 1990;336(8713):512.
14. Wiatrak BJ, Myer CM III, Cotton RT. Cystic fibrosis presenting with sinus disease in children. *Am J Dis Child* 1993;147(3):258–260.

15. Stern RC, Boat TF, Doershuk CF. Obstructive azoospermia as a diagnostic criterion for the cystic fibrosis syndrome. *Lancet* 1982;I(8286):1401–1404.

16. Adams GL, Hilger P, Warwick WJ. Cystic fibrosis. *Arch Otolaryngol* 1980;106:127–132.

17. Cepero R, Smith RJH, Catlin FI, Bressler KL, Furuta G, Shandera KC. Cystic fibrosis—an otolaryngologic perspective. *Otolaryngol Head Neck Surg* 1987;97:356–360.

18. Shwachman H, Kowalski M, Khaw K-T. Cystic fibrosis: a new outlook. 70 patients above 25 years of age. *Medicine* 1977;56:129–149.

19. Levine MR, Kim Y-d, Witt W. Frontal sinus mucopyocele in cystic fibrosis. *Ophthal Plast Reconstr Surg* 1988;4(4):221–225.

20. Sharma GD, Doershuk CF, Stern RC. Erosion of the wall of the frontal sinus caused by mucopyocele in cystic fibrosis. *J Pediatr* 1994;(5 pt 1)124:745–747.

21. Stern RC, Boat TF, Wood RE et al. Treatment and prognosis of nasal polyps in cystic fibrosis. *Am J Dis Child* 1982;136:1067–1070.

22. Wald ER, Milmoe GJ, Bowen A, et al. Acute maxillary sinusitis in children. *N Engl J Med* 1981;304(13):749–754.

23. Neely JG, Harrison GM, Jerger JF, Presberg H. The otolaryngologic aspects of cystic fibrosis. *Trans Am Acad Ophthalmol Otolaryngol* 1972;76(2):313–324.

24. Rulon JT, Brown HA, Logan GB. Nasal polyps and cystic fibrosis of the pancreas. *Arch Otolaryngol* 1963;78(1):192–199.

25. Tos M, Mogensen C, Thomsen J. Nasal polyps in cystic fibrosis. *J Laryngol Otol* 1977;91(10):827–835.

26. Miller CH, Hatem F, Metlay LA, et al. Can histologic criteria of nasal polyps be used to screen for cystic fibrosis. *Pediatr Asthma Allergy Immunol* 1994;8:51–56.

27. Oppenheimer EH, Rosenstein BJ. Differential pathology of nasal polyps in cystic fibrosis and atopy. *Lab Invest* 1979;40(4):445–449.

28. Wang EEL, Prober CG, Manson B, et al. Association of respiratory viral infections with pulmonary deterioration in patients with cystic fibrosis. *N Engl J Med* 1984;311:1653–1658.

29. Slavin RG. Recalcitrant asthma: have you looked for sinusitis? *J Respir Dis* 1986;7:61–65.

30. Slavin RG. Sinusitis in adults and its relation to allergic rhinitis, asthma, and nasal polyps. *J Allergy Clin Immunol* 1988;82:950–956.

31. Jaffe BF, Strome M, Khaw K-T, et al. Nasal polypectomy and sinus surgery for cystic fibrosis—a 10 year review. *Otolaryngol Clin North Am* 1977;10(1):81–90.

32. Crockett DM, McGill TJ, Healy GB, Friedman EM, Salkeld LJ. Nasal and paranasal sinus surgery in children with cystic fibrosis. *Ann Otol Rhinol Laryngol* 1987;96:367–372.

33. Stammberger H, Posawetz W. Functional endoscopic sinus surgery: concept, indications and results of the Messerklinger technique. *Eur Arch Otorhinolaryngol* 1990;247:63–76.

34. Cuyler JP. Follow-up of endoscopic sinus surgery on children with cystic fibrosis. *Arch Otolaryngol Head Neck Surg* 1992;118:505–506.

35. Duplechain JK, White JA, Miller RH. Pediatric sinusitis: the role of endoscopic sinus surgery in cystic fibrosis and other forms of sinonasal disease. *Arch Otolaryngol Head Neck Surg* 1991;117:422–426.

36. Jones JW, Parson DS, Cuyler JP. The results of functional endoscopic sinus (FES) surgery on the symptoms of patients with cystic fibrosis. *Int J Pediatr Otorhinolaryngol* 1993;28:25–32.

37. Nishioka GJ, Barbero GJ, Konig P, et al. Symptom outcome after functional endoscopic sinus surgery in patients with cystic fibrosis: a prospective study. *Otolaryngol Head Neck Surg* 1995;113(4):440–445.

38. Davidson TM, Murphy C, Mitchell M, et al. Management of chronic sinusitis in cystic fibrosis. *Laryngoscope* 1995;105(4):354–358.

39. Moss RB, King VV. Management of sinusitis in cystic fibrosis by endoscopic surgery and serial antimicrobial lavage: reduction in recurrence requiring surgery. *Arch Otolaryngol Head Neck Surg* 1995;121(5):566–572.

40. Lewiston N, King V, Umetsu D, et al. Cystic fibrosis patients who have undergone heart–lung transplantation benefit from maxillary sinus antrostomy and repeated sinus lavage. *Transplant Proc* 1991;23:1207–1208.

41. Davidson TM, Murphy C, Mitchell M, Smith C, Light M. Management of chronic sinusitis in cystic fibrosis. *Laryngoscope* 1995;105:354–358.

42. Hertz J, Cain WS, Bartoshuk LM, et al. Olfactory and taste sensitivity in children with cystic fibrosis. *Physiol Behav* 1975;14(1):89–94.

43. Lox CD, Davis JR, Christian CD, et al. Anosmic hypogonadotropic hypogonadism Kallman's syndrome—a case history complicated by cystic fibrosis. *Ariz Med* 1974;31(7):508–509.

Cystic Fibrosis in Adults,
edited by J. R. Yankaskas and M. R. Knowles,
Lippincott–Raven Publishers, Philadelphia, 1999.

11

New Therapeutic Strategies for Cystic Fibrosis Lung Disease

Larry G. Johnson and Michael R. Knowles

Cystic Fibrosis/Pulmonary Research and Treatment Center, Division of Pulmonary and Critical Care Medicine, University of North Carolina School of Medicine, Chapel Hill, North Carolina

The major morbidity and mortality in cystic fibrosis (CF) results from lung disease, and more than 95% of deaths result from respiratory failure. Defective airway epithelial ion transport (and other) cellular dysfunction reflects mutations in the cystic fibrosis transmembrane conductance regulator (CFTR) gene. The organ-level pathogenesis of CF lung disease reflects thick airway secretions associated with predisposition to bacterial infection early in life and subsequent chronic infection with *Staphylococcus aureus* and/or *Pseudomonas aeruginosa*. A defined cascade of pathogenic events has emerged from research over the past decade and offers the opportunity for multiple therapeutic strategies (Fig. 11–1).

Novel therapeutic approaches undergoing development include gene therapy, which currently is focused on pilot and feasibility studies to identify safe and effective vectors for transferring a normal copy of the CFTR gene into the defective airway epithelial cells in patients with CF. Better understanding of the pathobiology associated with the development and progression of lung disease in CF also has provided the opportunity for development of pharmacologic approaches that target different aspects of the pathogenic cascade (see Fig. 11–1). These therapeutic targets include: airway inflammation; altered local (airway) host defense and abnormal airway secre-

tions associated with the host response to chronic bacterial infection; defective processing to the plasma membrane of certain genetically defective species of the CFTR; mutant CFTR proteins, which may retain some residual function; and altered ion transport, which may respond to pharmacologic modification or bypass.

This chapter is designed to provide a conceptual framework of ongoing work in the areas of gene transfer and pharmacologic approaches to develop new therapies in CF (see Fig. 11–1). Only a brief review of the rationale for each type of therapeutic approach is provided because the genetic, cellular, and organ-level pathophysiology is discussed extensively in Chapters 1 through 6. The major goal of this chapter is to describe specific types of gene transfer vectors and pharmacologic agents that are being investigated. Although these approaches have not yet proven to be therapeutically beneficial and many are only in early stages of development, the broad spectrum of research activity offers testimony for the progress toward better therapy for this challenging disease.

GENE THERAPY

The increasingly rapid delineation of human genes linked to clinical disease has raised hopes for the development of specific genetic

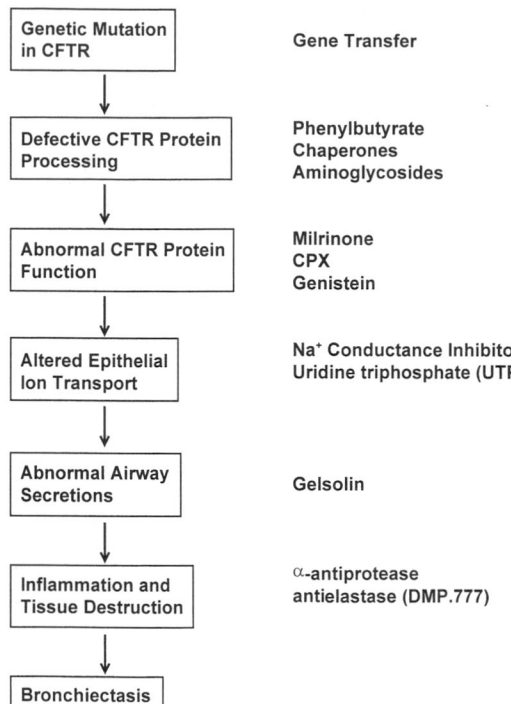

FIG. 11–1. Cellular and organ-level pathobiology of CF lung disease, and new therapeutic approaches that target specific aspects of the pathogenic cascade (see text for comments). CFTR, cystic fibrosis transmembrane conductance regulator; CPX, cyclopentyl-di-propylxanthine.

therapies for many inherited and acquired diseases. CF is a common inherited disorder with a high morbidity and mortality that makes it an attractive target for gene therapy. The autosomal inheritance pattern of this single gene (monogenic) disorder in which heterozygotes are phenotypically normal, combined with the relatively large numbers of patients available for clinical studies, has led to the establishment of CF as the prototypical disease for investigation of gene therapy in the lung. To date, more patients with CF have entered gene transfer clinical safety and efficacy trials than patients with any other inherited or acquired disorder. The lessons learned from the intense investigation of gene therapy as a clinical approach for the prevention of CF lung disease are reviewed.

Rationale and Targets for Cystic Fibrosis Gene Transfer

Because CF carriers (heterozygotes) are phenotypically normal, introduction of a single wild-type (normal) copy of the gene into defective CF epithelial cells should restore the normal phenotype. Consistent with this concept, introduction of a wild-type copy of the *CFTR* into CF airway epithelial cells *in vitro* using retrovirus, vaccinia virus, liposomes, and adenovirus vectors restores CFTR-mediated Cl⁻ transport function to these cells (1–6). Thus, gene therapy for CF may be feasible and warrants the intense investigation necessary to develop it for clinical application.

A key unknown in the development of gene therapy for CF is the appropriate cellular targets in human airways. Although the exact site where CF lung disease begins still is unknown, both the superficial columnar epithelial cells lining the lumen of the small airways and the serous cells of submucosal glands are possibilities. Where the disease begins is relevant because luminal (airway) delivery of gene transfer vectors targets the superficial columnar airway epithelium, whereas intravenous (blood) delivery targets the submucosal glands and possibly basal cells via the basolateral membrane. Basal cells are a potentially viable target because they possess the ability to differentiate into columnar epithelial cells. Current strategies primarily use the airway lumen to target the superficial airway epithelium.

Gene Transfer Vectors

Many naturally occurring viruses are known to cause human disease. These viruses introduce their own viral nucleic acid (DNA or RNA) into the host cell nucleus, where it can express viral genes that promote viral replication. Researchers have taken advantage of this unique ability of naturally occurring viruses to develop viral vectors that introduce and express therapeutic genes (cDNAs) in lieu of their viral structural genes, which have been deleted. Adenoviruses, adeno-associated viruses, and retroviruses are examples of viruses that have been altered to introduce therapeutic genes. Adenoviruses and adeno-associated viruses already are in clinical trials in patients with CF, and recent advances in retrovirus vector technology (see below) have raised hopes for their utility in CF as well. However, viral vectors potentially can induce a variety of immune and other adverse reactions that have made nonviral vectors an attractive alternative approach. Of the nonviral methods, only cationic liposomes have undergone sufficient investigation to enter initial clinical gene transfer safety and efficacy trials in CF. The characteristics of these vectors are summarized in Table 11–1.

Viral Vectors

Adenovirus Vectors

Adenoviruses are double-stranded DNA viruses, of which human serotypes 2 and 5 (which have 90% homology) provide the backbone for current adenovirus (Ad) vectors (7). Wild-type adenoviruses have a 36-kb genome consisting of a series of early genes that are responsible for virus replication, antigen presentation, and surveillance and a series of late genes that encode viral structural proteins (7–9). Several generations of Ad vectors have been developed (Fig. 11–2). First-generation vectors based on adenovirus serotype 5 (Ad5) have had the early region one (E1) genes deleted (7,10) to make the vector replication defective, whereas deletion of the E3 region creates sufficient room to insert the CFTR gene with a suitable promoter (see Fig. 11–2A). First generation Ad vectors encoding CFTR based on serotype 2 (Ad2) have only had the E1 gene deleted such that the vector genome actually may exceed the size of the wild-type virus genome (8), leading to less efficient packaging of Ad-DNA into viral particles and lower infectious titers (see Fig. 11–2A). E1-deleted second-generation vectors based on Ad5 have been developed in which the E2a region also has been mutated to form a temperature-sensitive mutant virus (see Fig. 11–2B). This mutant replicates in 293 cells at 32°C, but not at 39°C, potentially bringing an additional safety feature to this vector (11,12). E1-deleted second-generation vectors also have been developed with deletions in most [except for open reading frame six (ORF6)] or all of the E4 region (see Fig. 11–2B) in an attempt to limit late viral gene expression (13,14). Third-generation vectors also have been developed with deletions of all viral genes retaining only a small packaging signal and the inverted terminal repeats (see Fig. 11–2C) (15).

Adenoviruses enter cells by receptor-mediated endocytosis (16). They bind to high-affinity cell surface receptors [Coxsackie and adenovirus receptor (CAR)] (17) and subsequently are internalized through an integrin-mediated vesicular (endocytic) process. As a result of endosomolytic properties mediated by the Ad fiber protein, Ad can avoid lysosomal degradation such that efficient translocation of the

TABLE 11–1. *Characteristics of gene transfer vectors used in cystic fibrosis gene transfer trials*

Gene transfer vectors	cDNA insert size (kb)	Duration of expression	Transduces nondividing cells	Risk of insertional mutagenesis	Induction of cell-mediated immune response	Induction of humoral immune response
Adenovirus	7–8	Transient	Yes	?Slight	Yes	Yes
Adenoassociated virus	4.5	Long-term	Yes	Yes	No	No
Retrovirus						
MuLV[a]	7	Long-term	No	Yes	No	No
Lentivirus[b]	>7	Long-term	Yes	Yes	No	No
Cationic liposomes	>10	Transient	Yes	No	Rarely	No

[a]Derived from Moloney murine leukemia virus.
[b]Derived from human immunodeficiency virus. Experience with lentiviral vectors is limited.

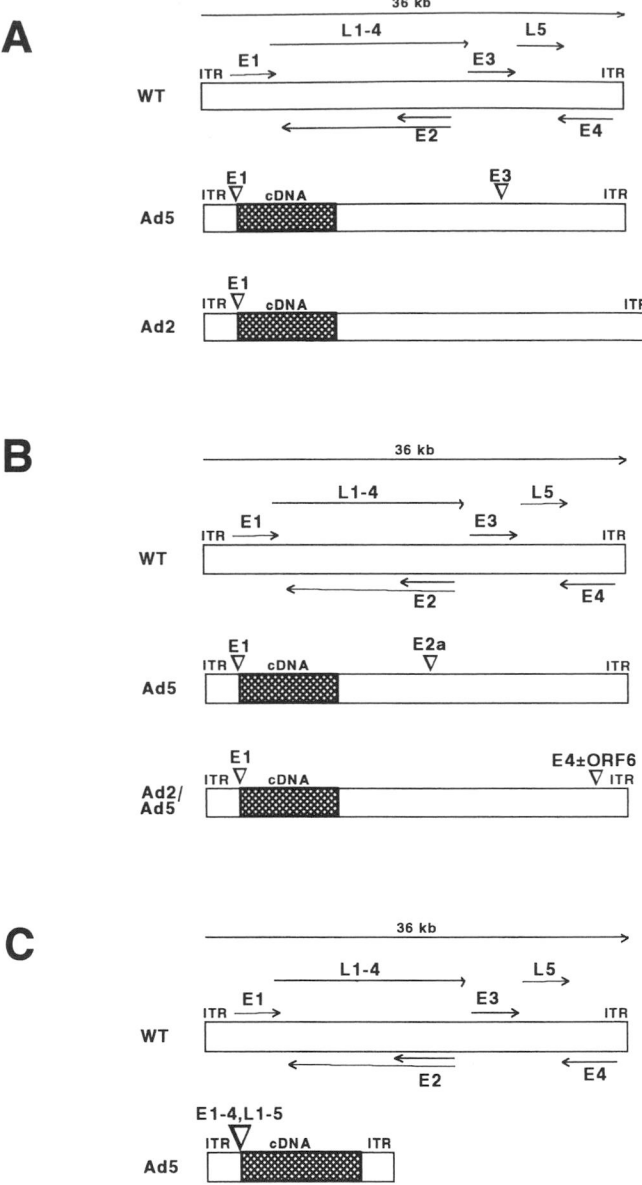

FIG. 11–2. Generations of adenovirus vectors from wild-type adenovirus. **(A),** First-generation vectors. **(B),** Second-generation vectors. **(C),** Third-generation vectors. Ad5, adenovirus serotype 5 vector; Ad2, adenovirus serotype 2 vector: E, early region viral genes; ITR, inverted terminal repeat; L, late region viral genes; WT, wild-type; ▽, deletion of an early or late region gene; ±, with or without. Arrows depict location of gene sequences and the direction of transcription.

DNA to the nucleus occurs where it exists as an episome (extrachromosomal DNA)-mediating expression of therapeutic genes (cDNAs). Because Ad vectors do not integrate at high frequencies, transient expression occurs such that repetitive administration is required (see Table 11–1).

Adeno-Associated Virus Vectors

Adeno-associated virus (AAV) vectors are attractive for gene therapy because they offer the possibility of long-term expression with a high degree of safety. They are derived from the naturally defective and nonpathogenic wild-type human parvoviruses, AAV2 and AAV3 (18–20). The life cycle of wild-type AAV is shown in Fig. 11–3A (20). AAV requires the presence of a helper virus to replicate or to cause a lytic infection. In the absence of a helper virus, AAV integrates into the host-cell genome and becomes latent. On a subsequent wild-type adenovirus or wild-type herpesvirus infection, the AAV genome can be rescued (excised) from the chromosome to generate a lytic infection.

The small AAV genome (~4.7 kb, see Fig. 11–3B) consists of the following: (a) inverted terminal repeats at the 5' and 3' ends of the molecule (19,20), which play a role in replication and are important for integration into the host-cell genome; and (b) the viral genes *rep* and *cap*, which mediate viral replication and nucleocapsid formation (see Fig 11–3B). Dele-

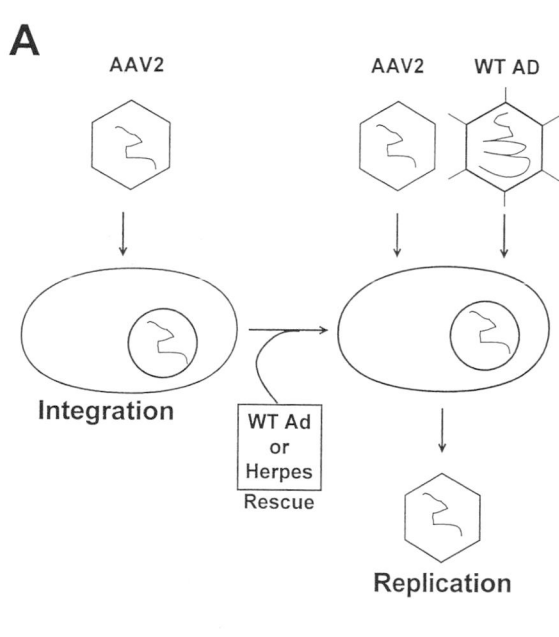

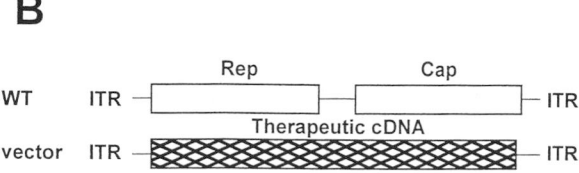

FIG. 11–3. Generation of adeno-associated virus (AAV) vectors. **(A)**, Life cycle of wild-type AAV. **(B)**, Map of wild-type AAV and an AAV vector. Ad, adenovirus; AAV-2, adeno-associated virus serotype 2; ITR, inverted terminal repeat; WT, wild-type.

tion of *rep* and *cap* creates an AAV vector with an insert size of approximately 4.5 kb, which limits the ability to insert the full-length wild-type CFTR (coding region of ~4.5 kb) with a suitable exogenous promoter. Hence, AAV vectors encoding the full-length wild-type CFTR cDNA may exceed the size of the wild-type genome (see Table 11–1), leading to inefficient packaging and subsequent difficulties with virus production.

Retrovirus Vectors

Retroviruses are RNA viruses whose genomes consist of two viral long terminal repeats (LTRs) that are important for cellular integration but also contain promoter elements, a packaging signal, and a series of structural genes, *gag*, *pol*, and *env* (Fig. 11–4). These structural genes encode the capsid protein, protease, reverse transcriptase and an integrase, and envelope glycoprotein, respectively. Deletion of *gag*, *pol*, and *env* creates space for insertion of therapeutic cDNAs (genes) into the retroviral genome, forming a replication defective retrovirus vector (21). Exogenous (internal) promoters also may be included in the sequences of the inserted gene, or alternatively, the viral 5 LTR may be used to drive transcription of the therapeutic gene.

The envelope glycoproteins of a wild-type retrovirus bind to cell-surface receptors to facilitate entry of the retrovirus into the cytoplasm, where the retroviral RNA is reverse-transcribed to form a cDNA, the provirus. This provirus is translocated to the nucleus, where it integrates into the host-cell chromosomes and, through the normal process of DNA transcription, encodes new viral proteins and new viral RNA, which are assembled at the cell surface into new viral particles. Replication-defective retrovirus vectors infect cells by a similar mechanism but unlike wild-type retroviruses, the integrated provirus from a retrovirus vector encodes the therapeutic gene and viral particles are not produced.

Retrovirus vectors are attractive as gene transfer vectors because integration of desired cDNAs into the host-cell genome offers the possibility of long-term expression. Previously, the low rates of epithelial cell proliferation in normal human airways combined with the relatively low titers of murine leukemia virus–derived vectors limited the utility of retrovirus vectors in lung epithelia *in vivo* because of their requirement for proliferating cells (22). Airway epithelial cells in patients with CF have been shown to have significantly higher rates of cell proliferation than rates measured in the airways of healthy subjects (23). Also, advances in the pseudotyping of retrovirus vectors (24) have led to the production of titers 1,000-fold (10^9 infectious units/mL) greater than previously achieved with amphotropic murine leukemia–derived vectors (~ 10^6 infectious units/mL). The successful expression of the *lacZ* reporter gene in rat neurons mediated by a pseudotyped human lentiviral [human immunodeficiency virus (HIV)-derived] vector (see Table 11–1) has raised hopes for the use of retrovirus vectors in patients with CF (25).

Nonviral Vectors

Cationic Liposomes

Cationic liposomes are composed of cationic lipids mixed in varying molar ratios with cholesterol and dioleylphosphatidylethanolamine

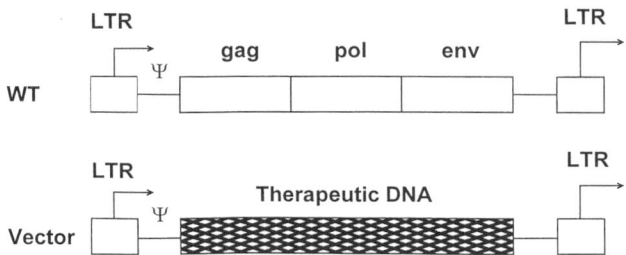

FIG. 11–4. Maps of wild-type murine leukemia retrovirus and a replication defective retrovirus vector. LTR, long terminal repeat; WT, Wild-type; ψ, viral packaging signal.

(DOPE), a neutral phospholipid. Commonly used cationic lipids for gene transfer include N[1-(2,3-dioleoxy)propyl] N,N,N trimethylammonium (DOTMA), 1,2-dimyristyloxypropyl-3-dimethylhydroxyethylam-monium bromide (DMRIE), or 3ß[N-N',N'-dimethylamino ethane-carbamoyl] cholesterol (DC-Chol) and N[1-(2,3-dioleoxy)propyl] N,N,N trimethylammonium methyl sulfate (DOTAP). Cationic liposomes bind to negatively charged plasmid DNA to form DNA-liposome complexes that may, under conditions of excess molar DNA, have a net negative charge. DNA-liposome complexes enter cells primarily by endocytosis (26,27), although the mechanism and specificity of binding to the cell surface, given the potential for negatively charged complexes, have not been delineated clearly. Cationic liposomes also promote the release of plasmid DNA from the endosome into the cytoplasm (27). Like adenoviruses, cationic liposomes do not integrate into the host-cell genome such that expression may be lost with cell division. Thus, repetitive administration of DNA-liposome complexes will be required for gene therapy.

Preclinical Studies

The goal of gene therapy in patients with CF is highly efficient airway gene transfer with a high degree of efficacy and safety. Significant preclinical data have been published regarding the ability of the various gene transfer vectors under investigation to achieve these goals. Data obtained from these studies are reviewed, and how each of the vectors performs with regard to the aforementioned goals is examined. Because retrovirus vectors have not yet proceeded to clinical investigation, they are not included in this discussion.

Efficiency

Efficiency of gene transfer refers to the percent or fraction of cells transduced. Correction of as few as 6% to 10% of CF airway epithelial cells within an epithelium may be sufficient to restore maximal CFTR-mediated Cl⁻ transport function to the entire epithelium (28). Re-

cently, it has been suggested that correction of 10% to 15% of CF cells within the epithelium also may restore antibacterial activity mediated by antibacterial peptides (defensins) to the airway surface fluid (29,30). In contrast, correction of all the cells in an epithelial sheet may be necessary to normalize Na⁺ hyperabsorption (31). A correlation between correction of the ion transport and/or other defects and the prevention of CF lung disease has not been studied. Therefore, transduction of all the columnar cells in the epithelium with a low level of endogenous CFTR, mimicking endogenous expression of the CFTR, may be the best strategy.

Adenovirus Vectors

Ad vectors have efficiently transferred genes to primary human airway epithelia *in vitro* and to cotton rat airway epithelia *in vivo* (4,5,8, 10,32). However, *in vivo* Ad-mediated gene transfer to the airway epithelia of nonhuman primates is inefficient (33). This observation may result from Ad-mediated transduction of different cell types *in vivo* with different efficiencies (34). Grubb et al. (34), using a model of mechanical injury, demonstrated that an Ad-*lacZ* vector efficiently transduced basal cells, the predominant cell type at the site of mechanical injury in human and mouse tracheal explants, whereas columnar cells in uninjured areas were resistant to gene transfer. This observation has been confirmed in model systems of well-differentiated rat and human airway epithelia and extended to human intrapulmonary (bronchial) airways (35). Furthermore, Dupuit et al. (36) performed parallel experiments in excised human airway specimens demonstrating preferential transduction of undifferentiated regenerating or wound repairing cells by Ad vectors, but not well-differentiated pseudostratified columnar epithelia. These studies contradict an earlier study by Mastrangeli et al. (37), who reported efficient *in vivo* transduction of columnar cells in cotton rats. This incongruity may have reflected either species differences or transduction of basal cells that subsequently differentiated into columnar cells.

Preliminary studies using radiolabeled Ad vectors have suggested that a low rate of vector internalization is the barrier to efficient gene transfer in well-differentiated columnar airway epithelial cells (38). This low rate of internalization correlates with a reduction in $\alpha_v\beta_3$ and $\alpha_v\beta_5$ integrin expression, which mediates cellular uptake of Ad in well-differentiated airway epithelial cells (39,40). A regional variation in $\alpha_v\beta_5$ integrin expression in the airways with low levels or absent expression occurring in more proximal airways and higher expression in more distal airways recently has been suggested (41). Surprisingly, increasing the duration of Ad vector incubation with well-differentiated epithelia *in vivo* may partially overcome the resistance of the epithelium to Ad-mediated gene transfer, presumably by increasing entry through nonspecific mechanisms (42,43).

In vivo Ad-mediated gene transfer to the airways of fetal animals may be more efficient than Ad gene transfer to adult airways. Efficient gene transfer to epithelial cells of airways and terminal saccules has been reported after instillation of an Ad-*lacZ* vector to major bronchi of 20- to 24-week gestation human fetal lungs (44). Infection of airway explant cultures from these fetal lungs demonstrated transgene expression primarily in the peripheral or wound-repairing type cells consistent with the findings of Dupuit et al. (36). Efficient Ad-mediated transduction of reporter genes (~18% of cells in the trachea) by Ad in fetal lamb airways after intratracheal administration *in utero* has been reported (45) but was limited by acute morphologic and inflammatory responses. Efficient Ad-mediated gene transfer to fetal rat airways after delivery into the amniotic fluid also has been reported (46).

The efficiency of gene transfer with repetitive administration of vector is an important issue for all transient (nonintegrating) expression vectors. Because the generation of neutralizing antibody after initial airway infection with adenovirus inhibits subsequent infection/transduction of susceptible cells (47–50), alternate administration of Ad vectors from different subgroups has been proposed as a strategy to circumvent the anti-Ad humoral response-inhibiting gene transfer with

repetitive administration (51). In these experiments, intratracheal administration of wild-type Ad5 (subgroup C)—but not wild-type Ad4 (subgroup E) or wild-type Ad30 (subgroup D)—prevented subsequent gene transfer mediated by intratracheal administration of an Ad5-*CAT* or Ad5-*lacZ* vector (subgroup C) 7 days later. Recently, Mack et al. (52) demonstrated that alternate administration of Ad vectors of different serotypes (Ad2 and Ad5), but within the same subgroup (subgroup C), also can circumvent the anti-Ad humoral response. Another strategy to enable consistent gene transfer with repetitive administration of Ad vectors is the inhibition of neutralizing antibody production by immunosuppressive therapy. Yang et al. (53) reported that intratracheal and/or intraperitoneal delivery of interleukin (IL)-12 and interferon-gamma (IFN-γ) markedly reduced (60-fold) production of vector-specific neutralizing and immunoglobulin A (IgA) antibodies in bronchoalveolar lavage (BAL) fluid of mice infected with an Ad5 vector and permitted successful gene transfer 28 days after initial intratracheal dosing with an Ad vector.

Adeno-Associated Virus Vectors

Efficient dose-dependent gene transfer to transformed airway epithelial cells has been reported with this vector (54,55). However, AAV vectors have been shown to transduce primary airway epithelia much less efficiently than immortalized airway cells because of persistence as single-stranded episomes that are converted inefficiently to double-stranded DNA, a requirement for transgene expression (56,57). Similar observations have been made in preliminary studies of well-differentiated airway epithelia in the human bronchial xenograft model (58). Further studies are needed to clearly delineate whether such phenomena occur *in vivo*.

Cationic Liposomes

Of the nonviral vectors, only cationic liposomes have undergone sufficient investigation to permit use in human clinical studies. Efficient cationic liposome-mediated gene transfer has been reported *in vitro* in a variety of cell types (59–64). However, several undifferentiated cell lines or cell types are resistant to transfection by cationic liposomes. Studies in these nontransfectable undifferentiated cells have identified nuclear entry as the rate limiting factor for efficient liposome-mediated gene transfer (65). In contrast, gene transfer to well-differentiated airway epithelial cells is limited by failure of DNA-liposome complexes to enter the cell (66). This inability to enter differentiated airway epithelial cells arises from a loss of phagocytic entry mechanisms in combination with decreased cell surface binding in differentiated columnar airway epithelial cells (66).

Efficacy

In preclinical studies, functional correction of the CFTR-mediated Cl⁻ permeability defect in CF cells transduced by wild-type CFTR has been used as a working definition of efficacy. Detection of CFTR protein by immunohistochemistry and transduced mRNA by *in situ* hybridization and reverse transcription-polymerase chain reaction (RT-PCR) are important confirmatory measures of gene expression, especially when gene transfer is below the level of detection by functional assays.

Adenovirus Vectors

Ad-mediated transduction of the CFTR can restore normal Cl⁻ transport function to primary human CF airway epithelia at low multiplicities of infection (MOI) or numbers of infectious particles per cell (4,31,67). In contrast, correction or normalization of raised Na⁺ transport in primary CF airway epithelia by Ad vectors requires a high MOI for transduction of all the cells within the CF epithelial sheet (31). These data are consistent with a report of Ad-mediated *CFTR* gene transfer in a mouse model of CF (34). In this model, partial correction (~50%) of the Cl⁻ transport defect and no correction of Na⁺ transport was detected in the nasal epithelium after *in vivo* Ad-mediated *CFTR* gene transfer, despite a high MOI and repetitive daily administration (4 consecutive

days) of vector. Recently, prolonged dosing of an Ad2-*CFTR* vector has been shown to fully correct the Cl⁻ and Na⁺ transport defects in the nasal epithelium of a CF mouse model (43), consistent with increased entry by nonspecific (nonintegrin-mediated) mechanisms.

Adeno-Associated Virus Vectors

In vitro correction of the CF Cl⁻ permeability defect has been reported in CF airway epithelial cells using AAV vectors encoding full-length wild-type CFTR through the use of promoter elements in the inverted terminal repeats and/or truncated *CFTR* cDNAs using small promoters (68,69). Flotte and coworkers (70) also have reported expression of CFTR from an AAV vector for up to 6 months by immunohistochemistry and by RT-PCR after bronchoscopic delivery to rabbit lung.

Cationic Liposomes

Novel cationic lipids (GL-67) have been reported to correct the CFTR-mediated Cl⁻ transport defect in CF airway epithelia *in vitro* (6). The level of correction detected corresponds to an MOI of 10 in cells infected with an Ad-*CFTR* vector. Cationic liposome-mediated gene transfer also has been reported to restore CFTR-mediated Cl⁻ transport to airways in transgenic (knock-out) mouse models of CF (71,72). Cationic liposome-mediated gene transfer also has produced high-efficiency transduction of the *lacZ* cDNA of rat airways *in vivo* after direct airway instillation (73). Direct instillation of *CFTR* DNA complexed to cationic liposomes also has been shown to significantly enhance forskolin [cyclic adenosine monophosphate (cAMP)]-stimulated currents over baseline currents measured in control and *lacZ*-treated rat tracheas (73).

Safety

Adenoviruses

The immunogenic responses induced by Ad vectors are a major concern for Ad-mediated gene therapy of CF. Ad vectors induce a dose-related, lymphocyte-predominant inflammatory response in murine, cotton rat, and baboon lungs (11,74–79). The inflammatory response is mediated by cytotoxic (CD8) T-cells and may be induced, in part, by production of viral gene products. Despite the E1-deletion, first-generation vectors have been shown to express late gene products, for example, hexon. Second-generation E2a-defective vectors reduce late gene expression and inflammation extending the duration of transgene expression in nonhuman primates and in rodents, although the duration of the inflammation also is extended (11,77,78).

Second-generation E1-deleted Ad2 vectors with deletions of the E4 region, except for ORF6 (see Fig. 11–2B), also have been associated with cellular inflammation. Studies in nonhuman primates examining toxicity with repetitive administration (every 3 weeks for up to 11 doses) of these vectors suggests that histopathologic changes of inflammation are minimal at doses of up to 3×10^9 infectious units delivered to a single lobe of lung (79). However, doses of vector greater than 3×10^9 infectious units generated the expected histologic changes of inflammation. The immunogenic profile of vectors with complete deletions of E4 (14) and of vectors that have had all of the viral genes deleted (ΔrAd) are anxiously awaited (see Fig 11–2) (15). Complete removal of helper virus (E1-deleted virus used to produce ΔrAd) from ΔrAd vector is a current limitation to the widespread use of completely deleted vectors.

Fetal animals generally have been presumed to be immune-tolerant hosts. Surprisingly, Ad vectors have been shown to cause an inflammatory response in fetal animals. McCray et al. (45) demonstrated that intratracheal delivery of Ad2 vectors encoding *lacZ* and *CFTR* transgenes *in utero* was associated with reactive hyperplasia and squamous metaplasia 3 days after vector delivery, a mononuclear cell inflammatory infiltrate 7 days after vector delivery, and persistence of vector in amniotic fluid for up to 7 days after vector delivery, consistent with replication.

Humoral responses to Ad vectors include the development of mucosal and neutralizing antibodies. These antibodies bind Ad vector on subsequent dosing, inhibiting efficient gene transfer with repetitive administration. Antibodies to foreign transgenes (reporter genes), for example, anti-ß-gal antibodies to transduced *lacZ*, have been identified in rodents after administration of Ad vectors (47,52), potentially limiting the duration of transgene expression. Whether the transduced CFTR in either individuals with CF or CF mice functions as an antigen for the induction of anti-CFTR antibodies has not been determined.

Although humoral and cell-mediated immunogenic responses are the major current safety limitation to Ad vectors for CF gene transfer, other potential limitations exist, including (a) neurogenic inflammation, (b) ectopic expression of the CFTR (expression in cells that do not endogenously express the gene), (c) low-frequency integration into the host-cell genome, and (d) dose-dependent increases in apoptosis or programmed cell death. Intra-airway administration of E1- and E3-deleted Ad vectors induces a dose-dependent potentiation in capsaicin-stimulated vascular permeability in rat airways consistent with neurogenic inflammation (80). This dose-dependent effect can be reduced by ultraviolet (UV)-psoralen inactivation of the Ad vector, consistent with inhibition of viral gene expression, or by administration of a selective substance P (NK1) receptor antagonist (80). Ectopic expression of the CFTR in fibroblasts slows cell growth and alters (depolarizes) the membrane potential (81), whereas overexpression of the CFTR in respiratory epithelia of transgenic mice has shown no deleterious effects on lung development, somatic growth characteristics, or reproductive function (82). The presence of Ad (E1a) sequences in low copy numbers (< 1/cell) in 13% of airway samples from patients with CF and 21% of airway samples from individuals who do not have CF raises concerns that integration of Ad sequences in airway epithelia potentially could complement E1-deleted vectors (83,84). Low-frequency integration (1 in 2,000) of full-length vectors also has been described (85) such that a theoretical risk of insertional mutagenesis exists with Ad vectors. Finally, dose-dependent induction of apoptosis and cell cycle alterations occurring after Ad infection of airway cells may be harmful to the reparative responses in CF airways (86).

Adeno-Associated Virus Vectors

Because *in vitro* studies demonstrate that AAV vectors integrate into multiple random sites (87), a risk of insertional mutagenesis persists with this vector. To date, immunogenic and inflammatory responses have not been reported in preclinical studies in the lungs of animals dosed with AAV vectors (20). However, recent studies in primates suggest that a theoretical risk for vector shedding with wild-type infection of helper virus (Ad or herpes) can occur *in vivo* (88).

Cationic Liposomes

Liposomes generally have been associated with a good safety profile *in vivo*. Canonico et al. (89) have examined the toxicity profile of cationic liposome-mediated expression of the human α_1-AT gene in rabbit lung *in vivo* after both aerosol and intravenous delivery using the cationic liposome DOTMA/DOPE (Lipofectin, Gibco BRL, Gaithersburg, MD) complexed to 500µg of α_1-AT plasmid DNA in a 1:5 (w/w) DNA:lipid ratio. No adverse effects of weekly aerosol or intravenous administration of 500 µg of a human α_1-AT plasmid complexed to 2,500 µg of Lipofectin were detectable by lung histology, lung compliance, and resistance measurements, or measurements of gas exchange over 4 weeks with either method of delivery. This study confirms the notion that conventional cationic lipids used in human clinical studies are safe. However, the low-toxicity profile (90), which generally has made liposome-mediated gene transfer attractive, may not be a feature of the newer lipids. In preliminary studies, these lipids induce an acute dose-dependent neutrophil predominant inflammatory response after intratracheal administration

to murine lung (91). Although aerosol delivery may reduce the degree of inflammation (92), the *in vivo* toxicity of these lipids in nonrodent lungs needs to be addressed.

Clinical Trials

Clinical gene transfer safety and efficacy trials of Ad, AAV, and cationic liposomes in airway epithelia of patients with CF have been initiated. Initial phase I trials evaluated single administration of Ad-*CFTR* vectors to the nasal and/or lower airway epithelia of patients with CF. Subsequent trials have evaluated the feasibility of repetitive dosing of Ad vectors and the safety and efficacy of aerosolized adenovirus vector administration. Recently, trials of cationic liposomes complexed to CFTR plasmid DNA have increased rapidly, and two trials of AAV-mediated gene transfer to CF airways have been initiated.

Adenovirus Vectors

The results of several trials (Table 11–2) evaluating single, aerosolized, or repetitive administration of Ad-CFTR vectors have been published (93–98). Ad-mediated correction of the Cl⁻ transport defect in the nasal epithelium of three patients with CF (MOIs of 1, 3, and 25) and expression of CFTR by RNA-specific (RS)-PCR in two of the three subjects studied (MOIs of 3 and 25) initially was reported in an uncontrolled study by Zabner et al. (93). The major criticism of this study has been the failure of the investigators to include the low Cl⁻ maneuver (a very sensitive discriminator of CF airway from non-CF airway Cl⁻ secretory responses when performed in the presence of isoproterenol) in the nasal potential difference technique used to measure Cl⁻ secretion in their study (99).

Expression of mRNA by RT-PCR of bronchial brushings from one and of immunohistochemical detection of CFTR in bronchial brushings from another of four patients has been reported by Crystal and colleagues (94) in their study of Ad-mediated gene transfer to nasal airway epithelia followed 24 hours later by deliv-

TABLE 11–2. *Clinical gene transfer safety and efficacy trials of adenovirus vectors in cystic fibrosis (CF)*

Principal investigator(s)	Description of trial
Ronald Crystal (94,95)	A phase I study, in patients with CF, of the safety, toxicity, and biological efficacy of a single administration of a replication deficient, recombinant adenovirus carrying the cDNA of the normal human CFTR gene in the lung
Ronald Crystal	Evaluation of repeat administration of a replication deficient, recombinant adenovirus containing the normal CFTR cDNA to the airways of individuals with CF
Michael Welsh (93) Alan E. Smith	CF gene therapy using an adenovirus vector: *in vivo* safety and efficacy in nasal epithelium
Michael Welsh (98) Joseph Zabner	Adenovirus-mediated gene transfer of the CFTR to the nasal epithelium and maxillary sinus of patients with CF
James M. Wilson	Gene therapy of CF lung disease using E1-deleted adenoviruses: a phase I trial
Richard C. Boucher (96) Michael R. Knowles	Gene therapy for CF using E1-deleted adenovirus: a phase I trial in the nasal cavity
Robert W. Wilmott Jeffrey Whitsett	A phase I study of gene therapy of CF using a replication-deficient recombinant adenovirus vector to deliver the human CFTR cDNA to the airways
Henry L. Dorkin	Adenovirus-mediated gene transfer for CF: safety of single administration in the lung (lobar instillation)
Henry L. Dorkin	Adenovirus-mediated gene transfer for CF: safety of single administration in the lung (aerosol administration)
G. Bellon (97)	Aerosol administration of recombinant adenovirus-expressing CFTR to patients with CF: a phase I trial

CFTR, cystic fibrosis transmembrane conductance regulator.

ery to the bronchial epithelium. In one patient, a systemic inflammatory syndrome developed, characterized by headache, fatigue, fever, tachycardia, hypotension, pulmonary infiltrates, and a decrease in lung function 12 to 24 hours after Ad-*CFTR* administration [2×10^9 plaque-forming units (PFUs)] to the right lower lobe bronchus. Increased IL-6 levels relative to the levels of the other study subjects were detected in association with the onset of symptoms. Clinical signs and symptoms resolved by 14 days with broad-spectrum antibiotics, antipyretics, nasal oxygen, and intravenous fluids, but chest radiographic abnormalities persisted for up to 25 days and lung function did not return to baseline for 30 days. Subsequently, functional data from administration of Ad-*CFTR* ($2 \times 10^5 - 2 \times 10^{8.5}$ PFUs) to the nasal epithelium of nine patients with CF, including data from the first four patients discussed previously, was reported (95). Partial correction of both Na+ hyperabsorption and Cl− secretion (33% of that measured in non-CF individuals) was detected by the nasal potential difference (PD) technique when averaged over 14 days. A dose-dependent relationship was not apparent in this particular study.

Knowles and colleagues (96) detected transduced CFTR-mRNA by RT-PCR and/or *in situ* hybridization in five of the six patients at the highest doses (MOI = 100 and 1,000) and in one of six patients at lower MOIs (MOI = 10) in their double-blind, vehicle-controlled, dose escalation study in the nasal epithelium of CF subjects. No correction of defective CFTR-mediated Cl− transport or normalization of raised Na+ transport was detected using the nasal potential difference technique. Morphometric analysis of *in situ* hybridization studies of mucosal biopsies from these subjects demonstrated transduction of less than 1% of the cells consistent with the functional assessment. The development of mucosal inflammation in the Ad5-CB*CFTR*-dosed nostril in two of three patients at MOIs of 1,000 precluded further increases in the dose of vector instilled. *In vivo* studies in rats suggested that the mucosal inflammation may have reflected vector-induced neurogenic inflammation (80). A 15-fold increase in neutralizing antibody titer was detected in one of the high-dose patients.

The results of a trial evaluating aerosol administration of recombinant Ad-*CFTR* recently have been published (97). In a dose escalation study with cohorts of two patients each, six patients with CF were dosed with Ad-CFTR via nasal instillation followed 24 hours later by aerosol administration. The doses of vector for nasal instillation were 1×10^5, 1×10^7, and 4×10^8 PFUs in a volume of 0.4 mL and 1×10^7, 1×10^8, and 5.4×10^8 PFUs for aerosol administration with a volume of 1.6 mL in a breath-activated jet nebulizer (OPTINEB, Air Liquide, Paris, France). The estimated dose of vector delivered to the airways was 25% of the dose in the nebulizer or 2.5×10^6, 2.5×10^7, and 1.35×10^8 PFUs, respectively, for each cohort. Transduced CFTR mRNA was detected by RT-PCR in nasal brush specimens obtained from all six patients and in bronchial brush specimens from one of six subjects 1 to 15 days after Ad-CFTR administration but was not detected in either nasal or bronchial specimens obtained from subjects at baseline (before vector administration). *CFTR* expression by immunohistochemistry also was detected in nasal brush specimens from all six subjects after vector administration and in bronchial brush specimens obtained from two of six subjects after aerosolized vector administration. Remarkably, the fraction of cells transduced by immunohistochemistry from nasal brush specimens ranged from 1.5% to 14.6% (mean, 5.2%) after vector administration. Unfortunately, the authors of this study noted that the combination of spontaneous variation in basal nasal potential difference measurements, repetitive trauma to the nasal mucosa, and their failure to perfect the nasal PD technique before initiating their study, prevented them from *measuring* the functional correlates of their Ad-mediated *CFTR* gene transfer. No safety concerns were raised in this particular study (97).

Zabner et al. (98) reported their results from the repeat administration of a second-generation Ad2-*CFTR* vector to the nasal epithelia of six patients with CF. The study was double blind for the last four subjects. Vector (0.2 to 0.6 mL) was delivered over 30 minutes to the inferior turbinate of one nostril with an equal volume of placebo (saline) delivered to the contralateral nostril in each subject. Five doses

of vector were administered, with an average of 44 days between doses. The doses of vector delivered were as follows: 2×10^7, 2×10^8, 2×10^9, 6.6×10^9, and 1×10^{10} infectious units. No adverse clinical effects were detected. However, a fourfold increase in IgG antibody titer in three subjects at doses greater than or equal to 2×10^9 infectious units and a fourfold increase in neutralizing antibody in three subjects at a dose of 6.6×10^9 infectious units were detected. No increase in levels of IgA antibody in nasal lavage fluid could be detected after dosing. Importantly, no correction of sodium transport was measured, and only a partial correction of Cl$^-$ transport was present at 2 to 6×10^9 infectious units (primarily in 2 of 6 subjects).

These data would suggest that the efficiency of Ad-mediated transduction of CFTR in the nasal epithelium of patients with CF is low. Moreover, safety concerns have been raised in humans with this vector system. Further improvements in Ad-mediated gene transfer efficiency and safety likely will be required to safely achieve sufficient efficacy.

Adeno-Associated Virus Vectors

Two clinical safety and efficacy trials of AAV vectors for CF gene therapy are underway (Table 11–3) (100,101). No data have been reported from either of these studies, one of which examines the utility of AAV-CFTR vectors in the nasal and lower airway epithe-

TABLE 11–3. *Clinical gene transfer safety and efficacy trials of adeno-associated viral vectors in cystic fibrosis (CF)*

Principal investigator(s)	Description of trial
Terence R. Flotte	A phase I study of an adeno-associated virus-CFTR gene vector in adult patients with CF with mild lung disease
Phyllis Gardner	A phase I/II study of tgAAV-CF for the treatment of chronic sinusitis in patients with CF

CFTR, cystic fibrosis transmembrane conductance regulator.

lium whereas the other examines its potential utility in the maxillary sinus, which also is lined by respiratory (airway) epithelium.

Cationic Liposomes

Several trials of cationic liposome-mediated CFTR gene transfer to the nasal epithelium of patients with CF have been initiated or proposed (102–105) (Table 11–4). Caplen et al. (102) reported a double-blind, placebo-controlled trial in which nine subjects with CF received CFTR plasmid DNA (pSV-CFTR) complexed with DC-Chol/DOPE liposomes in a 1:5 (w/w) DNA-to-lipid ratio. Six subjects with CF received only DC-Chol/DOPE liposomes to the nasal epithelia. The doses of DNA used were 0.01, 0.1, and 0.3mg plasmid DNA delivered by nasal spray. The highest dose was delivered in 0.2-mg aliquots to each nostril every 10 minutes, requiring a total time of 7.5 hours. Nasal potential difference measurements revealed a mean hyperpolarization of the nasal potential difference (more negative potential difference) after low Cl^- perfusion in patients receiving the CFTR plasmid DNA-liposome complex that was approximately 20% of that measured in controls. No differences in nasal PDs between CF controls dosed with liposomes only, and patients with CF dosed with

DNA-liposome complexes were detected after treatment with isoprenaline, a cAMP-mediated agonist. RT-PCR detected vector-derived CFTR mRNA in nasal biopsies of five of eight patients who received the DNA liposome complex, but it also was positive in one of five patients who received placebo (liposomes only). Importantly, no toxicity was observed, and in a separate publication, DC-Chol/DOPE liposomes without plasmid DNA delivered to the nasal epithelium in six controls and three subjects with CF did not alter nasal ion transport parameters, lung function, or alter antibiotic sensitivities of CF sputum bacterial isolates (103).

Gill and coworkers (104) reported data from a double-blind, placebo-controlled trial of DC-Chol/DOPE liposomes complexed to CFTR plasmid under the transcriptional control of a respiratory syncytial virus (RSV) 3 LTR promoter. A unique feature of this trial was the use of an empty plasmid vector complexed to liposomes in two of the four placebo patients (the other 2 received buffer). The 12 patients in this study received either placebo (4 patients), 0.04mg DNA (4 patients), or 0.4mg DNA (4 patients) to each nostril delivered via direct instillation over 2 days. Hyperpolarization of the nasal PD into the range of non-CF individuals with superfusion of a low Cl^- solution plus amiloride was reported in two of eight subjects

TABLE 11–4. *Clinical gene transfer safety and efficacy trials of cationic liposomes in cystic fibrosis (CF)*

Principal investigator(s)	Lipid	Description of trial
Eric W.F.W. Alton (102) Duncan M. Geddes	DC-Chol/DOPE	Liposome-mediated CFTR gene transfer to the nasal epithelium of patients with CF
Stephen Hyde (104)	DC-Chol/DOPE	A placebo-controlled study of liposome-mediated gene transfer to the nasal epithelium of patients with CF
Michael J. Welsh Joseph Zabner	Lipid #67	Cationic lipid-mediated gene transfer of CFTR: safety of a single administration to the nasal epithelia
Eric W.F.W. Alton Duncan M. Geddes	Lipid #67	Safety and efficacy of lipid #67 in the airway epithelium of patients with CF
Eric J. Sorscher James L. Logan	DMRIE/DOPE	Gene therapy for CF using cationic liposome-mediated gene transfer: a phase I trial of safety and efficacy in the nasal airway
David Porteous (105) J.A. Innes	DOTAP	DOTAP liposome delivery of gene therapy for CF—a phase I trial in the human nose
Michael R. Knowles Peadar G. Noone	EDMPC	A double-blind placebo-controlled dose-ranging study to evaluate the safety and biological efficacy of a lipid-DNA complex in the nasal epithelium of adult patients with CF

CFTR, cystic fibrosis transmembrane conductance regulator.

dosed with vector (1 from each cohort receiving CFTR vector DNA), but not in placebo-treated subjects. Functional gene transfer was detectable at the single-cell level in five of eight patients by SPQ analysis. However, a positive SPQ signal did not predict a response in the nasal PD maneuver, which tests the function of the epithelium. No evidence for correction of the raised basal PD (a measure of Na^+ transport) was detected, and immunohistochemical and molecular analysis were not performed. In one high-dose (0.4 mg) patient, a transient earache developed on the evening of initial dosing, with an associated injected tympanic membrane for 15 days. Because rhinovirus was cultured from nasal lavage fluid on day 14, delineation of infection versus neurogenic inflammation (80) as the etiology of the earache and inflamed tympanic membrane was not feasible.

Porteous and colleagues (105) reported their experience with a single dose of 0.4 mg pCMV-CFTR/2.4 mg DOTAP in a double-blind, placebo-controlled trial in the nasal epithelium of 16 patients with CF (8 placebo and 8 DNA/lipid complexes). Vector-specific CFTR mRNA was detectable by RT-PCR in two of eight patients receiving DNA liposome complexes, but no significant CFTR-related functional changes were detectable either by the nasal potential difference technique or by SPQ analysis of cells obtained by nasal brushing.

Conclusions: Gene Therapy

Therapy using genetic material remains a potentially attractive approach for CF lung disease. Significant progress has been made in the development of strategies to target CF lung disease. However, for gene therapy to be successful in its design and implementation, further definition of the pathophysiologic mechanisms by which CFTR dysfunction causes disease is required. Defining the appropriate site (airways vs. glands) for targeting gene transfer also is crucial. Assuming that the superficial epithelium is the target, the initial human trials indicate that the transduction efficiency of current gene transfer vectors *in vivo* is low. However, they have been extremely useful in helping to identify barriers to efficient gene transfer *in vivo* (Table 11–5). A major focus of future research will be to define ways to overcome these barriers to efficient gene transfer and to incorporate these concepts into new vector design. In this process, each patient studied provides insight into factors affecting gene transfer efficiency and efficacy while illustrating the challenges that must be overcome for gene therapy of CF to become a clinical reality.

PHARMACOLOGIC APPROACHES

Potential new therapies for the airways disease in CF can target the genetic defect by gene transfer techniques, or target, by pharmacologic approaches, aspects of the pathogenic cascade that are downstream from the genetic mutation. These downstream targets can be secondary effects of chronic infection and inflammation, which also may perturb the rheology of mucus secretions or may involve more proximate abnormalities, which would include defective processing of mutated CFTR to the plasma membrane, the activation of a mutant CFTR, or modifying or bypassing defective ion

TABLE 11–5. *Barriers to efficient* in vivo *airway gene transfer*

Vector	Binding	Entry	Nuclear transport	Second strand synthesis
Adenovirus	Yes	Yes	No	N/A
Adeno-associated virus	Unknown	Unknown	No	Yes
Retrovirus				
MuLV	Unknown	Unknown	Yes	N/A
Lentivirus	Unknown	Unknown	No	N/A
Cationic liposomes	Yes	Yes	Yes	N/A

MuLV, murine leukemia virus-derived retrovirus vector; N/A, not applicable.

transport (see Fig. 11-1). Specifically, this section provides a brief overview of current pharmacologic approaches that are being explored to thin airway secretions, treat the adverse effects of excessive human neutrophil elastase activity in the airways, assist the processing of defective CFTR to the plasma membrane, and/or activate mutant CFTR Cl⁻ channels, and correct the ion transport abnormalities.

Abnormal Mucus Viscosity

The thickened and difficult-to-clear secretions in the airways of patients with CF reflect not only abnormal mucus viscoelastic properties but also the effects of DNA and filamentous actin in patients with chronic infection and inflammation. The presence of large amounts of DNA and filamentous actin in CF airway secretions reflects the mass of degenerating leukocytes associated with chronic bacterial infection (106,107). Recombinant DNase has been shown to improve symptoms and pulmonary function in patients with CF (108) (see Chapter 7). Recent reports suggest that filamentous actin may be another therapeutic target in CF (106,109,110) because sputum from patients with CF contains filamentous actin, with consequent adverse effects on rheology. The adverse effects of actin filaments appear to involve complex interactions between actin and DNA, that is, actin filaments mediate DNA fiber formation (106). Gelsolin, a protein that severs noncovalent bonds between monomers within an actin filament, decreases the viscosity of CF sputum samples *in vitro* (110). Thus, gelsolin and related analogues join recombinant DNase as having therapeutic potential for improving the viscoelastic properties of airway secretions in patients with CF and assisting clearance of retained secretions. Phase I/II studies currently are underway.

Antiinflammatory Drugs and Antiproteases

It long has been suggested that the inflammatory response to chronic bacterial infection, which is complex and multifaceted (see Chapter 6), significantly contributes to the damage in the CF lung. Early studies focused on the use of systemic steroids as antiinflammatory agents. Although initial studies were promising, the long-term side effects of chronic steroid therapy precluded their clinical use (111). More recently, systemic high-dose ibuprofen has been shown in a double-blind study to slow the decline in lung function in an age-dependent fashion. Specifically, ibuprofen markedly reduced (eightfold) the rate of loss of lung function in children with CF and currently is recognized as a standard therapeutic approach for many patients (107,112). Thus, the concept of treating with antiinflammatory agents has gained objective support, and efforts currently are underway to identify more effective and safe antiinflammatory agents.

Human neutrophil elastase is present in large amounts in the airway secretions of patients with CF with chronic bacterial infection, and it has a major adverse effect on host defense. The effects of neutrophil elastase are manifold (see Chapter 6) but contribute to airway destruction and the inflammatory response via several pathways. Thus, administration of antiproteases might limit airway destruction and reduce the inflammatory response. Initial studies focused on aerosolized dosing with the naturally occurring antiprotease, α_1-antitrypsin. This approach has been limited by the requirement to prepare human α_1-antitrypsin from pooled plasma and the difficulties of effective dosing via the aerosol route to diseased airways (113,114).

A novel approach to treat excessive elastase activity in the airways of patients with CF involves the use of a small molecule (DMP-777-Dupont Merck) given by the oral route, which acts as a specific inhibitor of human neutrophil elastase (115). This compound inhibits elastase in circulating neutrophils, and after release from the intracellular neutrophil compartment, it has been demonstrated to effectively inhibit elastase in small animals, without significant toxicity. Phase I safety studies are underway in patients with CF.

Processing the Defective Cystic Fibrosis Transmembrane Conductance Regulator to the Plasma Membrane

Several types of mutations in CFTR are associated with abnormal production of the full-length CFTR protein or abnormal processing of the mutant protein to the plasma membrane. For example, the ΔF508 mutation is retained and degraded in the endoplasmic reticulum, rather than trafficked to the cell surface (116). Because the ΔF508-CFTR has partial chloride channel function (117), the ability to promote trafficking of the ΔF508-CFTR beyond the endoplasmic reticulum might restore partial function at the cell surface. Recent studies indicate that phenylbutyrate induces CFTR chloride channel function *in vitro* (118), which prompted a pilot clinical study to seek evidence of a biological effect *in vivo*. The oral administration of phenylbutyrate to homozygous ΔF508 patients with CF over 1 week suggested an increase in the CFTR chloride conductance of nasal epithelium, as assessed by *in vivo* nasal potential difference studies (119). Although the effect was modest, the outcome of this randomized double-blind, placebo-controlled study implies that such agents may be useful in modulating the defective ΔF508-CFTR function. The mechanism for phenylbutyrate to increase the ΔF508-CFTR chloride conductance is not clear, although it may operate by increasing transcription or processing or function of ΔF508-CFTR. The pilot data from human studies are certain to stimulate further work in this area because 70% of patients with CF from Northern European populations carry at least one copy of this allele.

There also is a major effort under way to define chemical chaperones that may correct the mutant phenotype of the ΔF508 protein by assisting in the processing at the level of the endoplasmic reticulum. Because the ΔF508 CFTR protein is temperature sensitive (120), there has been intense focus on identifying chaperones to correct this abnormality. Several groups have identified potential candidates, including glycerol and other cellular osmolytes (121–124). Although these current candidates are not likely to be useful in a clinical sense, they demonstrate the feasibility of attacking the ΔF508 mutant in a novel and potentially important way because as many as 70% of patients with CF carry this allele and might benefit from this therapeutic capability.

Another type of genetic mutation that may benefit from pharmacologic agents is premature stop mutations. Specifically, these mutations lead to production of truncated, nonfunctional CFTR protein. It is recognized that premature stop mutations can be overcome in some circumstances with aminoglycosides (125). The ability to correct this type of genetic defect would be quite beneficial, that is, 10% of all U.S. patients have at least one premature stop mutation, and as many as 60% of CF chromosomes in Israeli patients have a premature stop mutation (126). Recent studies directly tested the capability of aminoglycoside antibiotics to restore CFTR function, and a dose-dependent increase in the expression of full-length CFTR from R553X mRNA occurred in response to the aminoglycoside derivative, G-418 (127). Quantification of the effect indicated that as much as 25% of the CFTR produced was full length. Functional studies using the SPQ assay also indicated that the full-length CFTR protein functions as a cAMP-stimulated Cl⁻ channel (127). Initial clinical studies are underway in patients with CF.

Activating the Mutant Cystic Fibrosis Transmembrane Conductance Chloride Channel

Although some mutations in CFTR reach the plasma membrane but do not work, or are processed to the plasma membrane in small quantities, approaches to activate mutant CFTR Cl⁻ channels are envisioned as another way to correct cellular abnormalities in CF. Several different approaches and classes of compounds currently are being studied. First, it is recognized that the CFTR is a cAMP-activated Cl⁻ channel, and efforts have been underway for several years to study the effects of phosphodiesterase inhibitors on intracellular cAMP levels and Cl⁻ channel activity. This approach first was reported in oocytes (117), but the specific agent used in that study (IBMX) was not active *in vivo* in human subjects (128). More recent studies for testing this mechanism have focused on milrinone, a class III phosphodiesterase inhibitor (129,130). *In vitro* studies demonstrate that Cl⁻ efflux can be stimulated 40% above baseline in transformed CF cells homozygous for the ΔF508 mutation. Studies *in vivo* in murine nasal epithelium reveal that forskolin, an activator of adenylate cyclase, together with milrinone, activate the ΔF508 CFTR, whereas neither agent was active when used alone (130). Studies of milrinone in patients with CF are expected to be initiated soon.

A related xanthine [cyclopentyl-di-propylxanthine (CPX)] has been shown to induce Cl⁻ efflux in pancreatic (CFPAC) cells bearing the ΔF508 CFTR mutation (131–133). Although several mechanisms of actions have been suggested (131–134), the most recent explanation suggests that binding of CPX to the CFTR molecule, perhaps in the region of the first nucleotide-binding fold, is the mechanism of activating CFTR (134). Phase I/II studies of the effect of CPX in nasal epithelium are underway in patients with CF.

Another possibility for increasing cAMP levels and activating the mutant CFTR is by preventing dephosphorylation of the CFTR with phosphatase inhibitors. This approach has been effective *in vitro* (135). A separate series of studies has focused on genistein, a tyrosine kinase inhibitor, which has been noted to activate the CFTR *in vitro* (136,137). The most recent interpretation of the mechanism of action suggests that genistein activates the CFTR by inhibiting a protein phosphatase, rather than inhibiting a tyrosine kinase. This compound currently is being tested in Phase I/II studies of patients with CF bearing the ΔF508 mutation.

Modify or Bypass Defective Ion Transport

A better understanding of the role of airway epithelial ion transport as an important pulmonary host-defense mechanism has allowed better definition of the role of defective ion transport in the pathogenesis of CF airways disease (138). Also, clarification of the biological mechanisms and cellular ion transport elements involved in these processes offers the opportunity to target abnormal ion transport with pharmacologic agents.

Under basal circumstances, active Na⁺ absorption is the dominant ion transport function in airway epithelia and provides the driving force for isotonic volume absorption of airway surface liquid (139–141). The transport of Na⁺ involves entry into the cell through an epithelial Na⁺ channel on the apical membrane, which is sensitive to inhibition by amiloride (142). The major counterion is Cl⁻, which probably is absorbed across the paracellular pathway (143,144). There is no net Cl⁻ secretion under basal conditions because of an unfavorable electrochemical driving force, which implies the role of the Cl⁻ conductance in normal airway epithelia is unclear under basal circumstances. Normal airway epithelia have at least two Cl⁻ conductances in the apical membrane, that is, the cAMP-mediated CFTR Cl⁻ channel and an alternative calcium-activated Cl⁻ channel (Cl_a^-) (138,145–147).

In CF, an accelerated rate of Na⁺ absorption is the dominant abnormality of ion transport, and the relatively water permeable state of airway epithelia suggests that the excessive Na⁺ transport is associated with excessive isotonic volume absorption (140,141,148,149). We now recognize the mechanism for accelerated Na⁺ transport in CF. Under normal circumstances, the CFTR exerts an inhibitory influence on Na⁺ transport in airway epithelia, but the mutant CFTR in CF does not inhibit Na⁺ transport (150–153). Regarding Cl⁻ transport, CF airway epithelia have a limited (or no) activation of the mutant CFTR protein, but an alternative Cl⁻ conductance remains intact (145,147,154). Taken together, the accelerated Na⁺ absorption, coupled to the defective CFTR Cl⁻ channel, likely contributes to excessive volume absorption and impairment of airway surface liquid rheologic properties (155).

A recent alternative hypothesis has been advanced regarding airway epithelial host defense. Under that paradigm, normal airway epithelia absorb ions, but not volume (similar to the transport properties of the sweat duct) and generate a hypotonic airway surface liquid (29,156). In CF, this hypothesis implies that airway epithelia are unable to absorb Cl⁻ (like the defect in the CF sweat duct), which would result in a higher concentration of Cl^- (relative to normal) and inhibition of salt-sensitive antibacterial factors (possibly defensins) on airway surfaces (29,30). Although it has been postulated that this defect promotes infection in the CF lung, available data do not show a difference of ion composition in airway surface liquid of CF versus healthy subjects (155, 157,158).

The initial studies designed to modulate abnormal ion transport in CF focused on the accelerated rate of Na^+ transport. Amiloride, a Na^+ channel blocker, inhibits Na^- absorption when applied to the luminal surface of airway epithelia (139,140,159–161). Early studies testing the biological effect of aerosolized amiloride demonstrated that acute mucociliary clearance was improved in patients with CF (162,163). Three follow-up studies of acute dosing of amiloride also suggested beneficial effect on: (a) shortening the time for antibiotic cleanup, (b) increasing sputum volume, and (c) an improvement in forced expiratory volume in 1 second (FEV_1) (164–166). However, two subsequent acute studies of mucociliary clearance did not demonstrate benefit (167,168).

Regarding chronic therapy, initial studies in humans suggested that aerosolized amiloride slowed the decline of lung function in a small group of adult patients with CF over a 6-month period (169). However, subsequent studies of chronic aerosolized amiloride have not confirmed this initial report. Two of these chronic studies were small, and the protocols were designed to test whether amiloride provided additional benefit to standard therapies (170,171). A larger French study, assessed by a single measure of spirometry at beginning and after 6 months of aerosolized therapy, also showed no benefit (172). Finally, a large multicenter placebo-controlled trial sponsored by Glaxo-Wellcome Pharmaceuticals (Research Triangle Park, NC) did not demonstrate improved lung function (173).

The failure to find consistent outcomes regarding the effectiveness of amiloride aerosol may reflect several conceptual and functional possibilities. First, aerosolized amiloride would not be useful in CF if there is no hyperabsorp-

tion of Na^+ (and volume) of airway surface liquid. Second, if the traditional hypothesis is correct, the lack of efficacy may reflect the suboptimal drug specificity, dosing, and pharmacokinetics of amiloride (174). In that case, drugs with more specificity, or longer duration of action, such as benzamil, may be useful (175,176).

Recent attention has focused on bypassing the defective CFTR Cl^- conductance. Triphosphate nucleotides, including uridine triphosphate (UTP), activate an alternative Cl^- conductance in normal and CF airway epithelia *in vitro* and *in vivo* (145,147,154). The mechanism of action is via the extracellular 5'-nucleotide ($P2Y_2$) receptor, with the second-messenger signaling via increases in intracellular Ca^{++} (138,177). Whether activation of Cl_a^- induces Cl^- secretion (or absorption) depends on the electrochemical driving force. If the hypothesis about high concentrations of Cl^- in CF impairing antibacterial activity is correct, then UTP would work to drain the airway surface of excess Cl^-.

In addition to activating a Cl_a^- conductance, extracellular nucleotides also stimulate ciliary beat frequency and goblet cell degranulation (178,179). These effects suggest that the triphosphate nucleotides may play an important regulatory role in normal airway defense, and the natural agonist may be ATP, which is released from epithelia by mechanical stimulation (180–182).

In regard to treatment of CF airways disease with aerosolized UTP, initial studies demonstrated that the rate of mucociliary clearance in peripheral (small) airways of patients with CF was approximately half the rate of healthy subjects, and the combination of aerosolized UTP plus amiloride improved mucociliary clearance in peripheral airways to near normal levels (168,183). Although these data support the concept of UTP as a therapeutic agent, it may be necessary to use higher doses or more specific agonists, and current information is not available to indicate whether triphosphate nucleotides will be clinically beneficial as a single agent or whether it will need to be used in conjunction with a Na^+ conductance inhibitor. Ongoing studies are testing the safety and efficacy of aerosolized UTP and promising new analogues (184–186).

SUMMARY

The era following the discovery of the CF gene has allowed better definition of the pathobiology of CF lung disease at a cellular and organ level and has generated excitement about potential new therapies. Initial studies clearly have demonstrated that the transfer of a normal CFTR gene into an airway cell can be accomplished, and can correct the defective cellular function in CF *in vitro*. Although there has been steady progress at developing more efficient and safer gene transfer vectors, the application of these conceptual methodologies to *in vivo* gene transfer in the airways of patients with CF has been more difficult. The opportunity to attack the pathogenic cascade at several levels with pharmacologic agents also is exciting. Many Phase I and Phase II studies already are underway to explore the safety and therapeutic potential of such agents, and there is growing activity in the clinical research arena to develop study protocols that can more quickly link the biological effects of potential therapeutic agents to clinical benefit and allow rigorous testing of such drugs via the CF Therapeutic Development Center (TDC). Although the current approaches described in this chapter are unproven as therapeutic modalities, the broad range of therapeutic approaches that are being tested offer clear hope for better therapy to emerge from this ongoing research.

Note: M.R. Knowles is a founding scientist of Inspire Pharmaceuticals, which licensed the patent for aerosolized UTP from the University of North Carolina on March 10, 1995. M.R. Knowles and the University of North Carolina hold equity in Inspire Pharmaceuticals.

REFERENCES

1. Drumm ML, Pope HA, Cliff WH, et al. Correction of the cystic fibrosis defect *in vitro* by retrovirus-mediated gene transfer. Cell 1990;62(6):1227–1233.

2. Rich DP, Anderson MP, Gregory RJ, et al. Expression of cystic fibrosis transmembrane conductance regulator corrects defective chloride channel regulation in cystic fibrosis airway epithelial cells. *Nature* 1990; 347(6291):358–363.

3. Olsen JC, Johnson LG, Stutts MJ, et al. Correction of the apical membrane chloride permeability defect in polarized cystic fibrosis airway epithelia following retroviral-mediated gene transfer. *Hum Gene Ther* 1992;3(3):253–266.

4. Zabner J, Couture LA, Smith AE, et al. Correction of cAMP-stimulated fluid secretion in cystic fibrosis airway epithelia: efficiency of adenovirus-mediated gene transfer *in vitro. Hum Gene Ther* 1994;5(5):585–593.

5. Rosenfeld MA, Yoshimura K, Trapnell BC, et al. *In vivo* transfer of the human cystic fibrosis transmembrane conductance regulator gene to the airway epithelium. *Cell* 1992;68(1):143–155.

6. Lee ER, Marshall J, Siegel CS, et al. Detailed analysis of structures and formulations of cationic lipids for efficient gene transfer to the lung. *Hum Gene Ther* 1996;7(14):1701–1717.

7. Berkner KL. Development of adenovirus vectors for the expression of heterologous genes. *BioTechniques* 1988;6(7):616–629.

8. Rich DP, Couture LA, Cardoza LM, et al. Development and analysis of recombinant adenoviruses for gene therapy of cystic fibrosis. *Hum Gene Ther* 1993;4(4):461–476.

9. Ginsberg HS, Lundholm-Beauchamp U, Horswood RL, et al. Role of early region 3 (E3) in pathogenesis of adenovirus disease. *Proc Natl Acad Sci U S A* 1989;86(10):3823–3827.

10. Engelhardt JF, Stratford-Perricaudet LD, Yang Y, et al. Direct transfer of recombinant genes into human bronchial epithelia of xenografts with E1 deleted adenoviruses. *Nat Genet* 1993;4(1):27–34.

11. Yang Y, Nunes FA, Berencsi K, et al. Inactivation of E2a in recombinant adenoviruses improves the prospect for gene therapy in cystic fibrosis. *Nat Genet* 1994;7(3):362–369.

12. Engelhardt JF, Ye X, Doranz B, et al. Ablation of E2A in recombinant adenoviruses improves transgene persistence and decreases inflammatory response in mouse liver. *Proc Natl Acad Sci U S A* 1994;91(13):6196–6200.

13. Welsh MJ, Zabner J, Graham SM. Adenovirus-mediated gene transfer for cystic fibrosis: part A, safety of dose and repeat administration in the nasal epithelium; part B, clinical efficacy in the maxillary sinus. *Hum Gene Ther* 1995;6(2):205–218.

14. Wang Q, Jia XC, Finer MH. A packaging cell line for propagation of recombinant adenovirus vectors containing two lethal gene-region deletions. *Gene Ther* 1995;2(10):775–783.

15. Fisher KJ, Choi H, Burda J, et al. Recombinant adenovirus deleted of all viral genes for gene therapy of cystic fibrosis. *Virology* 1996;217(1):11–22.

16. FitzGerald DJP, Padmanabhan R, Pastan I, et al. Adenovirus-induced release of epidermal growth factor and *Pseudomonas* toxin into the cytosol of KB cells during receptor-mediated endocytosis. *Cell* 1983;32 (2):607–617.

17. Bergelson JM, Cunningham JA, Droguett G, et al. Isolation of a common receptor for Coxsackie B

viruses and adenoviruses 2 and 5. *Science* 1997;275: 1320–1323.

18. Blacklow NR, Hoggan MD, Kapkian AZ, et al. Epidemiology of adeno-associated virus infection in a nursery population. *Am J Epidemiol* 1968;88(3): 368–378.

19. Carter BJ. Parvoviruses as vectors. In: Tijssen PL, ed. *Handbook of parvoviruses*. Vol. 2. Boca Raton: CRC Press, 1990:247–284.

20. Flotte TR, Carter BJ. Adeno-associated virus vectors for gene therapy. *Gene Ther* 1995;2(6):357–362.

21. Miller AD, Rosman GJ. Improved retroviral vectors for gene transfer and expression. *BioTechniques* 1989;7(9):980–990.

22. Miller DG, Adam MA, Miller AD. Gene transfer by retrovirus vectors occurs only in cells that are actively replicating at the time of infection. *Mol Cell Biol* 1990;10(8):4239–4242.

23. Leigh MW, Kylander JE, Yankaskas JR, et al. Cell proliferation in bronchial epithelium and submucosal glands of cystic fibrosis patients. *Am J Respir Cell Mol Biol* 1995;12(6):605–612.

24. Burns JC, Friedmann T, Driever W, et al. Vesicular stomatitis virus G glycoprotein pseudotyped retroviral vectors: concentration to very high titer and efficient gene transfer into mammalian and nonmammalian cells. *Proc Natl Acad Sci U S A* 1993;90(17): 8033–8037.

25. Naldini L, Blomer U, Gallay P, et al. *In vivo* gene delivery and stable transduction of nondividing cells by a lentiviral vector. *Science* 1996;272(5259):263–267.

26. Legendre JY, Szoka FC, Jr. Delivery of plasmid DNA into mammalian cell lines using pH-sensitive liposomes: comparison with cationic liposomes. *Pharm Res* 1992;9(10):1235–1242.

27. Zhou X, Huang L. DNA transfection mediated by cationic liposomes containing lipopolylysine: characterization and mechanism of action. *Biochim Biophys Acta* 1994;1189(2):195–203.

28. Johnson LG, Olsen JC, Sarkadi B, et al. Efficiency of gene transfer for restoration of normal airway epithelial function in cystic fibrosis. *Nat Genet* 1992;2(1): 21–25.

29. Smith JJ, Travis SM, Greenberg EP, et al. Cystic fibrosis airway epithelia fail to kill bacteria because of abnormal airway surface fluid. *Cell* 1996;85(2): 229–236.

30. Goldman MJ, Anderson GM, Stolzenberg ED, et al. Human beta-defensin-1 is a salt-sensitive antibiotic that is inactivated in cystic fibrosis. *Cell* 1997;88 (4):553–560.

31. Johnson LG, Boyles SE, Wilson J, et al. Normalization of raised sodium absorption and raised calcium-mediated chloride secretion by adenovirus-mediated expression of cystic fibrosis transmembrane conductance regulator in primary human cystic fibrosis airway epithelial cells. *J Clin Invest* 1995;95(3):1377–1382.

32. Rosenfeld MA, Siegfried W, Yoshimura K, et al. Adenovirus-mediated transfer of a recombinant α1-antitrypsin gene to the lung epithelium *in vivo. Science* 1991;252(5004):431–434.

33. Engelhardt JF, Simon RH, Yang Y, et al. Adenovirus-mediated transfer of the CFTR gene to lung of non-human primates: biological efficacy study. *Hum Gene Ther* 1993;4(6):759–769.

34. Grubb BR, Pickles RJ, Ye H, et al. Inefficient gene transfer by adenovirus vector to cystic fibrosis airway epithelia of mice and humans. *Nature* 1994;371 (6500):802–806.

35. Pickles RJ, Barker PM, Ye H, et al. Efficient adenovirus-mediated gene transfer to basal but not columnar cells of cartilagenous airway epithelia. *Hum Gene Ther* 1996;7(8):921–931.

36. Dupuit F, Zahm JM, Pierrot D, et al. Regenerating cells in human airway surface epithelium represent preferential targets for recombinant adenovirus. *Hum Gene Ther* 1995;6(9):1185–1193.

37. Mastrangeli A, Danel C, Rosenfeld MA, et al. Diversity of airway epithelial cell targets for *in vivo* recombinant adenovirus-mediated gene transfer. *J Clin Invest* 1993;91(1):225–234.

38. Pickles RJ, McCarty D, Randell SH, et al. A low rate of adenoviral vector internalisation is responsible for inefficient gene transfer to well differentiated airway epithelia. *Pediatr Pulmonol Suppl* 1996;13:287 (abstract).

39. Wickham TJ, Mathias P, Cheresh DA, et al. Integrins alpha$_v$beta3 and alpha$_v$beta5 promote adenovirus internalization but not virus attachment. *Cell* 1993;73(2): 309–319.

40. Goldman MJ, Wilson JM: Expression of alpha v beta 5 integrin is necessary for efficient adenovirus-mediated gene transfer in the human airway. *J Virol* 1995;69(10):5951–5958.

41. Goldman M, Su Q, Wilson JM. Gradient of RGD-dependent entry of adenoviral vector in nasal and intrapulmonary epithelia: implications for gene therapy of cystic fibrosis. *Gene Ther* 1996;3(9):811–818.

42. Pilewski JM, Engelhardt JF, Bavaria JE, et al. Adenovirus-mediated gene transfer to human bronchial submucosal glands using xenografts. *Am J Physiol* 1995;268(4 Pt 1):L657–L665.

43. Zabner J, Zeiher BG, Friedman E, et al. Adenovirus-mediated gene transfer to ciliated airway epithelia requires prolonged incubation time. *J Virol* 1996;70 (10):6994–7003.

44. Ballard PL, Zepeda ML, Schwartz M, et al. Adenovirus-mediated gene transfer to human fetal lung *ex vivo. Am J Physiol* 1995;268(5 Pt 1):1839–1845.

45. McCray PB Jr, Armstrong K, Zabner J, et al. Adenoviral-mediated gene transfer to fetal pulmonary epithelia *in vitro* and *in vivo. J Clin Invest* 1995;95(6): 2620–2632.

46. Sekhon HS, Larson JE. *In utero* gene transfer into the pulmonary epithelium. *Nat Med* 1995;1(11):1201–1203.

47. Van Ginkel FW, Liu C, Simecka JW, et al. Intratracheal gene delivery with adenoviral vector induces elevated systemic IgG and mucosal IgA antibodies to adenovirus and beta-galactosidase. *Hum Gene Ther* 1995;6(7):895–903.

48. Kaplan JM, St. George JA, Pennington SE, et al. Humoral and cellular immune responses of nonhuman primates to long-term repeated lung exposure to Ad2/CFTR-2. *Gene Ther* 1996;3(2):117–127.

49. Dong JY, Wang D, Van Ginkel FW, et al. Systematic analysis of repeated gene delivery into animal lungs with a recombinant adenovirus vector. *Hum Gene Ther* 1996;7(3):319–331.

50. Yei S, Mittereder N, Tang K, et al. Adenovirus-mediated gene transfer for cystic fibrosis: quantitative

evaluation of repeated *in vivo* vector administration to the lung. *Gene Ther* 1994;1(3):192–200.

51. Mastrangeli A, Harvey BG, Yao J, et al. "Seroswitch" adenovirus-mediated *in vivo* gene transfer: circumvention of anti-adenovirus humoral immune defenses against repeat adenovirus vector administration by changing the adenovirus serotype. *Hum Gene Ther* 1996;7(1):79–87.

52. Mack CA, Song WR, Carpenter H, et al. Circumvention of anti-adenovirus neutralizing immunity by administration of an adenoviral vector of an alternate serotype. *Hum Gene Ther* 1997;8(1):99–109.

53. Yang Y, Trinchieri G, Wilson JM. Recombinant IL-12 prevents formation of blocking IgA antibodies to recombinant adenovirus and allows repeated gene therapy to mouse lung. *Nat Med* 1995;1(9):890–893.

54. Flotte TR, Solow R, Owens RA, et al. Gene expression from adeno-associated virus vectors in airway epithelial cells. *Am J Respir Cell Mol Biol* 1992; 7(3):349–356.

55. Flotte TR, Afione SA, Zeitlin PL. Adeno-associated virus vector gene expression occurs in nondividing cells in the absence of vector DNA integration. *Am J Respir Cell Mol Biol* 1994;11(5):517–521.

56. Halbert CL, Alexander IE, Wolgamot GM, et al. Adeno-associated virus vectors transduce primary cells much less efficiently than immortalized cells. *J Virol* 1995;69(3):1473–1479.

57. Ferrari FK, Samulski T, Shenk T, et al. Second-strand synthesis is a rate-limiting step for efficient transduction by recombinant adeno-associated virus vectors. *J Virol* 1996;70(5):3227–3234.

58. Goldman MJ, Weitzman MD, Fisher KJ, et al. Recombinant adeno-associated virus enters but does not transduce lung epithelium in a human bronchial xenograft model. *Pediatr Pulmonol Suppl* 1996; 13:256 (abstract).

59. Holmen SL, Vanbrocklin MW, Eversole RR, et al. Efficient lipid-mediated transfection of DNA into primary rat hepatocytes. *In Vitro Cell Dev Biol Anim* 1995;31(5):347–351.

60. Debs R, Pian M, Gaensler K, et al. Prolonged transgene expression in rodent lung cells. *Am J Respir Cell Mol Biol* 1992;7(4):406–413.

61. Jarnagin WR, Debs RJ, Wang SS, et al. Cationic lipid-mediated transfection of liver cells in primary culture. *Nucl Acids Res* 1992;20(16):4205–4211.

62. Felgner PL, Gadek TR, Holm M, et al. Lipofection: a highly efficient, lipid-mediated DNA-transfection procedure. *Proc Natl Acad Sci U S A* 1987;84(21): 7413–7417.

63. Lu L, Zeitlin PL, Guggino WB, et al. Gene transfer by lipofection in rabbit and human secretory epithelial cells. *Pflugers Arch* 1989;415(2):198–203.

64. Stribling R, Brunette E, Liggitt D, et al. Aerosol gene delivery *in vivo*. *Proc Natl Acad Sci U S A* 1992; 89(23):11277–11281.

65. Zabner J, Fasbender AJ, Moninger T, et al. Cellular and molecular barriers to gene transfer by a cationic lipid. *J Biol Chem* 1995;270(32):18997–19007.

66. Matsui H, Johnson LG, Randell SH, et al. Loss of binding and entry of liposome-DNA complexes decreases transfection efficiency in differentiated airway epithelial cells. *J Biol Chem* 1997;272(2): 1117–1126.

67. Johnson LG, Pickles RJ, Boyles SE, et al. *In vitro* assessment of variables affecting the efficiency and efficacy of adenovirus-mediated gene transfer to cystic fibrosis airway epithelia. *Hum Gene Ther* 1996;7(1): 51–59.

68. Egan M, Flotte T, Afione S, et al. Defective regulation of outwardly rectifying Cl⁻ channels by protein kinase A corrected by insertion of CFTR. *Nature* 1992;358(6387):581–584.

69. Flotte TR, Afione SA, Solow R, et al. Expression of the cystic fibrosis transmembrane conductance regulator from a novel adeno-associated virus promoter. *J Biol Chem* 1993;268(5):3781–3790.

70. Flotte TR, Afione SA, Conrad C, et al. Stable in vivo expression of the cystic fibrosis transmembrane conductance regulator with an adeno-associated virus vector. *Proc Natl Acad Sci U S A* 1993;90(22): 10613–10617.

71. Hyde SC, Gill DR, Higgins CF, et al. Correction of the ion transport defect in cystic fibrosis transgenic mice by gene therapy. *Nature* 1993;362(6417): 250–255.

72. Alton EWFW, Middleton PG, Caplen NJ, et al. Noninvasive liposome-mediated gene delivery can correct the ion transport defect in cystic fibrosis mutant mice. *Nat Genet* 1993;5(2):135–142.

73. Logan JJ, Bebok Z, Walker LC, et al. Cationic lipids for reporter gene and CFTR transfer to rat pulmonary epithelium. *Gene Ther* 1995;2(1):38–49.

74. Yang Y, Li Q, Ertl HC, et al. Cellular and humoral immune responses to viral antigens create barriers to lung-directed gene therapy with recombinant adenoviruses. *J Virol* 1995;69(4):2004–2015.

75. Simon RH, Engelhardt JF, Yang Y, et al. Adenovirus-mediated transfer of the CFTR gene to lung of nonhuman primates: toxicity study. *Hum Gene Ther* 1993;4(6):771–780.

76. Yei S, Mittereder N, Wert S, et al. *In vivo* evaluation of the safety of adenovirus-mediated transfer of the human cystic fibrosis transmembrane conductance regulator cDNA to the lung. *Hum Gene Ther* 1994;5(6):731–744.

77. Goldman MJ, Litzky LA, Engelhardt JF, et al. Transfer of the CFTR gene to the lung of nonhuman primates with E1-deleted, E2a-defective recombinant adenoviruses: a preclinical toxicology study. *Hum Gene Ther* 1995;6(7):839–851.

78. Engelhardt JF, Litzky L, Wilson JM. Prolonged transgene expression in cotton rat lung with recombinant adenoviruses defective in E2a. *Hum Gene Ther* 1994;5(10):1217–1229.

79. St. George JA, Pennington SE, Kaplan JM, et al. Biological response of nonhuman primates to long-term repeated lung exposure to Ad2/CFTR2. *Gene Ther* 1996;3(2):103–116.

80. Piedimonte G, Pickles RJ, Lehmann JR, et al. Replication-deficient adenoviral vector for gene transfer potentiates airway neurogenic inflammation. *Am J Respir Cell Mol Biol* 1997;16(3):250–258.

81. Stutts MJ, Gabriel SE, Olsen JC, et al. Functional consequences of heterologous expression of the cystic

fibrosis transmembrane conductance regulator in fibroblasts. *J Biol Chem* 1993;268(27):20653–20658.

82. Whitsett JA, Dey CR, Stripp BR, et al. Human cystic fibrosis transmembrane conductance regulator directed to respiratory epithelial cells of transgenic mice. *Nat Genet* 1992;2(1):13–20.

83. Eissa NT, Chu C, Danel C, et al. Evaluation of the respiratory epithelium of normals and individuals with cystic fibrosis for the presence of adenovirus E1a sequences relevant to the use of E1a- adenovirus vectors for gene therapy for the respiratory manifestations of cystic fibrosis. *Hum Gene Ther* 1994; 5(9):1105–1114.

84. Hayashi S, Gonzalez S, Kuwano K, et al. Adenovirus E1A DNA is present in lungs of patients with cystic fibrosis. *Pediatr Pulmonol Suppl* 1996;13:269 (abstract).

85. Olsen JC, Huang W, Johnson LG, et al. Persistence of adenoviral vector gene expression in CF airway cells is due to integration of vector sequences into chromosomal DNA. *Pediatr Pulmonol Suppl* 1994;10: 230 (abstract).

86. Teramoto S, Johnson LG, Huang W, et al. Effect of adenoviral vector infection on cell proliferation in cultured primary human airway epithelial cells. *Hum Gene Ther* 1995;6(8):1045–1053.

87. Kearns WG, Afione SA, Fulmer SB, et al. Recombinant adeno-associated virus (AAV-CFTR) vectors do not integrate in a site-specific fashion in an immortalized epithelial cell line. *Gene Ther* 1996;3(9):748–755.

88. Afione SA, Conrad CK, Kearns WG, et al. *In vivo* model of adeno-associated virus vector persistence and rescue. *J Virol* 1996;70(5):3235–3241.

89. Canonico AE, Plitman JD, Conary JT, et al. No lung toxicity after repeated aerosol or intravenous delivery of plasmid-cationic liposome complexes. *J Appl Physiol* 1994;77(1):415–419.

90. Ledley FD. Nonviral gene therapy: the promise of genes as pharmaceutical products. *Hum Gene Ther* 1995;6(9):1129–1144.

91. Garlick DS, Nichols M, Vaccaro C, et al. Pulmonary toxicity associated with intranasal instillation of cationic lipid:DNA complexes in mice. *Pediatr Pulmonol Suppl* 1995;12:221 (abstract).

92. Akita GY, Lukason MJ, Murray HL, et al. The safety and efficacy of aerosolized cationic lipid:pDNA complexes. *Pediatr Pulmonol Suppl* 1996;13:262 (abstract).

93. Zabner J, Couture LA, Gregory RJ, et al. Adenovirus-mediated gene transfer transiently corrects the chloride transport defect in nasal epithelia of patients with cystic fibrosis. *Cell* 1993;75(2):207–216.

94. Crystal RG, McElvaney NG, Rosenfeld MA, et al. Administration of an adenovirus containing the human CFTR cDNA to the respiratory tract of individuals with cystic fibrosis. *Nat Genet* 1994;8(1):42– 51.

95. Hay JG, McElvaney NG, Herena J, et al. Modification of nasal epithelial potential differences of individuals with cystic fibrosis consequent to local administration of a normal CFTR cDNA adenovirus gene transfer vector. *Hum Gene Ther* 1995;6(11): 1487–1496.

96. Knowles MR, Hohneker KW, Zhou Z, et al. A controlled study of adenoviral vector-mediated gene transfer in the nasal epithelium of patients with cystic fibrosis. *N Engl J Med* 1995;333(13):823–831.

97. Bellon G, Michel-Calemard L, Thouvenot D, et al. Aerosol administration of a recombinant adenovirus expressing CFTR to cystic fibrosis patients: a phase I clinical trial. *Hum Gene Ther* 1997;8(1):15–25.

98. Zabner J, Ramsey BW, Meeker DP, et al. Repeat administration of an adenovirus vector encoding cystic fibrosis transmembrane conductance regulator to the nasal epithelium of patients with cystic fibrosis. *J Clin Invest* 1996;97(6):1504–1511.

99. Knowles MR, Paradiso AM, Boucher RC. *In vivo* nasal potential difference: techniques and protocols for assessing efficacy of gene transfer in cystic fibrosis. *Hum Gene Ther* 1995;6(4):447–457.

100. Flotte T, Afione S, Beck S, et al. Phase I trial of AAV-CFTR gene transfer in adult CF patients with mild disease. *Pediatr Pulmonol Suppl* 1996;13:275 (abstract).

101. Wagner JA, Moran ML, Messner AH, et al. Safety of delivery of adeno-associated virus mediated gene transfer of CFTR in the maxillary sinus of CF patients with antrostomies. *Pediatr Pulmonol Suppl* 1996;13:276 (abstract).

102. Caplen NJ, Alton EWFW, Middleton PG, et al. Liposome-mediated CFTR gene transfer to the nasal epithelium of patients with cystic fibrosis. *Nat Med* 1995;1(1):39–46.

103. Middleton PG, Caplen NJ, Gao X, et al. Nasal application of the cationic liposome DC-Chol:DOPE does not alter ion transport, lung function or bacterial growth. *Eur Respir J* 1994;7(3):442–445.

104. Gill DR, Southern KW, Mofford KA, et al. A placebo-controlled study of liposome-mediated gene transfer to the nasal epithelium of patients with cystic fibrosis. *Gene Ther* 1997;4(3):199–209.

105. Porteous DJ, Dorin JR, McLachlan G, et al. Evidence for safety and efficacy of DOTAP cationic liposome mediated CFTR gene transfer to the nasal epithelium of patients with cystic fibrosis. *Gene Ther* 1997; 4(3):210–218.

106. Sheils CA, Kas J, Travassos W, et al. Actin filaments mediate DNA fiber formation in chronic inflammatory airway disease. *Am J Pathol* 1996;148(3): 919–927.

107. Ramsey BW. Management of pulmonary disease in patients with cystic fibrosis. *N Engl J Med* 1996; 335(3):179–188.

108. Fuchs HJ, Borowitz DS, Christiansen DH, et al. Effect of aerosolized recombinant DNase on exacerbations of respiratory symptoms and on pulmonary function in patients with cystic fibrosis: the Pulmozyme Study Group. *N Engl J Med* 1994;331(10): 637–642.

109. Janmey PA, Hvidt S, Kas J, et al. The mechanical properties of actin gels: elastic modulus and filament motions. *J Biol Chem* 1994;269(51):32503–32513.

110. Vasconcellos CA, Allen PG, Wohl ME, et al. Reduction in viscosity of cystic fibrosis sputum by gelsolin. *Science* 1994;263(5149):969–971.

111. Rosenstein BJ, Eigen H. Risks of alternate-day prednisone in patients with cystic fibrosis. *Pediatrics* 1991;87:245–246.

112. Konstan MW, Byard PJ, Hoppel CL, et al. Effect of high-dose ibuprofen in patients with cystic fibrosis. *N Engl J Med* 1995;332(13):848–854.

113. McElvaney NG, Hubbard RC, Birrer P, et al. Aerosol α1-antitrypsin treatment for cystic fibrosis. *Lancet* 1991;337(8738):392–394.

114. Berger M, Konstan M, Hilliard J. Aerosolized prolastin (alpha₁-protease inhibitor) in CF. *Pediatr Pulmonol* 1995;20:(6)421 (abstract).

115. Anonymous. *Phase I Study of DMP 777.* 1997; Cystic Fibrosis Foundation. http://www.cff.org/DMP777.htm.

116. Cheng SH, Gregory RJ, Marshall J, et al. Defective intracellular transport and processing of CFTR is the molecular basis of most cystic fibrosis. *Cell* 1990;63(4):827–834.

117. Drumm ML, Wilkinson DJ, Smith LS, et al. Chloride conductance expressed by delta F508 and other mutant CFTRs in Xenopus oocytes. *Science* 1991; 254(5039):1797–1799.

118. Rubenstein RC, Zeitlin PL. Phenylbutyric acid stimulates functional correction of cAMP-mediated chloride secretion in cystic fibrosis epithelial cells. *Pediatr Pulmonol Suppl* 1995;12:234 (abstract).

119. Rubenstein RC, Zeitlin PL. A pilot clinical trial of oral sodium 4-phenylbutyrate (Buphenyl) in Δ F508-homozygous cystic fibrosis patients: partial restoration of nasal epithelial CFTR function. *Am J Respir Crit Care Med* 1998;157(2):484–490.

120. Denning GM, Anderson MP, Amara JF, et al. Processing of mutant cystic fibrosis transmembrane conductance regulator is temperature-sensitive. *Nature* 1992;358:761–764.

121. Brown CR, Hongbrown LQ, Biwersi J, et al. Chemical chaperones correct the mutant phenotype of the delta-F508 cystic fibrosis transmembrane conductance regulator protein. *Cell Stress Chaperones* 1996;1(2):117–125.

122. Jensen TJ, Loo MA, Pind S, et al. Multiple proteolytic systems, including the proteasome, contribute to CFTR processing. *Cell* 1995;83(1):129–135.

123. Pind S, Riordan JR, Williams DB. Participation of the endoplasmic reticulum chaperone calnexin (p88, IP90) in the biogenesis of the cystic fibrosis transmembrane conductance regulator. *J Biol Chem* 1994;269(17):12784–12788.

124. Sato S, Ward CL, Krouse ME, et al. Glycerol reverses the misfolding phenotype of the most common cystic fibrosis mutation. *J Biol Chem* 1996; 271(2):635–638.

125. Delaney SJ, Wainwright BJ. New pharmaceutical approaches to the treatment of cystic fibrosis. *Nat Med* 1996;2(4):392–393.

126. Welsh MJ, Tsui L, Boat TF, et al. Cystic fibrosis. In: Scriver CR, Beaudet AL, Sly WS, et al., eds. *The metabolic and molecular bases of inherited disease.* 7th ed. New York: McGraw-Hill, 1995:3799–3876.

127. Howard M, Frizzell RA, Bedwell DM. Aminoglycoside antibiotics restore CFTR function by overcoming premature stop functions. *Nat Med* 1996;2(4): 467–469.

128. Grubb B, Lazarowski E, Knowles M, et al. Isobutyl-methylxanthine fails to stimulate chloride secretion in cystic fibrosis airway epithelia. *Am J Respir Cell Mol Biol* 1993;8:454–460.

129. Kelley TJ, al-Nakkash L, Cotton CU, et al. Activation of endogenous deltaF508 cystic fibrosis transmembrane conductance regulator by phosphodiesterase inhibition. *J Clin Invest* 1996;98(2):513–520.

130. Kelley TJ, Thomas K, Milgram LJH, et al. In vivo activation of the cystic fibrosis transmembrane conductance regulator mutant delta F508 in murine nasal epithelium. *Proc Natl Acad Sci U S A* 1997;94:2604–2608.

131. McCoy DE, Schwiebert EM, Karlson KH, et al. Identification and function of A1 adenosine receptors in normal and cystic fibrosis human airway epithelial cells. *Am J Physiol* 1995;268:1520–1527.

132. Haws CM, Nepomuceno IB, Krouse ME, et al. DeltaF508-CFTR channels: kinetics, activation by forskolin, and potentiation by xanthines. *Am J Physiol* 1996;270:C1544–C1555.

133. Eidelman O, Guay-Broder C, van Galen PJ, et al. A1 adenosine-receptor antagonists activate chloride efflux from cystic fibrosis cells. *Proc Natl Acad Sci U S A* 1992;89:5562–5566.

134. Cohen BE, Lee G, Jacobson KA, et al. 8-Cyclopentyl-1,3-dipropylxanthine and other xanthines differentially bind to the wild-type and deltaF508 mutant first nucleotide binding fold (NBF-1) domains of the cystic fibrosis transmembrane conductance regulator. *Biochemistry* 1997;36:6455–6461.

135. Becq F, Jensen TJ, Chang XB, et al. Phosphatase inhibitors activate normal and defective CFTR chloride channels. *Proc Natl Acad Sci U S A* 1994;91(19): 9160–9164.

136. Illek B, Fischer H, Santos GF, et al. cAMP-independent activation of CFTR Cl channels by the tyrosine kinase inhibitor genistein. *Am J Physiol* 1995;268: C886–C893.

137. Illek B, Fischer H, Machen TE. Alternate stimulation of apical CFTR by genistein in epithelia. *Am J Physiol* 1996;270:C265–C275.

138. Boucher RC. Human airway ion transport: part 2. *Am J Respir Crit Care Med* 1994;150(2):581–593.

139. Knowles M, Murray G, Shallal J, et al. Bioelectric properties and ion flow across excised human bronchi. *J Appl Physiol* 1984;56:868–877.

140. Boucher RC, Stutts MJ, Knowles MR, et al. Na⁺ transport in cystic fibrosis respiratory epithelia: abnormal basal rate and response to adenylate cyclase activation. *J Clin Invest* 1986;78(5):1245–1252.

141. Jiang C, Finkbeiner WE, Widdicombe JH, et al. Altered fluid transport across airway epithelium in cystic fibrosis. *Science* 1993;262(5132):424–427.

142. Oh YS, Benos DJ. Amiloride-sensitive sodium channels. In: Cragoe EJ Jr, Kleyman TR, Simchowitz L, eds. *Amiloride and its analogs unique cation transport inhibitors.* New York: VCH Publishers Inc, 4, 1992:41–56.

143. Willumsen NJ, Boucher RC. Shunt resistance and ion permeabilities in normal and cystic fibrosis airway epithelium. *Am J Physiol* 1989;256(5 Pt 1):C1054–C1063.

144. Willumsen NJ, Davis CW, Boucher RC. Intracellular Cl⁻ activity and cellular Cl⁻ pathways in cultured human airway epithelium. *Am J Physiol* 1989;256(5 Pt 1):C1033–C1044.

145. Mason SJ, Paradiso AM, Boucher RC. Regulation of transepithelial ion transport and intracellular calcium

by extracellular adenosine triphosphate in human normal and cystic fibrosis airway epithelium. *Br J Pharmacol* 1991;103:1649–1656.

146. Clarke LL, Grubb BR, Yankaskas JR, et al. Relationship of a non-CFTR mediated chloride conductance to organ-level disease in CFTR(-/-) mice. *Proc Natl Acad Sci U S A* 1994;91(2):479–483.

147. Clarke LL, Boucher RC. Chloride secretory response to extracellular ATP in normal and cystic fibrosis nasal epithelia. *Am J Physiol* 1992;263:C348–C356.

148. Boucher RC, Cotton CU, Gatzy JT, et al. Evidence for reduced Cl⁻ and increased Na⁺ permeability in cystic fibrosis human primary cell cultures. *J Physiol (Lond)* 1988;405:77–103.

149. Folkesson HG, Matthay MA, Frigeri A, et al. Transepithelial water permeability in microperfused distal airways: evidence for channel-mediated water transport. *J Clin Invest* 1996;97(3):664–671.

150. Stutts MJ, Canessa CM, Olsen JC, et al. CFTR as a cAMP-dependent regulator of sodium channels. *Science* 1995;269:847–850.

151. Mall M, Hipper A, Greger R, et al. Wild type but not delta F508 CFTR inhibits Na⁺ conductance when co-expressed in Xenopus oocytes. *FEBS Lett* 1996; 381:47–52.

152. Ismailov II, Awayda MS, Jovov B, et al. Regulation of epithelial sodium channels by the cystic fibrosis transmembrane conductance regulator. *J Biol Chem* 1996;271(9):4725–4732.

153. Stutts MJ, Rossier BC, Boucher RC. CFTR inverts PKA-mediated regulation of ENaC single channel kinetics. *J Biol Chem* 1997;272:14037–14040.

154. Knowles MR, Clarke LL, Boucher RC. Activation by extracellular nucleotides of chloride secretion in the airway epithelia of patients with cystic fibrosis. *N Engl J Med* 1991;325:533–538.

155. Knowles MR, Robinson JM, Wood RE, et al. Ion composition of airway surface liquid of patients with cystic fibrosis as compared to normal and disease-control subjects. *J Clin Invest* 1997;100(10):2588–2595.

156. Quinton PM. Viscosity versus composition in airway pathology (editorial). *Am J Respir Crit Care Med* 1994;149(1):6–7.

157. Smith JJ, Travis SM, Greenberg EP, et al. Erratum. *Cell* 1996;87(2): unnumbered page following 355.

158. Hull J, Skinner W, Robertson C, et al. Elemental content of airway surface liquid from infants with cystic fibrosis. *Am J Respir Crit Care Med* 1998; 157(1):10–14.

159. Knowles MR, Gatzy J, Boucher R. Increased bioelectric potential difference across respiratory epithelia in cystic fibrosis. *N Engl J Med* 1981;305: 1489–1495.

160. Knowles MR, Stutts MJ, Spock A, et al. Abnormal ion permeation through cystic fibrosis respiratory epithelium. *Science* 1983;221:1067–1070.

161. Knowles M, Gatzy J, Boucher R. Relative ion permeability of normal and cystic fibrosis nasal epithelium. *J Clin Invest* 1983;71:1410–1417.

162. Kohler D, App E, Schmitz-Schumann M, et al. Inhalation of amiloride improves the mucociliary and the cough clearance in patients with cystic fibrosis. *Eur J Respir Dis* 1986;69(Suppl 146):319–326.

163. App EM, King M, Helfesrieder R, et al. Acute and long-term amiloride inhalation in cystic fibrosis lung disease: a rational approach to cystic fibrosis therapy. *Am Rev Respir Dis* 1990;141:605–612.

164. Bowler IM, Kelman B, Worthington D, et al. Nebulized amiloride in respiratory exacerbations of cystic fibrosis: a randomised controlled trial. *Arch Dis Child* 1995;73(5):427–430.

165. Hofmann T, Senier I, Bittner P, et al. Aerosolized amiloride: dose-effect on nasal bioelectric properties, pharmacokinetics, and effect on sputum expectoration in patients with cystic fibrosis. *J Aerosol Med* 1997;10(2):147–158.

166. Visca A, Bignamini E. Concentration of inhaled amiloride in cystic fibrosis. *Lancet* 1996;347:1126.

167. Robinson M, Regnis JA, Bailey DL, et al. Effect of hypertonic saline, amiloride, and cough on mucociliary clearance in patients with cystic fibrosis. *Am J Respir Crit Care Med* 1996;153(5):1503–1509.

168. Bennett WD, Olivier KN, Zeman KL, et al. Effect of uridine 5'-triphosphate plus amiloride on mucociliary clearance in adult cystic fibrosis. *Am J Respir Crit Care Med* 1996;153(6):1796–1801.

169. Knowles MR, Church NL, Waltner WE, et al. A pilot study of aerosolized amiloride for the treatment of lung disease in cystic fibrosis. *N Engl J Med* 1990;322(14):1189–1194.

170. Graham A, Hasani A, Alton EWFW, et al. No added benefit from nebulized amiloride in patients with cystic fibrosis. *Eur Respir J* 1993;6(9):1243–1248.

171. Robinson M, Donnelly PM, Donnelly J, et al. Effect of long-term inhalation of amiloride on lung function and exercise capacity in adults with cystic fibrosis. *Am J Respir Crit Care Med* 1995;151:(4)A20 (abstract).

172. Pons G, Marchand MC, Foucard C, et al. French multicentre randomized double-blind placebo-controlled trial on nebulized amiloride in cystic fibrosis patients. *Pediatr Pulmonol Suppl* 1995;12:193 (abstract).

173. Church NL, Burroughs SM, Wisniewski ME, et al. The effect of amiloride on the decline of pulmonary function in cystic fibrosis patients 10 years of age and older. *Pediatr Pulmonol Suppl* 1996;13:279–280 (abstract).

174. Knowles MR, Church NL, Waltner WE, et al. Amiloride in cystic fibrosis: safety, pharmacokinetics, and efficacy in the treatment of pulmonary disease. In: Cragoe EJ Jr, Kleyman TR, Simchowitz L, eds. *Amiloride and its analogs: unique cation transport inhibitors.* New York: VCH Publishers Inc. 1992:301–316.

175. Hofmann T, Ziersch A, Senier I, et al. Benzamil and amiloride in CF nasal epithelium: time course of the effects on nasal potential difference *in vivo. Pediatr Pulmonol Suppl* 1996;13:280 (abstract).

176. Blank U, Clauss W, Weber WM. Effects of benzamil in human cystic fibrosis airway epithelium. *Cell Physiol Biochem* 1995;5:385–390.

177. Brown HA, Lazarowski ER, Boucher RC, et al. Evidence that UTP and ATP regulate phospholipase C through a common extracellular 5'-nucleotide receptor in human airway epithelial cells. *Mol Pharmacol* 1991;40:648–655.

178. Lansley AB, Sanderson MJ, Dirksen ER. Control of the beat cycle of respiratory tract cilia by Ca²⁺ and cAMP. *Am J Physiol* 1992;263:L232–L242.

179. Lethem MI, Dowell ML, Van Scott M, et al. Nucleotide regulation of goblet cells in human airway epithelial explants: normal exocytosis in cystic fibrosis. *Am J Respir Cell Mol Biol* 1993;9(3):315–322.

180. Grygorczyk R, Hanrahan JW. CFTR-independent ATP release from epithelial cells triggered by mechanical stimuli. *Am J Physiol* 1997;272:C1058–C1066.

181. Donaldson SH, Boucher RC, Knowles MR. In vivo regulation of ATP levels in human nasal epithelia. *Pediatr Pulmonol Suppl* 1996;13:289 (abstract).

182. Donaldson SH, Stutts MJ, Boucher RC, et al. Adenosine triphosphate levels in nasal surface liquid. *Am J Respir Crit Care Med* 1996;153:(4 Pt 2)A854 (abstract).

183. Olivier KN, Bennett WD, Hohneker KW, et al. Acute safety and effects on mucociliary clearance of aerosolized uridine 5'-triphosphate amiloride in normal human adults. *Am J Respir Crit Care Med* 1996;154(1):217–223.

184. Regnis JA, Lazarowski ER, Foy CE, et al. Uridine 5'-triphosphate metabolism by human nasal epithelial cells, whole blood and plasma *in vitro*. *Am J Respir Crit Care Med* 1996;153:(Suppl 4,2)A779 (abstract).

185. Lazarowski ER, Watt WC, Stutts MJ, et al. Enzymatic synthesis of UTPgammaS, a potent hydrolysis resistant agonist of P_{2U}-receptors. *Br J Pharmacol* 1996;117:203–209.

186. Shaffer C, Jacobus K, Foy C, et al. Controlled clinical studies indicate that INS316 (uridine 5'-triphosphate), a $P2Y_2$ receptor agonist stimulates mucuciliary clearance and enhances sputum expectoration. *Am J Rospir Crit Care Med* 1998;157(3): A796 (abstract).

SECTION III

Gastrointestinal

Cystic Fibrosis in Adults,
edited by J. R. Yankaskas and M. R. Knowles,
Lippincott–Raven Publishers, Philadelphia, 1999.

12

The Exocrine Pancreas

Peter R. Durie and Gordon G. Forstner

Department of Pediatrics, Faculty of Medicine, University of Toronto, and Division of Gastroenterology/Nutrition, The Research Institute, The Hospital for Sick Children, Toronto, Ontario, Canada

Cystic fibrosis (CF) was first described in the late 1930s on the basis of clinical evidence of both pancreatic and pulmonary disease. Before this time, numerous citations describe infants and children with neonatal intestinal obstruction due to meconium ileus, and descriptions of characteristic pancreatic and pulmonary disease date back several centuries. Dorothy Anderson (1) first provided extensive description of the clinical manifestations of CF and coined the term "cystic fibrosis of the pancreas" to characterize the condition. CF was segregated from other "celiac" syndromes, and the relationship between pancreatic and lung lesions were defined in Germany by Fanconi et al. (2) and in the United States by Anderson (1). The presence of pancreatic insufficiency in young infants was the key to the clinical diagnosis until di Sant'Agnese and colleagues (3) recognized that patients with CF have high concentrations of sodium and chloride in sweat. In 1950, Gibbs and colleagues (4) were the first to recognize that steatorrhea caused by pancreatic insufficiency was not present in all patients with CF. Subsequently, it has been recognized that clinical expression of the disease can be extremely variable. Since the early days, comprehensive and aggressive approaches to the symptomatic care of patients with CF have given rise to steady improvements in survival; it currently is commonplace for patients with CF to reach adulthood and enjoy remarkably good health and a productive life.

This chapter outlines the current understanding of clinical characteristics of the pancreas in CF and provides insights regarding its pathogenesis in this multisystem disease.

PATHOLOGIC FEATURES OF THE EXOCRINE PANCREAS IN CYSTIC FIBROSIS

The pancreas is abnormal in almost all patients with CF. When severely affected, the characteristic postmortem features of the CF exocrine pancreas include widespread loss of acinar cells, and the areas of destruction are replaced by fibrous tissue and fat (5,6). Intraluminal calcification may be present which may be noted sonographically or on x-ray imaging (7). Small, isolated cysts are seen, or occasionally, true macrocysts with an epithelial lining (which generally represent dilated ducts) (7,8). Severe morphologic changes within the exocrine pancreas, which have been described primarily in patients with relatively long-standing disease, probably reflect secondary pathologic events occurring over many years. However, the pancreatic lesions that have been reported vary considerably in severity; the pancreas is histologically normal at autopsy in some patients who die in infancy (9).

To develop a clear understanding of the pathologic processes that occur in the CF pancreas, early changes within the gland must be identified and compared with the early development of the normal pancreas. Normal prenatal and early postnatal development of the exocrine pancreas involves a clear pathway of maturation and differentiation of the acinar cells and epithelial ductal system (10). Acinar maturation is reflected by an increased ratio of acinar cells to connective tissue. Zymogen granules appear within acini at 14 to 16 weeks' gestation, and their number and size increase steadily up to birth. The main ductal system branches successively to form interlobular and intralobular ducts. Intercalated ducts arise as branches of the intralobular ducts and extend into the acini. The ductal system of the mature pancreas, which accounts for less than 5% of the volume of the entire pancreas, plays a vital role in fluid and electrolyte secretion.

Imrie and colleagues (11) performed a careful morphologic study of the postnatal development of the pancreas in infants with CF using comparative age-matched controls. They studied a series of 60 autopsy specimens from infants younger than 4 months of age at death, including 29 control subjects and 31 subjects with CF (24 with a history of meconium ileus). Quantitative microscopy was used to analyze the volumes of acinar tissue, connective tissue, ducts, and duct lumina. In control subjects, the volume of exocrine acinar tissue increased linearly with development age. As a result, the acinar:connective tissue ratio increased fourfold from birth to 4 months of age. In contrast, in subjects with CF, there was a deficiency in normal acinar development; the ratio of acinar:connective tissue showed progressive diminution with age. The failure of acinar development was similar for subjects who died of complications of meconium ileus and those who died of other causes.

The pancreatic ductal system of the controls occupied less than 5% of the total volume of the exocrine pancreas, whereas the intraluminal duct volume was less than 0.5% of the total exocrine pancreatic tissue. Because the lumen volume increased proportionately with acinar proliferation, there was no significant net increase in net luminal volume as a percentage of exocrine tissue volume with age. In striking contrast, the duct luminal volume of the ex-

ocrine pancreas from patients with CF was increased significantly, exceeding 4% of the total pancreatic volume. In more than 80% of the CF subjects, duct luminal volume exceeded that of the control subjects and volume did not alter with age. These authors (11) also demonstrated accumulation of secretory material within the pancreatic ducts, which previously had been recognized as a characteristic early feature of the exocrine pancreas in CF. This obstructive process within ducts, therefore, appears to cause dilation of the duct and acinar lumina, together with progressive degradation and atrophy of acini. Similar changes have been described by King et al. (9) in premature infants dying of CF. Focal dilatation of the small pancreatic ductules were described as the earliest changes, progressing to widespread involvement of the glands with flattening of the epithelium and plugging of ductules and acini by inspissated secretions. Some infants showed acinar atrophy and severe periductal and interacinar fibrosis at a very early age.

Obviously, the functional status of the exocrine pancreas was not determined by these postmortem studies, and because of their early death and the existence of meconium ileus, probably only patients with severe pancreatic disease were evaluated. To our knowledge, no studies have evaluated the histologic findings of patients with CF and pancreatic sufficiency. However, based on information from imaging studies and tests of exocrine pancreatic function, the majority of these patients can be expected to have morphologic changes that, because of genetic factors (see genotype studies), are less advanced. Because a significant percentage of patients with pancreatic sufficiency experience recurrent bouts of acute pancreatitis, some of the morphologic changes could be the result of the secondary effects of pancreatic inflammation. In this regard, the histologic findings can be corroborated by *in vivo* evaluation of exocrine pancreatic function of affected patients. As will be described, pancreatic secretions from patients with CF contain significantly higher concentrations of protein in comparison with controls; hyperconcentration of secretory proteins appear to result from a pri-

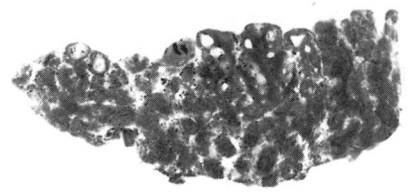

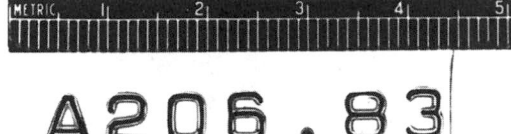

FIG. 12–1. Gross specimen of a portion of the pancreas from an adult patient with cystic fibrosis and pancreatic insufficiency. Multiple macronodular cysts (1 to 5 mm in diameter) are seen. Microscopic examination (not shown) revealed true cysts lined with cuboidal epithelium and ducts containing inspissated material.

mary deficit of ductal fluid secretion that predisposes the CF pancreas to intraductal precipitation of secreted protein and obstruction of small pancreatic ducts. Duct obstruction in turn results in progressive changes in pancreatic pathology.

The observation of pancreatic cyst formation and ductal calcification in older patients with CF (Fig. 12–1) may be the result of a similar pathologic process (7,8). True cysts with an epithelial lining commonly are seen with a diameter of 2 to 3 mm, but on occasion, cysts may be up to 50 mm in diameter. In our view, pancreatic cysts develop as a result of increased fluid pressure proximal to obstructed ducts.

IMAGING FEATURES OF THE EXOCRINE PANCREAS IN CYSTIC FIBROSIS

Several imaging modalities may be used to evaluate pancreatic involvement in CF (12–14). The pancreas rarely shows calcification on plain-film radiographs, but if present, calcification appears in a focal or more diffuse pattern; occasionally large calcific loci are seen. Calcific deposits also can be visualized by sonography and computerized tomography (CT).

On sonography, the CF pancreas usually is echo dense. There may be evidence of dilatation of pancreatic ducts. The size of the pancreas varies according to the stage of the pathologic process. Rarely, the pancreas can be larger than normal because of fatty infiltration or ductal dilatation, but it usually is quite small in adult patients with CF with pancreatic insufficiency. CT appearances generally reflect the aforementioned pathologic changes, that is, decreased attenuation due to fatty replacement. Calcification, cysts, or duct dilatation also may be observed in the occasional patient by this imaging modality (Fig. 12–2).

Recently, magnetic resonance imaging (MRI) has been used to evaluate pancreatic involvement in CF (14). Magnetic resonance (MR) images of 27 pancreatic-insufficient patients revealed a variety of patterns. Almost half the patients exhibited diffuse hyperintensity with residual lobulation; this corresponded to complete or nearly complete fatty replacement of the organ. In a small number of patients, a homogenous hyperintensity without lobulation was noted, and this also was believed to repre-

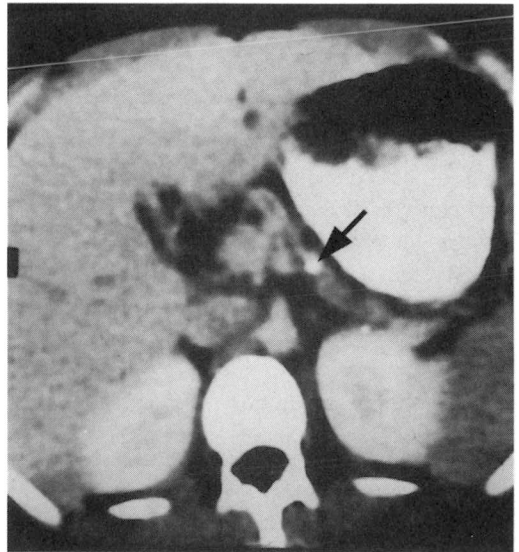

FIG. 12–2. Computerized tomography scan of a 17-year-old girl with cystic fibrosis and pancreatic insufficiency. The pancreas appears shrunken with calcification in the body *(arrow)*.

sent a complete fatty replacement with more severe destruction of the pancreatic parenchyma. In three patients, focal areas of hypointensity were detected within a hyperintense parenchyma. This was believed to represent partial replacement of the organ by adipose tissue. In 10 patients, no structural or signal intensity changes were detected, but because of the volume reduction in the body of the pancreas, it appeared to represent glandular atrophy without fat replacement. Although quantitative details concerning the severity of pancreatic disease were lacking, the investigators suggested a correlation existed between the specific MR images (T1 parameters) and the severity of pancreatic insufficiency; lower T1 values appeared to be seen in patients with marked pancreatic involvement. The investigators failed to evaluate the MR images in relation to age, which is important because the subjects ranged in age from 5 to 34 years. It is possible, therefore, that some of the observed variations in MRI correlated with the evolution of pancreatic disease.

FUNCTIONAL FEATURES OF THE EXOCRINE PANCREAS IN CYSTIC FIBROSIS

Approximately 85% of patients with CF exhibit signs and symptoms of pancreatic maldigestion, and in most cases, these symptoms are present at diagnosis (15). The remaining 15% of patients exhibit a variable degree of pancreatic dysfunction. Patients with CF who have documented evidence of maldigestion obviously have pancreatic insufficiency (PI). Those who absorb nutrients usually are defined less easily. They often are described as having "normal" pancreatic function, but in the majority of patients, quantitative evaluation of the exocrine pancreas demonstrates abnormal acinar and ductular function. For pragmatic reasons, it is useful to consider patients who lack pancreatic maldigestion as a single group. The operational term *pancreatic sufficiency* (PS) has been coined to designate patients with CF who have normal nutrient assimilation. However, this term does not imply that the func-

tional capacity of exocrine pancreas (i.e., ability to secrete zymogen, fluid, and electrolytes) is normal.

The exocrine pancreas has a large functional capacity; more than 98% of the pancreatic acinar reserve must be lost before signs and symptoms of maldigestion are evident (16,17). This was demonstrated by comparing fecal fat losses, obtained from 72-hour stool collections, with pancreatic secretion of enzymes obtained after direct pancreatic intubation studies. It generally is accepted that stool fat losses exceeding 7% of fat intake represents the threshold for developing pancreatic insufficiency. Healthy adult controls secreted pancreatic colipase (the essential coenzyme necessary for lipolysis) at a rate of approximately 10,000 units/kg body weight/hour. Patients with CF and PI were found to secrete very little colipase, usually less than 100 units/kg body weight/hour. Enzyme output among patients with CF with PS was extremely variable, spanning a 250-fold range. As can be seen in Figure 12–3, a few patients with CF with PS were capable of secreting normal quantities of colipase

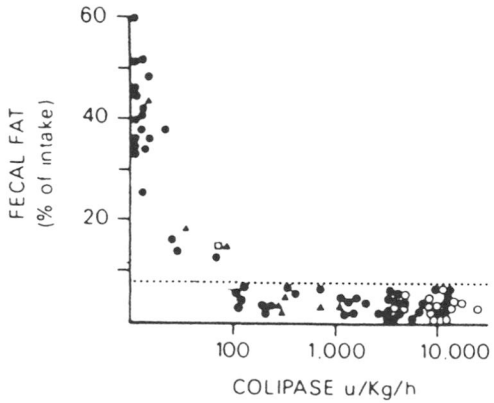

FIG. 12–3. Fecal fat losses, expressed as a percentage of fat intake plotted against pancreatic colipase secretion. Dotted horizontal line indicates 7% fat losses (upper limits of normal). Open circles, control subjects; closed circles, CF subjects; closed triangles, Shwachman syndrome; open square, patient with pancreatic hypoplasia. (Reprinted with permission from reference 17.)

when expressed as a percentage of the mean for normal control volunteers; the majority of patients with CF with PS secreted enzyme at or below the lower limit of the normal range or below. Thus, very little residual pancreatic function is required to prevent nutrient maldigestion—approximately 1% and 2% of residual pancreatic colipase and total lipase secretion, respectively.

PATHOPHYSIOLOGY OF PANCREATIC DISEASE IN CYSTIC FIBROSIS

In vivo studies of pancreatic secretions provide additional insights concerning the characteristics of pancreatic fluid and electrolyte secretions in both pancreatic-insufficient and pancreatic-sufficient patients with CF. Early studies performed by Hadorn et al. (18) showed evidence of deficient water and bicarbonate secretion from the pancreas of patients with CF after hormonal stimulation with intravenous secretin. Other investigators suggested that pancreatic secretions from patients with CF were rich in protein, particularly albumin (19). Unfortunately, these early studies were hampered by the fact that patients with CF were compared with normal controls and it was difficult to determine whether the observed secretory abnormalities were the result of an underlying primary CF defect or secondary to pathologic damage to the pancreas. We investigated a large number of patients with CF with a wide range of pancreatic function and compared pancreatic protein and water secretion in

patients with CF with matched non-CF subjects who had similar levels of pancreatic acinar function (20). Pancreatic acinar function in both groups extended from those with a severe deficit of function, within the pancreatic insufficient range, up to values within the normal range. We compared protein concentrations in three groups of patients with CF and non-CF patients—those with low, intermediate, and normal pancreatic function, which was defined by their ability to secrete pancreatic trypsin. Deficient fluid secretion was apparent in patients with CF in all three functional groups in comparison with matched non-CF controls. Total protein output (and albumin output) were not increased in CF in comparison with matched non-CF controls, but as a result of deficient fluid secretion, the protein concentration of the pancreatobiliary secretions was increased significantly in all three CF subgroups (Fig. 12–4). We demonstrated a significant correlation between protein and fluid secretion in the patients with CF, most of whom had fluid output below the lowest values obtained for the non-CF patients (less than 4.2 mL/kg body weight/hour).

A significant linear relationship existed between fluid and enzyme secretion in both the patients with CF and the non-CF controls (Fig. 12–5). No significant difference was observed in the slope of the regression lines, but at any given level of enzyme secretion, fluid secretion among subjects with CF was approximately 40% less than the corresponding non-CF value. Because data from patients with CF with se-

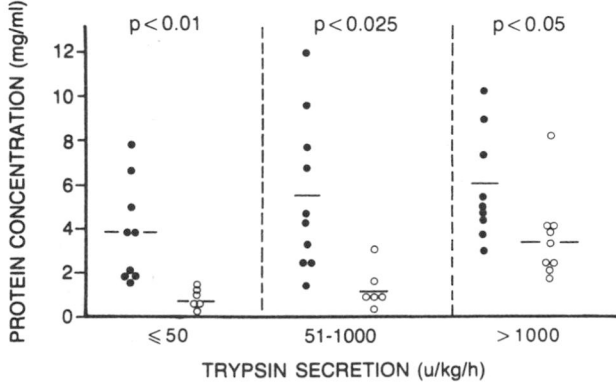

FIG. 12–4. Protein concentration of pancreaticobiliary secretions in patients with cystic fibrosis (solid circles) and controls (open circles) according to subgroups with low (< 50 units/kg/hour), intermediate (51 to 1,000 units/kg/hour), and normal (> 1,000 units/kg/hour) trypsin secretion. (Reprinted with permission from reference 20.)

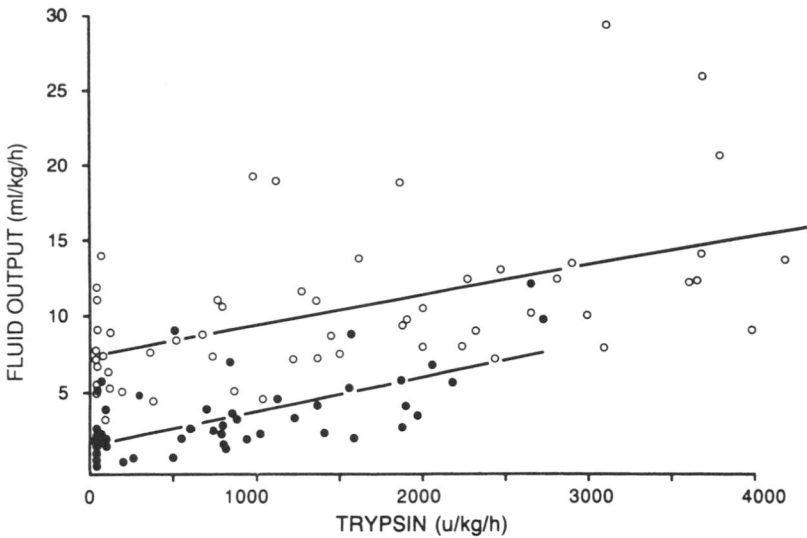

FIG. 12–5. Secretion of pancreaticobiliary fluid and trypsin in 56 patients with cystic fibrosis (closed circles) and 56 non-CF controls (open circles). There is a significant linear correction between fluid and trypsin output in the patients with CF and non-CF patients. The slopes of the two regression lines are not different. Mean fluid secretion in subjects with CF is significantly less than the non-CF controls. At any given level of trypsin secretion, patients with CF secrete less fluid (40% below non-CF values). (Reprinted with permission from reference 24.)

vere pancreatic damage could be affected by secondary pancreatic pathology, further analysis was performed in pancreatic-sufficient patients with CF, all of whom had trypsin output greater than the lower limits of the control range (> 1,000 units/kg body weight/hour). As shown in Table 12–1, acinar capacity (trypsin output) was identical in the CF and non-CF subgroups, but mean fluid secretion in the subjects with CF was diminished significantly.

Thus, from a pathophysiologic perspective, exocrine pancreatic disease in CF appears to develop as a result of deficient ductal fluid se-

TABLE 12–1. *Fluid secretion in CF and non-CF subjects with normal trypsin output (1000–2695 units/kg/hr)*

	CF	Non-CF	*P*
Trypsin (units/kg/hr)	1628 ± 459	1759 ± 491	NS
Fluid (mL/kg/hr)	6.08 ± 2.9	11.56 ± 4.3	<0.001

NS, not significant.

cretion coupled to normal protein load derived from acinar cell secretion, which leads to pancreatic protein hyperconcentration within the pancreatic ducts (Fig. 12–6). This process, in turn, predisposes to protein precipitation and obstruction within the pancreatic ducts leading to the well-recognized aforementioned secondary pathologic features. Indeed, the microscopic changes described in infants with CF with proteinaceous obstruction of dilated pancreatic ducts, and of cyst formation in some of older patients, clearly reflects this pathophysiologic process.

Physiologic studies of normal pancreatic ducts suggest that secretin-dependent bicarbonate secretion is the major driving force for fluid output (21). Isolated perfused pancreatic preparations provide good evidence of a chloride-dependent component of bicarbonate secretion (22). Because our studies suggested that impaired pancreatic fluid secretion is a primary phenomenon of CF, we examined the possibility that the CF pancreas is affected in a similar way to other epithelial tissue, particu-

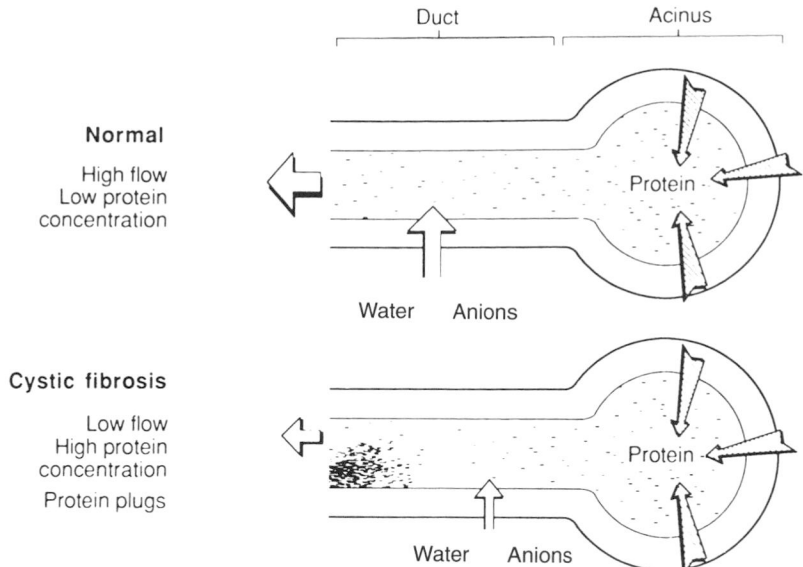

FIG. 12–6. Pancreatic pathophysiology in cystic fibrosis when ductal secretion is reduced because of decreased anion secretion; the protein concentration in the duct increases. High protein concentration increases susceptibility to precipitation and obstruction of duct lumina.

larly with respect to anion secretion. In this regard, fluid secretion likely is the consequence of net transport of electrolyte in the pancreatic duct. We demonstrated that both bicarbonate and chloride secretion was reduced significantly in CF, at all levels of acinar function (23,24). Both bicarbonate and chloride appear to be determinants of fluid secretion; at any given level of bicarbonate or chloride output, subjects with CF secreted significantly less fluid than control subjects. Thus, deficient fluid secretion in the pancreas of subjects with CF appears to be caused by reduced chloride and bicarbonate secretion, which almost certainly arise as a result of deficient or dysfunctional cystic fibrosis transmembrane conductance regulator (CFTR) chloride channel function in the apical surface of pancreatic ductal epithelia. Physiologic studies have demonstrated that chloride secretion in the pancreatic duct is required for ductal bicarbonate secretion. Specifically, luminal chloride is exchanged with intracellular bicarbonate at the ductal epithelial surface to promote bicarbonate secretion. Of interest, there was no difference in the ratio of these two anions between subjects with CF and

control subjects when patients with the same level of pancreatic acinar function were compared (25). This observation demonstrates that the lower fluid output in subjects with CF was not related to the chloride:bicarbonate ratio, but closely links chloride transport with bicarbonate transport in pancreatic ductal cells. In CF, impaired chloride secretion into the pancreatic duct, which is a prerequisite for chloride/bicarbonate exchange, accounts for the reduction in both chloride and bicarbonate secretion.

Histochemical studies of the normal human pancreas have localized the CFTR protein to intralobular duct cells and to pancreatic centroacinar cells (26). Antibodies to the CFTR protein appeared to be localized to the apical portion of these cells. These findings, therefore, suggest that small-duct epithelia play an important role in CF pathophysiology. Similar observations were made by Foulkes and Harris (27), who analyzed human fetal tissue by *in situ* hybridization using antisense RNA probes. High CFTR gene expression was observed in the epithelium of intralobular and small interlobular ducts. Kopelman et al. (28) applied

CFTR antisense oligonucleotides to pancreatic duct cells in tissue culture (PANC I) to demonstrate specific inhibition of cyclic adenosine monophosphate (cAMP)-activated conductance. Taken together, these studies confirm the key role of the CFTR in ductal epithelia of the pancreas.

PATIENTS WITH PANCREATIC INSUFFICIENCY

Exocrine Disease

Patients with the pancreatic insufficient phenotype are more likely to be diagnosed in infancy or childhood. In our experience, approximately 60% of patients are diagnosed before the age of 1 year and 85% before the age of 5 years. Growth failure and signs and symptoms of maldigestion, with or without pulmonary symptoms, are the frequent hallmarks of this condition in infancy and young children. The traditional stereotype, however, of a child with CF with wasting, abdominal protuberance, finger clubbing, a persisting cough, and foul, greasy, frequent stools is a relatively uncommon finding at diagnosis. In fact, chest symptoms may be absent or mild, and patients diagnosed in infancy or even at an older age may not experience failure to thrive. Hypoalbuminemia is a common finding in infancy (29,30). Edema and anemia, which are hallmarks of profound malnutrition, are less common, with a peak incidence at 3 to 4 months of age. Because edema may produce falsely low sweat chloride concentrations, it is wise to repeat a negative sweat test in such circumstances. Rectal prolapse occurs in 20% of patients, most commonly in those between 1 and 3 years of age (31). In up to half the cases, episodes of prolapse precede and should even suggest the diagnosis. Rectal prolapse, which is a self-limiting symptom, is extremely rare in adulthood. Remarkably, few patients with signs and symptoms of pancreatic insufficiency elude the diagnosis of CF in childhood.

The diagnosis of pancreatic insufficiency can be documented with the use of one or several indirect and/or direct tests of pancreatic function (see section on pancreatic function tests). Quantitative determination of fat losses over a 3- to 5-day period is perhaps the favored method of establishing the presence or absence of steatorrhea. Fecal fat losses are surprisingly variable from patient to patient. A small amount of residual endogenous secretion of enzymes (within the pancreatic insufficient range) partially accounts for this variability (17). A baseline fecal fat measurement, before commencing enzyme replacement therapy, may provide useful clinical information for the patient who fails to respond appropriately to enzyme supplements. In such circumstances, a second fecal fat study, while the patient is receiving enzyme therapy, may provide a useful guide before dosing adjustments or adjuvants are considered (see section on enzyme therapy).

A small percentage of patients are pancreatic sufficient at diagnosis but will progress to PI after varying periods of time (32,33). This is more likely to occur in infancy. Newborn screening studies reveal that a significant percentage of asymptomatic infants are pancreatic sufficient initially, only to progress to pancreatic-insufficient status within the first year or two of life (34). Approximately 15% of patients diagnosed conventionally, on the basis of suggestive signs and symptoms, remain pancreatic sufficient. As will be discussed in more detail subsequently, the pancreatic-insufficient and pancreatic-sufficient phenotypes are determined genetically on the basis of specific CFTR gene mutations. In most individuals who carry mutations that confer the pancreatic-insufficient phenotype, significant pancreatic damage develops at a very early age, usually beginning *in utero*. Thus, genotyping provides useful prognostic information about pancreatic exocrine status in adult subjects with CF. Individuals with two PI mutations almost without exception will have the PI phenotype at diagnosis or will progress to PI at a relatively early age. Those with one or two PS mutations are more likely to maintain a PS phenotype.

At diagnosis, fat-soluble vitamin deficiencies are a common biochemical observation, but clinical manifestations are rare (35). Bruising or intracranial hemorrhage have been reported during the neonatal period due to vitamin K deficiency (36). Biochemical evidence of vitamin E deficiency is common at diagnosis (37). Clinical sequelae, including ophthalmoplegia, absent deep tendon reflexes, hand tremors, and ataxia, have been reported in late adolescents and adult patients with CF, which suggests that vitamin E deficiency occurs as a late sequela of malabsorption (38). Most patients with clinical evidence of vitamin E deficiency have had significant CF-associated liver disease as well, possibly exacerbating vitamin E malabsorption. Vitamin A status of patients tends to mirror that of vitamin E. Signs and symptoms of rickets are rare, but older children and adults, particularly those with chronic malnutrition, have evidence of bony demineralization (see Chapter 18) (39). Vitamin B12 may be malabsorbed in untreated pancreatic-insufficient patients, but megaloblastic anemia has not been reported in treated patients, because pancreatic enzyme supplements facilitate B12-intrinsic factor binding. Most patients with PI have low plasma and tissue levels of linoleic acid, but symptomatic essential fatty acid deficiency is rare (40).

Endocrine Disease

Diabetes mellitus, which was first recognized as a complication of CF in the 1950s, previously was believed to be an uncommon complication (41). This probably reflected poor survival among patients with CF in earlier decades. Subsequently, in direct association with a dramatic improvement in survival, the prevalence of CF-related diabetes (CFRD) has increased (42,43). A 5-year prospective study of 191 patients with CF demonstrated the cumulative incidence of CFRD is 24% in patients aged 20 years and 76% in those aged 30 years (43). Although not well documented in this study, only patients with PI appear to be at increased risk of developing CFRD. Among 307 patients attending the Toronto Adult CF Clinic, 53 developed or had CFRD over a preceding 5-year period. All 53 patients were pancreatic insufficient (D. Wilson et al., unpublished observation, 1997).

CFRD differs from type 1 (insulin-dependent) or type 2 (non-insulin-dependent) diabetes mellitus, with respect to both etiology and clinical presentation (see Chapter 18). It is speculated that glucose intolerance is caused by a deficiency of insulin as a result of a reduction in the beta cell mass in pancreatic islets (44). In keeping with this supposition is the age-related increase in prevalence of CFRD, together with its strong association with pancreatic insufficiency. From a pathologic perspective, the pancreas becomes fibrotic with disruption of pancreatic architecture, which with time may cause disorganization and strangulation of the islets. Pathologic studies show reduction in the density of pancreatic islets in patients with CF compared with diabetic patients without CF; patients with CFRD have an even greater reduction in pancreatic islet cell density (44). Interestingly, glucose intolerance occurs in CFRD with less severe beta cell destruction than in type 1 diabetes. However, cells that produce other regulatory hormones, such as glucagon, somatostatin, and pancreatic polypeptide, which are located in the periphery of the islets, appear to be relatively preserved in CFRD. Islet cell antibodies are present in the occasional patients with CFRD but not to the same extent as seen in type 1 diabetes.

Clinical signs and symptoms of diabetes due to CFRD usually are quite mild and controlled easily with small doses of insulin. High basal and postglucose-stimulated gastric inhibitory peptide levels are found once carbohydrate intolerance develops. Hyperglycemia due to diabetes is known to have detrimental effects on the nutritional status, including derangement in protein metabolism (45). Furthermore, it is becoming recognized increasingly that well-controlled patients with CFRD are at risk of developing all the well-known complications associated with long-standing diabetes mellitus, including retinopathy, nephropathy, neuropathy, and hypertension.

Unlike the typical signs and symptoms of type 1 diabetes, which are easily recognized clinically, patients with CFRD frequently deny symptoms. In a recent study of 50 patients with CF, no clinical or biochemical parameter reliably established a diagnosis of CFRD other than a formal oral glucose intolerance test. This was confirmed by a prospective study of 191 Danish patients in whom symptoms of glycosuria, fasting hyperglycemia, or increased levels of glycosylated hemoglobin failed to reliably identify patients with CFRD (43).

PATIENTS WITH PANCREATIC SUFFICIENCY

Cross-sectional analysis of large CF populations of a heterogeneous ethnic background reveal that approximately 10% to 15% of patients possess sufficient pancreatic exocrine function (PS) for normal digestion (15). In this subgroup of patients, relentless progression of pancreatic disease either does not occur or seems to be retarded for many decades. Pancreatic morphology has been studied in very few of these patients, but available evidence suggests that many of these patients do possess significant pancreatic damage. Portions of the pancreas may become atrophic, and, in areas of relative preservation, there appears to be plugging within large and small ducts and variable amounts of fibrosis. In approximately 50% of these patients, however, pancreatic enzyme secretion is within the normal range, suggesting that the pathologic damage is minimal. Quantitative pancreatic function studies also show evidence of a primary defect of anion secretion (Cl^- and HCO_3^-) and reduced fluid secretion (see above, "Pathophysiology of Pancreatic Disease").

Our studies of exocrine pancreatic function of conventionally diagnosed patients with CF have helped delineate specific clinical characteristics of this disease among patients with the pancreatic-insufficient and pancreatic-sufficient phenotypes. Clearly, the presence or absence of exocrine PS plays a significant role in determining overall prognosis. Those with pancreatic sufficiency are diagnosed at a later age, experience milder symptoms and, as a group, far superior overall prognosis than their counterparts with PI (15). Specifically, patients with CF with PS have lower mean sweat chloride concentrations, maintain better pulmonary function with age, and are less likely to have chronic pulmonary

colonization with *Pseudomonas aeruginosa* or *Burkholderia cepacia* infections. This fascinating subgroup of patients grow normally in childhood and as a general rule do not experience nutritional difficulties in adulthood. Survival is far superior to those with PI. Between 1970 and 1982, there were 123 deaths from CF in the Toronto clinic; only 3 of these patients had pancreatic sufficiency. Two of these patients were in extremely good health, with essentially normal pulmonary function before death, but succumbed after acute sepsis and pulmonary invasion with *B. cepacia*. Other common gastrointestinal complications often recognized in patients with CF, including hepatobiliary disease and distal intestinal obstruction syndrome (meconium ileus equivalent), rarely are encountered in patients with PS. Acute recurrent pancreatitis, conversely, is a relatively common clinical complication (46,47). This is not too surprising because of the preservation of pancreatic acinar tissue which, together with the underlying tendency to intrapancreatic ductal obstruction, could lead to recurrent episodes of pancreatic inflammation. In our experience, and in the experience of others, up to 10% of patients with CF with the pancreatic-sufficient phenotype will experience this complication. Not infrequently, acute recurrent pancreatitis is the presenting symptom at diagnosis, particularly in adolescence and adulthood (48–50).

GENOTYPE STUDIES

Before the discovery of the CFTR gene, family studies suggested that genetic factors may influence the degree of pancreatic disease and possibly its rate of progression. An analysis of 63 families with more than one sibling with CF demonstrated that individuals within families were highly concordant for pancreatic function status (51). Specifically, in 46 families, all siblings had documented PI requiring oral enzyme replacement therapy, and in 9 families, all siblings had PS. Pancreatic function status was discordant in siblings from eight families at diagnosis, but five of these families became concordant with time. In at least one of the siblings who had pancreatic sufficiency at diagnosis, pancreatic insufficiency developed at a late stage. The remarkable agreement of pancreatic function test data within families suggested that pancreatic status (PS or PI) represented distinct phenotypic expression of CF, possibly reflecting different mutations in the CFTR gene. This was confirmed by genetic investigation of the haplotype distribution of DNA probes closely linked to the CF locus (52), which showed a different distribution of haplotypes among CF chromosomes from pancreatic-sufficient patients in comparison with those from patients with PI.

Since the CFTR gene was cloned in 1989 (53–55), more extensive genotype–phenotype correlations have been made, which shed further light on these clinical observations. When the most common CFTR gene mutation (ΔF508) was identified, a hypothesis was proposed that "mild" and "severe" CFTR mutations exist; patients with the PI phenotype would be expected to carry two "severe" CFTR gene mutations, whereas those with one or two "mild" mutations would have the PS

phenotype (55). The most common mutation, ΔF508, would be classified as a "severe" mutation because 98% of patients homozygous for this mutation were pancreatic insufficient (56). Unlike other manifestations of CF disease, the exocrine pancreas exhibits a remarkable correlation between genotype and phenotype. Because 85% of patients with CF have PI, it is estimated that more than 90% of the CF chromosomes carry mutations (including ΔF508) that are severe, whereas approximately 10% have mutations that are "mild" with respect to the pancreas. In general, all mutations classified as nonsense, frameshift, and amino acid deletions and some missense and splice site mutations will be considered severe and therefore confer the PI phenotype (57). However, some missense mutations and splice site defects may be associated with PS (Table 12–2). The majority of patients carrying one or two "mild" mutations maintain PS for many years, even decades. However, pancreatic-sufficient patients require close monitoring of pancreatic status.

TABLE 12–2. *Examples of "mild" and "severe" cystic fibrosis transmembrane conductance regulator gene mutations*

Mutations	Severe	Mild
Missense	I148T	G91R
	G480C	E92K
	V520F	R117H
	G551D	P205S
	A599T	R334W
	R560T	R347P
	G1242E	R347H
	S1255P	A455E
	N1303K	G551S
	G1349D	Y563N
		P574H
Amino acid deletion	ΔF508	
	ΔI507	
Stop codon	Q493X	
	G542X	
	R553X	
	R1162X	
	W1282X	
Splice junction	621 + 1G → T	2789 + 5G → A
	1717 − 1G → T	3849 + 10kbC → T
Frame shift	556delA	
	1078delT	
	3659delC	
	3905insT	

Modified from reference 57.

A small subset of patients carrying "severe" CFTR gene mutations may be pancreatic sufficient initially, then may develop PI. This observation is especially true at an early age, especially if patients are diagnosed by neonatal screening. Waters et al. (34) showed that up to 38% of screened infants with CF are pancreatic sufficient on the basis of fecal studies. In the majority, however, PI develops at an early age. In our experience, the majority of pancreatic-sufficient patients in whom PI develops carry "severe" mutations. Quantitative analysis of pancreatic secretions in these patients, however, reveal that they have an extremely low pancreatic reserve (33). The occasional patient with a "mild" CFTR gene mutation on one or both alleles may suffer recurrent bouts of pancreatitis. Acute pancreatitis, in turn, may induce progressive pancreatic damage, and PI may ensue over many years.

MOLECULAR MECHANISMS OF CYSTIC FIBROSIS TRANSMEMBRANE CONDUCTANCE REGULATOR DYSFUNCTION AND THE EXOCRINE PANCREAS

Mutations in the gene-encoding CFTR could produce a loss of chloride channels or their dysfunction in a variety of ways. Tsui (58) was the first to categorize CFTR mutations into specific classes according to their presumed functional properties as a small conductance chloride channel. It was recognized that this classification system does not account for the possibility that CFTR may have additional intracellular roles, such as acid–base control within organelles, and additional cell membrane effects, such as an influence on sodium reabsorption.

In this classification system, mutations are grouped into five general classes (Fig. 12–7) (58,59). Class I CFTR mutations result from ineffective synthesis of a full-length normal CFTR polypeptide. Nonsense and frameshift mutations or aberrant splicing of mRNA would be examples of Class I mutations. Class II mutations include those in which there is intracellular arrest of the mature protein. Intracellular protein trafficking and maturation is an extremely complex, poorly understood process,

but it is not too surprising that several CFTR mutations behave in such a way. ΔF508, the most common CFTR gene mutation, is an example of a Class II mutation. The ΔF508 protein becomes mislocalized within epithelial cells because of improper folding. The efficiency of intracellular processing is temperature sensitive; at low temperature, the protein moves through the endoplasmic reticulum normally and after glycosylation in the Golgi apparatus reaches the apical membrane, where it functions normally as a chloride channel. Mutant CFTR proteins belonging to Class III include those that are processed appropriately and localized within the apical membrane but are unable to respond to agonists and therefore function as chloride channels. Perhaps the most common example of a Class III mutation is the missense mutation G551D. Many Class III mutations possess amino acid alterations that affect adenosine triphosphate (ATP) binding. Because CFTR mutations belonging to Classes I, II, and III lack chloride channel activity in the apical membrane, it is possible to predict that they all confer a "severe" pancreatic phenotype. Indeed, to date, all patients carrying mutations on both alleles belonging to these three functional classes possess the pancreatic-insufficient phenotype.

A number of CFTR mutations have been classified as Class IV mutations. The majority carry mutations that are located in areas corresponding to the transmembrane segments; these appear to cause alterations in conductance and/or gating properties of the chloride channel. The most common CFTR gene mutation in this group is R117H, which shows reduced conductivity *in vitro*. Class IV mutations, recognized to date, confer the pancreatic sufficient phenotype in the majority of patients. Class V mutations are associated with reduced synthesis of the normal CFTR. CFTR mutations in this class might include promoter mutations, those that promote alternate splicing of the CFTR transcript, or missense mutations that affect protein maturation. Currently, most CFTR mutations identified as Class V mutants are the result of alternatively spliced mRNA. Clearly, the relative amount of normal mRNA and protein that is made can be quite variable from one individual to another;

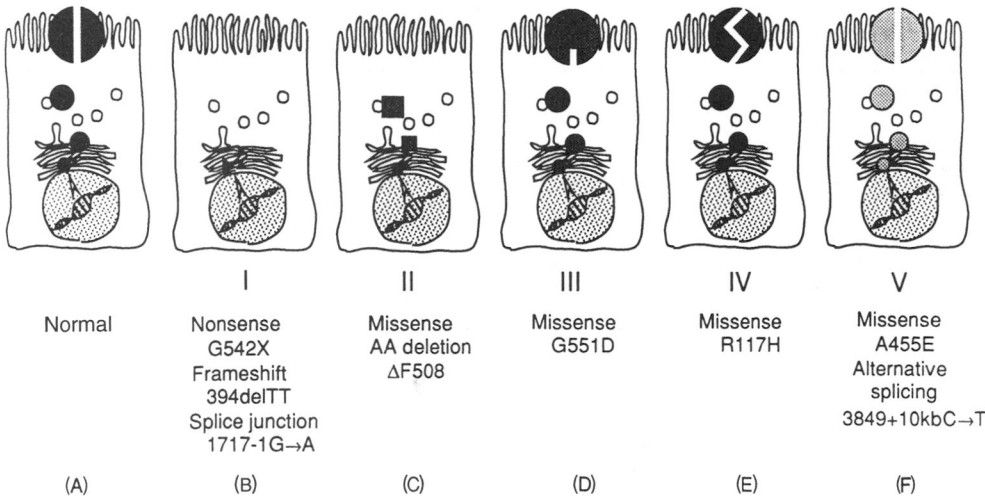

FIG. 12–7. CFTR gene mutations classified according to functional properties of the protein product. **(A),** Normal CFTR is positioned correctly at the apical membrane of an epithelial cell and functions as a chloride channel. **(B),** Class I: no CFTR mRNA or CFTR protein is found (e.g., nonsense frameshift of splice site mutation). **(C),** Class II: trafficking defect; CFTR mRNA formed but protein fails to traffic to the cellular membrane. **(D),** Class III: regulation defect; CFTR protein reaches the apical membrane but fails to respond to stimulation by cAMP. **(E),** Class IV: channel defect; CFTR functions as a chloride channel but with altered properties. **(F),** Class V: synthesis defect; reduced synthesis or defective processing of CFTR protein; chloride channel properties are normal.

consequently, symptoms might vary considerably as well. The most common alternative splicing mutation in this class is 3849 + 10KB C → T. Individuals with this mutation have been known to have either the pancreatic-insufficient or the pancreatic-sufficient phenotype. A few missense mutations, notably A455E and P574H, appear to have normal chloride channel-gating properties and so it is assumed that the mutant protein is processed ineffectively. Although the majority of patients with this mutation are pancreatic sufficient, some individuals have the pancreatic-insufficient phenotype. The variable phenotype may be explained by variations in the efficiency of protein maturation from individual to individual.

PANCREATIC FUNCTION TESTS

In patients with CF, pancreatic function assessment is required in several clinical circumstances. Pancreatic function status (PS or PI) of all newly diagnosed patients must be assessed. Those with PS require systematic longitudinal monitoring of pancreatic function. The re-

sponse to pancreatic enzyme therapy of pancreatic-insufficient patients will need assessment if persistent maldigestion is suspected. Finally, in rare cases, where the diagnosis of CF remains uncertain, certain pancreatic function tests are of some value as a diagnostic tool.

Because the pancreas and its secretions are anatomically inaccessible, exocrine pancreatic function is difficult to quantitate. All currently available tests have drawbacks—at least one, and in most cases, several. As shown in Table 12–3, pancreatic function tests may be categorized into three general groups (60). Direct tests are largely invasive techniques that permit direct sampling of pancreatic secretions. Indirect tests rely on some secondary effect of pancreatic dysfunction. Blood tests are dependent on the fact that small quantities of pancreatic enzymes (or pancreatic hormones) are detectable in the circulation.

Direct Tests

Direct tests permit the pancreatic functional reserve to be assessed. Under physiologic con-

TABLE 12–3. *Tests of exocrine pancreatic function*

Direct tests	Indirect tests	Blood tests
Exogenous stimulants	Stool	Isoamylase
Secretin	Microscopy—fat, meat fibers	Lipase
Cholecystokinin[a]	Steatocrit	Cationic/anionic trypsinogen
Cerulein[a]	Fecal balance studies	Pancreatic polypeptide
Bombesin	Dual radiolabelled fat	
	Trypsin, chymotrypsin, elastase	
Nutrient stimulants		
Lundh test meal	Breath	
Fatty acids	^{14}C-lipids	
Amino acids	^{13}C-lipids	
Hydrochloric acid	^{14}C-cholesterol octanoate	
Bile salts	Starch breath hydrogen tests	
	Urine/plasma markers	
	Bentiromide	
	Fluorescein dilaurate (pancreolauryl)	
	Oral tolerance tests (fat and vitamins)	
	Dual-label Schilling test	
	Urinary lactulose	

[a]Used in various dose combinations with or without secretin.

ditions, ingestion of a meal induces the exocrine pancreas to secrete fluid and ions in response to several hormonal and neural stimuli. These include hormone release [cholecystokinin (CCK) and secretin] from the proximal intestine and neural stimulation via a rich supply of vagal afferents that act on muscarinic receptors. Direct pancreatic function testing uses one or both of these pathways by supplying either exogenous hormones or intestinal nutrients and duodenal aspiration of pancreatic secretions under stimulated conditions. Successful quantitation of human pancreatic secretions, therefore, relies on the ability to quantitatively collect both acinar and ductal secretions.

There is no standard method for administration of exogenous hormones to stimulate the exocrine pancreas (60). The dose and nature of hormones used, the mode of administration (intravenous bolus or constant intravenous infusion), and the duration of infusion varies from center to center; in the case of combined hormones, the sequence of administration also may differ. Synthetic preparations of secretin and CCK may be preferable to animal extracts because they are not contaminated with other gut-derived peptides and are less allergenic. Other investigators have used CCK-like hormones such as cerulein or bombesin.

The test established in our unit is based on methodologies developed by investigators at the Mayo Clinic in 1970 (61). As shown in Figure 12–8, the technique involves nasoduodenal intubation with a double lumen tube containing two ports: one port is positioned opposite the ampulla of Vater to permit a constant perfusion of an isotonic, nonabsorbable marker solution; a second port, situated distally at the ligament of Treitz, is used for collection, by aspiration, of mixed pancreatic secretions and marker solution. A separate gastric tube removes gastric contents to avoid contamination of the duodenal contents and to assess for evidence of duodenogastric reflux of the nonabsorbable marker.

Losses of pancreatic juice from the distal duodenal collection port are accounted for by calculating the percent recovery of the infused marker. After a period of equilibration, mixed pancreatic and biliary secretions are collected for 1 hour (three 20-minute collection periods) while continuously infusing with intravenous CCK and secretin. Each hormone is provided at a dose sufficient to induce maximal pancreatic stimulation. When carefully performed, this test provides precise information regarding pancreatic enzyme, fluid, and electrolyte secretion. It is particularly useful for precisely

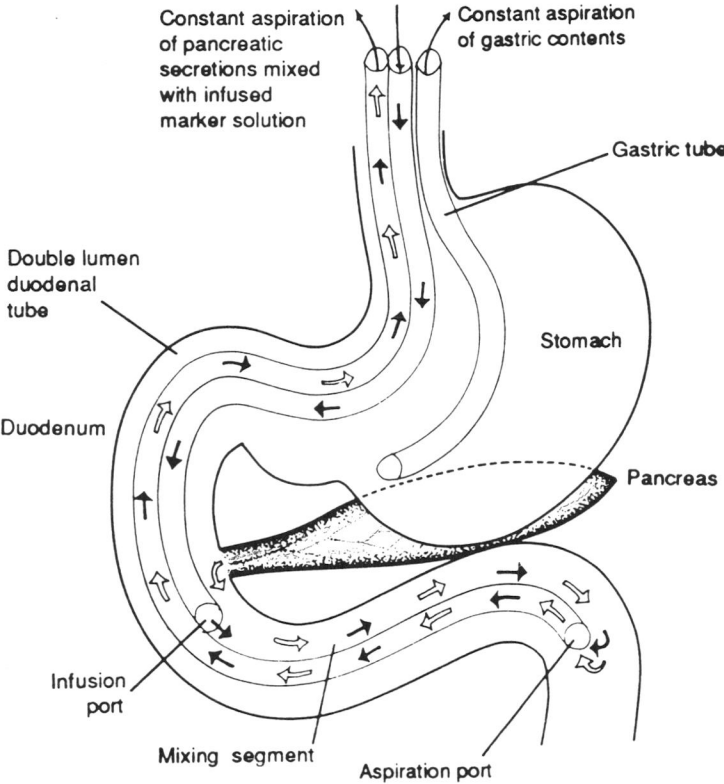

FIG. 12–8. Schematic diagram of the direct quantitative pancreatic function test. Gastric secretions are removed via a nasogastric tube. A nonabsorbable marker is perfused at a constant rate, in an isoosmotic solution, via the proximal port of a double lumen nasoduodenal tube. The proximal port is situated at the ampulla of Vater. After a period of equilibration, pancreatic secretions are stimulated maximally with intravenous hormones [cholecystokinin (CCK) and/or secretin]. Pancreatic secretions mix with the infused marker solution in the duodenum, and the mixture is aspirated over a defined period of time via the distal port. The distal port is situated close to the ligament of Treitz.

defining pancreatic reserve in a patient suspected of PS and in some instances is a useful aid for confirming the diagnosis of CF (17). Unfortunately, the complex, time-consuming, and invasive nature of the test severely limits its utility for routine clinical assessment.

An alternative, semiquantitative direct method of assessing exocrine pancreatic function uses nutrients to endogenously stimulate the pancreas. The most-used method, the Lundh meal, involves ingestion of a liquid test meal composed of dry milk, vegetable oil, and dextrose (62). This approach is more physiologic be-cause it relies on endogenous release of hormones as well as vagal stimuli. Unfortunately, the presence of nutrients in the collections render enzymatic determination difficult in the laboratory. In addition, lack of a duodenal marker perfusate, coupled with the presence of salivary and gastric secretions in the aspirate, makes this test relatively qualitative. Other nutrients have been used. The most potent nutrient stimuli are essential amino acids, particularly phenylalanine, but methionine, valine, and tryptophan also have been shown to stimulate pancreatic secretions (63). Amino acids may be given as a duodenal infusion, together with a nonabsorbable marker. Because amino acids do not interfere with enzymatic determinations, more accurate quantitation is to be expected. Alternative approaches have used dilute hydrochloric acid and bile acids as stimulants, but these approaches have not gained wide acceptance.

Indirect Tests

A variety of indirect tests are available, all of which rely on the secondary effects of pancreatic dysfunction (see Table 12–3). Some rely on measurement of fecal products of maldigestion, whereas others depend on the ability of pancreatic enzymes to cleave specific substrates, which generate measurable end-products that are detectable in breath, blood, or urine. Most of these tests cannot reliably assess exocrine pancreatic reserve of pancreatic-sufficient patients. In addition, nonpancreatic causes of malabsorption and/or maldigestion may be difficult to exclude. However, many indirect tests offer the advantage of being relatively cheap to perform and are noninvasive; others, for example, fecal fat determination, can be used to evaluate the efficacy of pancreatic enzyme supplementation in subjects with PI.

Microscopic stool examination is a useful, qualitative test (64). In pancreatic-insufficient patients, meat fibers or neutral fat droplets may be detected. The presence of neutral fat droplets in fecal specimens do not differentiate pancreatic from nonpancreatic causes of maldigestion. Several stains can be used to identify neutral fat, although fat droplets can be seen readily without staining. If stool is obtained by rectal examination, lubricants containing oil or petroleum jelly should be avoided. Although, somewhat crude, stool microscopy is a useful screening test to confirm the presence of PI in a newly diagnosed patient with CF.

The steatocrit method operates on the principle that stool within a hematocrit tube can be separated into lipid, liquid, and solid phases by centrifugation (65). Reference values and ranges have been established, and several modifications have been advocated to improve sensitivity. This test may be a useful adjunct in centers with limited technical expertise and provides a crude method for monitoring the response to pancreatic enzyme supplement therapy.

Perhaps the most widely used stool tests involve pooled fecal collections over a period of 72 to 96 hours. All major nutrients classes (fat, protein, and carbohydrate), or total energy content, may be measured (60). None of these tests discriminate patients with pancreatic and nonpancreatic causes of malabsorption. Unfortunately, the unpleasant nature of stool tests for both patients and laboratory technicians has limited their acceptance. Alternative tests using isotopic markers are expensive, are almost as inconvenient, and offer no real advantage. Fecal fat determination remains the most frequently used method. In adults, the test involves consuming a daily diet containing 100 g of fat. Stools are collected, pooled, and refrigerated. The accuracy of collection can be improved by using a nonabsorbable marker at the start and the end of the collection period. Steatorrhea is considered to be present if more than 7% of ingested fat is detected in the feces. The potential for error is great because of incomplete stool collections, inaccurate quantitation of intake, and, in the occasional patient, altered intestinal transit. Similar results are obtained by fecal determination of fecal energy, by bomb calorimetry, or by fecal nitrogen analysis.

The capacity to measure the fecal enzymes has existed for many years (66). A number of potential problems exist with these tests. Pancreatic enzymes are subject to proteolytic degradation by both pancreatic and bacterial proteases. Pancreatic chymotrypsin and a more recently established immunoassay method for detecting pancreatic elastase are favored because they are more resistant to inactivation by colonic bacteria. Chymotrypsin may be bound strongly to insoluble stool residue. However, a commercial test employs a detergent to solubilize fecal chymotrypsin stool (67). Fecal chymotrypsin is relatively stable at 18°C for up to 72 hours and thus can be sent, without refrigeration, to a reference laboratory. Because false-positive measurements will occur in patients receiving oral pancreatic enzymes, supplements should be discontinued at least 5 days before measurement (67). A recently described immunoassay method for detecting human pancreatic elastase is of potential value for assessment during enzyme therapy (68) because it does not cross-react with porcine elastase. At best, fecal enzymes are a useful screening tool for differentiating between pancreatic-insufficient and pancreatic-sufficient patients.

Breath tests rely on metabolism of an orally administered substrate that releases a freely diffusible gas that is excreted by the lungs. Substrate selection is based on the need for pancreatic digestion, and the exhaled gas may indicate either a deficiency or intactness of a digestive process. For example, ingested lipids are hydrolyzed predominantly by pancreatic lipases in the small intestine, absorbed as free fatty acids and monoglycerides, and transported to the liver where oxidative metabolism liberates CO_2. A radiolabelled breath test takes the advantage of this fact by using either [14]C- or ^{13}C-labelled triglycerides as substrate (69,70). Three triglycerides containing different carbon chain links length (trioctanoin, tripalmitate, and triolein) have been evaluated. All three substrates are capable of detecting fat malabsorption, but they vary in their ability to differentiate between pancreatic and nonpancreatic causes. Because trioctanoin is limited by lipolysis alone, it can be used to distinguish PI from hepatic or mucosal causes of malabsorption. Different lipid substrates used in sequence, for example, by testing with triolein and repeating the test with trioctanoin, may improve test specificity. An alternative approach is to perform a two-stage test using the same substrate, with and without administration of oral pancreatic enzymes. [14]C cholesterol octanoate, which is hydrolyzed by the pancreatic-specific cholesterol esterase, also has been used as a substrate (71). Starch also has been used successfully as a substrate using a [13]CO_2 breath test as a marker of pancreatic disease (72).

Nonradioactive breath tests have been developed, using expired hydrogen as the marker.

Dietary starch normally is cleaved enzymatically into oligosaccharides by pancreatic isoamylase before further cleavage by brush border disaccharidases. When pancreatic amylase secretion is impaired, undigested starch is consumed by colonic bacteria, generating hydrogen, which is excreted in the breath. A two-stage test, with and without adjunctive oral pancreatic enzymes, can help to distinguish pancreatic from nonpancreatic causes of steatorrhea (73). Unfortunately, the test is relatively cumbersome, requiring 2 days to complete. Furthermore, a significant percentage of healthy individuals do not harbor hydrogen-producing bacteria in the colon, particularly if patients are receiving antibiotic prophylaxis or recently have completed a course of antibiotics. At best, breath tests are qualitative measures of exocrine pancreatic function; very few have been adopted for routine clinical purposes.

An alternative approach involves the use of an orally ingested substrate, which is cleaved by a pancreatic enzyme, releasing a marker that is measured in plasma or urine. The most commonly used tests are bentiromide and the pancreolauryl test. The principles of the two tests are similar. In the case of bentiromide, a nonabsorbable synthetic peptide (*N*-benzoyl-l-tyrosyl-*p*-aminobenzoic acid), when given by mouth, is cleaved by pancreatic chymotrypsin in the upper small intestine, releasing the marker, paraaminobenzoic acid (PABA) (74). PABA is absorbed rapidly, conjugated in the liver, and excreted in the urine. PABA can be measured in both blood and urine by a colorimetric assay or by high-performance liquid chromatography (HPLC) (75,76). False abnormal results have been demonstrated in subjects with bowel, liver, or renal disease because of defects in absorption, conjugation, or excretion of PABA. Additionally, both intestinal bacteria in the intestinal brush border may demonstrate chymotrypsin-like activity, which in turn reduces specificity (77,78). Ingestion of a number of drugs and foods may result in elevated aromatic amines that interfere with the colorimetric determination of PABA. HPLC techniques are more specific for the detection of

PABA and its metabolites (76). If the urine test is used, a 500-mg dose of bentiromide is recommended with clear fluids (79). The urine recovery of PABA from a 6-hour collection is expressed as the percentage of the orally ingested PABA. Less than 50% PABA excretion purportedly reflects PI. To correct for potential problems with absorption, hepatic conjugation, or excretion of the drug, several modifications have been proposed, including a two-stage test with an equivalent dose of free PABA or coadministration of radiolabelled PABA, or a free structural analogue of PABA, such as p-amino salicylic acid (PAS) (80,81). Experience in both children and adults suggest that the test is best conducted by measuring PABA in plasma (75,82). This obviates the need for lengthy urine collections, and most studies demonstrate improved sensitivity (Fig. 12–9). Test sensitivity may be improved further by administering bentiromide with a liquid meal.

The pancreolauryl test uses oral fluorescein dilaurate, which is capable of being hydrolyzed by pancreatic cholesterol esterase (60). The marker fluorescein is liberated, readily absorbed in the small intestine, partially conjugated in the liver, and excreted in the urine, predominantly as fluorescein diglucuronide. In adults, fluorescein dilaurate is ingested with a standard meal, and urine is collected over a 10-hour period (83–85). Some investigators advocate a second test with equimolar-free fluorescein to correct for differences in intestinal absorption. A more convenient serum test has been developed. The pancreolauryl test has similar advantages and disadvantages to the bentiromide test.

Blood Tests

Pancreatic enzymes are detectable in small quantities in the circulation of healthy individ-

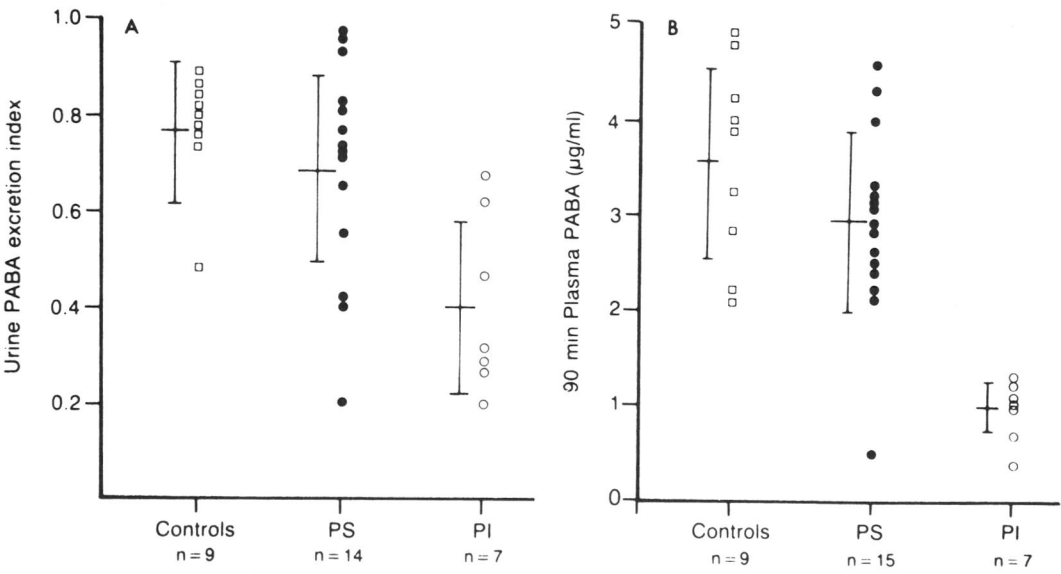

FIG. 12–9. (A), Urine paraaminobenzoic acid (PABA) excretion index is shown for controls, patients with pancreatic sufficiency (PS), and patients with pancreatic insufficiency (PI). The mean PABA excretion index for the patients with PI is significantly lower than means for controls and subjects with PS ($P < 0.001$). However, there are numerous false-positive and false-negative results. **(B),** Plasma PABA levels obtained in the same subjects at the same time as the urine collection. Mean plasma PABA concentration is significantly lower than the means for controls and subjects with PS ($P < 0.0001$). Only one false-positive result was observed in a patient who had low pancreatic function at the threshold for developing PI. (Reprinted from reference 75.)

uals. Some enzymes, such as pancreatic lipase and amylase, are present in the circulation as active enzymes, whereas most proteases (e.g., trypsinogen and chymotrypsinogen) are present in the inactive or proenzyme form (60,86). High concentrations of circulating pancreatic enzymes are recognized in three clinical situations: acute pancreatitis, pancreatic ductal obstruction, and impaired renal function. In acute pancreatitis, enzymes are released from acinar cells directly into the circulation as a consequence of pancreatic acinar cell injury. Renal disease will result in increased concentrations of circulating pancreatic enzymes because of reduced clearance. In pancreatic ductal obstruction, high circulating enzyme concentrations are believed to be the result of the regurgitant release of enzymes from acini or ducts. CF is a good example of the latter mechanism because obstruction is believed to be a primary complication of pancreatic disease due to inspissated secretions. Low circulating pancreatic enzyme concentrations, conversely, would

be expected if pancreatic acinar cell mass is reduced greatly because of atrophy.

Previously, the lack of specificity of biochemical determinations of enzymes limited their usefulness for assessing pancreatic disease. Currently, highly specific immunoassay techniques are available that are capable of detecting nanogram concentrations of enzymes. In CF, immunoassays for human cationic trypsin(ogen) has received the most attention. In 1979, Crossley and colleagues (87) first noted that infants with CF had high circulated concentrations of immunoreactive trypsin(ogen). This observation led to the development of the serum trypsinogen [immunoreactive trypsin (IRT)] test for newborn screening of CF. This technique also has been used to assess pancreatic dysfunction, but in CF, there are significant age-related limitations (88). Serum trypsinogen concentrations are many-fold elevated in both pancreatic-sufficient and pancreatic-insufficient infants with CF. This probably reflects the presence of ductal obstruction of dis-

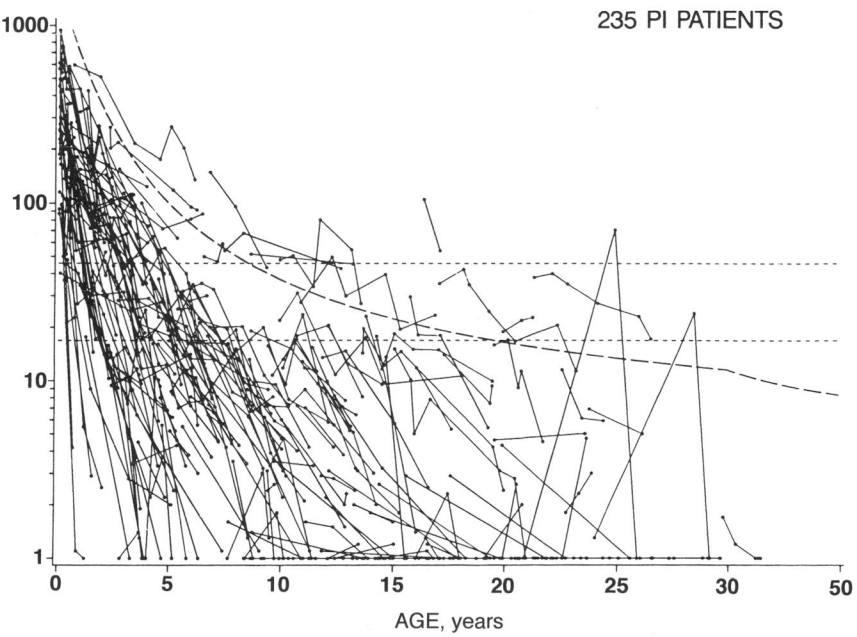

FIG. 12–10. Serial measurements of serum immunoreactive trypsinogen in 233 patients with CF with pancreatic insufficiency. Parallel dotted lines indicate the normal range of values. The dashed line indicates the upper limit of the 95% confidence interval for measurements obtained from cross-sectional data.

tal to functional acinar tissue. In subjects with PI, serum trypsinogen values decrease rapidly, reaching low or undetectable values by 5 to 7 years of age (Fig. 12–10). After 7 years of age, 95% of patients with PI have serum trypsinogen levels two standard deviations below the mean for a control population. This almost certainly reflects progressive acinar atrophy. In contrast, 96% of patients with PS have trypsinogen levels within or above the non-CF range at all ages. Serial assessment of pancreatic-sufficient patients with CF show widely fluctuating trypsinogen concentrations ranging from normal to values well above the normal range (Fig. 12–11) (32). Patients who progress from PS to PI exhibit a pattern different from those who maintain PS (32). This small patient group exhibited a progressive decrease in serum trypsinogen levels after a similar but delayed pattern as that observed in the patients with PI at diagnosis. Thus, despite its obvious limitations in infancy, measurement of serum enzymes provides a useful screening method for defining pancreatic function status in older patients with CF and for monitoring pancreatic function status in subjects with PS.

PANCREATIC ENZYME REPLACEMENT THERAPY

Patients with documented PI require regular meal-time supplementation with pancreatic enzymes. Although far from ideal, current management remains the most important method of attempting to correct the nutritional effects of maldigestion. For a variety of reasons, complete correction of malabsorption is unlikely to occur in the majority of patients. In the past, restriction of dietary fat was seen as a method of improving symptoms of bloating, abdominal pain, and bulky malodorous stools. Currently, there is good evidence that fat restriction results in caloric deprivation, which contributes significantly to malnutrition and disease morbidity (89). In this regard, early studies in CF showed a direct association between the sever-

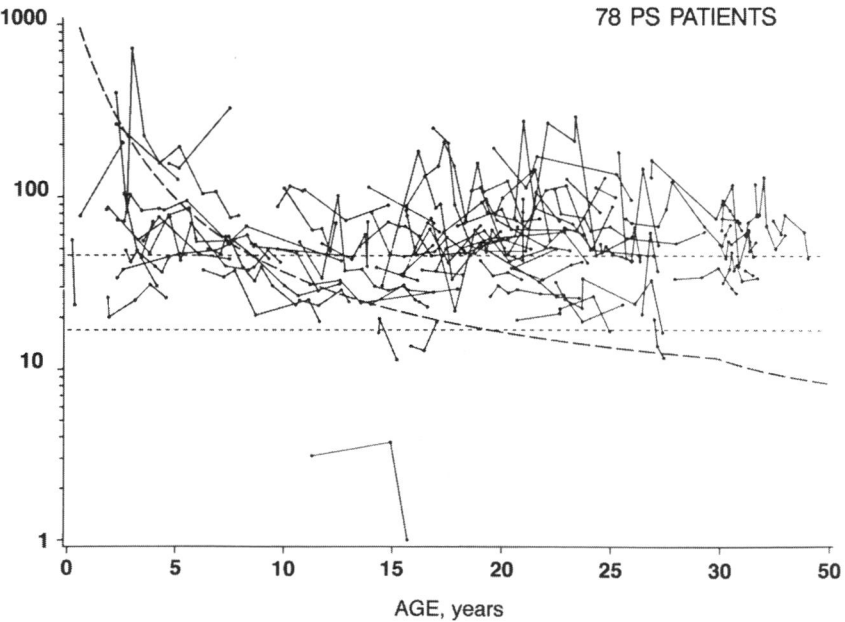

FIG. 12–11. Serial measurement of serum trypsinogen in 78 patients with pancreatic sufficiency. Parallel dotted lines indicate the normal range of values. The dashed line indicates the upper limit of the 95% confidence interval for pancreatic insufficiency measurements, which are shown in Figure 12-10.

ity of malnutrition and survival. Currently, malnutrition due to iatrogenic nutrient deprivation is an unacceptable practice. Therefore, a normal, or even high-fat diet, in conjunction with optimal pancreatic enzyme replacement therapy is indicated to optimize total energy absorption (see Chapter 13).

Pancreatic extracts from various mammalian sources have been available for more than 80 years. Most current commercial enzyme preparations are of porcine origin. Because of their biologic nature, these products have a relatively short shelf-life and are susceptible to accelerated deterioration under adverse conditions, such as exposure to sunlight, high temperature, and high humidity. Individual products vary considerably in their lipase, protease, and amylase activities. Regulations governing product inserts require description of the minimum enzyme activities of lipase and protease during the shelf-life of a product. The actual enzyme activity usually is considerably higher, sometimes up to 200% greater than the stated activity (90). Products are available as loose powder, pancreatic powder contained in gelatin capsules, or preparations coated with a pH-sensitive coating. The latter products are available as variable-sized microspheres or uniformly sized microtablets. Enzymatic activity (amylase, lipase, and protease) varies considerably; for example, ranging from 4,000 to 25,000 lipase units per capsule. Therefore, care should be taken to ensure that the patient is knowledgeable about the precise dose taken per meal or snack, particularly when prescribing a new product or the same commercial product with a different potency. Dissolution properties also vary somewhat from product to product but in most cases, the coating dissolves at a slightly acidic pH (range 5.1 to 6). Products with pH-resistant coatings offer a theoretical advantage because the harsh gastric environment, which contains acid and pepsin, is known to irreversibly denature ingested enzymes before they enter the duodenum (91). Pancreatic lipase is particularly sensitive to acid-peptic denaturation, and it has been estimated that more than 90% of the ingested enzyme is destroyed irreversibly before entering the duodenum. Nevertheless, for a variety of reasons, pH-resistant products are far from optimal. Individual requirements are extremely variable; some patients show correction of maldigestion with relatively small amounts of enzymes whereas others continue to have significant maldigestion on extremely high doses.

The various factors that are known to influence the efficacy of enzyme therapy are summarized in Table 12–4. Poor compliance probably is a more frequent problem than generally is appreciated. Enzymes should be administered throughout the meal to maximize mixing with chyme as it enters the duodenum (92). In practice, patients should be advised to take their enzyme dose in one-third allotments—at the beginning of the meal, at midmeal, and toward the end of the meal.

Patients with CF with PI tend to have gastric acid hypersecretion, which may adversely effect the small intestine milieu (93). Furthermore, patients with severe steatorrhea may experience delayed gastric emptying because of the so-called "ileal break" mechanism (94). The rate of gastric emptying of enteric-coated products will vary according to particle size (95), which in turn may affect the degree of mixing with chyme. Smaller particles will empty first, whereas larger ones are retained

TABLE 12–4. *Potential drug and host factors influencing enzyme therapy*

| | Host factors | | |
Drug factors	Gastric	Intestinal	Hepatobiliary
Dose	Acid/peptic inactivation	Intraluminal pH	Bile acid deficiency
Potency	Gastric emptying	Motility	Bile acid precipitation
Product (powder, coating)	Mixing with gastric contents	Bacterial overgrowth?	
Compliance		Intestinal mucins?	
Timing of ingestion		Intestinal resection	

selectively in the stomach. Theoretically, variable-sized microspheres will empty more evenly throughout the entire process of gastric emptying.

Under physiologic conditions, ingestion of a meal triggers a series of carefully timed intestinal events. As gastric content enters the duodenum, it mixes with pancreaticobiliary fluid rich in pancreatic enzymes, bicarbonate, and bile salts. The alkaline milieu establishes an appropriate environment for enzymes to act and maintains bile acids in the aqueous phase above the critical micellar concentration. Digestion and absorption of macronutrients is complete within the first third of the small intestine. In treated patients with CF and PI, several factors adversely influence this process. There is diminished secretion of alkali into the duodenum because of the CF defect in the pancreatic ducts and secondary pancreatic and biliary pathology. Intraluminal pH may remain low, which in turn may prevent or delay dissolution of the pH-resistant coating (96,97). If enzyme dissolution is delayed, enzyme release may occur in the distal small intestine, or even in the colon. A relatively acidic intestinal environment may irreversibly inactivate pancreatic enzymes or may be below the pH optimum for enzyme activity (98). Furthermore, ingested proteases may inactivate susceptible enzymes, such as pancreatic lipase. An acidic intestinal milieu will enhance bile acid precipitation (98). Patients with CF-associated liver disease or impaired bile acid absorption [because of ileal resection for meconium ileus (MI)] may have a depleted bile acid pool. Patients who have required intestinal resection for meconium ileus or other intestinal complications may be prone to difficulties with intestinal stasis because of disordered intestinal motility. Small bowel bacterial overgrowth may, in turn, adversely affect enzyme therapy and/or induce small intestinal mucosal damage. Altered physical and biochemical characteristics of intestinal mucins in patients with CF may interfere with intraluminal digestion and nutrient absorption.

Thus, for a variety of reasons, enzyme efficacy will vary considerably from patient to patient. Consideration should be given to the amount of active ingredient in a particular product and the type and quantity of the meal that is to be consumed. Theoretically, malabsorption will be abolished if the amount of enzyme in the duodenum exceeds 5% to 10% of the quantities normally secreted by the pancreas after a meal. On the assumption that there is no inactivation of enzymes in the stomach, it is estimated that a healthy adult requires approximately 30,000 units of lipase for an average meal. In reality, the enzymes dose will be much higher if the various deleterious factors are considered. Accordingly, doses should be titrated according to each individual's response but should not exceed the current dosing guidelines (Table 12–5).

Several approaches may be considered to improve the efficiency of enzyme replacement therapy. Adjuvant therapy focuses primarily on gastric and intestinal acidity. In the case of powdered products, antacids or H_2-receptor antagonists have been used with some success to increase gastric pH, thereby reducing the degree of gastric inactivation of pancreatic enzymes (99,100). Enteric-coated products rely on a luminal pH of greater than 5.2 to 6 for effective dissolution of the protective coating. In theory, adjuvant agents designed to inhibit gastric acid secretion will raise proximal intestinal pH, thereby increasing the rate of dissolution. Under such conditions, bile acids will remain in the aqueous phase and enzyme activity will be optimized. In a study of adult patients with CF with PI, postprandial jejunal pH was less than 5 for a considerably longer period of time compared with healthy subjects (98). There was a significant reduction in lipase activity and a decrease in aqueous phase lipid concentrations, together with increased bile acid precipitation. Suppression of gastric acid secretion significantly reduced bile acid precipitation and improved lipolysis. Supportive data in adolescents show a direct correlation between the severity of steatorrhea and postprandial pH within the proximal intestine (96,97). Patients with extended postprandial periods of duodenal pH less than 4 experienced severe steatorrhea despite adequate doses of exogenous enteric-coated enzymes. Thus, selective patients

TABLE 12–5. *Current enzyme dosing guidelines for adults with cystic fibrosis[a]*

	Meals	Snacks
Starting dose	500 lipase units/kg	250 lipase units/kg
Maximum dose[b]	2500 lipase units/kg	1250 lipase units/kg

Data from reference 107.

[a]Guidelines are based on enteric coated microspheres. When powdered enzymes are used, the dose may be doubled.

[b]If the maximum dose is exceeded, further investigation is indicated and other causes of malabsorption/maldigestion should be excluded.

will benefit from measures designed to increase small intestinal pH. Several drugs have been used with apparent success, including histamine antagonists, prostaglandin inhibitors and more potent gastric acid inhibitors, such as omeprazole (101–103).

There are several notable side effects of enzyme replacement therapy. These products are, in essence, concentrated packages of potent proteolytic, lipolytic, and amylolytic enzymes. Therefore, it is not surprising that they will cause severe mucosal excoriation if chewed or held in the mouth too long, and with rapid intestinal transit, anal excoriation has been observed. Hyperuricemia and hyperuricosuria, believed to result from the high purine content of the conventional enzyme preparations, appear to be dose-related effects (104,105). These side effects are unlikely to occur if enzymes are used within the recommended dosing guidelines. The powdered products may produce allergic responses, including bronchospasm, nasal irritation, and repeated coughing, not only in patients, but also in susceptible care givers and relatives. Severe, potentially life-threatening attacks of acute anaphylaxis have been reported, but this complication is more likely to occur with release of the contents of powdered enzymes into the air.

In 1994, Smyth and colleagues (106) in the United Kingdom described a new intestinal complication in patients with CF, stricture of the ascending colon, which occurred in association with the use of extremely high doses of high-potency enzymes. Shortly thereafter, additional case reports emanated from other CF centers in the United States and Europe. Initial reports described patients with signs and symp-

toms of intestinal obstruction with evidence of a "colonic stricture" in the proximal colon. This complication temporally was associated with introduction of large doses of high-strength enteric-coated pancreatic enzymes. A spectrum of intestinal pathology primarily affecting the colon has been described. The term *fibrosing colonopathy* has been coined to include both the prestricture state and the presence of true strictures (107). Pathologically, the colonic lesion is characterized by mild to moderate mucosal and submucosal inflammation affecting all or part of the colon. More severe changes are evident in the submucosa, which is characterized by a circular band of fibrosis and luminal narrowing that may be limited to a focal area or extend throughout the colon. Clinically, patients present with signs and symptoms of colitis with or without intestinal obstruction.

In an attempt to understand the relationship between enzyme therapy and this complication, case control studies have been conducted in the United Kingdom and the United States (108, 109). Individual case reports and the more extensive case control studies showed that fibrosing colonopathy occurred primarily in infants and young children. There have been no reported cases in adults; the oldest reported patient was 14 years of age at diagnosis. Case control studies in both the United Kingdom and the United States showed a highly significant association between this complication and the amount of enzyme ingested per meal. The U.K. case control study also suggested a direct association with high-strength enzymes and specific commercial products (108). However, the U.S. study showed that this complication occurred with both high-strength and low-strength products; the total daily dose of enzyme (expressed in units of enzyme activity/kg body weight/day) was the most important independent risk factor for the occurrence of fibrosing colonopathy, which appeared to be unrelated to product potency and product type (109). The risk appeared to increase exponentially with increasing dose.

The mechanism of injury causing fibrosing colonopathy is unknown. Pancreatic enzymes are crude extracts that contain high concentrations of a mixture of digestive enzymes and also other unmeasured components such as growth factors and hormones. Although the case control studies have provided several answers concerning dosage, they cannot address questions concerning pathophysiology. The fact remains that administration of high doses of pancreatic enzyme, beyond those recommended in the recent consensus report, are quite unnecessary and are potentially harmful.

SUMMARY

In this chapter, we provided a general overview of the nature and range of severity of exocrine pancreatic disease in patients with CF. We have attempted to underline the observation that the exocrine pancreas is abnormal in almost all cases, from a functional point of view, but the severity of pancreatic disease is highly variable. The variability in severity of pancreatic disease can be attributed largely to the functional effects of mutations in the gene-encoding CFTR. In general terms, patients with CF with the pancreatic-insufficient phenotype have the worst prognosis, with respect to morbidity and survival. Although pancreatic enzyme replacement therapy for patients with PI is a key component of daily therapy, currently available drugs fail to completely correct pancreatic maldigestion in a large percentage of patients.

REFERENCES

1. Anderson D. Cystic fibrosis of the pancreas and its relation to celiac disease. *Am Dis Child* 1938;56: 344–399.
2. Fanconi G, Uehlinger E, Knauer C. Das coelioksyndrom bei angeborener zystisher pankreas fibromatose and bronchicktasis. *Wein Med Wochensch* 1936;86: 753.
3. di Sant'Agnese PA, Darling RC, Pevierra GA, Shea E. Abnormal electrolyte composition of sweat in cystic fibrosis of the pancreas. *Pediatrics* 1953;12:549–563.
4. Gibbs GE, Bostick WL, Smith PM. Incomplete pancreatic deficiency in cystic fibrosis of the pancreas. *J Pediatr* 1950;37:320.
5. Oppenheimer E, Esterly J. Cystic fibrosis of the pancreas. *Arch Pathol* 1973;96(3):149–154.
6. Kopito LE, Shwachman H, Vawter GF, Edlow J. The pancreas in cystic fibrosis: chemical composition and comparative morphology. *Pediatr Res* 1976;10(8): 742–749.
7. Liu P, Daneman A, Stringer DA, Durie PR. Pancreatic cysts and calcification in cystic fibrosis. *J Can Assoc Radiol* 1986;37(4):279–282.
8. Grand RJ, Schwartz RH, di Sant'Agnese PA, Gelderman AH. Macroscopic cysts of the pancreas in a case of cystic fibrosis. *J Pediatr* 1966;69(3):393–398.
9. King A, Mueller RF, Heeley AF, et al. Diagnosis of cystic fibrosis in premature infants. *Pediatr Res* 1986;20(6):536–541.
10. Grand RJ, Watkins JB, Torti FM. Development of the human gastrointestinal tract. *Gastroenterology* 1976; 70(5 Part 1):790–810.
11. Imrie J, Fagan D, Sturgess J. Quantitative evaluation of the development of the exocrine pancreas in CF and control infants. *Am J Pathol* 1979;95(3):697–707.
12. The pancreas. In: DA Stringer, ed. *Pediatric gastrointestinal imaging.* Toronto/Philadelphia: BC Decker Inc, 1989:585–609.
13. Daneman A, Gaskin K, Martin DJ, Cutz E. Pancreatic changes in cystic fibrosis: CT and sonographic appearances. *Am J Radiol* 1983;141(4):653–655.
14. Richenel TO, Tjon AT, Heijerman HGM, et al. Cystic fibrosis: MR imaging of the pancreas. *Radiology* 1991;179:103.
15. Gaskin K, Gurwitz D, Durie P, et al. Improved respiratory prognosis in CF patients with normal fat absorption. *J Pediatr* 1982;100(6):857–862.
16. Gaskin KJ, Durie P, Hill RE, Lee M, Forstner GG. Colipase and maximally activated pancreatic lipase in normal subjects and patients with steatorrhea. *J Clin Invest* 1982;69(2):427–434.
17. Gaskin KJ, Durie P, Lee L, Hill R, Forstner GG. Colipase and lipase secretion in childhood onset of pancreatic insufficiency: delineation of patients with steatorrhea with relative colipase deficiency. *Gastroenterology* 1984;86(1):1–7.
18. Hadorn B, Johansen PG, Anderson CM. Pancreozymin secretin test of exocrine pancreatic function in cystic fibrosis. *Can Med Assoc J* 1968;98:377.
19. Knauff RE, Adams JA. Proteins and mucoproteins in the duodenal fluids of cystic fibrosis and control subjects. *Clin Chim Acta* 1968;19:245.
20. Kopelman HR, Durie P, Gaskin KJ, Weizman Z, Forstner GG. Pancreatic fluid and protein hyperconcentration in cystic fibrosis. *N Engl Med J* 1985; 312(6):329–334.
21. Case RM, Scratcherd T, Wynn RD. The origin and secretion of pancreatic juice bicarbonate. *J Physiol* 1970;210(2):1–15.

22. Case RM, Halz J, Hudson D, Scratcherd T, Wynn RDA. Electrolyte secretion by the isolated cat pancreas during replacement of extracellular bicarbonate by organic anion and chloride by inorganic anions. *J Physiol* 1979;286:563–576.

23. Gaskin KJ, Durie P, Corey M, Wei P, Forstner GG. Evidence of a primary defect of bicarbonate secretion in cystic fibrosis. *Pediatr Res* 1982;16(7):554–557.

24. Kopelman HR, Corey M, Gaskin KJ, Durie P, Forstner GG. Impaired chloride secretion, as well as bicarbonate secretion underlies the fluid secretory defect in the cystic fibrosis pancreas. *Gastroenterology* 1988;95(2):349–355.

25. Kopelman H, Forstner G, Durie P, Corey M. Origins of chloride and bicarbonate secretory defect in the cystic fibrosis pancreas, as suggested by pancreatic function studies in control and CF subjects with preserved pancreatic function. *Clin Invest Med* 1989;12(3):207–211.

26. Marino C, Matovcik LM, Gorelick FS, Cohn JA. Localization of the cystic fibrosis transmembrane conductance regulator in pancreas. *J Clin Invest* 1991;88(2):712–716.

27. Foulkes AG, Harris A. Localization of expression of the cystic fibrosis gene in human pancreatic development. *Pancreas* 1993;8(1):3–6.

28. Kopelman H, Gauthier C, Bornstein M. Antisense oligodeoxynucleotide to the cystic fibrosis transmembrane conductance regulator inhibits cyclic AMP-activated but not calcium-activated cell volume reduction in a human pancreatic duct cell line. *J Clin Invest* 1993;91(3):1253–1257.

29. Lee P, Roloff D, Howat W. Hypoproteinemia and anemia in infants with cystic fibrosis. *JAMA* 1974; 228(5):585–588.

30. Reisman J, Petrou C, Corey M, et al. Hypoalbuminemia at initial examination in patients with cystic fibrosis. *J Pediatr* 1989;115(5 Part 1):755–758.

31. Stern RC, Izant RJ, Boat TF, et al. Treatment and prognosis of rectal prolapse in cystic fibrosis. *Gasteroenterology* 1982; 82(4):707–710.

32. Couper RTL, Corey M, Durie PR, et al. Longitudinal evaluation of serum trypsinogen measurement in pancreatic-insufficient and pancreatic-sufficient patients with cystic fibrosis. *J Pediatr* 1995;127(3): 408–413.

33. Couper RTL, Corey M, Moore J, et al. Decline of exocrine pancreatic function in cystic fibrosis patients with pancreatic sufficiency. *Pediatr Res* 1992;32(2):179–182.

34. Waters DL, Dorney SFA, Gaskin KJ, et al. Pancreatic function in infants identified as having cystic fibrosis in a neonatal screening program. *N Engl J Med* 1990;322(5):303–308.

35. Sokol RJ, Reardon MC, Accurso FJ, et al. Fat-soluble-vitamin status during the first year of life in infants with cystic fibrosis identified by screening of newborns. *Am J Clin Nutr* 1989;50(5):1064–1071.

36. Torstenson OL, Humphrey GB, Edson JR. Cystic fibrosis presenting with severe hemorrhage due to vitamin K malabsorption: a report of three cases. *Pediatrics* 1970;45:857.

37. Farrell PM, Bieri JG, Fratanloni JF, et al. The occurrence and effects of human vitamin E deficiency: a study in patients with cystic fibrosis. *J Clin Invest* 1977;60(1):233–241.

38. Elias E, Muller DPR, Scott J. Association of spinocerebellar disorders with cystic fibrosis or chronic childhood cholestasis and very low serum vitamin E. *Lancet* 1981;2(8259):1319–3121.

39. Reiter EO, Brugman SM, Pike JW, et al. Vitamin D metabolites in adolescents and young adults with cystic fibrosis. *J Pediatr* 1985;106(1):21–26.

40. Hubbard VS, Dunn GD, di Sant'Agnese PA. Abnormal fatty acid composition of plasma lipids in cystic fibrosis. *Lancet* 1977;2(8052–8053):1302–1304.

41. Shwachman H, Leubher H, Catzel P, et al. Mucoviscidosis. *Adv Pediatr* 1955;7:249.

42. Lanng S, Thorsteinsson B, Lund-Andersen C, et al. Diabetes mellitus in Danish cystic fibrosis patients: prevalence and late diabetic complications. *Acta Paediatr* 1994;83(1):72–77.

43. Lanng S, Hansen A, Thorsteinsson B, et al. Glucose tolerance in patients with cystic fibrosis: five year prospective study. *Br Med J* 1995;311(7006): 655–659.

44. Soejima K, Landing BH. Pancreatic islets in older patients with cystic fibrosis with and without diabetes mellitus: Morphometric and immunocytologic studies. *Pediatr Pathol* 1986;6(1):25–46.

45. Gougeon R, Pencharz PB, Marliss EB. Protein metabolism in diabetes mellitus: Implications for clinical management. In: Cowett RM, ed. *Diabetes*. New York: Raven Press, 1995:241–258.

46. Shwachman H, Lebenthal E, Khaw K-T. Recurrent acute pancreatitis in patients with cystic fibrosis with normal pancreatic enzymes. *Pediatrics* 1975;55(1): 86–95.

47. Weizman Z, Durie PR. Acute pancreatitis in childhood. *J Pediatr* 1988;113(1 Part 1):24–29.

48. Masaryk TJ, Achkar E. Pancreatitis as initial presentation of cystic fibrosis in young adults: a report of two cases. *Dig Dis Sci* 1983;28(10):874–878.

49. Gross V, Schoelmerich J, Denzel K, et al. Relapsing pancreatitis as initial manifestation of cystic fibrosis in a young man without pulmonary disease. *Int J Pancreatol* 1989;4(2):221–228.

50. Atlas AB, Orenstein SR, Orenstein DM. Pancreatitis in young children with cystic fibrosis. *J Pediatr* 1992; 120:756.

51. Corey M, Durie PR, Moore D. Familial concordance of pancreatic function in cystic fibrosis. *J Pediatr* 1989;115(3):274–277.

52. Kerem BS, Buchanan JA, Durie PR, et al. DNA marker haplotype association with pancreatic sufficiency in cystic fibrosis. *Am J Hum Genet* 1989;44(6):827–834.

53. Rommens JM, Iannuzzi MC, Kerem B, et al. Identification of the cystic fibrosis gene: chromosome walking and jumping. *Science* 1989;245(4922): 1059–1065.

54. Riordan JR, Rommens JM, Kerem B, et al. Identification of the cystic fibrosis gene: cloning and characterization of complementary DNA. *Science* 1989; 245(4922):1066–1072.

55. Kerem B, Rommens JM, Buchanan JA, et al. Identification of the cystic fibrosis gene: genetic analysis. *Science* 1989;245(4922):1073–1080.

56. Kerem E, Corey M, Kerem B-S, et al. The relation between genotype and phenotype in cystic fibrosis—

analysis of the most common mutation (ΔF508). *N Engl J Med* 1990;323(22):1517–1522.

57. Kristidis P, Bozon D, Corey M, et al. Genetic determination of exocrine pancreatic function in cystic fibrosis. *Am J Hum Genet* 1992;50(6):1178–1184.

58. Tsui L-C. The spectrum of cystic fibrosis mutations. *Trends Genetics* 1992;8(11):392–398.

59. Wilschanski M, Zielenski J, Markiewicz D, et al. Correlation of sweat chloride concentration with classes of the cystic fibrosis transmembrane conductance regulator mutations. *J Pediatr* 1995;127(5):705–710.

60. Couper R. Pancreatic function tests. In: Walker WA, Durie PR, Watkins JB, Walker-Smith JS, Hamilton JR, eds. *Pediatric gastrointestinal disease: pathophysiology, diagnosis, management.* 2nd ed. Philadelphia: Mosby, 1996:1621–1635.

61. Go VLW, Hofmann AF, Summerskill WHJ. Simultaneous measurements of total pancreatic, biliary and gastric outputs in man using a perfusion technique. *Gastroenterology* 1970;58(3):321–328.

62. Lundh G. Pancreatic exocrine function in neoplastic and inflammatory disease: a simple and reliable new test. *Gastroenterology* 1962;42:275.

63. Go VLW, Hofmann AF, Summerskill WHJ. Pancreozymin bioassay in man based on pancreatic enzyme secretion: potency of specific amino acids and other digestive products. *J Clin Invest* 1970;49(8):1558–1564.

64. Khouri MR, Huang G, Shiau YF. Sudan stain of fecal fat: new insight into an old test. *Gastroenterology* 1989;96(2 Part 1):421–427.

65. Colombo C, Maiavacca R, Ronchi M, et al. The steatocrit: a simple method for monitoring fat malabsorption in patients with cystic fibrosis. *J Pediatr Gastroenterol Nutr* 1987;6(6):926–930.

66. Durie PR, Goldberg DM. Biochemical tests of pancreatic function in infancy and childhood. *Adv Clin Enzymol* 1986;4:77.

67. Kaspar P, Möller G, Wahlefeld A. New photometric assay for chymotrypsin in stool. *Clin Chem* 1984;30(11):1753–1757.

68. Stein J, Jung M, Sziegoleit A, et al. Immunoreactive elastase I: clinical evaluation of a new noninvasive test of pancreatic function. *Clin Chem* 1996;42(2):222–226.

69. Mills PR, Horton PW, Watkinson G. The value of the ^{14}C breath test in the assessment of fat absorption. *Scand J Gastroenterol* 1979;14(8):914–920.

70. Watkins JB, Klein PD, Scholler DA, et al. Diagnosis and differentiation of fat malabsorption in children using ^{13}C-labelled lipids: trioctanoin triolein and palmitic acid breath tests. *Gastroenterology* 1982;82: 911.

71. Cole SG, Rossi S, Stern A, Hofmann AF. Cholesteryl octanonate breath test: preliminary studies on a new noninvasive test of human pancreatic exocrine function. *Gastroenterology* 1987;93(6):1372–1380.

72. Hiele M, Ghoss Y, Rutgeerts PJ, Vantrappen GR. Starch digestion in normal subjects and patients with pancreatic disease using $^{13}CO_2$ breath tests. *Gastroenterology* 1989;96(2 Part 1):503–509.

73. Kerlin P, Wong L, Harris B, Capra S. Rice flour, breath hydrogen and malabsorption. *Gastroenterology* 1984;87(3):578–585.

74. Imondi AR, Stradley RP, Wolgemuth R. Synthetic peptides in the diagnosis of exocrine pancreatic insufficiency in animals. *Gut* 1972;13(9):726–731.

75. Weizman Z, Forstner GG, Gaskin KJ, et al. Bentiromide test for assessing pancreatic dysfunction using analysis of para-aminobenzoic acid in plasma and urine studies in cystic fibrosis and Shwachman's syndrome. *Gastroenterology* 1985;89(3):596–604.

76. Durie PR, Yung-Jato LY, Soldin SJ, et al. Bentiromide test using liquid chromatographic measurement of p-aminobenzoic acid and its metabolites for diagnosing pancreatic insufficiency in children. *J Pediatr* 1992;121(3):413–416.

77. Sterchi EE, Green JR, Lentz MJ. Non pancreatic hydrolysis of *N*-benzoyl-l-tyrosyl-*p*-aminobenzoic acid (PABA-peptide) in the human small intestine. *Clin Sci* 1982;62(5):557–560.

78. Gyr K, Felsenfeld O, Imondi AR. Chymotrypsin-like activity of some intestinal bacteria. *Dig Dis Sci* 1978;23(5):413–416.

79. Toskes PP. Bentiromide as a test of exocrine pancreatic function in adult patients with pancreatic exocrine insufficiency: determination of appropriate dose and urinary collection interval. *Gastroenterology* 1983;85(3):565–569.

80. Mitchell CJ, Humphrey CS, Bullen AW, et al. Improved diagnostic accuracy of a modified oral pancreatic function test. *Scand J Gastroenterol* 1979;14(6):737–741.

81. Hoek FJ, van den Berg FAJTM, Klein Elhorst JT, et al. Improved specificity of the PABA test with p-aminosalicylic acid (PAS). *Gut* 1987;28(4):468–473.

82. Delchier J-C, Soule J-C. BT-PABA test with plasma PABA measurements: evaluation of sensitivity and specificity. *Gut* 1983;24(4):318–325.

83. Malis F, Fric P, Kasahrek E, Slaby J. Comparative study of the estimation of exocrine pancreatic function using p-(*N*-acetyl-l-tyrosyl) and p-(*N*-benzoyl-l-tyrosyl) aminobenzoic acid. *Acta Hepatogastroenterol* 1983;30(3):99–101.

84. Scharpé 82 S, Iliano L. Two indirect tests of exocrine pancreatic function evaluated. *Clin Chem* 1987;33(1):5–12.

85. Lankisch PG, Brauneis J, Otto et al. Pancreolauryl and NBT-PABA tests: are serum tests a more practicable alternative to urine tests in the diagnosis of exocrine pancreatic insufficiency? *Gastroenterology* 1986;90(2):350–354.

86. Goldberg DM, Durie PR. Biochemical tests in the diagnosis of chronic pancreatitis and in the evaluation of pancreatic insufficiency. *Clin Biochem* 1993;26(4):253–275.

87. Crossley JR, Elliott RB, Smith PA. Dried-blood spot screening for cystic fibrosis in the newborn. *Lancet* 1979;1(8114):471–474.

88. Durie PR, Forstner GG, Gaskin KJ, et al. Age-related alterations of immunoreactive pancreatic cationic trypsinogen in sera from cystic fibrosis patients with and without pancreatic insufficiency. *Pediatr Res* 1986;20(3):209–213.

89. Pencharz PB, Durie PR. Nutritional management of cystic fibrosis. *Annu Rev Nutr* 1993;13:111–136.

90. Kraisinger M, Hochhaus G, Stecenko A, et al. Clinical pharmacology of pancreatic enzymes in cystic fibrosis and in vitro performance of microencapsulated formulation. *J Clin Pharm* 1994;34(2):158–166.

91. DiMagno EP, Malagelada JR, Go VLW, et al. Fate of orally ingested enzymes in pancreatic insufficiency. *N Engl J Med* 1977;296(23):1318–1322.

92. Cleghorn GJ. Pharmacologic treatment of pancreatic insufficiency. In: Walker WA, Durie PR, Hamilton JR, Walker-Smith JA, Watkins JB, eds. *Pediatric gastrointestinal disease.* 2nd ed. Philadelphia: Mosby, 1996:2011–2016.

93. Cox KL, Isenberg JN, Ament NE. Gastric acid hypersecretion in cystic fibrosis. *J Pediatr Gastroenterol Nutr* 1982;1(4):559–565.

94. Read NW, McFarlane A, Kinsman RJ, et al. Effect of infusion of nutrient solutions into the ileum on gastrointestinal transit and plasma levels of neurotensin and enteroglucagon. *Gasteroenterology* 1984;86(2):274–280.

95. Meyer JH, Elashoff J, Porter-Fink V, Dressman J, Amidon GL. Human postprandial gastric emptying of 1–3 millimeter spheres. *Gastroenterology* 1988;94(6):1315–1325.

96. Robinson PJ, Smith AL, Sly PD. Duodenal pH in cystic fibrosis and its relationship to fat malabsorption. *Dig Dis Sci* 1990;35(6):1299–1304.

97. Barraclough M, Taylor CJ. Twenty-four hour ambulatory gastric and duodenal pH profiles in cystic fibrosis effect of duodenal hyperacidity on pancreatic enzyme function and fat absorption. *J Pediatr Gastroenterol Nutr* 1996;23(1):45–50.

98. Zentler-Munro PL, Fitzpatrick WJF, Batten JC, et al. Effect of intrajejunal acidity in aqueous phase bile acid and lipid concentrations in pancreatic steatorrhea due to cystic fibrosis. *Gut* 1984;25(5):500–507.

99. Durie PR, Bell L, Linton W, et al. Effect of cimetidine and sodium bicarbonate on pancreatic replacement therapy in cystic fibrosis. *Gut* 1980;21(9):778–786.

100. Boyle BJ, Long WB, Balistreri WF, et al. Effect of cimetidine and pancreatic enzymes on serum and fecal bile acids and fat malabsorption in cystic fibrosis. *Gastroenterology* 1980;78(5 Part 1):950–953.

101. Gow R, Bradbear R, Francis P, et al. Comparative study of varying regimens to improve steatorrhea and azotorrhea in cystic fibrosis: effectiveness of an enteric-coated preparation with and without antacids and cimetidine. *Lancet* 1981;2(8255):1071–1074.

102. Heijerman HG, Lamers CB, Dijkman JH, et al. Ranitidine compared with the dimethyl prostaglandin E_2-analogue emprostil as adjunct pancreatic enzyme replacement in cystic fibrosis. *Scand J Gastroenterol* 1990;178:26–31.

103. Heijerman HG, Lamers CB, Bakker W. Omeprazole enhances the efficacy of pancreatin (pancrease) in cystic fibrosis. *Ann Intern Med* 1991;114(3):200–201.

104. Stapleton FB, Kennedy J, Nousia-Arvanitakis S. Hyperuricemia due to high dose pancreatic extract therapy in cystic fibrosis. *N Engl J Med* 1976;295(5):246–248.

105. Davidson GP, Hassel FM, Crozier D, et al. Iatrogenic hyperuricemia in children with cystic fibrosis. *J Pediatr* 1978;93(6):976–978.

106. Smyth RL, van Velzen D, Smyth AR, et al. Strictures of the ascending colon in cystic fibrosis and high-strength pancreatic enzymes. *Lancet* 1994;343(8889):85–86.

107. Borowitz DS, Grand RJ, Durie PR, the Consensus Committee. Use of pancreatic enzyme supplements for patients with cystic fibrosis in the context of fibrosing colonopathy. *J Pediatr* 1995;127(5):681–684.

108. Smyth RL, Ashby D, O'Hea U, et al. Fibrosing colonopathy in cystic fibrosis: results of a case-control study. *Lancet* 1995;346(8985):1247–1251.

109. FitzSimmons SC, Burkhart GA, Borowitz D. High dose pancreatic enzyme supplements and fibrosing colonopathy in children with cystic fibrosis. *N Engl J Med* 1997;336(18):1283–1289.

Cystic Fibrosis in Adults,
edited by J. R. Yankaskas and M. R. Knowles,
Lippincott–Raven Publishers, Philadelphia, 1999.

13

Nutrition

Daina Kalnins, *Cynthia Stewart, *†Elizabeth Tullis, and ††Paul B. Pencharz

*Division of Respiratory Medicine, Department of Pediatrics and The Research Institute, The Hospital for Sick Children; *Adult Cystic Fibrosis Program, St. Michael's Hospital; †Division of Respirology, Department of Medicine, University of Toronto; and ††Division of Gastroenterology and Nutrition, The Hospital for Sick Children, and University of Toronto, Toronto, Ontario, Canada*

BASIS FOR THE DISEASE

The predominant clinical feature of cystic fibrosis (CF) is respiratory tract involvement, in which airway obstruction by sticky mucus gives rise to chronic infection, especially with *Pseudomonas* species, and eventual bronchiectasis. Most patients experience gastrointestinal difficulties; 85% show pancreatic insufficiency due to obstruction in the small pancreatic ducts, which in turn leads to pancreatic fibrosis and atrophy (1). In the newborn period, more than 10% of affected patients present with bowel obstruction from meconium ileus (2). Overt liver disease develops in up to 5% of patients, frequently in adolescence or adulthood. Infertility in males is virtually universal (3). Undernutrition is an important cause of morbidity in affected children, adolescents, and young adults (4–7). In this chapter, the pathogenesis of the various factors that contribute to an energy deficit is addressed and approaches to nutritional evaluation and therapy are described.

As information about the variety of CF mutations has accumulated, we have gained considerable insight into its genotype–phenotype relationships. From the clinical and nutritional viewpoint, CF mutations can be grouped into those that cause pancreatic insufficiency and those that permit pancreatic sufficiency (1).

The term pancreatic sufficiency is an operational one, describing patients who almost always have pancreatic disease but retain enough pancreatic function to permit normal digestion and absorption of nutrients. Pancreatic-sufficient patients, who constitute approximately 15% of the patient population, usually have much milder disease expression, which is characterized by diagnosis at a later age (presumably because of milder symptoms), better growth, and a far superior survival rate than that found in patients with pancreatic insufficiency. The rate of progression of lung disease usually is slower than that seen in pancreatic-insufficient patients.

We have proposed that mutations in the cystic fibrosis transmembrane conductance regulator (CFTR) gene can be divided into two categories—severe and mild—according to the status of pancreatic function (8). Our data show that pancreatic insufficiency develops in patients with two severe mutations, whereas those with one or two mild alleles have pancreatic sufficiency; exceptions to this rule are few. There currently is a growing understanding (9) of the molecular consequences of the different classes of CF mutations, which range from no synthesis of CFTR, through blocks in processing and regulation, to altered conductance and reduced synthesis (see Chapter 2). Thus, the relationship between genotype and phenotype is becoming clearer. With respect to nutrition issues, those with pancreatic sufficiency (i.e., those with a milder genetic defect) better maintain their nutritional status.

OVERVIEW OF NUTRITIONAL PROBLEMS

Chronic undernutrition with significant weight retardation and linear growth failure long has been recognized as a general problem among the CF patient populations. Some researchers believed that it was an inherent consequence of the disease, whereas others argued that it resulted from physiologic adaptation to advanced pulmonary disease. Some early studies of patients with CF (5,7), however, showed a good correlation between the degree of malnutrition and the severity of pulmonary disease, which in turn adversely affected the survival rate. Although a causal association between these two factors has been postulated, it is not clear whether prevention of malnutrition and of growth failure would slow the progression of lung disease and improve survival rates. The past decade has seen renewed interest in evaluating the multiple interdependent variables that cause chronic malnutrition and growth failure. In most CF centers around the world, nutritional support currently is viewed as an integral part of the multidisciplinary care of patients, and aggressive programs have been instituted to prevent malnutrition.

Growth retardation in patients with CF is recognized as being caused by an unfavorable energy balance rather than being inherent to the disease. More than 10 years ago, reports from Toronto (4,10) indicated that most patients attending the CF clinic at The Hospital for Sick Children conformed to the normal distribution of growth in the general population. Cross-sectional data from the Toronto clinic (10) showed a normal distribution of height percentiles in males and females. Although weight distribution was skewed toward the lower percentiles in females, particularly after adolescence, weight retardation was far less evident than that reported from other centers.

In a comparative study of two CF clinic populations of similar size and age distribution (Boston and Toronto in 1982), Corey et al. (11) found a marked difference in median ages of survival: 21 years in Boston versus 30 years in Toronto (Table 13–1). Furthermore, after 10 years of age, there was a dramatic separation in survival curves between the two centers. Pulmonary function was no different in the two clinic populations. Males and females attending the Toronto clinic, however, were taller than those in the Boston clinic, and males in Toronto were heavier. With the exception of nutritional management, the general approach to patient care, particularly pulmonary care, was similar in the two clinics. It was suggested that the higher survival rate in the Toronto CF population could be attributed to superior nutritional status.

An examination of dietary practices in the two clinics revealed a striking difference in philosophy. The approach in Boston (12), which closely resembled that of most centers in the 1980s, was to prescribe a low-fat, carbohydrate-rich diet, with the rationale that reduction in dietary fat would improve bowel symptoms and reduce stool bulk. Recognizing the problem of maldigestion and poor absorption of long-chain triglycerides, many centers advocated the use of artificial diets, including protein hydrolysates and substituting medium-chain triglycerides (MCTs) for long-chain fats (13). However, other reports (14) showed no long-term benefits to growth when protein hydrolysates and MCTs were used as supplements or substitutes. The effect was to provide

TABLE 13–1. *Characteristics of 1982 cystic fibrosis clinic populations in Boston and Toronto*

	Boston	Tóronto
Number of patients	499	534
Male/female (%)	57/43	58/42
Age:		
Mean ± SD (yrs)	15.9 ± 9.6	15.2 ± 8.3
Range (yrs)	0–45	0–43
Median (50%)		
survival (yrs)	21	30

Adapted from reference 11.

patients with CF with a restrictive, unpalatable diet and to exclude them from the many energy-rich foods that compose some of the tastier choices in the usual Western diet. Fortunately, these supplements rarely are advocated currently, for reasons of cost, poor compliance, and unpalatability. Chronic malnutrition from reduced energy intake appears to have been an unfortunate iatrogenic effect in most CF programs throughout the world.

Since the early 1970s, the Toronto group advocated a calorically enriched diet by encouraging rather than restricting dietary fat and recommending additional enzyme supplements to enhance digestion (15,16). Fat is the most energy-rich, economic, and appetizing energy source, so patients were encouraged to eat larger portions than their peers, to add fat in the form of butter or untrimmed meat, and to eat high-calorie snacks between meals and before bed. Fat malabsorption occurred; but with additional and more potent pancreatic enzyme supplements, net absorbed energy increased and better growth resulted. Coincidentally, the primary objective of nutritional management generally is accepted to be achieving normal nutrition and growth in children and maintaining goal weight in adults. This view is reflected in this statement from a Consensus Conference (17) on Nutritional Assessment and Management in Cystic Fibrosis, organized by the U.S. Cystic Fibrosis Foundation, "There is no reason to accept nutritional failure and/or impaired growth in any individual with CF."

PATHOGENESIS OF ENERGY IMBALANCE

A variety of complex factors, both related and unrelated, may give rise to energy imbalance in patients with CF. The net effect on growth potential varies considerably from patient to patient, according to marked differences in disease expression and with progression of the disease. In simple terms, an energy deficit results from an imbalance between energy needs and intake (Table 13–2) (18) and is determined by three factors: energy losses, energy expenditure, and energy intake.

TABLE 13–2. *Energy imbalance in cystic fibrosis*

Increased needs	Reduced intake
Increased intestinal losses	Reduced intake
Pancreatic insufficiency	Iatrogenic fat restriction
Bile salt metabolism	Anorexia
Hepatobiliary disease	Feeding disorders
Regurgitation from reflux	Depression
Increased urinary losses	Esophagitis (secondary to reflux)
Diabetes mellitus	
Increased energy expenditure	
Pulmonary disease	
Primary defect?	
Pregnancy, lactation	

Adapted from reference 18.

Energy Losses

Fecal nutrient losses from maldigestion/malabsorption are known to contribute to energy imbalance. Only 1% to 2% of residual pancreatic capacity for secreting enzyme is required to prevent maldigestion (19); however, in most patients with CF (approximately 85%), evidence of pancreatic failure is present at diagnosis. In those who exhibit maldigestion, strong correlations exist between residual pancreatic function (colipase secretion) and the severity of fat malabsorption (Fig 13–1). Patients with documented steatorrhea, therefore, have variable but very limited residual pancreatic function (see Chapter 12).

This observation only partially explains why some patients with pancreatic insufficiency digest nutrients better than others when given pancreatic enzyme supplements with meals. Despite improvements in the enzymatic potency and intestinal delivery of ingested pancreatic enzyme supplements, many patients continue to have severe steatorrhea and azotorrhea, even when they receive what are considered to be adequate amounts of enzyme supplements, that is, 1,800–2,500 units of lipase/g fat (20,21). In the absence of adequate pancreatic bicarbonate secretion (22), gastric acid entering the duodenum may lower intestinal pH until well into the jejunum. The acid-resistant coating of the newer enzyme preparations may not dissolve in the proximal intestine. Pancre-

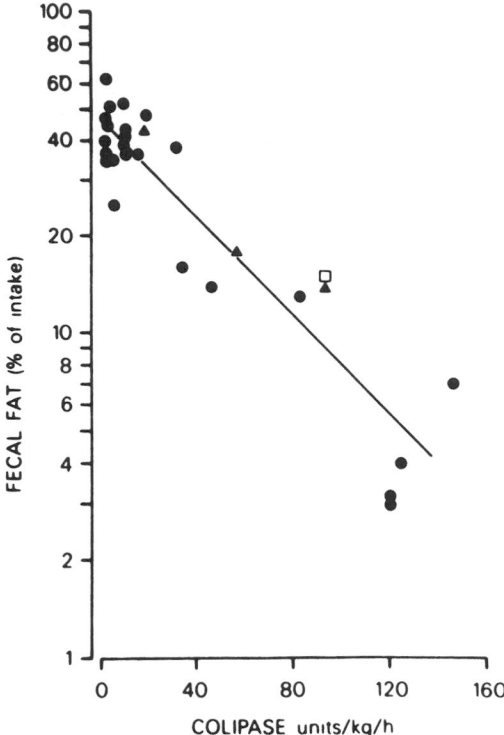

FECAL FAT (% of intake)

COLIPASE units/kg/h

FIG. 13–1. Comparison of fecal fat excretion (percentage of fat intake) with pancreatic colipase secretion in 28 patients with steatorrhea due to pancreatic insufficiency. ●, patients with cystic fibrosis; ▲, patients with Shwachman syndrome; □, patients with congenital pancreatic hypoplasia ($r = 0.92$, $P < 0.001$). Normal excretion is less than 7%. (From reference 19.)

testinal mucus, with altered physical properties, may have a harmful effect on the thickness of the intestinal unstirred layer, further limiting nutrient absorption.

Two additional factors, more prevalent in adolescents and adult patients with CF, may contribute to energy losses. CF-related diabetes (CFRD), if not adequately controlled, may increase caloric losses because of glycosuria. Advanced liver disease with multifocal biliary cirrhosis may result in inadequate bile-salt secretion, which in turn causes severe fat malabsorption.

Energy Intake

It has been widely accepted that energy intake should exceed normal requirements; it has been suggested (6) that patients may require 120% to 150% of the recommended daily allowance (RDA) for age and gender. However, when we accurately evaluated the nutrient intake of a group of otherwise healthy adolescents with CF, we were surprised to learn that energy intakes were close to the normal range for age, body weight, and gender (25). Patients with normal growth percentiles for height and weight did show higher energy intakes than those whose growth was retarded. More recently, a study completed at our clinic (26) revealed that adolescent males and females with normal growth percentiles consumed 110% of the RDA. Other CF centers that have developed more liberal attitudes to fat consumption have noted a corresponding improvement in energy intake and growth (27,28). Other reports (29) found nutrient intakes in patients with CF to be close to the normal range.

Patients with CF are especially prone to complications that might limit oral intake. Esophagitis induced by acid reflux is common in patients with advanced pulmonary disease and frequently is associated with pain, anorexia, and vomiting after bouts of coughing (DIOS) (30,31). Distal intestinal obstruction syndrome, an unusual form of subacute obstruction within the distal ileum and proximal colon, is seen in some adolescents and adults with pancreatic failure (32); it frequently causes recurrent,

atic lipase is denatured readily at pH less than 2; even if it is not denatured, enzymatic activity is reduced considerably at a low pH. Bile acids are precipitated readily in an acid milieu (23), and duodenal bile-acid concentration may fall below the critical micellar concentration, thereby exacerbating fat maldigestion. Precipitated bile salts also appear to be lost from the enterohepatic circulation in greater quantities, thus reducing the total bile salt pool and altering the glycocholate:taurocholate ratio. Bile salt losses are aggravated by the binding of salts to unabsorbed protein or neutral lipid. Oral taurine supplements have been reported (24) to benefit some patients. Viscid, thick in-

crampy abdominal pain that often is aggravated by eating. This syndrome may result from poor compliance with enzyme therapy. Other abdominal symptoms, including extrahepatic biliary obstruction, cholangitis, advanced liver disease, and severe constipation, are less likely to be associated with a prolonged reduction in dietary intake. Encouraging compliance with enzyme therapy and adequate fluid intake sometimes can help relieve these abdominal symptoms and prevent recurrence.

Respiratory problems usually cause restricted oral intake because of anorexia, resulting in acute weight loss. With improvement in respiratory symptoms, patients with mild pulmonary disease can be expected to show a rapid catch-up in weight. In the terminal stages of pulmonary disease, however, chronic anorexia is a consistent feature. Furthermore, patients with severe chronic disease are prone to bouts of clinical depression, which in the adolescent or adult may lead to severe anorexia.

Oral supplements often are prescribed for adolescents and adults with poor eating habits due to busy school or work schedules. However, their efficacy must be evaluated during treatment because preliminary results from one study (33) indicate that oral supplements do not improve nutritional status. Gastrostomy or jejunostomy tubes have been used for supplemental enteral feedings, usually with satisfactory nutritional results. In some patients, this nutritional support method has reduced anxiety arising from poor weight gain; in others, however, poor compliance has resulted in less use and limited or no weight gain (see Nutritional Support section).

Energy Expenditure and Metabolism

Several studies have examined the rates of energy expenditure in patients with CF. In 1984, Pencharz and colleagues (34) evaluated the relationship between heart rate and energy expenditure, using an exercise cycle with graded workloads. Simultaneous measurements of oxygen consumption and carbon dioxide production were taken by means of a closed-circuit indirect calorimeter and heart-rate telemetry. The subjects were malnourished and had moderate to advanced pulmonary disease. They were receiving nutritional rehabilitation by continuous nasogastric tube feeding with a semi-elemental diet. Absorbed energy intake was calculated by subtracting stool energy content from the energy content of the feed. The energy needs of the patients were shown to be 25% to 80% higher than those of healthy persons of the same age, gender, and size. It was hypothesized that energy expenditure was increased because of the increased work of breathing in patients with advanced lung disease. These patients might be unable to ingest sufficient calories to meet energy needs, resulting in energy imbalance and weight loss.

In a subsequent study (35), resting energy expenditure (REE) was measured by continuous computerized open-circuit indirect calorimetry in 71 patients (8.9 to 35.5 years of age) who did not have an acute respiratory infection. Nutritional status and pulmonary function were studied simultaneously. REE was found to be above normal (range, 95% to 153% of predicted values) for age, gender, and weight and was correlated negatively with pulmonary function and nutritional status (percentage of body fat). Consistent with the observations of others (5), pulmonary function was correlated positively with nutritional status. These findings since have been confirmed by Buchdahl and colleagues (36), who demonstrated that patients with CF had an REE of 9% greater than body weight and 7% greater than lean body mass, respectively, compared with healthy controls.

These two studies (35,36) hinted that the CF gene may have a direct effect on basal metabolism. Feigal and Shapiro (37) had earlier reported that mitochondria from fibroblasts cultured from CF homozygotes and heterozygotes had increased oxygen consumption associated with calcium transport. Rates of consumption in the homozygote were twice those of controls, and in the heterozygote they were one and one-half times those of controls. In a subsequent study of CF nasal epithelium, oxygen consumption exceeded that found in control tissue by two to three times (38).

Shepherd et al. (39) investigated total daily energy expenditure by the double-labeled water method in clinically well, adequately nourished infants with CF without clinical evidence of lung disease and compared the results with those in studies of healthy infants. This methodology permitted measurement of total energy expenditure in unrestricted subjects. Infants with CF were reported to have rates of energy expenditure 25% higher per kilogram of body weight than values obtained in healthy infants matched for age, but total daily energy expenditure was not increased (40). Over the next 2 years, when additional subjects were evaluated, even the differences per unit weight between the infants with CF and controls disappeared. When the gene responsible for CF was identified (41), it was speculated that the gene product might be involved directly in the regulation of ion transport across membranes (42) because the CFTR shared structural similarity with several other transport systems involving transmembrane regions and adenosine triphosphate (ATP)-binding domains. Further studies (42) strongly suggested that the CFTR is a cyclic adenosine monophosphate (cAMP)-regulated chloride channel, providing further evidence that the genetic defect may affect basal metabolism directly.

O'Rawe and coworkers (43) reported preliminary results that supported the hypothesis that the genetic defect has such an effect. REE was increased by 25% in subjects homozygous for the most common CF mutation (ΔF508) and by 10% in those with ΔF508 on one chromosome and an undefined CF gene mutation on the other. However, their study did not control for lung function or nutritional status, both important determinants of REE (35). We also have shown that primary undernutrition results in a decreased REE (44). In a study (45) in which we controlled for both these confounding variables, we noted little if any increase in REE in healthy, normally nourished males with CF with good lung function. Furthermore, we were unable to demonstrate any difference in REE in patient groups with different genotypes. Thus, if there is a primary genetic cause for increased REE in patients with CF, its effects must be minimal. Conversely, once forced expiratory volume in 1 second (FEV$_1$) decreased to less than 75% of predicted values, the subject's REE

increased in a curvilinear (quadratic) fashion (Fig. 13–2) (45). Therefore, deteriorating lung function appears to be the major factor associated with an increase in REE.

O'Rawe et al. (46) examined REE and patient genotype while controlling for nutritional status but not lung function. The FEV$_1$ data for their homozygous group (ΔF508/ΔF508) was 48% to 64% of that predicted (mean, 56%); for their heterozygous group (ΔF508/other), it was 52% to 74% (mean, 63%). Therefore, it is not surprising, considering the pulmonary function versus REE data shown in Figure 13–2, that the REE data in each group were 121% and 109% of predicted values, respectively. The authors did attempt to correct for the effects of lung function, using analysis of covariance; however, their data are open to the alternative explanation, namely that the increased REE is secondary to reduced lung function.

Protein synthesis is believed to be responsible for up to 25% of REE (47). We therefore measured REE and whole-body protein synthesis in healthy control subjects, in undernourished patients with CF, and in patients with anorexia nervosa matched to the patients with CF by nutritional status (48). There were no significant differences in protein synthesis be-

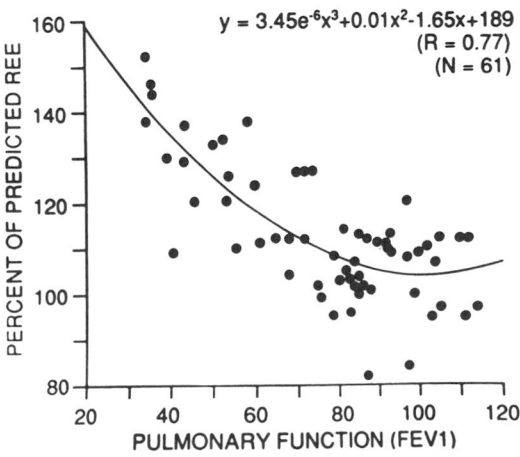

FIG. 13–2. Resting energy expenditure (percentage of predicted) vs. pulmonary function in normally nourished males with cystic fibrosis. (From reference 45.)

tween the three groups. However, the patients with anorexia nervosa had lower REE than controls, and the patients with CF had higher REE. When we measured protein synthesis and REE in patients with CF during renourishment with nocturnal supplemental feedings, REE increased significantly with refeeding, but protein synthesis did not change (44). The increase in REE with refeeding provides evidence that patients with CF adapt to a negative energy balance just as patients with self-imposed food restriction do (49). Following refeeding, patients with anorexia nervosa increased their REE in a pattern similar to that of the undernourished patients with CF (44,49).

Thus, at least two factors appear to affect REE in the undernourished patient with CF with impaired lung function. The first is a normal response to a negative energy balance; the second appears to be related to the severity of lung function impairment. The precise causes of increased REE in patients with CF with moderate to severe lung disease remain to be elucidated. However, the evidence is compelling that alterations in protein metabolism are not responsible (44,48).

REE also can be increased by drugs used in the management of CF lung disease. Before chest physiotherapy, for example, many patients use inhaled bronchodilators, usually sympathomimetic amines. One of these, the β-agonist salbutamol, has been shown to be absorbed through the respiratory tree and to cause a significant increase in REE (approximately 10%) over a period of 3 hours (50).

In practical terms, energy requirements should be determined by assessing total daily energy expenditure. A significant increase probably would result in a negative energy balance, which, if left untreated, would lead to undernutrition. Patients with moderate lung impairment adapt to an increased REE by reducing their activity levels, thereby maintaining total daily energy expenditure at levels comparable to controls (51).

Pregnancy and lactation in females with CF increase the daily energy needs of females by 300 to 500 kcal/day. These factors are discussed later in this chapter.

Pathogenesis of an Energy Deficit

We have proposed a model to explain the cause of the energy deficit in patients with CF (Fig 13–3). This model helps to define the web of interdependent variables giving rise to

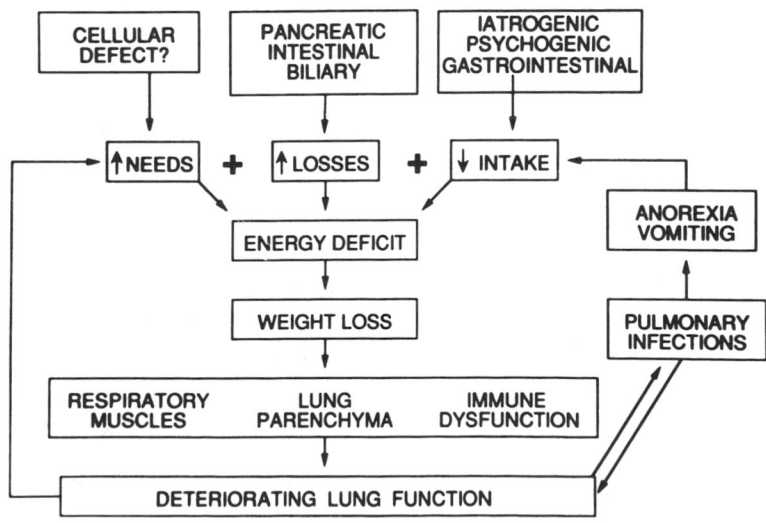

FIG. 13–3. Interdependent factors that may give rise to progressive energy deficit and weight loss as lung function deteriorates. (From reference 18.)

chronic malnutrition and growth failure in these patients. It must be reemphasized, however, that most patients with CF can maintain normal growth velocity and nutritional status by voluntary intake of calories, particularly when lung function remains relatively unimpaired (16). Expressed another way, most patients are capable of compensating for the factors that contribute to an energy deficit. We and others have speculated that malnutrition and decline in pulmonary function are interrelated closely, but a cause-and-effect relationship remains to be proven.

As lung disease worsens, most commonly in older adolescents and young adults, several factors come into play that might predispose the patient to an energy deficit. The frequency and severity of pulmonary infections may increase, inducing anorexia. Chest infections often cause vomiting, which may reduce intake further. These factors, in combination with the increase in REE that accompanies advancing lung disease, may lead to an energy deficit. Weight loss will result, initially causing a substantial loss of adipose tissue and, with time, a loss of lean tissue along with muscle wasting. Wasting of the respiratory muscles would adversely affect respiratory mechanics and reduce effectiveness, thereby further contributing to the deterioration of lung function. Malnutrition is known to adversely affect lung elasticity and a variety of aspects of immune function (52). Taken together, these factors appear to contribute to progressive deterioration of lung function. In essence, a vicious cycle is established, leading inevitably to end-stage pulmonary failure and death.

DEFICITS OF MICRONUTRIENTS

Deficits of essential micronutrients can occur as a result of primary malnutrition or secondary features of the disease, such as pancreatic failure (53,54).

Water-Soluble Vitamins

With the exception of vitamin B12, water-soluble vitamins are well absorbed by patients with CF, and there is no evidence of clinically significant deficiencies in well-nourished patients. In pancreatic-insufficient patients, vitamin B12 absorption can be normalized with adequate pancreatic-enzyme replacement therapy. Vitamin B12 administration is unnecessary, except for patients with meconium ileus who have undergone extensive ileal resection and show biochemical evidence of B12 deficiency.

Fat-Soluble Vitamins

Deficiencies of vitamins A, D, E, and K have been demonstrated at diagnosis (53–55). Supplements of the fat-soluble vitamins are a necessary part of the nutritional care of patients with CF with pancreatic insufficiency or severe liver disease. Vitamins A and E are of the greatest concern, particularly in patients with severe malabsorption or liver disease. Vitamin D deficiency is more of a concern among those with inadequate sunlight exposure (56) or advanced cholestatic liver disease. The most recent evidence suggests that subclinical vitamin K deficiency is more common than currently believed (57). Current recommendations for supplementation with fat-soluble vitamins were provided in the proceedings of a recent consensus conference on nutrition assessment and management (17): 200 to 400 international units of vitamin E, 400 to 800 international units of vitamin D, and 5,000 to 10,000 international units of vitamin A. Vitamin E can be offered in a water-soluble form as a capsule, Aquasol E (Rover Pharmaceutical, Fort Washington, PA). Vitamins A and D are available in standard multiple vitamins at a dose of one to two tablets a day. The use of ADEK (Scandipharm, New York, NY) currently is being evaluated at our clinics; other researchers (58) have reported its successful use.

Trace Metals

No obvious defect of trace-metal absorption or metabolism has been observed in CF. Plasma zinc levels, for example, appear to be low only in patients with moderate to severe malnutrition, and the levels correlate directly with plasma proteins, retinol-binding protein, and vitamin A (59). Plasma levels of copper and ceruloplasmin may be elevated in patients with CF, but usually are in proportion to the severity of pulmonary disease-ceruloplasmin in an acute-phase reactant (59). There is no reliable evidence to support the clinical importance of selenium deficiency (60). Symptomatic hypomagnesemia, with evidence of a positive Trousseau sign, tremulousness, muscle cramps, and weakness, may develop in patients receiving aminoglycosides (61) and is reported to be a secondary complication in patients treated for distal intestinal obstruction syndrome with repeated oral doses of N-acetylcysteine.

Iron-deficiency anemia with low serum ferritin frequently is seen in patients with advanced pulmonary disease (53) but also may occur in stable patients (62). In patients with pulmonary insufficiency, polycythemia seems to occur less commonly with other pulmonary disorders of comparable severity, suggesting that these patients have a relative anemia. However, hemoglobin values do respond to nutritional repletion of the undernourished patient (63). The precise mechanism of iron-deficiency anemia is poorly understood because there is no evidence of a defect of iron absorption or metabolism. In fact, some reports (64) demonstrated increased iron absorption in children with CF not receiving pancreatic extracts; these studies may have been performed in children with depleted iron stores.

Essential Fatty Acids

In infancy, particularly before diagnosis, clinical features of essential fatty acid deficiency can appear, including desquamating skin lesions, increased susceptibility to infection, poor wound healing, thrombocytopenia, and growth retardation. In older patients who are treated adequately, clinical evidence of this deficiency is rare. Most patients with pancreatic insufficiency nevertheless have biochemical abnormalities of blood and tissue lipids (65). Changes include decreased linoleic and

increased palmitoleic, oleic, and eicosatrienoic acids. One report (66) suggested that these biochemical abnormalities reflect an underlying defect of fatty acid metabolism, whereas another (67) argued that the low plasma and tissue levels are the result of increased metabolic usage in undernourished patients. In a survey of 32 patients, we found that low essential fatty acid levels in the plasma were confined to patients with less than 5% of pancreatic function (68). Furthermore, Parsons et al. (69) concluded that suboptimal caloric intake and undernutrition are important determinants in the development of essential fatty acid deficiency. Tissue levels were restored by providing malnourished patients with CF with caloric supplements via nasogastric tube feeding.

NUTRITIONAL ASSESSMENT

Clinical

Nutritional support is an integral part of the care of patients with CF and requires close clinical evaluation of nutritional status and appropriate dietary counseling. Evaluations for newly diagnosed patients should include a 72-hour fecal fat collection and serum levels of vitamins A and E, bentiromide, and trypsinogen (see Biochemical section). If patients are pancreatic insufficient, the importance of enzyme therapy cannot be overemphasized. During routine follow-up visits, weight should be monitored, enzyme therapy reviewed, and dietary counseling provided as required. Patients with CF being transferred to an adult facility should receive a complete review of enzyme and vitamin therapy, diet history, and 3-day fecal fat collection, if necessary. Patients then become familiar with a new dietitian and begin to develop a trusting relationship. Patients who receive an adequate diet can be expected to maintain normal nutritional status until impeded by advanced respiratory disease. Patients who lose weight deserve closer evaluation, particularly those with advancement in their pulmonary disease.

Clinical assessment of nutritional status is done primarily by anthropometry, namely of height, weight, midarm circumference, and triceps skinfolds. Normative data are available for these measurements in adults (70). Our preference is to express the patient's weight as a percentage of ideal weight for height, age, and gender, as detailed in the consensus report on nutritional assessment and management in CF (17). This approach is used extensively with children and adolescents. For adults older than 18 years of age, the body mass index (BMI) (weight/height^2 in kg/m^2), originally developed for use in studies of obesity, also is used for studies of undernutrition. The normal range is 20 to 25 kg/m^2 and is independent of age and gender in adults. In the adult with CF, concern should be shown for a patient whose BMI is decreasing, particularly if it decreases to less than 19.

BMI does not reflect body composition, as is evident by its independence of gender; for this reason, triceps skinfolds (reflecting fat mass) and midarm muscle circumference (reflecting muscle mass) are useful adjuncts to height and weight measurements (70). Other clinical techniques to measure body composition, such as bioelectrical impedance analysis, still must be validated fully (71).

Close involvement of a qualified, experienced dietitian is invaluable. Compliance with pancreatic enzyme supplements and energy intake requires ongoing evaluation. The 72-hour fecal fat test should be considered a part of the routine assessment of enzyme therapy, particularly for those with poor weight gain or poor weight maintenance or with malabsorption symptoms. This requires documentation of weighed nutrient intake as well as enzyme dose. Enzyme dosage may require adjustment with or without the use of agents to inhibit or neutralize gastric-acid secretion. Redistribution or an increase in the total dose of enzymes may help relieve malabsorption symptoms. The enzyme dose should not exceed 4,000 units of lipase per gram of fat/day (20) or 2,500 units of lipase per kg/meal (72). High-strength enzymes should be provided only if the total daily dose does not exceed recommended safe levels. (See Chapter 12 for discussion of different enzymes.)

Patients with mild pulmonary disease often will lose weight after an acute respiratory infection but generally catch up after recovery. Those with recurrent abdominal pain due to distal intestinal obstruction syndrome often reduce caloric intake to control their symptoms. In these cases, aggressive treatment may be necessary and, in our experience, is best achieved by intestinal lavage with a balanced electrolyte solution containing polyethylene glycol (73). Similarly, signs of esophageal reflux and esophagitis (30,31) must be considered and aggressive treatment instituted because severe symptoms will reduce caloric intake. Generally, patients with hepatic disease will grow normally, except in rare instances of severe cholestasis or hepatic decompensation.

The diet must be calorically adequate for individual needs. Actual energy requirements of patients with CF vary extensively, for the aforementioned reasons. Dietary intake may be affected by a patient's level of self-esteem and general feeling of well-being. It therefore is essential that patients who have nutritional difficulties receive psychological support, especially in adolescence and adulthood. Exercise programs aimed at improving physical capacity are important. Improved muscle mass may lead to a sense of accomplishment and stimulate an interest in providing nutritional support for physical goals.

As a general rule, protein intakes of patients with CF are more than adequate (25), but nitrogen balance may be particularly sensitive to insufficient total energy intake. Provided that the latter is adequate, we recommend that protein intake equal the recommended daily allowance for age, gender, and weight. The use of fat, previously discussed in detail, provides an excellent supply of palatable, energy-rich calories. The limited reserves of essential fatty acids in patients with CF and the vulnerability of malnourished patients to essential fatty acid deficiency require specific attention. Although there is no evidence to suggest that biochemical essential fatty acid deficiency has any major clinical impact, we recommend a diet that contains adequate quantities of linoleic acid to maintain normal or close-to-normal fatty-acid profiles. There is no known defect in the transport of monosaccharides, and some investigators even have suggested enhanced glucose absorption. Complex carbohydrates are tolerated quite well and are good sources of energy.

Biochemical

Biochemical evaluation at diagnosis requires a careful assessment of pancreatic and nutritional status. To determine pancreatic status and the need for pancreatic enzymes, we recommend quantitative evaluation of fecal fat losses with accurate measurement of fat intake. Alternatively, recent modifications to the oral bentiromide test (N-benzyl-tyrosyl-aminobenzoic acid) provide a less costly and time-consuming method of evaluating pancreatic function (74). Poor substitutes include documentation of fat on stool microscopy, stool trypsin or chymotrypsin activity, serum carotene, and vitamin A and E levels; many of these tests are useful, however, for monitoring response to treatment on return visits. Serum levels of immunoreactive trypsinogen may be reduced in the patient with pancreatic insufficiency, but only after the age of 7 to 8 years (75). The most accurate method of assessing pancreatic function is the direct pancreatic stimulation test (19), but this invasive, difficult test should be reserved for patients with pancreatic sufficiency to better define reserve exocrine function.

Routine laboratory studies of nutritional status in patients with CF recently were reviewed, and a consensus report was published (17). It was recommended that a complete blood count be taken and levels of plasma retinol and α-tocopherol performed at diagnosis and yearly as a part of routine care. If low levels of retinol or α-tocopherol are detected, the patients need a more comprehensive evaluation of their fat absorption and liver function and an increase in the dosage of vitamins A and E. If there is evidence of iron deficiency on routine hematologic studies, then iron status must be measured more accurately, that is, serum iron, transferrin, and ferritin.

Electrolytes, acid–base status, and serum albumin should be measured at diagnosis. Subsequently, serum albumin is indicated only if there is weight loss or clinical deterioration. Proteins with a short half-life, such as transferrin, retinol-binding protein, and prealbumin, are unnecessary because they offer no advantage over serum albumin combined with anthropometry. Electrolytes and acid–base measurements are indicated with prolonged fever or during the summer heat. In hot climates or during periods of strenuous exercise, sports drinks (containing additional electrolytes) are encouraged. Salt tablets are not necessary, but the liberal use of table salt is encouraged.

STANDARD NUTRITION AND DIETARY SUPPLEMENTATION

Standard guidelines for the nutritional evaluation and care of patients with CF must be modified according to individual needs, the age and gender of the patient, and specific complications of the disease. Patients should be encouraged to follow what used to be considered a standard North American diet, with 35% to 40% of energy in the form of fat. Some patients are concerned because a lower-fat diet is recommended to prevent atherosclerosis; however, the main priority for patients with CF is prevention of a negative energy balance. As the proportion of dietary energy derived from fat decreases, so does the total number of calories ingested. Clearly, this reduction in calories is inappropriate. However, if a patient has pancreatic sufficiency and a family history of hyperlipidemia, blood lipid levels should be monitored.

Another potential problem is that of dietary fiber. Because some patients with CF become constipated, a moderate amount of dietary fiber is recommended, provided that there is adequate fluid intake. However, a high-fiber diet can be low in energy and may exacerbate distal ileal obstructive syndrome; therefore, diets high in fiber should be avoided.

With the patient who loses weight, we approach diagnosis from the perspective of energy balance. Key factors are energy intake, absorption, and expenditure. Energy and enzyme intake is determined from 3-day food records. Absorption is measured by 72-hour stool collection combined with a 72-hour food record, which will permit the coefficient of fat absorption to be calculated. Energy expenditure is measured by open-circuit indirect calorimetry (35). We recognize that most centers will not have access to indirect calorimetry; therefore, on the basis of our experience, we have suggested a way of estimating the REE of a patient with CF based on normal standards, lung function, age, and gender (17). Estimated REE enables the calculation of daily energy needs. The reader is referred to Appendix A of the consensus report (17) for further details. Generally, a close estimate of energy requirements can be calculated using the basal metabolic rate $\times$ 1.1 (for malabsorption) $\times$ an activity factor (1.5 to 1.7) + 200 to 400 kcal/day.

The first step in managing the patient who has lost weight, after ensuring that enzyme therapy is optimized, is to augment the fat content of the diet and include snacks in the meal plan. The dietitian, using results of 3-day food records, can suggest ways to increase the energy value of the meal plan. Homemade milkshakes may be recommended for some patients, whereas others prefer to use commercially prepared high-energy beverages and foods. However, as reported earlier (33), we are concerned that oral supplements may replace food intake and question their efficacy. Conversely, in gastrostomy-supplemented patients, although food intake was suppressed by 20%, total daily energy intake was increased and nutritional status was improved (44).

NUTRITIONAL SUPPORT

In patients in whom dietary intervention and oral supplementation do not resolve their negative energy balance, a variety of nutritional support approaches have been tried, including nasogastric and enterostomy feeding and parenteral nutrition. The hope is that restoration of nutritional status may provide easier control of chest infections, ameliorate the rate of decline in respiratory function, and extend survival.

We have reviewed critically the current literature on the subject.

Short-Term Studies

A variety of short-term parenteral and enteral feeding techniques have been used with malnourished patients with CF. Shepherd et al. (76) evaluated malnourished patients with CF (mean age, 5.43 years) 6 months before and after a 3-week period of parenteral nutrition. During the pretreatment period, while receiving "conventional" dietary management, the patients showed inadequate growth velocity; however, 6 months after the short period of intravenous nutrition, they exhibited continuing catch-up growth, suffered fewer pulmonary infections, and showed a significant improvement in clinical score.

Other studies have failed to show lasting improvement after short-term nutritional support. The improved nutritional status in the patients in the study by Shepherd and colleagues (76) could be explained by aggressive pulmonary management during hospitalization. In addition, the very young age of their patients suggests that closer attention to voluntary nutrition may well have prevented the problem at the outset.

Mansell et al. (77), who evaluated older malnourished patients with CF (aged 10 to 17 years), also demonstrated improvement in nutritional status after a 1-month period of supplemental parenteral nutrition when patients were provided with 120% of their energy needs. Immediately after this supplementation, body weight, triceps skinfold thickness, and midarm muscle circumference increased significantly. Maximum inspiratory airway pressure also increased, suggesting improvement in respiratory muscle strength; however, none of the indices of lung function improved. One month after parenteral nutrition, however, the patients were once again malnourished, decreasing to levels similar to those seen before treatment.

In a study from Montreal (78), supplemental feeding by nasogastric tube was instituted while patients were in the hospital and was continued at home for 4 weeks. Patients showed substantial weight gain, attributable to increased caloric intake, but the nutritional changes were transient and not accompanied by long-term improvement in growth.

Pencharz et al. (34) evaluated body composition, nutritional status, and energy needs of six undernourished adolescents and adults with CF. Lean body mass was preserved, but there was significant wasting of adipose tissue. After a brief period of nasogastric feeding with a semielemental diet, the effects of refeeding on body composition were reassessed: body weight, body fat, and total body potassium increased significantly, but fat-free body mass and total body nitrogen did not change. None of the subjects was able to continue the feeding for longer than 2 to 3 months because of nasal irritation and coughing up the tube.

Thus, the benefits of brief periods of supplemental nutrition do not produce long-term improvement in growth or function. This result is not surprising when one considers the pathogenesis of the energy imbalance (see Fig 13–3) because the underlying causative factors are not reversed.

Long-Term Studies

Because the effects of brief periods of energy supplementation on chronically malnour-ished CF patients were transient, long-term approaches clearly were necessary to achieve and maintain normal nutrition in patients unable to meet their own energy needs. In addition, it was believed that reversal of malnutrition might influence favorably the course of pulmonary disease and, consequently, the rate of survival.

Several investigators have studied the effect of parenteral nutrition in patients with CF and malnutrition, delivered over periods varying from 4 months (79) to more than 1 year (80). Once sufficient energy was delivered, all the patients improved their weight and nutritional status. However, no change was seen in their pulmonary status; once total parenteral nutrition was discontinued, all patients reverted progressively to their former state of malnutrition (79,80). In the longest-term study (80), central-line complications were significant, and there was an increased need for intravenous antibiotics.

As shown in Table 13–3, three major studies (63, 82–83) have addressed the problem by using forms of nocturnal enteral supplements. In a study from Toronto (63), patients were given nocturnal supplemental feeding of a semielemental formula by gastrostomy tube for an average period of 1 year. The adolescent and adult patients were suffering from moderate to severe lung disease, and all were markedly

TABLE 13–3. *Long-term enteral feeding of malnourished patients with cystic fibrosis*

Variable	Toronto	Ottawa	Brisbane
Patients (male/female)	14 (5/9)	10 (5/5)	10 (5/5)
Age			
Mean (yrs)	12.9	13.6	8.9
Range (yrs)	5–22	6–21	3–13
Study design			
Enteral route	Gastrostomy	Jejunostomy	Nasogastric/gastrostomy
Supplement type	Semielemental	Intact	Semielemental
Duration (yrs)	1.1	1.6	1.0
Controls	Concurrent	Retrospective	Prospective
Patient characteristics			
Weight as % of height[a]	82 ± 10	80 ± 9	No data
FEV_1 (%)	47 ± 15	No data	66 ± 16
Forced vital capacity (%)	53 ± 13	64 ± 18	84 ± 12

[a]Weight was expressed as deviation from the reference standard (i.e., Z-score).
FEV_1, forced expiratory volume in 1 second.
Adapted from reference 18.

wasted or stunted. Gastrostomy tubes were placed endoscopically using local anesthesia. A contemporary group of patients with CF (matched for age, gender, nutritional status, and pulmonary function) drawn from the clinic's computerized data bank were pair-matched to the study group. In a second Canadian study (82), 10 malnourished patients with CF (mean age, 13.6 years) with moderate to severe lung disease were provided with nocturnal supplemental feeding of an intact formula by a needle jejunostomy tube for periods of 10 to 36 months. Pancreatic enzyme supplements were added to the formula. In the third study, from Australia, Shepherd et al. (83) evaluated 10 undernourished patients with CF (mean age, 8.9 years) who were unable to maintain normal growth by oral means. They were followed during a 1-year course of nutritional supplement with a balanced-peptide or a semielemental formula given overnight by nasogastric or gastrostomy feeding. These patients were compared concurrently with patients receiving conventional nutritional therapy and matched for height, gender, and pulmonary function. In all three studies, normal activity and regular meals were permitted during daytime hours.

In each study, long-term enteral supplemental feeding produced a significant improvement in catch-up growth and positive changes in body composition (Table 13–4). There appeared to be beneficial effects on pulmonary function, but the effect on survival remains unanswered. In the two Canadian studies

(81,82), nutritional supplements appeared to slow the rate of deterioration of pulmonary function. In the study by Shepherd and associates (83), respiratory function deteriorated in the control group but appeared to improve in the patient group; however, the patients were considerably younger than those in the two Canadian studies.

After our initial publication of the results of long-term gastrostomy supplemental feeding (63), we established a multidisciplinary approach to the evaluation and care of the failing patient (Table 13–5). This approach uses the services of dietitians, nutrition support nurses, social workers, and physicians. Patients identified as having an energy problem are seen first by the dietitian. If diet counseling and/or voluntary supplements are not effective, the patient is referred for assessment for long-term gastrostomy feeding. It includes both a family and social evaluation and a medical/nutritional assessment. Once the multidisciplinary team has considered the factors for and against nutritional intervention, the patient and family are brought into the decision-making process.

Currently, only 10 of the 300 patients attending the adult CF clinic at St. Michael's Hospital are receiving supplementary gastrostomy feeds. Because their energy needs remain elevated, few patients have been able to discontinue gastrostomy feeding completely; they have, however, been able to maintain an appropriate weight. Some have been able to decrease the frequency of feedings to 4 to 5 nights per week

TABLE 13–4. *Effects of long-term enteral feeding in malnourished patients with cystic fibrosis*

Variable	Toronto	Ottawa	Brisbane
Nutritional status			
ΔWeight (kg)	+	+	+
ΔHeight (cm)	+	+	+
ΔWeight as % of height (%)	+	+	+
Total body potassium (g)	+	No data	No data
Body fat (%)	+	No data	No data
Midarm muscle circumference	No data	+	No data
Protein synthesis	No data	No data	+
Respiratory function			
Patients	Unchanged	Unchanged[a]	Improved
Controls	Deteriorated	Deteriorated[a]	Deteriorated

[a]Compared with year before intervention.
Adapted from reference 18.

TABLE 13–5. *Approach to nutritional treatment of patients with cystic fibrosis*

Encourage good feeding habits early
In patients with growth failure, assess
  Energy intake
  Absorptive function
  Gastrointestinal complications that might reduce
    intake
  Energy expenditure
  Psychological/family dysfunction
Provide voluntary supplements and/or modify
  enzyme therapy
Consider invasive methods of nutritional
  supplementation before severe undernutrition
  occurs
Avoid invasive methods in patients with end-stage
  pulmonary failure because these only will prolong
  the agony of dying

while maintaining an appropriate weight. In the past 4 to 5 years, we have shifted from percutaneous, endoscopically placed gastrostomy tubes to placement by an interventional radiologist guided by diagnostic imaging (84). This procedure is well tolerated, and patients are discharged 3 to 5 days after gastrostomy insertion. A full description of our enterostomy program has been published (85).

Parenteral nutrition, as described earlier, can improve weight gain in the short term but is not used routinely with our adult patients because it is expensive, yields minimal benefits, and poses higher risks of infection (80). In some situations, lipids alone may be used to help maintain or promote weight gain in hospitalized patients who are not able to meet their energy requirements with oral intake alone.

When close attention is paid to the individual's energy needs and nutritional status, undernutrition can be prevented or treated promptly. In the majority of patients, normal weight and nutrition can be attained with the rational use of a normal high-energy diet. However, in a small group of patients with CF, advanced lung disease causes an increase in energy expenditure; energy imbalance may result. At this stage, long-term, invasive methods of nutritional support should be considered. In patients with more advanced lung disease who are candidates for a lung transplant, prior maintenance of nutritional status is an important prognostic factor.

However, aggressive nutritional therapy should not be initiated during the terminal stages, when the patient is suffering from end-stage cardiopulmonary failure (81).

SPECIAL CONSIDERATIONS

Cystic Fibrosis-Related Diabetes

Recent studies suggest that 8% to 15% of patients with CF may suffer from CFRD (86). Prevalence has increased because adults with CF are living longer (80); the mean age of onset is 18 to 20 years (87–90). CFRD differs from type 1 or type 2 diabetes mellitus because patients are nonketotic and the diet management is different (see Chapter 18). The definition of diagnosis of CFRD is described in a consensus report (91), which also provides guidelines on its management and on normal energy needs for weight gain or weight maintenance. Although additional calories may be required to restore weight lost before diagnosis of CFRD, treatment with insulin (1 or 2 daily injections) often is adequate to restore normal weight.

Dietary management of this second disease, along with insulin treatment, may seem overwhelming to the patient with CF newly diagnosed with diabetes. Patients are encouraged to maintain a normal- to high-fat (35% to 40% of total energy) intake, with normal carbohydrate and protein consumption. Monosaccharides or simple sugars need not be avoided as long as they are not consumed as isolated snacks. Simple-sugar foods can be consumed with meals and can be substituted for foods of similar carbohydrate content. A list of complex and simple carbohydrate foods with sample serving sizes can help the patient replace foods in the diet to ensure similar amounts of carbohydrate are taken with meals and snacks. Insulin is adjusted to the usual meal schedule. Special attention is given to patients receiving gastrostomy tube feedings; they are taught to decrease and adjust insulin if feeds are not taken regularly.

The importance of consistent timing of meals and snacks with insulin therapy must be stressed. Unless the meal plan before diagnosis of CFRD already was inappropriate, insulin is adjusted to the usual intake, and consistency in timing and quality and quantity of foods is reviewed. The recommended frequency of glucose testing is based on individual lifestyle. The dietitian reviews the patient's usual intake, encourages consistency, and emphasizes the importance of enzyme compliance. Patients always should have an easily accessible source of sucrose in case of unexpected hypoglycemia. This can include hard candies, sugar packets, or glucose tablets or gels. Sugars should be monitored before and after exercise, and increased calories should be consumed before any exercise.

Because patients with CF are living longer, complications such as nephropathy, retinopathy, and other diabetes-related sequelae have been reported. Strict control of blood sugars has not been advocated routinely for CFRD. This practice needs to be reassessed because patients are living longer and complications associated with CFRD may occur.

Pregnancy and Lactation

Some women with CF can become pregnant and carry a child to term. An ideal weight before becoming pregnant, which is associated with a better outcome for mother and child (92,93), is encouraged. Women with CF should follow RDA guidelines for pregnancy. A dietitian can help the patient with a higher-energy meal plan to support the growing fetus. In most cases, appetite increases naturally with pregnancy. Special attention must be paid to the patient with severe vomiting because of morning sickness; parenteral nutrition may be recommended. Usually, vitamin supplementation is advised, with an additional prenatal vitamin taken daily.

As in pregnancy, energy needs increase during lactation. However, depending on her clinical condition, the woman who chooses to breastfeed may find it difficult to maintain increased intake because of the increased demands of caring for an infant. If she is unable to maintain an ideal weight or if her health status is compromised, a commercial infant formula may be recommended to supplement or replace breast milk. At our clinic, four women have breastfed their infants, including one who breast fed for 2½ years.

Limited data are available on the breast milk of mothers with CF (94). The nutrient content of breast milk of a woman with CF may be altered, but it is adequate to support an infant's nutritional needs. One woman with CF who gave birth to two healthy infants recommended small, energy-packed meals taken frequently throughout the day, rather than three larger meals, to maintain appropriate weight gain. She said that regaining lost weight during a viral illness was especially difficult, so she used high-energy milkshakes to supplement intake. She found breastfeeding her infants fairly successful, although supplementation with a formula was necessary for her first baby.

Liver Disease

No specific nutritional restrictions or alterations in the diet are required for patients with documented liver disease. It is recommended that these patients take a vitamin K supplement daily.

LIVING WITH CYSTIC FIBROSIS: FITTING GOOD NUTRITION INTO AN ADULT LIFESTYLE

Although patients with CF who reach adulthood have been counseled frequently about the importance of good nutrition and enzyme compliance, nutritional assessment must continue. Despite a lifelong routine practice, some adults still claim that they forget to take their enzymes. A survey recently conducted at our clinic (D. Kalnins, unpublished data, 1995) revealed that 16% of adult patients (n = 32) missed taking enzymes with some meals, and 12% missed taking them with some snacks. Busy school schedules and type of work also can have negative effects on nutritional intake, possibly resulting in weight loss. One patient reported that a more stable lifestyle (since marriage) helped him improve weight gain and maintain a healthier clinical status. For adults with CF with busy schedules, suggestions from clinic staff on ways to increase oral intake are helpful.

A problem manifested in many young female adults is the desire to be thin, a result of society's preference for slender female models. The CF dietitian may find it difficult to counsel these patients, especially those who decrease intake or compliance with enzyme therapy to lose weight. The CF clinic team must convey the same message to these patients, explaining the rationale and informing them of the potential consequences of their actions. Significant weight loss should be prevented before pulmonary status is affected.

Adults with CF read news reports about recommendations for the public to decrease fat and salt in the diet and can become concerned about their own diet. No restrictions on fat or salt are necessary. Patients with a family history of heart disease or hyperlipidemia may have blood lipid levels monitored, but to date there have been no reports of elevated levels in patients with CF. As lung function deteriorates and sickness occurs more frequently, smaller, more frequent meals should be emphasized to try to avoid significant weight loss. Finally, adults with CF can help educate the CF care giver about the problems they have encountered and the solutions they used to solve them. In this way, the patient and clinician can work together to achieve optimum care for the patient.

ACKNOWLEDGMENTS

Much of the work from our units referred to in this chapter has been made possible through the generous support of the Canadian Cystic Fibrosis Foundation. We thank Kevin Taylor and Sue McKellar for sharing their experiences. This chapter was prepared with the assistance of Editorial Services, The Hospital for Sick Children, Toronto, Ontario, Canada.

REFERENCES

1. Gaskin K, Gurwitz D, Durie P, et al: Improved respiratory prognosis in patients with cystic fibrosis with normal fat absorption. *J Pediatr* 1982;100:857–862.
2. Kerem E, Corey M, Kerem B, et al. Clinical and genetic comparisons of patients with cystic fibrosis, with or without meconium ileus. *J Pediatr* 1989;114:767–773.
3. Scott-Jupp R, Lana M, Tanner MS. Prevalence of liver disease in cystic fibrosis. *Arch Dis Child* 1991;66:698–701.
4. Gurwitz D, Corey M, Francis PWJ, et al. Perspectives in cystic fibrosis. *Pediatr Clin North Am* 1979;26:603–615.
5. Kraemer R, Rodeberg A, Hadorn B, et al. Relative underweight in cystic fibrosis and its prognostic value. *Acta Paediatr Scand* 1978;67:33–37.
6. Roy CC, Darling P, Weber AM. A rational approach to meeting macro- and micronutrient needs in cystic fibrosis. *J Pediatr Gastroenterol Nutr* 1984;3(Suppl 1):S154–S162.
7. Sproul A, Huang N. Growth patterns in children with cystic fibrosis. *J Pediatr* 1964;65:664–676.
8. Kerem E, Corey M, Kerem B-S, et al. The relation between genotype and phenotype in cystic fibrosis—analysis of the most common mutation (delta F508). *N Engl J Med* 1990;323:1517–1522.
9. Zielenski J, Tsui L-C. Cystic fibrosis: genotypic and phenotypic variations. *Ann Rev Genetics* 1995;29:777–807.
10. Corey M. Longitudinal studies in cystic fibrosis. In: Sturgess JM, ed. *Perspectives in cystic fibrosis: proceedings of the 8th International Congress on Cystic Fibrosis.* Toronto, Ontario: Canadian Cystic Fibrosis Foundation, 1980:264–255.
11. Corey M, McLaughlin FJ, Williams M, et al. A comparison of survival, growth, and pulmonary function in patients with cystic fibrosis in Boston and Toronto. *J Clin Epidemiol* 1988;41:583–591.
12. Shwachman H. Therapy of cystic fibrosis of the pancreas. *Pediatrics* 1960;25:155–163.
13. Allan JD, Mason A, Moss AD. Nutritional supplementation in treatment of cystic fibrosis of the pancreas. *Am J Dis Child* 1973;126:22–26.
14. Gracey M, Burke V, Anderson CM. Assessment of medium-chain triglyceride feeding in infants with cystic fibrosis. *Arch Dis Child* 1969;44:401–403.
15. Crozier DN. Cystic fibrosis: a not-so-fatal disease. *Pediatr Clin North Am* 1974;21:935–950.
16. Pencharz PB. Energy intakes and low-fat diets in children with cystic fibrosis (editorial). *J Pediatr Gastroenterol Nutr* 1983;2:400–402.
17. Ramsey BW, Farrell PM, Pencharz P, the Consensus Committee. Nutritional assessment and management in cystic fibrosis: a consensus report. *Am J Clin Nutr* 1992;55:108–116.
18. Durie PR, Pencharz PB. A rational approach to the nutritional care of patients with cystic fibrosis. *J R Soc Med* 1989;82(Suppl 16):11–20.
19. Gaskin KJ, Durie PR, Lee L, et al. Colipase and lipase secretion in childhood-onset pancreatic insufficiency: delineation of patients with steatorrhea secondary to relative colipase deficiency. *Gastroenterology* 1984;86:1–7.
20. Kalnins D, Durie PR, Ellis L. Pancreatic enzymes: evaluation of current practice in a large CF clinic. *Pediatr Pulmonol Suppl* 1995;12:266 (abstract).
21. Kalnins D, Ellis L, Corey M, Pencharz PB, Durie PR. Extreme variability of response to enzyme treatment of patients with cystic fibrosis. *Pediatr Pulmonol Suppl* 1997;14:309 (abstract).

22. Gaskin KJ, Durie PR, Corey M, et al. Evidence for a primary defect of pancreatic HCO_3^- secretion in cystic fibrosis. *Pediatr Res* 1982;16:554–557.

23. Zentler-Munro PL, Fine DR, Batten JC, et al. Effect of cimetidine on enzyme inactivation, bile acid precipitation, and lipid solubilisation in pancreatic steatorrhea due to cystic fibrosis. *Gut* 1985;26:892–901.

24. Belli DC, Levy E, Darling P, et al. Taurine improves the absorption of a fat meal in patients with cystic fibrosis. *Pediatrics* 1987;80:517–523.

25. Bell L, Linton W, Corey ML, et al. Nutrient intakes of adolescents with cystic fibrosis. *J Can Diet Assoc* 1981;42(1):62–71.

26. Bentur L, Kalnins D, Levison H, et al. Dietary intakes of adolescent males and females—is there a difference? *J Pediatr Gastroenterol Nutr* 1996;22:254–258.

27. Daniels L, Davidson GP, Martin AJ. Comparison of the macronutrient intake of healthy controls and children with cystic fibrosis on low fat or nonrestricted fat diets. *J Pediatr Gastroenterol Nutr* 1987;6:381–386.

28. Parsons HG, Beaudry P, Dumas A, et al. Energy needs and growth in children with cystic fibrosis. *J Pediatr Gastroenterol Nutr* 1983;2:44–49.

29. MacDonald A, Holden C, Harris G. Nutritional strategies in cystic fibrosis: current issues. *J R Soc Med Vol* 1991;84(Suppl 18):28–35.

30. Feigelson J, Girault F, Pecau Y. Gastro-oesophageal reflux and esophagitis in cystic fibrosis. *Acta Paediatr Scand* 1987;76:989–990.

31. Scott RB, O'Laughlin EV, Gall DG. Gastroesophageal reflux in patients with cystic fibrosis. *J Pediatr* 1985;106:223–227.

32. Rosenstein BJ, Langbaum TS. Incidence of distal intestinal obstruction syndrome in cystic fibrosis. *J Pediatr Gastroenterol Nutr* 1983;2:299–301.

33. Kalnins D, Durie P, Corey M, et al. Are oral dietary supplements effective in the nutritional management of adolescents and adults with CF? *Pediatr Pulmonol Suppl* 1996;13:314 (abstract).

34. Pencharz P, Hill R, Archibald E, et al. Energy needs and nutritional rehabilitation in undernourished adolescents and young adult patients with cystic fibrosis. *J Pediatr Gastroenterol Nutr* 1984;3(Suppl 1):S147–S153.

35. Vaisman N, Pencharz PB, Corey M, et al. Energy expenditure of patients with cystic fibrosis. *J Pediatr* 1987;111:496–500.

36. Buchdahl RM, Cox M, Fulleylove C, et al. Increased resting energy expenditure in cystic fibrosis. *J Appl Physiol* 1988;64:1810–1816.

37. Feigal R, Shapiro BL. Mitochondrial calcium uptake and oxygen consumption in cystic fibrosis. *Nature* 1979;278:276–277.

38. Stutts MJ, Knowles MR, Gatzy JT, et al. Oxygen consumption and ouabain binding sites in cystic fibrosis nasal epithelium. *Pediatr Res* 1986;20:1316–1320.

39. Shepherd RW, Holt TL, Vasques-Velasquez L, et al. Increased energy expenditure in young children with cystic fibrosis. *Lancet* 1988;i:1300–1303.

40. Pencharz PB, Berall G, Vaisman N, et al. Energy expenditure in children with cystic fibrosis. *Lancet* 1988;ii:513–514.

41. Rommens JM, Iannuzzi MC, Kerem B-S, et al. Identification of the cystic fibrosis gene: chromosome walking and jumping. *Science* 1989;245:1059–1065.

42. Riordan JR, Rommens JM, Kerem B-S, et al. Identification of the cystic fibrosis gene: cloning and characterization of complementary DNA. *Science* 1989;245:1066–1073.

43. O'Rawe A, Dodge JA, Redmond AOB, et al. Gene/energy interaction in cystic fibrosis. *Lancet* 1990;335:552–553.

44. Vaisman N, Clarke R, Pencharz PB. Nutritional rehabilitation increases resting energy expenditure without affecting protein turnover in patients with cystic fibrosis. *J Pediatr Gastroenterol Nutr* 1991;13:383–390.

45. Fried MD, Durie PR, Tsui L-C, et al. The cystic fibrosis gene and resting energy expenditure. *J Pediatr* 1991;119:913–916.

46. O'Rawe A, McIntosh I, Dodge JA, et al. Increased energy expenditure in cystic fibrosis is associated with specific mutations. *Clin Sci* 1992;82:71–76.

47. Summers M, McBride BW, Milligan LP. Components of basal energy expenditure. In: Dobson A, Dobson M, eds. *Aspects of digestive physiology in ruminants: proceedings of a satellite symposium of the 30th International Congress of the International Union of Physiological Sciences.* Ithaca, NY: Cornell University Press, 1988:257–285.

48. Vaisman N, Clarke R, Rossi M, et al. Protein turnover and resting energy expenditure in patients with undernutrition and chronic lung disease. *Am J Clin Nutr* 1992;55:63–69.

49. Vaisman N, Rossi M, Corey M, et al. Effect of refeeding on the energy metabolism of adolescent girls who have anorexia nervosa. *Eur J Clin Nutr* 1991;45:527–537.

50. Vaisman N, Levy LD, Pencharz PB, et al. Effect of salbutamol on resting energy expenditure in patients with cystic fibrosis. *J Pediatr* 1987;111:137–139.

51. Spicher V, Roulet M, Schutz Y. Assessment of total energy expenditure in free-living patients with cystic fibrosis. *J Pediatr* 1991;118:865–872.

52. Chandra RK, Newberne PM. *Nutrition, immunity and infection: mechanisms of interaction.* New York: Plenum Press, 1977.

53. Chase PM, Long MA, Lavin MH. Cystic fibrosis and malnutrition. *J Pediatr* 1979;95:337–347.

54. Congden PJ, Bruce G, Rothburn MM, et al. Vitamin status in treated patients with cystic fibrosis. *Arch Dis Child* 1981;56:708–714.

55. Sokol RJ, Reardon MC, Accurso FJ, et al. Fat-soluble-vitamin status during the first year of life in infants with cystic fibrosis identified by screening of newborns. *Am J Clin Nutr* 1989;50:1064–1071.

56. Reiter EO, Brugman SM, Pike JW, et al. Vitamin D metabolites in adolescents and young adults with cystic fibrosis: effects of sun and season. *J Pediatr* 1985;106:21–26.

57. Rashid M, Durie P, Kalnins D, et al. Prevalence of vitamin K deficiency in children with cystic fibrosis. *Pediatr Pulmonol Suppl* 1996;13:313 (abstract).

58. Eid NS, Eddy M, Greer P, et al. Water-soluble vitamins in cystic fibrosis. *Pediatr Pulmonol Suppl* 1993;9:281 (abstract).

59. Solomons NW, Wagonfeld JB, Rieger C, et al. Some biochemical indices of nutrition in treated cystic fibrosis patients. *Am J Clin Nutr* 1981;34:462–474.

60. Castillo R, Landon C, Eckhardt K, et al. Selenium and vitamin E status in cystic fibrosis. *J Pediatr* 1981;99:583–585.

61. Green CG, Doershuk CF, Stern RC. Symptomatic hypomagnesemia in cystic fibrosis. *J Pediatr* 1985;107:425–428.
62. Ater JL, Herbst JJ, Landaw SA, et al. Relative anemia and iron deficiency in cystic fibrosis. *Pediatrics* 1983;71:810–814.
63. Levy LD, Durie PR, Pencharz PB, et al. Effects of long-term nutritional rehabilitation on body composition and clinical status in malnourished children and adolescents with cystic fibrosis. *J Pediatr* 1985;107:225–230.
64. Heinrich HC, Bender-Gotze C, Gabbe EE, et al. Absorption of inorganic iron(^{59}Fe^{2+}) in relation to iron stores in pancreatic exocrine insufficiency due to cystic fibrosis. *Klin Wochenschr* 1977;55:587–593.
65. Farrell PM, Mischler EH, Engle MJ, et al. Fatty acid abnormalities in cystic fibrosis. *Pediatr Res* 1985;19:104–109.
66. Rogiers V, Dab I, Crokaert R, et al. Long chain non-esterified fatty acid pattern in plasma of cystic fibrosis patients and their parents. *Pediatr Res* 1980;14:1088–1091.
67. Hubbard VS, Dunn GD. Fatty acid composition of erythrocyte phospholipids from patients with cystic fibrosis. *Clin Chim Acta* 1980;102:115–118.
68. Forstner G, Durie P, Corey M. *Cystic fibrosis, progress in gastroenterology and nutrition.* 10th International Cystic Fibrosis Congress, Sydney, Australia. Excerpta Medica, Asia Pacific Congress, 1988;Series 74:154–160.
69. Parsons HG, O'Loughlin EV, Forbes D, et al. Supplemental calories improve essential fatty acid deficiency in cystic fibrosis patients. *Pediatr Res* 1988;24:353–356.
70. Frisancho AR. *Anthropometric standards for the assessment of growth and nutritional status.* Ann Arbor, MI: University of Michigan Press, 1990.
71. Azcue M, Fried M, Pencharz P. Use of bioelectrical impedance analysis to measure total body water in patients with cystic fibrosis. *J Pediatr Gastroenterol Nutr* 1993;16:440–445.
72. Borowitz DS, Grand RJ, Durie PR, the Consensus Committee. Use of pancreatic enzyme supplements for patients with cystic fibrosis in the context of fibrosing colonopathy. *J Pediatrics* 1995;127:681–684.
73. Cleghorn GJ, Stringer DA, Forstner GG, et al. Treatment of distal intestinal obstruction syndrome in cystic fibrosis with a balanced intestinal lavage solution. *Lancet* 1986;i:8–11.
74. Weizman Z, Forstner GG, Gaskin KJ, et al. Bentiromide test for assessing pancreatic dysfunction using analysis of para-aminobenzoic acid in plasma and urine: studies in cystic fibrosis and Shwachman's syndrome. *Gastroenterology* 1985;89:596–604.
75. Durie PR, Forstner GG, Gaskin KJ, et al. Age-related alterations of immunoreactive pancreatic cationic trypsinogen in sera from cystic fibrosis patients with and without pancreatic insufficiency. *Pediatr Res* 1986;20:209–213.
76. Shepherd R, Cooksley WGE, Domville Cooke WD. Improved growth and clinical, nutritional, and respiratory changes in response to nutritional therapy in cystic fibrosis. *J Pediatr* 1980;97:351–357.
77. Mansell AL, Andersen JC, Muttart CR, et al. Short-term pulmonary effects of total parenteral nutrition in children with cystic fibrosis. *J Pediatr* 1984;104:700–705.
78. Bertrand JM, Morin CL, Lasalle R, et al. Short-term clinical, nutritional, and functional effects of continuous elemental enteral alimentation in patients with cystic fibrosis. *J Pediatr* 1984;104:41–46.
79. Kirvela O, Stern RC, Askanazi J, et al. Long-term parenteral nutrition in cystic fibrosis. *Nutrition* 1993;9(2):119–126.
80. Allen ED, Mick AB, Nicol J, et al. Prolonged parenteral nutrition for cystic fibrosis patients. *Nutr Clin Prac* 1995;10:73–79.
81. Levy L, Durie P, Pencharz P, et al. Prognostic factors associated with patient survival during nutritional rehabilitation in malnourished children and adolescents with cystic fibrosis. *J Pediatr Gastroenterol Nutr* 1986;5:97–102.
82. Boland MP, Stoski DS, MacDonald NE, et al. Chronic jejunostomy feeding with a non-elemental formula in undernourished patients with cystic fibrosis. *Lancet* 1986;i:232–234.
83. Shepherd RW, Holt TL, Thomas BJ, et al. Nutritional rehabilitation in cystic fibrosis: controlled studies of effects on nutritional growth retardation, body protein turnover, and course of pulmonary disease. *J Pediatr* 1986;109:788–794.
84. Ho C-S, Gray RR, Goldfinger M, et al. Percutaneous gastrostomy for enteral feeding. *Radiology* 1985;156:349–351.
85. Grunow J, Chait P, Savoie S, et al. Gastrostomy feeding. In: David TJ, ed. *Recent advances in paediatrics.* New York: Churchill Livingstone, 1993;12:23–39.
86. Knowles MR, Fernald GW. Diabetes and cystic fibrosis: new questions emerging from increased longevity. *J Pediatr* 1988;112:415–416.
87. Dodge JA, Morrison G. Diabetes mellitus in cystic fibrosis: a review. *J R Soc Med* 1992;85 Suppl 19:25–28.
88. Rodman HM, Doershuk CF, Roland JM. The interaction of the two diseases: diabetes mellitus and cystic fibrosis. *Medicine* 1986;65:389–397.
89. Finkelstein SM, Wielinski CL, Elliott GR, et al. Diabetes mellitus associated with cystic fibrosis. *J Pediatr* 1988;112:373–377.
90. Reisman J, Corey M, Canny G, et al. Diabetes mellitus in patients with cystic fibrosis: effect on survival. *Pediatrics* 1990;86:374–377.
91. Zipf W. Consensus Conference on CF-related diabetes mellitus. In: *Concepts in care.* Vol. I, Section IV, Part 7. Bethesda, MD: Cystic Fibrosis Foundation, 1990:1–7.
92. Canny GJ, Corey M, Livingstone RA, et al. Pregnancy and cystic fibrosis. *Obstet Gynecol* 1991;77:850–853.
93. Palmer J, Dillon-Baker C, Tecklin JS, et al. Pregnancy in patients with cystic fibrosis. *Ann Intern Med* 1983;99:596–600.
94. Michel SH, Mueller DH. Impact of lactation on women with cystic fibrosis and their infants: a review of five cases. *J Am Diet Assoc* 1994;94:159–165.

Cystic Fibrosis in Adults,
edited by J. R. Yankaskas and M. R. Knowles,
Lippincott–Raven Publishers, Philadelphia, 1999.

14

Hepatobiliary System

Carla Colombo, *Andrea Crosignani, †Maria Luisa Melzi, †Stefania Comi,
††Giovanna Pizzamiglio, and †Annamaria Giunta

*Department of Pediatrics, University of Sassari, Sassari; *Istituto di Scienze Biomediche, San Paolo
Hospital; and Department of Pediatrics and ††Department of Internal Medicine, University of Milan,
Milan, Italy*

As the life expectancy of patients with cystic fibrosis (CF) improves, there is increasing awareness of the impact that extrapulmonary problems may have on morbidity and survival. In this respect, hepatobiliary complications have received increasing attention in the last few years. Severe liver disease that causes portal hypertension and bleeding esophageal varices is clinically evident and fortunately rare. The diagnosis and management of milder disease is complicated by inconsistencies between biochemical markers and clinical manifestations. The natural history of CF hepatic disease is poorly defined, and the long-term effects of most forms of therapy have not been established rigorously. Careful evaluation of the hepatobiliary system, its functions, and its responses to controlled interventions should increase our understanding of this important organ system and permit the development of more effective therapy. The aim of this chapter is to describe the epidemiology, natural history and novel therapeutic approaches for hepatobiliary complications of CF, particularly in adults.

EPIDEMIOLOGY

Liver Disease

The epidemiologic characteristics of CF-associated liver disease are still poorly defined. Information regarding its incidence and rate of progression is limited, probably because no universal criteria to assess the presence and severity of this condition currently are available. Thus, it is difficult to define on a clinical basis the incidence of the most characteristic lesion, focal biliary cirrhosis, because this initially is an exclusively histologic disorder, causing no symptoms and inconsistent abnormalities in serum liver enzymes (1,2). Conversely, histologic data obtained by means of liver biopsy during life are insufficient to provide reliable epidemiologic information. Data on the prevalence of clinically relevant liver disease also are unsatisfactory and not consistent, probably depending on the different criteria used for definition.

In a recent study performed to characterize the natural history of liver disease in CF, 183 patients who presented at the CF Center of Milan from 1980 to 1990 were assessed regularly through yearly clinical, biochemical and ultrasonographic follow-up (3). The age of this population was 15.1 ± 7.4 years [mean ± standard deviation (SD)] at the time of the report, and 35 were older than 18 years of age during the study. Liver disease was defined by the presence of at least two of the following for more than 1 year: clinical hepatomegaly, serum liver enzyme levels greater than 1.5 times the upper limit of normal, and ultrasound abnormalities, including hepatomegaly, increased or heterogeneous echogenicity, nodularity, irregular margins, and splenomegaly. In this patient population, liver disease developed in 35 patients (19%) over a mean follow-up period of 10 years. Mean age at diagnosis of liver disease was 6.2 years, ranging from 0.2 to 26.6 years. At the time of diagnosis of liver disease, 17% of patients were younger than 1 year of age and 17% of patients were older than 10 years of age; only one patient was an adult (3). Using this multifaceted approach, similar prevalence figures have been reported in other centers (4,5).

In contrast, using exclusively the clinical criteria of firm hepatomegaly, Scott-Jupp et al. (6) reported a prevalence of liver disease of 4.2% in a large British CF population. After reviewing the case notes of 1,100 patients with CF covering the entire age range, the incidence of CF-associated liver disease did not appear to increase steadily in adult life, as previously suggested by postmortem findings (7,8). In fact, the clinical presentation of liver disease was found to be relatively uncommon in young children; there was a peak during adolescence and a decrease in prevalence over the age of 20 years (6). A gender difference has been reported by several studies, males being affected on the average twice as much as females (3,6,9).

There are no conclusive data on the percentage of patients with CF with associated liver disease in whom portal hypertension and its complications develop. Data reported by the U.S. CF centers indicate that cirrhosis and portal hypertension were present in only 0.9 % of the total population (166 of 18,455 patients with CF) in 1994, although they accounted for almost 4.2% of total complications reported in the same year (166 of 3,950) (10). In addition, liver disease and liver failure were the second cause of death after cardiorespiratory problems, accounting for 2.2% of overall CF mortality.

Biliary Tract

The prevalence of biliary abnormalities also is not defined precisely. Radiolucent gallstones have been reported in a percentage of patients with CF ranging from 12% to 27.5% (2,8,11). According to the data reported by the U.S. CF

patient registry, gallbladder disease requiring surgery is a rare event in CF, affecting 0.3% of patients with CF seen in 1994 (10). A higher proportion of patients with CF shows morphologic and functional abnormalities of the gallbladder. Microgallbladder is detectable in up to 30%, whereas the finding of a nonopacifying gallbladder on oral cholecystography ranges from 8% to 18% of patients (11). Abnormalities in the biliary tree seem to be present in a consistent proportion of patients with CF with liver disease (12,13).

Conflicting data are given on the frequency of common bile duct stenosis in CF: the prevalence figure of 96% in patients with CF with liver disease reported by Gaskin et al. (14) in Australia has not been confirmed by other centers around the world (1.1% to 13%) (12,15).

PATHOGENESIS

The pathologic picture of CF-associated liver disease already had suggested that bile duct obstruction by amorphous eosinophilic, periodic acid Schiff (PAS)-positive, diastase-resistant material plays a major pathogenetic role, even if direct evidence of cholestasis rarely is present beyond the neonatal period (16). A clear association between cirrhosis and mucus plugs also has been reported by an autopsy survey (17).

Major advances in our understanding of the pathophysiology of CF-associated liver disease have been achieved recently by studies dealing with the basic defect within the liver. Studies performed in the rat (18), and more recently in man (19), have indicated that within the hepatobiliary system, the cystic fibrosis transmembrane conductance regulator (CFTR) is expressed uniquely in the apical domain of bile duct epithelial cells (cholangiocytes), and that it is not detectable in other cells of the liver, including hepatocytes. In isolated bile duct cells of the rat, it also has been shown that one of the two different chloride channels that participate in the control of fluid and electrolyte transport across biliary epithelium is associated with the endogenous expression of CFTR (19). Thus, the primary pathogenetic event in CF-associated liver disease seems to occur within the bile duct epithelium; this is in agreement with the electron microscopy observation that bile duct cell damage is almost universal in patients with CF, being present also in those without clinically apparent liver disease (20).

CF-associated liver disease therefore may become the first example of an inherited disease in which the primary abnormality is in biliary cells rather than hepatocytes, resulting in an exclusively ductular secretory insufficiency. In fact, dysfunction of the cyclic adenosine monophosphate (cAMP)-dependent chloride channel in the apical membrane of bile duct cells would impair chloride efflux, a process that is considered of major importance in generating negative intraluminal potential, paracellular movement of sodium and water, and ultimately, dilution of bile (19).

A model system for further investigations on the pathogenesis of CF-associated liver disease has been developed. Cell lines from human CF-affected intrahepatic biliary epithelial cells have been obtained and characterized (21): these cells do not express the CFTR chloride channel, suggesting that a disturbance of chloride transport in bile duct epithelium could explain the production of inspissated secretions. Obstruction of bile ductules may induce a series of secondary events, such as retention of hepatotoxic bile acids, release of inflammatory cytokines, production of free radicals, and lipid peroxidation, which may be responsible for the progression of liver damage. Oxidative injury to liver cell membrane also may occur through increased free radicals production (22). This may be favored by decreased lipid-soluble antioxidant activity because vitamin E and ß-carotene deficiencies have been documented in patients with CF. Mechanisms involved in the pathogenesis of CF-associated liver disease are summarized in Figure 14–1. Finally, in a few patients, the development of liver disease may be attributed to mechanical factors, such as distal stenosis of the common bile duct (12,14,15), lithiasis of bile ducts, or right heart failure.

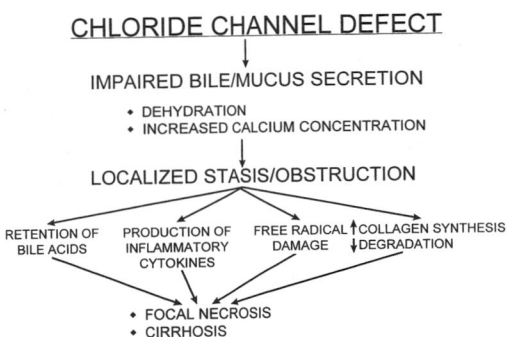

FIG. 14–1. Mechanisms involved in the pathogenesis of CF-associated liver disease.

GENETICS OF CYSTIC FIBROSIS–ASSOCIATED LIVER DISEASE

Currently, there is no explanation why liver disease develops in some patients with CF and not others. The possibility that one (or a few) specific mutation(s) of the CFTR gene may be associated with a greater severity of bile duct cell secretory insufficiency has been excluded. A series of studies from Europe and Canada have indicated the lack of specific genotype–phenotype relationship for clinical liver disease (23–26). Even in patients with severe liver disease undergoing liver transplantation, a specific pattern of CFTR mutations was not observed (27). Although in all these series, allele frequencies and genotype distribution were not significantly different in the two groups of patients with CF with and without liver disease (23–26), those with liver disease generally were found to carry the severe types of mutations that have been associated with pancreatic insufficiency and a more severe expression of the disease. In contrast, hepatic abnormalities were seldom detected in patients with CF carrying mild missense mutations associated with pancreatic sufficiency and mild lung disease, suggesting that liver disease may be less likely to develop in this group of patients, even though a specific association has yet to be established.

The role of histocompatibility antigens in determining a higher susceptibility for liver disease in patients with CF (28,29) is under investigation. A significant increase in the frequency of HLA-A2, B7, DR2, and DQw6 has been documented in British patients with CF with liver disease; HLA-DQw6 was present in 65% of patients with liver disease compared with 32% of those without liver disease. This suggests that a gene linked with HLA-DQ may control lymphocyte-mediated immune response, thus contributing to liver damage through stimulation of fibrogenesis (28).

RISK FACTORS FOR THE DEVELOPMENT OF LIVER DISEASE IN CYSTIC FIBROSIS

Identification of risk factors for the development of liver disease in patients with CF could specifically address careful monitoring of hepatic status in high-risk subjects, in whom prophylactic strategies also could be attempted (30). A relationship between cirrhosis and distal intestinal obstruction in the neonatal period or later in life has been documented by a retrospective autopsy study (17), and more recently by a clinical study, which has shown that the risk for the development of liver disease is almost fourfold higher in patients with a history of meconium ileus or distal intestinal obstruction syndrome (DIOS) than in patients with CF unaffected by these complications (23). The increased risk may be related to the production of particularly inspissated secretions at both the intestinal and hepatobiliary levels. It should be noted, however, that in other CF populations (British, Swedish), neonatal meconium ileus could not be associated with later development of CF-associated liver disease (6,31).

NATURAL HISTORY

The remarkable advances in the definition of the pathogenesis of CF-associated liver disease have not been accompanied by a parallel increase in the understanding of its natural history, which still is hampered by several problems. We still lack reliable markers of hepatobiliary status to be included in prognostic models because neither a standard parameter of liver function nor any specific clinical finding is satisfactory for this purpose. In addition, in the absence of extensive data on long-term follow-up of an adequate number of patients with CF with liver disease, most of the information available has been derived from cross-sectional clinical studies.

Autopsy data indicate that the prevalence of focal biliary cirrhosis tends to increase with age: the typical lesion was documented in 10%, 15%, and 27% of patients with CF who had died before 3 months of age, between 3 and 12 months of age, and after the first year of life, respectively (7). An autopsy study in adults has confirmed this trend because focal biliary cirrhosis was detected in more than 70% of patients with CF older than 20 years of age (8). Progression of hepatic lesions, from plugged bile ducts observed in infants during the first few months of life to cirrhosis in older children, has been documented, thus providing evidence that mucus trapped in the biliary portal ductules may be a precursor of focal biliary cirrhosis (5). Conversely, inspissated mucus in the biliary tree may be a reversible lesion in a substantial proportion of infants with CF [almost 50% of cases in the series reported by Oppenheimer and Esterly (7)], and this favorable evolution may be related to growth of the biliary tree with progressive establishment of multiple interductal connections (16).

The development of multilobular biliary cirrhosis with derangement of hepatic architecture and nodular regeneration is recognized as a subsequent stage of liver involvement in CF, which seems to occur in approximately 2% to 5% of patients with CF (1,2).

Indirect evidence from clinical studies indicates that, as in other chronic liver diseases mainly involving the biliary tree, liver disease associated with CF has a mild course and frequently is asymptomatic and slowly progressive (1). Although the hemodynamic consequences of cirrhosis often are prominent and severe, deaths from complications of portal hypertension and hepatocellular failure are relatively rare in patients with CF (32).

Data on long-term follow-up of hepatic status are limited. Follow-up of hepatic status in 450 patients observed over a 28-year period recently has been reported (9). In this group of untreated patients, multilobular biliary cirrhosis developed in 31 cases. Liver disease had its onset during childhood in most cases, with a relatively rapid progression to cirrhosis and portal hypertension; 6 patients died of complications of cirrhosis, but death was due to respiratory complications in another 10. Interestingly, improved survival has been reported by the same authors in the cirrhotic patients followed over the last 2 decades, and survival of more than 10 years after diagnosis of liver cirrhosis has been the prevalent feature. In this period, active search for liver disease has taken place, employing laboratory analyses and imaging techniques. This has led to increased recognition of asymptomatic patients with slowly progressive disease. Assessment of the long-term outcome of these patients remains a challenging problem for the future, in the light of novel therapeutic approaches and specifically, treatment with ursodeoxycholic acid (UDCA).

CLINICAL FEATURES OF HEPATOBILIARY DISEASE

Liver disease rarely is a clue leading to the diagnosis of CF. This has been reported in 1.5% of patients who first were diagnosed in the United States during 1994 (10), indicating that patients with unexplained cirrhosis should have a sweat test as part of the diagnostic evaluation.

The most frequent modalities of detection of CF-associated liver disease are the finding of hepatomegaly and/or enlarged spleen at physical examination or at ultrasonography during regular follow-up, and/or the finding of significant abnormalities in liver biochemistry. Only rarely, esophageal varices or ascites may be the initial signs of liver disease. Further diagnostic evaluation usually leads to the diagnosis of one of the classic pictures of fatty liver syndrome or biliary cirrhosis. The reported frequencies of different hepatobiliary manifestations in patients with CF are summarized in Table 14–1.

TABLE 14–1. *Reported frequency of hepatobiliary diseases in cystic fibrosis*

Disease	Frequency (%)
Neonatal liver disease	6–40
Neonatal cholestasis	?
Fatty liver	15–30
Isolated massive steatosis	5
Multilobular biliary cirrhosis	2–5
Gallbladder abnormalities (nonfunctional or small)	24–45%
Gallstones	4–12
Common bile duct stenosis	?

Fatty Liver

Isolated massive steatosis has been reported at the time of diagnosis in patients in poor nutritional status, with gradual resolution after institution of enzymatic therapy (33). This manifestation of CF is becoming less frequent because of earlier diagnosis and more appropriate nutritional care. Specific nutritional deficiencies also may have a pathogenetic role, as suggested by the substantial biochemical and ultrasonographic improvement in one infant with CF and massive steatosis after carnitine supplementation (34).

Steatosis of lower degree is frequently reported both at ultrasound and at histologic examination in patients with CF of any age, regardless of nutritional status. A variable degree of hepatomegaly, often associated with abnormal serum transaminase levels, may be present. Progression from steatosis to focal biliary fibrosis has been documented in a few patients in whom follow-up biopsies have been performed (33,35), suggesting that steatosis may represent the first step in the development of more severe hepatic lesions.

Focal or Multilobular Biliary Cirrhosis

Focal biliary cirrhosis generally is asymptomatic or may present with moderate hepatomegaly with or without abnormalities in serum liver enzyme levels; it is recognized most frequently during the school years, although it has been reported as early as in the neonatal period. Age at presentation of liver disease in patients with CF followed at the CF Center of Milan,

TABLE 14–2. *Age at presentation of liver disease in patients with cystic fibrosis followed at the CF Center of Milan (n = 53)*

Age (yrs)	No.	%
0–5	22	41
5–10	19	36
10–15	8	15
15–20	0	0
20–25	0	0
25–30	4	7

where prospective studies are performed on a regular basis and diagnosis often made in childhood, is reported in Table 14–2. The clinical characteristics of children and adults with CF-associated liver disease are similar, as observed in patients followed at our center (Table 14–3).

Even in the more advanced stage of multilobular biliary cirrhosis, serum liver enzyme levels may be completely normal, and long-standing preservation of liver function is characteristic (29). As previously mentioned, portal hypertension often is the major clinical problem causing splenomegaly and eventually upper gastrointestinal bleeding. Splenic enlargement of remarkable degree may occur and cause left upper quadrant pain or discomfort, dyspnea, and signs of hypersplenism (32).

Inspissated Bile Syndrome

Prolonged cholestatic jaundice during the first year of life rarely occurs in patients with CF (36,37), mostly in those with meconium ileus, as a result of viscous biliary secretions that block the extrahepatic bile ducts (inspissated bile syndrome) (7). Although biliary infusion therapy sometimes has been used successfully, spontaneous resolution generally occurs. There is no evidence of any relationship between inspissated bile syndrome and later development of focal biliary cirrhosis (1). Obstructive jaundice later in life, particularly in adults, may result from lithiasis, sclerosing cholangitis, or stenosis of the common bile duct (15,38).

Common Bile Duct Stricture

Stenosis of the intrapancreatic portion of the common bile duct due to pancreatic fibrosis may cause complete or partial biliary obstruction, with jaundice and/or biliary pain (14,38–40). The frequency of this complication in patients with CF has been the subject of controversy in recent years (12–14,41). Gaskin et al. (14) reported common bile duct lesions or tapering, diagnosed by scintigraphy and confirmed by cholangiography, in almost all patients with CF with liver disease, in the absence of common bile duct dilatation at ultrasonography. Therefore, stricture of the distal common bile duct has been suggested to play a major role in the pathogenesis of CF-associated liver disease, which therefore might benefit from surgical decompression. Interestingly, recurrent right upper quadrant abdominal pain was present in more than 50% of these patients, and in 14 patients who underwent

TABLE 14–3. *Clinical data of patients with cystic fibrosis and associated liver disease followed at the CF Center of Milan, based on age*

Abnormality	Age <18 yrs (n = 38)		≥18 yrs (n = 15)	
	No.	%	No.	%
Hepatomegaly	25	65	14	93
Splenomegaly	16	42	7	46
Biochemical abnormalities	27	71	11	73
Ultrasonography				
Inhomogeneous echoes	12	31	9	60
Steatosis	5	13	2	13
Cirrhosis	5	13	2	13
Portal hypertension	10	26	3	20
Microgallbladder	4	10	5	33
Gallstones or sludge	3	7	3	20

surgery, this symptom disappeared. However, the high frequency of common bile duct stricture could not be confirmed at cholangiography by two other studies in adults, despite the presence of suggestive scintigraphic abnormalities (12,15).

Sclerosing Cholangitis

Sclerosing cholangitis first was reported by Strandvik et al. (42) in four patients with CF, two of whom also had inflammatory bowel disease (42). Cholangiographic features suggestive for sclerosing cholangitis (with beading and stricturing involving mainly large intrahepatic ducts) have been detected in the majority of adult patients with CF-associated liver disease investigated thus far with cholangiography (12,15). In view of their frequency, these abnormalities may represent a possible evolution of CF-associated liver disease.

Gallbladder Abnormalities

Microgallbladder is an ultrasonographic finding in more than 20% of patients with CF (11); submucosal cysts, septate gallbladders, and adenomyomas also have been described (8). Cholelithiasis is an occasional finding in patients with CF; its prevalence has been shown to increase with age (8,43). Symptoms have been reported to occur in less than 4% of cases, again with an age-related trend of symptomatic gallbladder disease (43). In our series of 127 adults with CF, 20% were found to have gallstones; 7 of them (27%) were symptomatic.

Until recently, the composition of CF gallstones was considered mainly to be cholesterol (44), but one study has indicated calcium bilirubinate as the main component (45). This finding is in keeping with the recently reported failure of bile acid therapy to dissolve radiolucent gallstones in patients with CF (46). Bile stasis and abnormalities in biliary mucus may predispose to nidus formation. Intrahepatic stones (hepatolithiasis) also have been observed (47).

Motor abnormalities of the extrahepatic biliary tree (dyskinesia) also have been reported, and these may be associated with gallbladder distension and biliary pain (12).

DIAGNOSIS OF HEPTOBILIARY DISEASE

With the perspective of new and potentially effective therapeutic strategies for CF-related liver disease, early diagnosis is warranted because only early lesions are likely to be reversible. As previously mentioned, mutation analysis is of benefit for this purpose, by excluding patients with mild mutations from the high-risk group. Evidence of liver disease in patients with CF often is subtle, and appreciable symptoms and clinical signs tend to develop only when pathologic changes are more pronounced. At present, there are neither satisfactory methods nor universal criteria for its diagnosis, which generally is based on clinical examination, biochemical tests, and imaging techniques. For the asymptomatic patient, regular clinical examinations and annual serum enzyme studies may be appropriate screening methods. Consistent abnormalities should be evaluated further with selected imaging studies. These serve both to define anatomic abnormalities and to follow disease progression and responses to therapy. The currently available diagnostic tools are described below.

Clinical Examination

With regard to physical examination, remember that in patients with CF, a palpable liver simply may reflect pulmonary hyperinflation, and therefore, liver span assessment is required. Selective enlargement of the left lobe is characteristic, which becomes increasingly hard and palpable in the epigastrium (28,29). Clinical hepatomegaly has been found to be related to histologic findings of fibrosis (14), thus suggesting high specificity for such a clinical sign, which, however, is not sensitive for early-stage disease. Splenomegaly generally is associated with cirrhosis and portal hypertension. In patients with splenomegaly, the presence of esophageal varices should be assessed by endoscopic examination.

Liver Biochemistry

Standard serum liver enzyme levels have low sensitivity for the diagnosis of CF-associated liver disease. In fact, abnormalities of serum liver enzymes related to cholestasis and cytolysis may be mild or intermittent and do not correlate with the severity of hepatic lesions. In addition, minor and transient elevations of the transaminase levels frequently are observed during pulmonary exacerbation, antibiotic treatment, and hypoxemia (48); therefore, serial determinations should be performed. Of the different enzymes that have been measured, those that originate from the biliary epithelium (γ-glutamyl-transpeptidase, 5'-nucle-otidase, and the biliary isoenzyme of alkaline phosphatase) are the more specific for CF-associated liver disease (49). Most patients with CF with liver involvement do not have hyperbilirubinemia or abnormalities in indices of synthetic function, at least until end-stage liver disease.

With regard to fasting and postprandial serum bile acid concentrations, the presence of bile acid malabsorption in patients with CF with pancreatic insufficiency (50) may limit their diagnostic accuracy and probably explains the reported lack of correlation between fasting serum bile acid levels and histopathologic features (51).

Dynamic Tests of Liver Function

There are only limited data on the diagnostic value of dynamic tests of liver function, such as aminopyrine breath test, galactose elimination capacity, or caffeine tolerance test. Their sensitivity in early stages of CF-associated liver disease probably is limited by the focal distribution of hepatic lesions, as shown for caffeine tolerance test as an index of microsomal function (4). When serially performed, these tests may provide valuable information on disease progression, as shown in other cholestatic liver diseases (52).

Liver Biopsy

Liver biopsy has had a limited role in CF-associated liver disease, and this also is because of the heterogeneous distribution of hepatic lesions (1,2), with risk of sampling errors when needle liver biopsy is performed, particularly in early stages (14).

Imaging

Among imaging techniques, ultrasonography certainly is the most widely used to evaluate the presence of hepatobiliary problems in patients with CF (53). It is the technique of choice for the detection of stones within the gallbladder or the biliary tree and also permits detection of steatosis, cirrhosis, and portal hypertension. Ultrasonography is employed increasingly in the long-term follow-up of patients with CF with liver disease. For a better evaluation of portal hypertension, it has been used in association with Doppler studies of the portal vein (54). However, it has not yet been established whether this finding precedes the occurrence of clinical splenomegaly.

Recently, a simple ultrasound scoring system for the diagnosis of CF-associated liver disease has been developed and validated (55). The score, which is based on three simple echographic features (coarseness of liver parenchyma, nodularity of the liver edge, and increased periportal echogenicity), proved to correlate with a series of clinical and biochemical parameters and with ultrasound markers of portal hypertension (splenic size, splenic vein diameter, portal-systemic collaterals).

Hepatobiliary scintigraphy with new generation technetium-labelled iminodiacetic acid derivatives (^{99m}Tc-HIDA) represents a noninvasive means of assessing patency of the extrahepatic bile ducts and also of quantifying liver function and biliary secretion. A very high rate of scintigraphic abnormalities suggestive of biliary drainage impairment, with dilatation of the intra- and extrahepatic bile ducts and delayed excretion of the tracer, has been reported in patients with CF with liver disease (14,56–

58). This sometimes is consistent with common bile duct obstruction, but ultrasound examination very rarely demonstrates concomitant dilatation of the intra- and extrahepatic biliary tree (13,41). Nonvisualization of the gallbladder also is relatively common.

This spectrum of scintigraphic abnormalities, which also has been reported in a significant number of patients without overt liver disease, may fluctuate with time, suggesting an intermittent or reversible nature of liver involvement in early stages (57). Biliary stasis or adherence of the tracer to abnormal mucus within the biliary tree may be responsible for the prolonged retention of the isotope (15). Therefore, hepatobiliary scintigraphy is not considered a reliable diagnostic procedure in establishing common bile duct obstruction in patients with CF. If common bile duct obstruction is suspected, a cholangiographic study should be performed, which also can reveal features of intra- and extrahepatic cholelithiasis or sclerosing cholangitis. Computer-assisted tomography of the abdomen does not add much to ultrasound and physical examination, although it may provide a better global view of the abdomen (59). The use of magnetic resonance imaging, currently limited to the evaluation of patients with CF in the perspective of liver transplantation and to postoperative assessment of shunt patency (60), may be extended to evaluation of the biliary tree.

MANAGEMENT OF CYSTIC FIBROSIS LIVER DISEASE

As the mean age of survival of patients with CF is significantly increasing, treatment of liver disease in adult patients is becoming a relevant clinical issue. Until recently, clinical management of CF-associated liver disease was limited to treatment of complications of cirrhosis and portal hypertension. With the remarkable advances in the global treatment of patients with CF over the last 2 decades, the expectant management policy no longer is acceptable, especially in view of the fact that liver disease is the second cause of death, behind respiratory problems. Although CF-associated liver disease may be difficult to diagnose because of its variable clinical, biochemical, imaging, and histologic manifestations, bile acid therapy is relatively nontoxic and may provide significant benefits. Its more extensive use should be encouraged, pending the results of controlled clinical trials. In the following paragraphs, the different therapeutic strategies currently available or under evaluation are described.

Bile Acid Therapy

Because the treatment by gene therapy of the initial pathogenic processes of liver disease associated with CF is not yet feasible, therapeutic and prophylactic strategies should be aimed at counteracting the secondary pathogenic events of liver disease. Possible strategies include prevention of both bile plugging within the ductules and retention of detergent, hepatotoxic, endogenous bile acids, which are considered to have a prominent role in determining liver cell injury during cholestasis (61,62). In fact, the normal bile acid pool of patients with CF is relatively hydrophobic because dihydroxy bile acids predominate (63) and the conjugation profile, although variable, favors glycine (2) because these patients tend to be taurine deficient (64) as a result of bile acid malabsorption (50).

The hydrophilic, nontoxic UDCA has been employed largely in the treatment of chronic cholestatic liver diseases (65), such as primary biliary cirrhosis, primary sclerosing cholangitis, and several forms of pediatric cholestasis, including CF. The rationale underlying its use is to displace from the enterohepatic circulation detergent endogenous bile acids, which are retained in chronic cholestasis, by replacing them with a nontoxic compound (66). In addition, UDCA was suggested to exert a direct cytoprotective effect on the canalicular membranes (67). The role of the choleretic properties of UDCA in determining its effectiveness in chronic liver diseases remains to be established because the occurrence of a cholehepatic recycling of protonated UDCA with induction of a bicarbonate-rich hypercholeresis has been documented thus far only in experimental models at high doses (68); this mechanism of action may be particularly important in patients with CF with liver disease, in whom biliary drainage may be affected severely (56).

Increasing information is available on the effects of UDCA treatment in CF-associated liver disease from both open and controlled studies (5,56,69–78). A consistent and sustained improvement of biochemical indices related to cholestasis and cytolysis during UDCA treatment has been observed in all these studies. As reported for primary biliary cirrhosis (79), serum liver enzymes return to baseline levels after treatment discontinuation (71). The biochemical response to treatment, which was confirmed by two controlled multicenter trials (76,78), is dose dependent in patients with CF in whom daily doses of UDCA of 20 mg/kg body weight/day are needed to compensate for poor intestinal absorption (73). In fact, administration of the usual therapeutic dosages of UDCA (10 mg/kg) yield a biliary UDCA enrichment of approximately 25%, which is much lower than that typically found in other patients with liver disease (69). More recently, a dose-response study of orally administered UDCA, using doses ranging 20 to 40 mg/kg, demonstrated that no further biliary enrichment with UDCA could be achieved with doses higher than 20 mg/kg (80).

However, it should be highlighted that the dose-response relationship has been investigated only in pediatric patients (73) and no data presently are available from dose-response studies in adult patients with CF-associated liver disease. In young adults with CF-associated liver disease, a significant and substantial improvement of serum liver enzymes was found after the administration of UDCA at the daily dose of 15 to 20 mg/kg (70).

Data on the dose-response relationship during UDCA administration to adult patients with chronic cholestatic liver disease are limited to primary biliary cirrhosis and primary sclerosing cholangitis (81), and daily doses of 8 to 12 mg/kg and 12 to 15 mg/kg, respectively, were suggested. Because bile acid malabsorption does not occur in these two latter conditions, higher doses of UDCA are expected to be indicated for adult patients with CF. Therefore, it seems reasonable that the optimal dose of 20 mg/kg/day that was suggested for pediatric patients with CF also may be extrapolated for adults. In adult patients with CF-associated liver disease and pancreatic sufficiency, lower doses of UDCA may be required; however, again, no data from studies specifically aimed at addressing this issue are available.

Beneficial effects on different aspects of quantitative liver function (i.e., hepatic excretory function and microsomal reserve) have been documented also in adult patients (70). However, during treatment, such improvements were not maintained consistently, particularly in patients with more advanced liver disease (72). Improvement in hepatic excretory function and biliary drainage also has been documented by means of hepatobiliary scintigraphy (56,58), which has been indicated as a useful tool for monitoring the response to UDCA treatment. Only preliminary data on the effects of UDCA on liver histology presently are available; a study performed in a limited number of patients reported a marginal improvement in inflammation and fibrosis after 2 years of UDCA treatment (74).

The effects of UDCA on nutritional status seem to be restricted to more compromised patients; in fact, a significant increase in body weight, body mass index, urinary creatinine excretion, and prothrombin time value was documented only in young adults with CF and longstanding cholestasis associated with major nutritional problems (70). In contrast, none of the other studies available could document any significant effect on growth and nutrition in CF patients with and without liver disease (77,82). UDCA is known to form mixed micelles less efficiently than primary bile acids (83); therefore, deterioration of steatorrhea during chronic administration of UDCA may occur in patients with severe degree of pancreatic insufficiency. Nevertheless, no substantial modification in steatorrhea has been observed thus far (69–71,78).

The long-term benefit of UDCA treatment in preventing events related to morbidity and mortality in patients with CF with liver disease is under evaluation (75,84). This important information hopefully will be obtained by long-term studies performed on large cohorts of patients aimed at evaluating the effects on clinically relevant end-points, such as survival, need for liver transplantation, or occurrence of complications of cirrhosis and portal hypertension. In adult patients with primary biliary cirrhosis, UDCA was shown to significantly improve transplantation-free survival (85). Conversely, there are limited data on the occurrence of clinically relevant events during UDCA administration in adult patients with CF-associated liver disease. However, the impressive improvement of biliary secretion, as assessed by hepatobiliary scintigraphy (56), suggests that all patients with established diagnosis of liver disease should be treated with UDCA.

It previously was shown that taurine deficiency often is present in patients with CF (64) and that taurine supplementation can improve the efficiency of micellar solubilization of lipophilic products (86–88). Long-term administration of unconjugated UDCA may increase critically taurine need for bile acid conjugation and may aggravate the degree of taurine deficiency, with possible detrimental effects on the efficiency of fat digestion in patients with CF. Therefore, taurine supplementation has been recommended by some investigators during treatment with UDCA in CF-associated liver disease (69,71). More recently, the effects of this supplementation have been evaluated in a double-blind fashion (78). In patients with CF with liver disease who received taurine supplementation, with or without UDCA, there was a trend toward improvement of fat absorption and a significant increase in serum prealbumin levels. These data strongly suggest that taurine supplementation is advisable in patients with CF with pancreatic insufficiency and poor nutritional status during chronic administration of UDCA.

Guidelines for UDCA therapy with or without taurine are summarized in Table 14–4. Because the objective of such a treatment is to delay the progression of the disease, treatment should be started at an early stage. A daily dose

TABLE 14–4. *Guidelines for ursodeoxycholic acid (UDCA) therapy in adult patients with cystic fibrosis–associated liver disease*

Who should be treated?	All patients with diagnosis of liver disease
Timing for starting treatment	As soon as possible
Suggested dose	20 mg/kg/day
Treatment schedule	Multiple divided doses: at least three times per day
Taurine supplementation (30–40 mg/kg/day)	Indicated in patients with pancreatic insufficiency and poor nutritional status
Monitoring for compliance	Biliary enrichment in UDCA: at the steady state, 30–35% of total bile acids (HPLC)
Clinical monitoring	Serial determinations of serum liver enzymes (every 4–6 mos)

HPLC, high-pressure liquid chromatography.

of 20 mg/kg is recommended. Because high doses of UDCA undergo incomplete intestinal absorption (89), a therapeutic schedule based on multiple divided doses seems to be more appropriate. Taurine supplementation is indicated in the presence of pancreatic insufficiency and poor nutritional status. To test the compliance to treatment, biliary enrichment with UDCA should be evaluated by high-performance liquid chromotography (HPLC) after at least 8 weeks of treatment, when the steady state is expected to be reached (90). Serum concentration of UDCA was proved to be related only slightly to UDCA biliary enrichment (73,80) and therefore is not indicated to test the compliance. To test the efficacy of UDCA therapy, evaluation of indices of cholestasis and cytolysis should be performed every 4 to 6 months (80).

Complications of Cirrhosis

A clinically relevant complication of CF-associated liver disease is the presence of esophageal varices (29,32). Prophylactic treatment aimed at avoiding bleeding is indicated in various forms of liver cirrhosis (91). However, ß-receptor blockade should be avoided in patients with CF because of the increased risk of bronchoconstriction, even with the ß-1 selective agents (92). There is no evidence to support the use of prophylactic injection sclerotherapy for esophageal varices for patients with CF with liver disease as for any other form of liver disease causing portal hypertension. Conversely, variceal bleeding has been treated successfully by repeated injection sclerotherapy in patients with CF, although this procedure has not always relieved all portal hypertension-associated problems (93).

Surgical portocaval anastomosis may be considered only for those patients in whom sclerotherapy was not successful; the surgical risks are considerable, and in addition, portosystemic shunting may precipitate or worsen hepatic encephalopathy and also may render a subsequent liver transplantation more difficult. Selective distal splenorenal shunting is the most widely recommended procedure because it is associated with the lowest risk of encephalopathy (92). Partial splenectomy with conservation of the upper pole of the spleen has been performed successfully in patients with massive splenic enlargement (94).

Finally, transjugular intrahepatic portosystemic shunt (TIPS) can be employed as a short-term method for portal decompression in patients awaiting liver transplantation (95). Its usefulness in patients with CF with portal hypertension and recurrent variceal bleeding is suggested by a recent case report (96).

Liver Transplantation

Liver transplantation can be considered an effective treatment for those patients with CF with end-stage liver disease and mild pulmonary involvement (97–101). The outcome of liver transplantation reported thus far is consistent with medium-term survival rates ranging from 70% to 100%, with a good quality of life. In addition, a beneficial effect on lung function sometimes has been reported. Special attention to pulmonary status should be provided, with intensive care beginning in the pretransplant period. Postoperative management resembles that of other liver transplant recipients, with

the only exception of the dose of cyclosporine. As for other drugs (102), patients with CF often need higher doses and/or more frequent dosing intervals because of both intestinal malabsorption and altered drug metabolism. Therefore, they often need prolonged intravenous cyclosporine administration, and a careful monitoring of serum cyclosporine levels should be accomplished (103). The experience with combined liver–heart–lung transplantation currently is too limited to allow any conclusion on its indications; it has been suggested that problems with rejection may be less severe after the triple transplant than after liver graft only (101).

Treatment of Initial Pathogenic Processes

Specific therapy for CF-associated liver disease ultimately may require somatic gene transfer. Recent experimental studies have indicated that this approach may be feasible. In fact, recombinant adenoviruses expressing the human CFTR gene recently were delivered specifically to the rat biliary tract by means of endoscopic retrograde cholangiography (104), and successful gene expression in bile duct cells was demonstrated. Somatic gene therapy therefore could be attempted in patients with CF and may represent the ideal response to all liver-related problems in patients with CF. Drugs that modulate intracellular trafficking of newly synthesized proteins (e.g., ΔF508 CFTR to the apical membrane) or pharmacologic agents that modulate membrane ion channels (e.g., UTP) may be potential alternatives to somatic cell gene therapy.

SUMMARY

Hepatobiliary disease causes significant complications for some adults with CF, and liver failure causes about 2% of CF deaths. Liver disease, manifest by hepatosplenomegaly, abnormal liver function tests, and/or ultrasonographic abnormalities, has a peak incidence in adolescence and affects males more than females. Most patients with liver disease also have exocrine pancreatic insufficiency, but no specific genotype/phenotype correlations have been identified. The underlying mechanism of disease probably involves biliary cell dysfunction, leading to abnormal bile and secondary complications. Hepatic steatosis is common, and multilobular biliary cirrhosis, a pathology characteristic of CF liver disease, occurs in about 5% of adults. Synthetic hepatic functions tend to be preserved until late in the course of cirrhotic disease. Gall stones and microgallbladder are common biliary tract complications. Diagnostic and management approaches to these problems are similar to those for hepatobiliary diseases of other etiologies. UDCA treatment, to modify abnormal CF bile composition, may be effective at slowing the progression of hepatobiliary disease, and controlled clinical trials are under way. Liver transplantation has been effective therapy for severe CF-related cirrhosis. The incidence of hepatobiliary complications is likely to increase as the survival of adults with CF continues to improve. A more thorough understanding of the pathophysiological processes responsible for these problems, and carefully designed clinical studies, may lead to better ways to diagnose, prevent, and treat such important problems.

REFERENCES

1. Colombo C, Battezzati PM, Podda M. Hepatobiliary disease in cystic fibrosis. *Semin Liv Dis* 1994;14:259–269.
2. Roy CC, Weber AM, Morin CL et al. Hepatobiliary disease in cystic fibrosis: a survey of current issues and concepts. *J Pediatr Gastroenterol Nutr* 1982;1:469–478.
3. Colombo C, Battezzati PM, Comi S, Melzi ML, Giunta A. *Natural history of cirrhosis in cystic fibrosis.* Proceedings of the 12th International CF Conference, Jerusalem, 1996:S79–S80.
4. Weber AM, Lenaerts C, Smith L, Roy CC. Screening and diagnosis of cystic fibrosis-related liver disease. *Pediatr Pulmonol* 1989;Suppl 4:40–41.
5. Wong LTX, Davidson AGF, Jevon G, Peacock D, Gravelle A, Schmidt J. *Hepatobiliary disease in children with cystic fibrosis: a clinical and pathologic evaluation of the effect of ursodeoxycholic acid therapy.* Proceedings of the 12th International CF Conference, Jerusalem, 1996:S237 (abstract).
6. Scott-Jupp R, Lama M, Tanner MS. Prevalence of liver disease in cystic fibrosis. *Arch Dis Child* 1991;66:698–701.
7. Oppenheimer EH, Esterly JR. Hepatic changes in young infants with cystic fibrosis: possible relation to focal biliary cirrhosis. *J Pediatr* 1975;86:683–689.
8. Vawter GF, Shwachman H. Cystic fibrosis in adults: an autopsy study. *Pathol Ann* 1979;14:357–382.
9. Feigelson J, Anagnostopoulos C, Poquet M, Pecau Y, Munck A, Navarro J. Liver cirrhosis in cystic fibrosis: therapeutic implications and long-term follow-up. *Arch Dis Child* 1993;68:653–657.
10. FitzSimmons SC. *Cystic Fibrosis Foundation, Patient Registry 1994 Annual Data Report.* Bethesda, MD: Cystic Fibrosis Foundation, August 1995.
11. Jebbink MCW, Heijerman HGM, Masclee AAM, Lamers CBHW. Gallbladder disease in cystic fibrosis. *Neth J Med* 1992;41:123–126.
12. Nagel RA, Westaby D, Javaid A, et al. Liver disease and bile duct abnormalities in adults with cystic fibrosis. *Lancet* 1989;2:1422–1425.
13. Connon JJ. Gallbladder and biliary tract disease in cystic fibrosis: facts and fancy. *Pediatr Pulmonol* 1989;4:41–43.
14. Gaskin KJ, Waters DLM, Howman-Giles R, et al. Liver disease and common bile-duct stenosis in cystic fibrosis. *N Engl J Med* 1988;318:340–346.
15. O'Brien S, Keogan M, Casey M, et al. Biliary complications of cystic fibrosis. *Gut* 1992;33:387–391.
16. Sinaasappel M. Hepatobiliary pathology in patients with cystic fibrosis. *Acta Paediatr Scand* 1989;Suppl 363:45–51.
17. Maurage C, Lenaerts C, Weber AM, Brochu P, Yousef I, Roy CC. Meconium ileus and its equivalent as a risk factor for the development of cirrhosis: an autopsy study in cystic fibrosis. *J Pediatr Gastroenterol Nutr* 1989;9:17–20.
18. Fitz JG, Basavappa S, McGill J, Melhus O, Cohn JA. Regulation of membrane chloride currents in rat bile duct epithelial cells. *J Clin Invest* 1993;91:319–328.
19. Cohn JA, Strong TV, Picciotto MR, Nairn AC, Collins FS, Fitz JG. Localization of the cystic fibrosis transmembrane conductance regulator in human bile duct epithelial cells. *Gastroenterology* 1993;105:1857–1864.
20. Lindblad A, Hultcrantz R, Strandvik B. Bile duct destruction and collagen deposition: a prominent ultrastructural feature of the liver in cystic fibrosis. *Hepatology* 1992;16:372–381.
21. Grubman SA, Fang SL, Mulberg AE, et al. Correction of the cystic fibrosis defect by gene complementation in human intrahepatic biliary epithelial cell lines. *Gastroenterology* 1995;108:584–592.
22. Sokol RJ. Lipid peroxidation in cholestasis. In: Lentze MJ, Reichen J, eds. *Paediatric cholestasis: novel approaches to treatment.* Proceedings of the 63rd Falk Symposium. Lancaster, UK: Kluwer Academic Publishers, 1992:75–80.
23. Colombo C, Apostolo MG, Ferrari M, et al. Analysis of risk factors for the development of liver disease in CF. *J Pediatr* 1994;124:393–399.
24. Ferrari M, Colombo C, Sebastio G, et al. Cystic fibrosis patients with liver disease are not genetically distinct. *Am J Hum Gen* 1991;48:815–816 (letter).
25. Duthie A, Doherty DG, Williams C, et al. Genotype analysis for DF 508, G551D and R553X mutations in

children and young adults with cystic fibrosis with and without liver disease. *Hepatology* 1992;15:660–664.

26. Kovesi T, Corey M, Tsui L-C, Levison H, Durie P. The association between liver disease and mutations of the cystic fibrosis gene. *Pediatr Pulmonol* 1992; Suppl 8:244 (36) (abstract).

27. Mack DR, Traystman MD, Colombo JL, et al. Clinical denouement and mutation analysis of patients with cystic fibrosis undergoing liver transplantation for biliary cirrhosis. *J Pediatr* 1995;127:881–887.

28. Williams SGJ, Westaby D, Tanner MS, Mowat AP. Liver and biliary problems in cystic fibrosis. *Br Med Bull* 1992;48:877–892.

29. Tanner MS, Taylor CJ. Liver disease in cystic fibrosis. *Arch Dis Child* 1995;72:281–284.

30. Colombo C, Battezzati PM, Genoni S, Giunta A. *Prophylactic treatment with ursodeoxycholic acid in infants with CF at high risk for the development of liver disease: is a multicenter European study feasible?* Proceedings of the 19th European Cystic Fibrosis Conference, Paris, May 29–June 3, 1994.

31. Lindblad A, Hjelte L, Strandvik B. Incidence of liver disease in patients with cystic fibrosis and meconium ileus. *J Pediatr* 1995;125:155–156 (letter).

32. Tanner MS. Liver and biliary problems in cystic fibrosis. *J R Soc Med* 1992;85:20–24.

33. Isenberg JN. Cystic fibrosis: its influence on the liver, biliary tree, and bile salt metabolism. *Semin Liver Dis* 1982;2:302–313.

34. Treem WR, Stanley CA. Massive hepatomegaly, steatosis and secondary plasma carnitine deficiency in an infant with cystic fibrosis. *Pediatrics* 1989;83:993–997.

35. Isenberg J N, L'Heureux PR, Warwick WJ, Sharp HL. Clinical observations on the biliary system in cystic fibrosis. *Am J Gastroenterol* 1976;65:134–141.

36. Valman HB, France NE, Wallis PG. Prolonged neonatal jaundice in cystic fibrosis. *Arch Dis Child* 1971;46:805–809.

37. Evans JS, George DE, Mollit D. Biliary infusion therapy in the inspissated bile syndrome of cystic fibrosis. *J Pediatr Gastroenterol Nutr* 1991;12:131–135.

38. Lambert JR, Cole M, Crozier DN, Connon JJ. Intrapancreatic common bile duct compression causing jaundice in an adult with cystic fibrosis. *Gastroenterology* 1981;80:169–172.

39. Vitullo BB, Rochan L, Seemayer TA, Beardmore H, deBelle RC. Intrapancreatic compression of the common bile duct in cystic fibrosis. *J Pediatr* 1978;93:1060–1061.

40. Patrick MK, Howman-Giles R, De Silva M, Van Asperen P, Pitkin J, Gaskin KJ. Common bile duct obstruction causing right upper abdominal pain in cystic fibrosis. *J Pediatr* 1986;108:101–102.

41. Roy CC, Lenaerts C, Garel L, Patriquin H, Weber AM. Biliary disease in cystic fibrosis. *N Engl J Med* 1988;319:312 (letter).

42. Strandvik B, Hjelte L, Gabrielson N, Glaumann H. Sclerosing cholangitis in cystic fibrosis. *Scand J Gastroenterol* 1988;143(Suppl):121–124.

43. Stern RC, Rothstein FC, Doershuk CF. Treatment and prognosis of symptomatic gallbladder disease in patients with cystic fibrosis. *J Pediatr Gastroenterol Nutr* 1986;5:35–40.

44. Roy CC, Weber AM, Morin CL, Combes JC, Nusslé D, Megevand A, Lasalle R. Abnormal biliary lipid composition in cystic fibrosis: effect of pancreatic enzymes. *N Engl J Med* 1977;297:1301–1305.

45. Angelico M, Gandin C, Canuzzi P, et al. Gallstones in cystic fibrosis: a critical reappraisal. *Hepatology* 1991;14:768–775.

46. Colombo C, Bertolini E, Assaisso M, Bettinardi N, Giunta A, Podda M. Failure of ursodeoxycholic acid to dissolve radiolucent gallstones in patients with cystic fibrosis. *Acta Paediatr Scand* 1993;82:562–565.

47. Bass S, Connon JJ, Ho CS. Biliary tree in cystic fibrosis. *Gastroenterology* 1983;84:1592–1596.

48. Westaby D. Liver and biliary disease in cystic fibrosis. In: Hodson ME, Gadders DM, eds. *Cystic fibrosis.* London, 1995:281–293.

49. Shoenau E, Boeswald W, Wanner R, et al. High-molecular mass ("Biliary") isoenzyme of alkaline phosphatase and the diagnosis of liver dysfunction in cystic fibrosis. *Clin Chem* 1989;35(9):1988–1990.

50. Weber AM, Roy CC, Morin CL, et al. Malabsorption of bile acids in children with cystic fibrosis. *N Engl J Med* 1973;289:1001–1005.

51. Strandvik B, Samuelson K. Fasting serum bile acid levels in relation to liver histopathology in cystic fibrosis. *Scand J Gastroenterol* 1985;20(3):381–384.

52. Reichen J, Widmer T, Cotting J. Accurate prediction of death by serial determination of galactose elimination capacity in primary biliary cirrhosis: a comparison with the Mayo model. *Hepatology* 1991;14:504–510.

53. Graham N, Manhlre AR, Stead RJ, Lees WR, Hodson ME, Batten JC. Cystic fibrosis: ultrasonographic findings in the pancreas and hepatobiliary system correlated with clinical data and pathology. *Clin Radiol* 1985;36:199–203.

54. Vergesslich KA, Gatz M, Mostbeck G, Sommer G, Ponhold W. Portal venous blood flow in cystic fibrosis: assessment by duplex Doppler sonography. *Pediatr Radiol* 1989;19:371–374.

55. Williams SGJ, Evanson JE, Barrett N, Hodson ME, Boultbee JE, Westaby D. An ultrasound scoring system for the diagnosis of liver disease in cystic fibrosis. *J Hepatol* 1995;22:513–521.

56. Colombo C, Castellani MR, Balistreri WF, Seregni E, Assaisso ML, Giunta A. Scintigraphic documentation of an improvement in hepatobiliary excretory function after treatment with ursodeoxycholic acid in patients with cystic fibrosis and associated liver disease. *Hepatology* 1992;15:677–684.

57. Semih Dogan A, Conway JJ, Lloyd-Still JD. Hepatobiliary scintigraphy in children with cystic fibrosis and liver disease. *J Nucl Med* 1994;35:432–435.

58. O'Connor PJ, Southern KW, Bowler IM, Irving HC, Robinson PJ, Littlewood JM. The role of hepatobiliary scintigraphy in cystic fibrosis. *Hepatology* 1996;23:281–287.

59. Cunningham DG, Churchill RJ, Reynes CJ. Computed tomography in the evaluation of liver disease in cystic fibrosis patients. *J Comput Assist Tomogr* 1980;4(2):151–154.

60. Fiel SB, Friedman AC et al. Magnetic resonance imaging in young adults with cystic fibrosis. *Chest* 1987;91:2–6.

61. Hofmann AF, Popper H. Ursodeoxycholic acid for primary biliary cirrhosis. *Lancet* 1987;ii:398–399.

62. Attili AF, Angelico M, Cantafora A, Alvaro D, Capocaccia L. Bile acid induced liver toxicity: relation to the hydrophobic–hydrophylic balance of bile acids. *Med Hypotheses* 1986;19:57–69.

63. Nagakawa M, Colombo C, Setchell KDR. Comprehensive study of the biliary bile acid composition of patients with cystic fibrosis and associated liver disease before and after UDCA administration. *Hepatology* 1990;12:322–334.

64. Thompson GN. Excessive fecal taurine loss predisposes to taurine deficiency in cystic fibrosis. *J Pediatr Gastroenterol Nutr* 1988;7:214–217.

65. de Caestecker JS, Jazrawi RP, Petroni ML, Northfield TC. Ursodeoxycholic acid in chronic liver disease. *Gut* 1991;32:1061–1065.

66. Heuman DM. Hepatoprotective properties of ursodeoxycholic acid (editorial). *Gastroenterology* 1993;104:1865–1870.

67. Gulduduna S, Zimmer G, Imhof M, et al. Molecular aspects of membrane stabilization by ursodeoxycholate. *Gastroenterology* 1993;104:1736–1744.

68. Dumont M, Uchman S Erlinger S. Hypercholeresis induced by ursodeoxycholic acid and 7-ketolithocholic acid in the rat: possible role of bicarbonate transport. *Gastroenterology* 1980;79:82–89.

69. Colombo C, Setchell KDR, Podda M, Crosignani A, Roda A, Curcio L, Giunta A. The effects of ursodeoxycholic acid therapy in liver disease associated with cystic fibrosis. *J Pediatr* 1990;117:482–489.

70. Cotting J, Lentze M, Reichen J. Effects of ursodeoxycholic acid treatment on nutrition and liver function in patients with cystic fibrosis and longstanding cholestasis. *Gut* 1990;31:918–921.

71. Galabert C, Montet JC, Lengrand D, et al. Effects of ursodeoxycholic acid on liver function in patients with cystic fibrosis and chronic cholestasis. *J Pediatr* 1992;121:138–141.

72. Reichen J, Paumgartner G, Cotting J, Lentze MJ. Effect of long-term ursodeoxycholate on liver function, nutritional state and serum bile acids in cystic fibrosis with long-standing cholestasis. In: Paumgartner G, Stiehl A, Gerok W, eds. *Bile acids as therapeutic agents: from basic science to clinical practice*. Proceedings of the 58th Falk Symposium. Lancaster U.K.: Kluwer Academic Publishers, 1991: 335–344.

73. Colombo C, Crosignani A, Assaisso ML, et al. Ursodeoxycholic acid therapy in cystic fibrosis associated liver disease: a dose-response study. *Hepatology* 1992;16:924–930.

74. Lindblad A, Strandvik B. *Long-term study of the effect of ursodeoxycholic acid on liver morphology and liver function in patients with cystic fibrosis*. Proceedings of the 20th European Cystic Fibrosis Conference, 1995:89 (abstract).

75. Colombo C, Apostolo MG, Comi S, Giunta A. Long-term treatment with ursodeoxycholic acid in liver disease associated with cystic fibrosis. *J Pediatr Gastroenterol Nutr* 1995;19:470 (102) (abstract).

76. Bittner P, Posselt HG, Sailer T, et al. The effect of treatment with ursodeoxycholic acid in cystic fibrosis and hepatopathy: results of a placebo-controlled study. In: Paumgartner G, Stiehl A, Gerok W, eds. *Bile acids as therapeutic agents: from basic science to clinical practice*. Proceedings of the 58th Falk

Symposium, Freiburg, Germany, October 1990. Kluwer Academic Publishers, 1991:345–348.

77. O'Brien S, Fitzgerald MX, Hegarty JE. A controlled trial of ursodeoxycholic acid treatment in cystic fibrosis-related liver disease. *Eur J Gastroenterol Hepatol* 1992;4:857–863.

78. Colombo C, Battezzati PM, Podda M, Bettinardi N, Giunta A, the Italian Group for the Study of Ursodeoxycholic Acid in Cystic Fibrosis. Ursodeoxycholic acid for liver disease associated with cystic fibrosis: a double-blind multicenter trial. *Hepatology* 1996;23:1484–1490.

79. Leuschner U, Guldutuna S, Imhof M, Hubner K, Benjaminov A, Leuschner M. Effects of ursodeoxycholic acid after 4 and 12 years of therapy in early and late stages of primary biliary cirrhosis. *J Hepatol* 1994;21:624–633.

80. Crosignani A, Setchell KDR, Invernizzi P, Larghi A, Rodrigues CMP, Podda M. Clinical pharmacokinetics of therapeutic bile acids. *Clin Pharmacokinet* 1996;30:333–358.

81. Podda M, Ghezzi C, Battezzati PM, et al. Effect of different doses of ursodeoxycholic acid in chronic liver disease. *Dig Dis Sci* 1989;34:59S–65S.

82. Merli M, Bertasi S, Servi R, et al. Effect of a medium dose of ursodeoxycholic acid with or without taurine supplementation on the nutritional status of patients with cystic fibrosis: a randomized, placebo-controlled, crossover trial. *J Pediatr Gastroenterol Nutr* 1994;19:198–203.

83. Carey MC, Montet JC, Phillips MC, Armstrong MJ, Mazer NA. Thermodynamic and molecular basis for dissimilar cholesterol-solubilizing capacities by micellar solutions of bile salts: cases of sodium chenodeoxycholate and sodium ursodeoxycholate and their glycine and taurine conjugates. *Biochemistry* 1981;20:3637–3648.

84. Colombo C, Crosignani A, Apostolo MG, Marzano MT, Bettinardi N, Giunta A. Oral bile acids in cystic fibrosis-associated liver disease. *J R Soc Med* 1994;87(Suppl 21):20–24.

85. Poupon RE, Poupon R, Balkau B, the UDCA-PBC Study Group. Ursodiol for long-term treatment of primary biliary cirrhosis. *N Engl J Med* 1994;330:1342–1347.

86. Anonymous. Taurine supplementation in cystic fibrosis. *Nutr Rev* 1988;46:257–258.

87. Smith LJ, Lacaille F, Lepage G, Ronco N, Lamarre A, Roy CC. Taurine decreases fecal fatty acid and sterol excretion in cystic fibrosis: a randomized double-blind trial. *Am J Disease Children* 1991;145:1401–1404.

88. Colombo C, ArlatiS, Curcio L, et al. Effect of taurine supplementation on fat and bile acid absorption in patients with cystic fibrosis. *Scand J Gastroenterol* 1988;23(Suppl 143):151–156.

89. Walker S, Rudolph G, Raedsch R, et al. Intestinal absorption of ursodeoxycholic acid in patients with extrahepatic biliary obstruction and bile drainage. *Gastroenterology* 1992;102:810–815.

90. Bachrach WH, Hofmann AF. Ursodeoxycholic acid in the treatment of cholesterol cholelithiasis: part I. *Dig Dis Sci* 1982;27:833–856.

91. Sanyal AJ, Purdum PP, Luketic VA, Shiffman ML. Bleeding gastroesophageal varices. *Semin Liver Dis* 1993;13:328–342.

92. Bern EM, Grand RJ. Management of therapy for hepatobiliary disease in cystic fibrosis. *New Insights Cystic Fibrosis* 1996;4:4–8.

93. Stringer MD, Price JF, Mowat AP, Howard ER. Liver cirrhosis in cystic fibrosis. *Arch Dis Child* 1993; 69:407 (letter).

94. Louis D, Chazalette JP. Cystic fibrosis and portal hypertension: interest of partial splenectomy. *Eur J Pediatr Surg* 1993;3:22–24.

95. Rossle M, Haag K, Ochs A, et al. The transjugular intrahepatic portosystemic stent-shunt procedure for variceal bleeding. *N Engl J Med* 1994;330:165–171.

96. Berger KJ, Schreiber RA, Tchervenkov J, Kopelman H, Brassard R, Stein L. Decompression of portal hypertension in a child with cystic fibrosis after transjugular intrahepatic portosystemic stent-shunt placement. *J Pediatr Gastroenterol Nutr* 1994;19:322–325.

97. Noble-Jamieson G, Barnes ND, Jamieson N, Friend P, Caine R. Liver transplantation for hepatic cirrhosis in cystic fibrosis. *J R Soc Med* 1996;89(Suppl 27):31–37.

98. Cox KL, Ward RE, Furgiuele TL, Cannon RA, Sanders KD, Kurland G. Orthotopic liver transplantation in patients with cystic fibrosis. *Pediatrics* 1987;80:571–574.

99. Cox K. The role of liver transplantation in cystic fibrosis patients. *Pediatr Pulmonol* 1990;Suppl 6:78–79.

100. Mieles LA, Orenstein D, Teperman L, Podesta L, Koneru B, Starzl TE. Liver transplantation in cystic fibrosis. *Lancet* 1989;i:1073.

101. Noble-Jamieson G, Valente J, Barnes ND, et al. Liver transplantation for hepatic cirrhosis in cystic fibrosis. *Arch Dis Child* 1994;71:349–352.

102. Prandota J. Drug disposition in cystic fibrosis: progress in understanding pathophysiology and pharmacokinetics. *Pediatr Infect Dis J* 1987;6:1111–1126.

103. Cooney GF, Fiel SB, Shaw LM, Cavarochhi NC. Cyclosporin bioavailability in heart–lung transplantation candidates with cystic fibrosis. *Transplantation* 1990;49:821–823.

104. Yang Y, Raper SE, Cohn JA, Engelhardt JF, Wilson JM. An approach for treating the hepatobiliary disease of cystic fibrosis by somatic gene transfer. *Proc Natl Acad Sci U S A* 1993;90:4601–4605.

Cystic Fibrosis in Adults,
edited by J. R. Yankaskas and M. R. Knowles,
Lippincott–Raven Publishers, Philadelphia, 1999.

15

Intestines

Kevin John Gaskin

*Department of Paediatrics, James Fairfax Institute of Paediatric Nutrition, Royal Alexandra
Hospital for Children, Westmead, Sydney, New South Wales, Australia*

The predominant gastrointestinal symptomatology in cystic fibrosis (CF) is related to the presence of pancreatic insufficiency and subsequent maldigestion and malabsorption of nutrients (see Chapter 12). The range of specific gastrointestinal problems experienced by patients with CF are outlined in Table 15–1. Some of these problems, including rectal prolapse, meconium ileus (MI), and the distal intestinal obstruction syndrome (DIOS), are the result of the effects of pancreatic insufficiency and the underlying gut secretion anomaly, whereas the etiology of other complications, including gastroesophageal reflux, Crohn's disease, and colonic strictures, is less certain but likely secondary to the disease or therapy received.

Meconium ileus is a neonatal phenomenon and rectal prolapse a problem experienced by young children and rarely seen in patients older than 5 years of age (1). However, the other gastrointestinal problems, ranging from esophagitis to DIOS, occur during childhood and are recognized complications during adolescence and adulthood (1). Although they very rarely cause mortality, these complications and the difficulties often encountered in their diagnosis—for instance, in differentiating DIOS from appendiceal disease, Crohn's disease, or intussusception—can lead to considerable morbidity for the individual patient. In this chapter, recent work on the underlying pathophysiology of gut disease in CF is discussed, and the major gut complications in adults with CF are highlighted.

PATHOPHYSIOLOGY

The major advances over the last decade in defining the molecular pathogenesis of CF are described in Section I, pertaining to the CF gene structure and function, the cystic fibrosis transmembrane conductance regulator (CFTR), the relationship with impaired epithelial electrolyte transport, and the influence of different CFTR mutations on cell function and phenotypic expressions of the disease. Over the same interval, investigation of the gastrointestinal anomalies have focused on chloride transport abnormalities in small and large intestine, intestinal absorption, and the role of gut hormones and motility problems in contributing to the genesis of gut disease.

Chloride Transport Abnormalities
in the Gut

Ion transport abnormalities have been demonstrated in intestinal tissue from patients with CF by both *in vivo* colonic transepithelial potential difference studies (2,3) and *in vitro* studies of chloride transport in biopsy tissue from the small intestine (4,5), and rectum (6,7). In experiments using biopsy tissue from CF jejunum mounted in Ussing chambers, a range of secretagogues, including the phosphodiesterase inhibitor isobutylmethylxanthine, dibutyryl cyclic adenosine monophosphate (cAMP), phorbol dibutyrate, and the calcium ionophore A23187, failed to induce chloride secretion

TABLE 15–1. *Gastrointestinal disease in cystic fibrosis*

Esophagus	Gastroesophageal reflux
	Esophagitis
	Barrett's esophagus
	Stricture formation
Stomach/duodenum	Gastric ulcer
	Gastritis
	Duodenal ulcer
Small intestine	Giardiasis
	Crohn's disease
	Celiac disease
	Meconium ileus
	Distal intestinal obstruction syndrome (meconium ileus equivalent)
	Intussusception (ileocolic)
	Volvulus
	Ileal adenocarcinoma
Appendix	Acute appendicitis
	Appendiceal abscess
	Perforation
	Mucocele
Colon	Fecal impaction
	Constipation
	Megacolon
	Inflammatory bowel disease
	Crohn's disease
	Fibrosing colonopathy
	Rectal prolapse
	Carcinoma

(8). These observations were made in both ΔF508 patients with pancreatic insufficiency and also in one ΔF508 homozygous pancreatic-sufficient patient with nearly 50% of normal colipase secretion. The data differed from those of a later study of CF rectal suction biopsies (9) in which residual rectal Cl^- secretion correlated with the degree of preservation of pancreatic function, that is, patients with zero rectal Cl^- secretion were pancreatic insufficient, but those with higher residual Cl^- secretion were pancreatic sufficient.

The occurrences of neonatal MI or DIOS in older patients with CF have been compared with the protein hyperconcentration observed in pancreatic secretions from patients with CF (10). This is not an unreasonable comparison given the similarities of transport processes in intestinal crypt and pancreatic duct epithelia, notably that both contain apical membrane Cl^- channels and Cl^-/HCO_3^- exchangers (10). Defects in crypt Cl^- and fluid secretion in CF may contribute to the formation of viscous intestinal contents, and in this regard, the localization of the CFTR in intestinal crypt cells is supportive of this theory (11). Of interest, CFTR recently also has been localized to normal jejunal villous cells (12), and others have characterized villous cells with CFTR expression specifically as having an absence of the brush border disaccharidases sucrase and lactase (13). The exact role of these specialized villous cells remains unclear, but they may have an important transport function, as indicated by the marked basolateral expression of Na^+, K^+ ATPase.

The chloride secretion anomaly in the gut, coupled with failure to hydrate intestinal contents, no doubt contributes to the genesis of both MI and distal intestinal obstruction syndrome. If so, certain genotypes might predispose to the development of these intestinal complications. The CF Genetic Consortium data suggest that there is little difference in the incidence of these complications in ΔF508 homozygotes or most compound ΔF508 heterozygotes (14). However, of note, MI did not occur in patients with the R117H/ΔF508 genotype and appeared less common in the W1282X/ΔF508 genotype and in the non-ΔF508 compound heterozygotes or homozygotes. The R117H mutation is associated with pancreatic sufficiency, that is, with the milder form of pancreatic disease (15). In future studies, intestinal chloride secretion in these patients should be assessed to determine whether the chloride secretion defect is milder, similar to the findings in pancreatic-sufficient patients (9), thus accounting for the lack of occurrence of MI in these patients.

Mucus Secretion

Although the thick inspissated secretions in CF probably are the result of poor hydration of secretions, many have observed intestinal mucus producing glands in patients with CF to show hyperplasia and hypertrophy (16). Mucin produced from CF colon appears more dense, sulphated, and glycosylated, and ileal mucus shows abnormal fucosylation (17,18). Whether these abnormalities are primary and related to the underlying abnormality or are secondary to complications of the disease—for instance, pancreatic insufficiency—is uncertain. Evidence for the former relates to recent studies suggesting that the CFTR may have an important role as an intracellular chloride channel in the regulation of the pH of intracellular compartments (19,20) and the subsequent demonstration of defective acidification of the Golgi complex, lysosomes, and endosomes in CF cells. The latter defect may interfere with the intracellular processing of glycoproteins by inhibiting modifying enzymes such as sialyltransferase. Further evidence for the role of the CFTR in processing mucus glycoproteins has been demonstrated in bronchial xenograft studies (21); however, mucus sulfation appeared uncorrelated to CFTR function. Other evidence supporting the role of CFTR in mucin secretion has been demonstrated in submandibular cells *in vitro*, where antibodies raised against the CFTR inhibited mucin secretion in response to beta-adrenergic stimulation, replicating the abnormality observed in CF (22). Further work is necessary to define the variant roles of the CFTR to provide a more complete understanding of its role in mucin processing and secretion.

Alternatively, some of the intestinal mucin abnormalities could be the result of secondary complications of the disease as, for example, defective degradation associated with pancreatic insufficiency. Degradation of intestinal mucins involves desialation, increasing susceptibility to proteolysis by pancreatic proteases, lysosomal glycosidases, and colonic bacterial proteases and glycosidases (23). Pancreatic proteases cleave some peptide bonds in the mucin molecules and also may cleave nonglycosylated peptides that cross-link mucin fibrils and therefore aid mucin dispersal. In the absence of adequate pancreatic enzyme secretion in pancreatic-insufficient patients, mucin proteolysis would not occur, thus contributing to the development of viscous inspissated secretions.

Lessons from the Cystic Fibrosis Mouse Model

The major intestinal complications of CF, namely neonatal MI and DIOS, are considered to have a multifactorial etiology, including defective enterocyte chloride secretion, pancreatic insufficiency, and prolonged intestinal transit time. Pancreatic insufficiency appears to be a significant component contributing to the genesis of DIOS because the latter has been linked to noncompliance with or to inadequate pancreatic enzyme replacement therapy. Moreover, MI or DIOS rarely have been reported in appropriately proven pancreatic-sufficient patients. However, it also is apparent that MI and DIOS are not observed in other non-CF diseases associated with pancreatic insufficiency, for example, Shwachman syndrome (24), suggesting that severe pancreatic disease alone cannot cause MI or DIOS.

The aforementioned data suggest that both pancreatic insufficiency and the intestinal chloride secretion defect are important in the genesis of MI and DIOS. However, in the Dutch study of ion transport in rectal biopsies from patients with CF, residual chloride secretion was correlated directly with pancreatic function, that is, patients without detectable intestinal chloride secretion were pancreatic insufficient and those with relatively high chloride secretion were pancreatic sufficient (9). In relation to the occurrence of MI or DIOS, these data could suggest that the underlying intestinal secretion defect is the major contributing factor and the severity of the pancreatic disease merely is incidental, reflecting the severity of the underlying secretion defect. This hypothesis would explain the lack of occurrence of MI or DIOS in most pancreatic-sufficient patients who have a milder secretion defect and, conversely, their occurrence in pancreatic-insufficient patients or the rare pancreatic-sufficient patients who have a severe intestinal chloride secretion defect.

The recent development of the CF mouse model has provided further insight into the development of the intestinal complications. In the model developed by disruption of the CFTR gene, a high rate of intestinal complications occurred in the absence of severe histologic changes in the exocrine pancreas (25). Although perinatal deaths were attributed often to non-CF problems, those that died between

12 and 40 days had intestinal obstruction and, commonly, intestinal perforation with fecal peritonitis. Intraluminal, "putty-like" masses were found in the distal intestine, similar to human patients. Histologically, the major changes occurred in the crypts of Lieberkuhn and were more severe in the distal intestine.

Inspissated eosinophilic secretions were found confined to the crypt bases proximal to the intraluminal obstruction, but distal to the obstruction there was dilatation of the crypts and formation of concretions and cast-like structures. Crypt mucus distension also was seen in animals without intestinal obstruction, suggesting that the abnormality was related to the underlying intestinal secretion problem.

In another mouse model produced by other investigators, a milder intestinal lesion occurred, but again, in the absence of discernible pancreatic pathology (26). The findings in both models of intestinal disease in the absence of pancreatic pathology suggest that the neonatal intestinal complications of CF result mainly from the primary intestinal secretion deficit. What remains unknown is whether the additional feature of pancreatic insufficiency increases the severity of the intestinal complication or contributes to the development of DIOS in older patients.

Intestinal Absorption Problems

The major factor causing malabsorption in CF is maldigestion due to pancreatic insufficiency. Patients with pancreatic insufficiency have less than 1% and 2% of average normal colipase and lipase secretion, respectively (27), and consequently malabsorb up to 80% of ingested triglyceride. Similarly, nitrogen malabsorption results from poor pancreatic protease output and protein maldigestion and azotorrhea of up to 50% of nitrogen intake may occur (28). The crucial role of the pancreas in patients with CF, in terms of absorption, is further evident in those with preservation of pancreatic function (pancreatic sufficiency), where even as little as 1% of normal colipase output maintains normal absorption of ingested triglyceride (27). These observations suggest that the

underlying intestinal secretion problem in CF has minimal effects on fat absorption. In keeping with this concept, histologic examination of the small intestine in patients with CF, although demonstrating hyperplasia and hypertrophy of mucus-secreting glands, usually demonstrates normal villous structure and normal or even high disaccharidase activity, indicating the normal maturation of villous cells (1).

Among large groups of pancreatic-insufficient patients, it also is evident, however, that fat malabsorption is quite variable, ranging from 10% to 80% of fat intake (29). Although some of this variability (up to 25% to 30%) of fat malabsorption may be explained by the small amount of residual pancreatic colipase and lipase secretion (27), other factors likely contribute to this variability. Lipolytic activity has, for example, been found in gastric secretions of healthy subjects and in pancreatic-insufficient patients with CF; lingual lipase is increased (30) and may account for up to 90% of the lipolytic activity in the duodenum of these patients. Although the exact role of this specific nonpancreatic lipase is undefined, it may account for some of the variability in fat digestion and absorption seen in such patients. Variable fat absorption also may be related to poor micelle formation due to low bile acid concentrations in the small intestine. In malabsorption, bile acids bind to food residues, with sequestration in the lumen, decreased reabsorption in the terminal ileum, and excessive fecal losses. In addition, the limitation of taurine availability for conjugation leads to a preponderance of glycine conjugated bile acids that, in the more acidic environment of the CF upper small intestine, precipitate out or are protonated, leading to significant passive absorption in the upper small intestine. In this regard, taurine conjugates are protonated very minimally in an acidic environment, and therefore, oral taurine supplements possibly could correct this anomaly (30). However, there is conflicting evidence from the results of different studies on the effect of taurine on fat absorption in patients with CF. Dietary and biliary phospholipids also may interfere with fat digestion because their amphipathic properties lead to their adherence onto the surface of fat droplets, interfering with lipase activity (30). In the absence of phospholipase A_2 due to pancreatic insufficiency, the undegraded phospholipids could impede fat digestion and absorption, but their exact effect remains to be quantitated.

Monosaccharide absorption appears to be enhanced in patients with CF. Studies have demonstrated, for instance, that patients with CF given D-xylose in conjunction with a test meal had significantly higher D-xylose blood levels than controls (31,32). In addition, significantly enhanced glucose absorption, particularly at low glucose concentrations encountered under physiologic conditions, was demonstrated in patients with CF during intestinal perfusion studies (33). Higher glycine and fructose absorption was observed in some patients, and net water absorption was increased when enhanced glucose absorption was evident. The same study demonstrated a significantly thinner unstirred water layer in CF, and it was postulated that the increased glucose absorption was caused by a decrease in the diffusion barriers, possibly caused by abnormal mucus. Another study of the same phenomenon reported an enhanced rate of sodium glucose cotransport (34), but this finding has not been confirmed by other *in vitro* studies of human CF tissue (5,8), nor in the mouse model (35).

Intestinal Permeability and Motility Abnormalities

Increased intestinal permeability has been demonstrated in patients with CF using a variety of nonmetabolizable probe molecules, including lactulose, L-rhamnose, and edetic acid (EDTA) labelled with chromium 51 (36,37). The increased permeability has been attributed to a number of mechanisms, including abnormal mucus overlying the intestinal wall, bacterial contamination of the small intestine, and mucosal injury from hypersecretion of gastric acid. However, in a more recent study, the same phenomenon was found in patients with Shwachman syndrome with pancreatic insufficiency (38). Moreover, the same study demonstrated that urinary lactulose excretion was correlated inversely with duodenal trypsin output, such that pancreatic-sufficient patients with adequate trypsin output had low urinary lactulose excretion, and conversely, pancreatic-insufficient patients had higher urinary lactulose. These results suggested the increased intestinal permeability to these probe molecules was related to pancreatic insufficiency and not to a primary transport problem in the intestine. The authors proposed that as lactulose permeates paracellularly, the loss of intestinal barrier integrity in the presence of pancreatic insufficiency increased lactulose intestinal absorption and subsequent urinary excretion.

The aforementioned studies with oral lactulose also were designed to determine orocecal transit times as an assessment of intestinal motility and demonstrated that patients with CF have prolonged transit compared with controls (37,38). However, in the CF group, prolonged transit did not relate to the degree of exocrine pancreatic dysfunction because there was no difference in transit between patients with and without steatorrhea (38). The mechanism of the altered intestinal motility in CF thus remains enigmatic and requires further investigation. Because intestinal motility is regulated partially by the action of circulating gut peptides, these parameters have been studied in patients with CF. In fasting subjects receiving a liquid test meal with lactulose, fasting serum levels of peptide YY and postprandial serum levels of motilin, enteroglucagon, neurotensin, and peptide YY all were significantly elevated in patients with CF versus controls (39). Such changes, however, were not observed if oral enzyme supplements were given at the time of administration of the test meal. Others have demonstrated a loss of vasoactive intestinal peptide immunoreactivity in small intestinal tissue from patients with CF but normal staining for substance P, leu-enkephalin, somatostatin, or neuropeptide (40). It is conceivable that the variable delay in orocecal transit relates to variable circulating or tissue levels of gut peptides with consequent variable modulation of intestinal motility.

DISEASE IN THE GASTROINTESTINAL TRACT

As indicated in Table 15–1, there is a wide range of problems affecting the gastrointestinal tract in CF. Some, including MI and DIOS, probably are primary—being directly related to CFTR dysfunction. Others, particularly gastroesophageal reflux with or without esophagitis, Barrett's esophagus, or stricture formation, would appear unrelated to CFTR dysfunction and can be designated as secondary occurrences. Fibrosing colonopathy also is associated with excessive ingestion of pancreatic enzyme replacement therapy and thus can be regarded as a secondary complication. Whether appendiceal disease, inflammatory bowel disease, or malignancy of the small or large intestine is primary and related to CFTR dysfunction or secondary to the disease or therapy given for the disease over time remains to be evaluated.

Salivary Glands

Enlargement due to hyperplasia and hypertrophy of the submandibular salivary glands has been reported in up to 90% of patients with CF (41). Eosinophilic plugging and proximal dilatation of ducts is evident histologically in all the mucus-secreting glands, including the sublingual, submucosal, and submandibular glands. The formation in the duct system of insoluble complexes consisting of undissolved zymogen granules and hydroxyapatite crystals may contribute to this process.

There is conflicting evidence concerning parotid gland involvement in CF. Some consider the duct system normal based on sialographic studies (42), but others have described atrophic acini and ductal distension associated with inspissation of ductal contents (43). Certainly, both submandibular and parotid secretions of some patients with CF form an insoluble calcium–phosphate protein complex in the presence of high salivary calcium concentrations, which have been reported in patients with CF. The same phenomenon may explain the propensity of dental calculus to develop on the teeth of patients with CF, adjacent to the duct outlets of the submandibular and parotid glands (43). Salivary gland involvement, however, rarely causes serious clinical problems in either children or adults with CF.

Gastroesophageal Reflux Disease

Over the past decade, there has been increasing recognition of the occurrence of gastroesophageal reflux disease (GERD) in CF, particularly in older patients with moderate to severe lung disease. Up to 25% of patients experience GERD (44), and one report has indicated that esophagitis (45) will develop in more than 50% of patients with GERD, with the propensity to develop esophageal strictures (46).

Symptoms of GERD are outlined in Table 15–2. Although many of the symptoms are specific, for example, heartburn, water brash, epigastric pain, and hematemesis, others, including anorexia, growth failure, and chest symptoms, could be attributed to nonesophageal complications of this disease. Many patients with CF appear to accept GERD symptomatology simply as part of their underlying disease. As such, careful history taking is required to elicit these symptoms, which the patient otherwise would not have volunteered spontaneously.

The etiology of GERD likely is multifactorial. It often is present in patients with moderate to severe lung disease (45), and thus, an inter-

TABLE 15–2. *Symptoms and complications of gastroesophageal reflux*

Heartburn
Chest pain
Water brash
Regurgitation
Vomiting
Epigastric pain
Hematemesis
Anemia
Anorexia
Weight loss
Growth failure
Cough
Recurrent chest infections
Deteriorating lung function

relationship of these entities is highly probable. Increased abdominothoracic pressure gradients occurring during coughing, wheezing, forced expiration during chest physiotherapy, and tilting during postural drainage may contribute to the problem. Chest hyperinflation with flattening of the diaphragm may disturb the anatomy and function of the diaphragm, interfering with the hiatus and bronchodilator medication, including theophylline derivatives, and beta-adrenergic agents will cause lower esophageal sphincter relaxation and predispose to GERD. Gastric emptying also may be impaired. Although scintigraphic studies of gastric emptying using liquid test meals have not shown prolonged gastric emptying times, studies need to be performed using solid test meals. Persistently low lower esophageal sphincter pressure and/or increased gastric pressure no doubt could contribute to GERD, but in studies of patients with CF combining both gastric and esophageal manometry with esophageal pH monitoring, the most common cause of GERD appears to be inappropriate lower esophageal sphincter relaxation (47).

The link between GERD and the development of pulmonary disease remains speculative. It is possible that GERD and subsequent aspiration will exacerbate lung disease, but equally, lung disease and/or therapy for lung disease could induce GERD. It may not be possible to determine cause and effect, but GERD should be considered in those patients who experience exacerbation of lung disease when commencing nocturnal intragastric tube feeding regimens.

Investigation of GERD involves a number of procedures. A barium swallow and meal is relatively noninvasive and will determine the presence of anatomic abnormalities, including hiatal hernia and malrotation. In addition, it will demonstrate obvious esophageal strictures. Twenty-four hour esophageal pH monitoring can determine the duration and severity of acid reflux, but some patients with severe coughing and respiratory disease will not tolerate this procedure for prolonged periods. Given the reported high incidence of esophagitis, esophagoscopy should be considered for all patients with symptoms of GERD, unexplained anorexia, or growth failure. However, this recommendation should be tempered depending on the severity of lung disease and whether the patient will tolerate intravenous sedation or general anesthetic for the procedure.

GERD without esophagitis is managed conservatively with posture and agents that promote gastric emptying, including cisapride. Patients with esophagitis will require therapy with gastric acid suppression agents using either the H_2 receptor antagonists (cimetidine, ranitidine, famotidine, or nizatidine) or the proton-pump inhibitors (omeprazole). Most will require maximal therapy for 12 weeks and follow-up maintenance therapy. H_2-receptor antagonist therapy for esophagitis has met with variable success in non-CF adults with esophagitis, healing the esophagitis in 40% to 66% of patients over 6 to 12 weeks (48), and in maintenance studies with only minor advantages compared with placebo regimens (49). Omeprazole clearly is the superior drug, healing esophagitis in most studies in more than 80% of patients by 12 weeks (50). Unfortunately, the majority of the patients relapse on cessation of the drug, and thus, prolonged maintenance therapy is required. There is ongoing concern about profound suppression of gastric acid secretion, and the induction of hypergastrinemia, which in long-term animal studies has been associated with the development of gastric endocrine cell hyperplasia and gastric retinoid tumors (51). The alternative to prolonged drug therapy is surgical fundoplication. Although the latter may be acceptable to patients with mild lung disease, it is not a consideration for those with severe lung disease, and drug therapy should be continued in the latter to ameliorate their symptoms, hopefully improving their quality of life and nutritional intake before possible lung transplantation.

Peptic Ulcer Disease

There have been anecdotal reports of duodenal ulcer disease in both children and adults with CF. Given the reported hypersecretion of gastric acid reported in one study (52) and the known low pancreatic bicarbonate output (53) in CF, one might have expected ulcer disease to be more common.

In the preendoscopy era, the diagnosis of ulcer disease was dependent on barium meal examinations. Despite the likelihood of overdiagnosis of ulcer disease through misinterpretation of the increased duodenal folds and thick mucus adhering to the duodenal mucosa, ulcer disease was not reported commonly. Moreover, after the advent of endoscopy, ulcer disease rarely has been recognized. Ulcer disease has been intensely researched in non-CF adult patients, particularly in relation to *Helicobacter pylori* infection. This organism originally was associated with the development of antral gastritis and duodenitis, and although its role in the causation of ulcer disease was controversial, it was linked directly to recurrence of ulcer disease. Subsequent information indicates that *H. pylori* is the most common cause of ulcer disease in adults and that treatment should be aimed at both healing the ulcer and eradicating the organism (54). The lower incidence of ulcer disease in CF could relate to a lower incidence of *H. pylori* infection, but anecdotal data suggest that this is not the case (1). Thus, one would have to suspect that somehow patients with CF were protected from the effects of this organism. Although the protection mechanism has not been investigated, it could relate to excessive mucoprotein secretion, modification of mucoproteins, and/or the excessive viscosity of secretions. Investigation of this area may well be very important in the understanding of the pathogenesis of ulcer disease in the healthy population.

Patients suspected of having ulcer disease should undergo endoscopy to prove the diagnosis and to test for the presence or absence of *H. pylori*. If *H. pylori*–associated peptic ulcer disease is demonstrated, H_2 receptor antagonist or omeprazole with a single or double antibiotic regimen is recommended (55). In the absence of *H. pylori*, H_2 receptor antagonists or omeprazole can be used as single therapy, and they may be required for long-term maintenance therapy if there is recrude-scence of the ulcer after initial cessation of therapy.

Distal Intestinal Obstruction Syndrome

DIOS originally was designated as meconium ileus (MI) equivalent. However, the latter term was confusing because older patients do not have meconium, neonatal MI does not necessarily predispose to DIOS, and it is unclear whether there is a unifying mechanism causing these complications. DIOS, by definition, is impaction of inspissated intestinal contents (mainly mucofeculent material) in the terminal ileum, cecum, and proximal colon. Clinically, the term has encompassed simple fecal impaction, patients with recurrent colicky abdominal pain associated with a palpable mass in the right lower quadrant, and others who present with intestinal obstruction, abdominal distension, and bilious vomiting. Unfortunately, these symptoms and signs are not entirely specific and can occur in patients with appendicitis, periappendiceal abscesses, intussusception, Crohn's disease, colonic strictures, and volvulus, all of which have been described in CF populations. Some of these complications occur simultaneously, for example, DIOS and intussusception, thus making diagnosis and management even more complex.

DIOS is considered more common in adolescent and adult patients with CF. In the two original reviews of adult patients with CF, the incidence of DIOS was high, reported in 17% and 24% of patients, respectively (56,57). However, these reviews occurred before the advent of microspheric enzyme replacement therapy and the introduction of normal fat diets in most CF clinics. In a recent reevaluation of this complication, it was reported in only 4% of patients, with all but one case occurring after 15 years of age (58). The age-related incidence increased from 7.5 cases/1,000 patient years in the 15- to 20-year-old age group to 35.5 cases/1,000 in the 20- to 25-year-old group but declined thereafter, possibly because of the small number of surviving patients.

As indicated previously, the etiology of DIOS remains unclear. With few exceptions, it appears to occur in patients with pancreatic insufficiency and can be precipitated by noncompliance to enzyme therapy. Impairment of intestinal chloride and fluid secretion likely is a major contributing factor, producing poorly hydrated intestinal contents and thus increasing the risk of impaction. In addition, the CF enterocyte demonstrates enhanced glucose and amino acid absorption and subsequent increased fluid absorption. Administration of high-carbohydrate low-fat diets thus could contribute further to the hydration problems of the gut contents. Other factors include administration of opiate derivatives, the enhanced viscosity of intestinal mucus—which may relate partially to pancreatic insufficiency and lack of proteolysis (23), and the presence of prolonged orocecal transit times (37,38).

In terms of diagnosis, DIOS should be suspected when a patient presents with colicky abdominal pain and a mass in the right lower quadrant. A plain abdominal radiograph will demonstrate the impacted fecal mass. In the absence of clinical or radiographic signs of obstruction or clinical evidence of peritoneal inflammation, oral washout therapy can be commenced. However, if obstructive or peritoneal signs are present, oral therapy is inappropriate. The patient may require nasogastric aspiration and intravenous fluid therapy before diagnostic investigations. If obstructive signs are present, one must consider a variety of diagnoses, including intussusception, fibrosing colonopathy, Crohn's disease, malignancy, or, if there is evidence of previous abdominal surgery, localized volvulus. Peritoneal signs could suggest either appendiceal disease or Crohn's disease. In the aforementioned circumstances, the sequence of imaging investigations often is determined by the presenting features and the clinician's previous experience. Ultrasound examination followed by a water-soluble contrast enema is a reasonable course. Ultrasound will recognize intussusception and appendiceal disease, and the follow-up water soluble contrast enema examination will diagnose DIOS, intussusception, and strictures and will help to treat DIOS and intussusception. If there is a suggestion of fibrosing colonopathy or malignancy, colonoscopy and biopsy are required for histologic diagnosis of the lesion. Rarely, after these investigations, the diagnosis will remain uncertain, and surgical exploration may be required.

Therapy for DIOS is somewhat empirical. Simple impaction without obstruction often can be relieved with large doses of mineral or paraffin oil (50 to 100 mL twice a day) or with the nonabsorbable sugar lactulose, although the latter has the disadvantage of excessive flatulence. The balanced iso-osmotic polyethylene glycol-containing colonoscopy preparations, for example, *Go-lytely* (Braintree Laboratories, Inc., Braintree, MA), have proven very useful in treating oil-resistant cases of DIOS (59). Adult patients may require up to 5 L of this solution over a 4- to 5-hour period to obtain a thorough evacuation of the mass, and the procedure may have to be repeated in 24 to 48 hours if the mass is not removed entirely.

If DIOS is associated with partial or complete intestinal obstruction with bilious vomiting, intravenous fluids and nasogastric tube aspiration should be commenced. Water-soluble contrast enemas using meglumine diatrizoate (Gastrografin) or the less expensive combination of diatrizoate meglumine + sodium diatrizoate (Urografin) and polysorbate (Tween 80) nearly always will clear the obstruction and then allow a nasogastric infusion of *Go-lytely* to ensure complete evacuation. Only rarely is surgery required for an uncomplicated DIOS. In a recent report (60) of a child with CF and chronic DIOS resistant to conservative measures, a gastrostomy button was inserted through the appendiceal stump, which permitted frequent washout procedures to relieve the impaction. This is a novel approach; however, considering the limited experience, this should be considered only for the rare patient who fails to respond to conservative measures. The prophylactic use of either oral paraffin oil or lactulose has been recommended for those with recurrent DIOS, but the value of such therapy is unknown. Compliance with and the adequacy of enzyme replacement therapy should be questioned before introducing prophylactic therapy.

Constipation and Megacolon

Constipation is a common occurrence in adults with CF and is up to three times more frequent than DIOS (1). Generally, the patient responds to the administration of common laxatives, especially mineral or paraffin oil. Resistant patients may have DIOS and require more intensive therapy with intestinal lavage, or even water-soluble contrast enemas. Some adult patients may present with quite marked distension of their colon, suggestive of megacolon. This complication usually results from longstanding malabsorption and the sheer bulk of the stool, but it also could be the result of intestinal dysmotility.

Intussusception

Intussusception is a well-recognized but uncommon complication of CF. In non-CF populations, it is a disease of young children; however, within CF populations, it most commonly is found in older patients (1). Its occurrence has been related to inspissated secretions adhering to the mucosa and acting as a lead point. Most reports have indicated that the intussusception is ileocolic in location. As mentioned previously, intussusception may occur simultaneously with either DIOS, fecal impaction, or appendiceal disease, and in the latter situation, the appendix may act as the lead point. In one adult series, intussusception was reported in 5% of patients overall and in 20% of patients presenting with intestinal obstruction that was attributed most commonly and incorrectly to DIOS (57). The intussusception was recurrent, and was more frequent in males older than 15 years of age, and all patients were pancreatic insufficient. Of particular interest, none had hematochezia, which typically is present in young children with intussusception who do not have CF.

One must consider this entity in every patient who presents with colicky abdominal pain and a palpable abdominal mass. Because this presentation most likely is caused by DIOS, an abdominal ultrasound or contrast enema are needed to distinguish the two entities. If intussusception is recognized, reduction can be attempted hydrostatically at the time of the enema. Indications for laparotomy include failure to reduce the intussusception, suspected complications, for example, appendiceal disease, or for recurrence of the problem.

Intestinal volvulus also has been described in patients with CF and usually is related to previous surgical intervention. This entity needs to be considered in patients presenting with intestinal obstruction and a history of surgery.

Appendiceal Disease

There are several reports describing the occurrence of appendicitis in CF (61,62,63). Most have emphasized that this is an unusual complication but also have alluded to the difficulty and delay in diagnosis and management, and thus, the high incidence of complications, including appendiceal abscess and perforation. In a retrospective review over a 10-year period, one clinic reported appendicitis in 9 of 803 patients, and in 4 of these patients, diagnosis was delayed for up to 56 days after the onset of symptoms (62). An appendiceal abscess developed in all four of these patients. The authors noted that eight of the nine patients were receiving long-term antibiotics, and this factor may have modified the presentation. These findings confirmed those of a preceding report where over a 15-year period, 19 of 1,220 (1.8%) patients had classic appendicitis over a wide age range, including adult patients (61). In 13 of these patients, perforation was present. In the same series, a further seven patients presenting with chronic intermittent right lower quadrant pain underwent laparotomy and were found to have tensely distended appendices with inspissated mucus, but without inflammation.

The occurrence of acute appendicitis in both series of between 1% to 2% is considerably lower than the commonly accepted 7% rate of non-CF populations. The lower incidence in CF is difficult to explain, considering that at postmortem, the appendix lumen often is obstructed by inspissated eosinophilic secretions and the appendix may be swollen and tense, as described previously. Others also have observed these findings in older patients, and the large, distended appendix may act as a lead point for an intussusception. Coughlin et al. (61) also alluded to this phenomenon: in four patients with recurrent intussusception, exploration revealed tensely distended appendices, and appendicectomy resulted in complete resolution of the patients' symptoms. The occurrence of intussusception of the appendix in CF has been emphasized further by others as a cause of recurrent lower abdominal pain and rectal bleeding (64).

The difficulty in diagnosing appendiceal disease in CF is evident in nearly all of the aforementioned reports. The diagnosis may be masked by concomitant antibiotic therapy, and the presenting symptoms and signs are similar to those observed in DIOS, intussusception, and Crohn's disease. Patients with these disorders can present with a mass lesion, abdominal tenderness, and recurrent colicky abdominal pain; thus, these disorders are confounding factors that interfere with direct diagnosis of appendiceal disease. Rebound tenderness and guarding in the right iliac fossa are useful physical signs predicting localized appendiceal inflammation. In addition, the presence of a limp may signify appendicitis, with perforation and the formation of a psoas abscess. Investigations, including plain abdominal x-ray, ultrasound, computed tomography (CT) scan, and even gallium or leukocyte scans, may aid diagnosis, but often they are unhelpful. In the presence of guarding, tenderness, and a mass lesion with or without fever, one must consider a laparotomy to exclude appendicitis. In these circumstances, even if the ultrasound or CT scan are suggestive of fecal impaction, one cannot dismiss the possibility of appendicitis because these entities may occur simultaneously.

Giardiasis

There have been several reports of giardiasis in adults with preexistent pancreatic or hepatic disease who do not have CF (65,66). This has led to the hypothesis that these diseases may predispose to infestation with *Giardia*, but this issue has not been studied. However, if this contention is correct, it perhaps is surprising that the coexistence of *Giardia* and CF has been reported infrequently considering the known pancreatic and hepatic components of this disease. After the recognition of two cases of *Giardia* and CF with intractable gastrointestinal symptoms, one group investigated this association in some 107 patients with CF and 64 normal household contacts of the patients with CF (67). *Giardia* infestation was present in 28% of the patients with CF, and of relevance in the current text, the prevalence appeared to increase with age, with 44% of patients older than 20 years of age positive for *Giardia*. In contrast, 11% of controls younger than 5 years of age and none older than 10 years were positive for *Giardia*, consistent with the known propensity of *Giardia* to affect young children who do not have CF. The authors acknowledged the possibility that the high prevalence of *Giardia* could have been related to their detection technique, namely, counterimmunoelectrophoresis (CIE), against fecal *Giardia* antigens. Single microscopic examination confirmed the presence of *Giardia* cysts in only 44.1% and 42.9% in the CF and control groups, respectively, who were positive for fecal antigens. The investigators assessed whether the CIE technique cross-reacted with other antigens, but were not able to demonstrate such reactions. The observation of the high prevalence of giardiasis in CF patients potentially is important, but the study did not demonstrate any relationship with gastrointestinal symptoms, and indices of malabsorption were not assessed. Thus, follow-up studies are needed, not only to confirm the observation, but also to determine whether *Giardia* infestation in CF causes functional abnormalities in relation to absorption of nutrients or simply is an incidental parasite with either mild or no clinical sequelae.

Crohn's Disease

For a period of 40 years after the original description of CF, there were only three reports of the coexistence of Crohn's disease and CF (68). Thus, it appeared likely that these were chance occurrences. However, in the past decade, there have been multiple single reports of the occurrence of Crohn's disease in CF, suggesting that the coexistence of these two disorders was more than a coincidence (68). These observations prompted a survey of 52 U.S. CF clinics involving some 11,321 patients and comparison with rates of inflammatory bowel disease in the general population of the United States and Europe (69). The preliminary results of this survey demonstrated that 28 patients had inflammatory bowel disease, 25 (89%) with Crohn's disease, with an average age of 15.6 years. The prevalence of Crohn's in this series of 1 in 404 cases was 11 times that expected from published data in the United States or Europe for a comparably aged non-CF control group. However, this is the only publication to date indicating this relationship and because it is preliminary and was not a true case control study, the high prevalence of Crohn's disease in CF reported in the study requires confirmation.

The clinical and pathologic findings of Crohn's disease in patients with CF are identical to those for the non-CF population (68). Patients present with a history of anorexia, diarrhea, hematochezia, weight loss, and, consistently, abdominal pain. They may have fistula formation, perianal disease, and extra gastrointestinal manifestations of their disease, including arthritis. Some are anemic, because of blood loss, and have hypoproteinemia. However, of note, in most cases there has been undue delay in diagnosis because the clinical symptoms and signs are not necessarily specific and could be present in other complications, including DIOS and appendiceal masses. Our own clinic has identified two patients, one who presented with arthritis and later partial intestinal obstruction and the other with recurrent lower abdominal pain and bowel obstruction. The first 12-year-old patient demonstrated narrowing of the proximal colon (Fig. 15–1) and at colonoscopy was found to have granulomatous inflammation, ulcers, pseudopolyps, and cobblestoning of the entire proximal colon. In the other 22-year-old patient

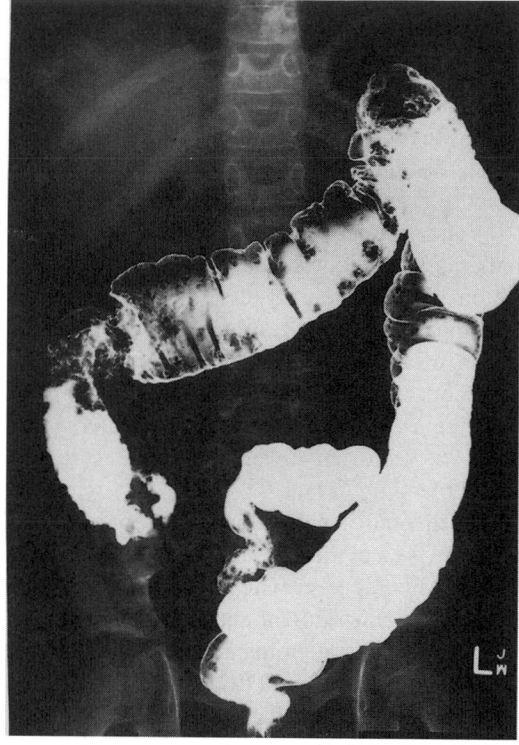

FIG. 15–1. Barium enema from a patient with cystic fibrosis and Crohn's disease. There are two areas of narrowing in the cecum and proximal transverse colon. Cobblestoning of the mucosa and irregularity of the mucosa of the ascending colon are evident.

who required exploration for intestinal obstruction, and macroscopic features of Crohn's disease with creeping fat around the colon extending from the terminal ileum to the hepatic flexure were demonstrated. At histologic examination, there clearly was granulomatous inflammation, as demonstrated in Figure 15–2. Of interest in both cases was the marked pseudopolyp formation, which is considered uncommon in Crohn's disease.

The occurrence of Crohn's disease in CF as described previously, raises the important question as to whether CF predisposes patients to the development of Crohn's disease. Among the CF patients with Crohn's disease, there is a preponderance who are ΔF508 homozygotes, all have been pancreatic insufficient and have required enzyme replacement

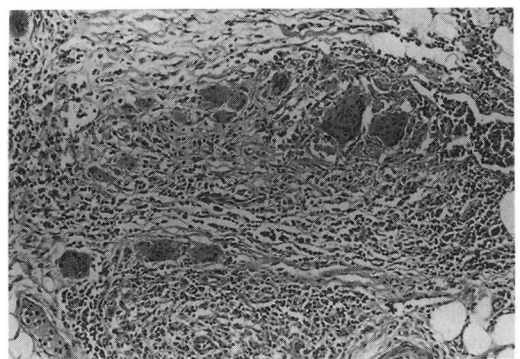

FIG. 15–2. Histologic examination of biopsies from ascending colon revealing a chronic inflammatory infiltrate with noncaseating granulomata consistent with Crohn's disease.

therapy, and all have received varying antibiotic therapy for lung disease. How these various factors interact to predispose the patient to Crohn's disease is enigmatic. Speculatively, nontuberculous mycobacteria, hypergammaglobulinemia, increased receptors for bacterial adherence, abnormal clearance mechanisms related to dysmotility and viscous mucus, and the development of immune complexes may contribute. The increased reporting of Crohn's disease has occurred after the advent of the microspheric enzyme preparations, and it will be important to determine whether, like fibrosing colonopathy, there is a relationship between Crohn's disease and the excessive use of these enzyme preparations.

The latter does raise the issue as to whether the occurrence of Crohn's disease or fibrosing colonopathy in patients with CF is a distinct entity or a disease spectrum. Because there is no absolute diagnostic test, the entities currently are distinguished by their clinical presentation and radiologic and pathologic findings. Both conditions commonly are located to the right colon, have inflammatory and fibrosing components, and can present with bloody diarrhea. However, Crohn's disease can be located elsewhere in the gut, including perianally; there usually is an intense inflammatory component; and, of importance, the inflammation usually is granulomatous—features not currently described in fibrosing colonopathy. Furthermore, the clinical features of protein loss with hypoproteinemia and extragastrointestinal manifestations, for example, arthritis, are recognized features of Crohn's disease but not fibrosing colonopathy. These features may assist in diagnosis, but ultimately, colonoscopy and histologic examination of the lesion are essential for diagnosis.

Fibrosing Colonopathy

In 1994, anecdotal reports of colonic strictures first were published in Britain. The cases appeared temporally related to the introduction of high-strength pancreatic enzyme supplements (70,71). Subsequent analysis of data from the U.S. Cystic Fibrosis Foundation revealed a total of 35 cases (72), and a further 14 cases were reported from the U.K. CF registry (73).

In general, patients have been young (< 15 years of age), presenting with intestinal obstruction, abdominal pain, bloody diarrhea, poor weight gain, and/or chylous ascites. The diagnosis was suspected in patients consuming more than 6,000 lipase units/meal for more than 6 months and in those with a previous history of abdominal surgery. Abdominal ultrasound examination may suggest the diagnosis, particularly if chylous ascites is present, but a contrast enema is the investigation of choice, demonstrating the presence of a colonic stricture, usually in the proximal colon. Ultimately, the diagnosis will be made surgically or by colonoscopy and histologic examination of biopsy specimens. Typically, at surgery fusiform, long segment stenoses are found. Histologically, biopsies demonstrate fibrosis in the lamina propria, with varying degrees and quite often minimal nongranulomatous inflammation.

The British case control study suggests a strong temporal relationship between the introduction of high-dose lipase enzyme replacement therapy and the occurrence of fibrosing colonopathy, with an average lipase intake of 46,200 units/kg/day (73). The U.S. Consensus Meeting noted that lipase doses in excess of 6,000 units/kg/meal were associated with fibrosing colonopathy, regardless of whether standard or high-dose lipase preparations were taken (72). For doses between 2,500 and 6,000 units/kg/meal, the risk was uncertain, and the committee recommended that all patients consume less than 2,500 units/kg/meal to avoid the complication.

To date, the complication rarely has been reported in adult patients. This observation may relate to more appropriate use of enzyme preparations by the older population, but the aforementioned report certainly cautions those involved in adult CF care to avoid excessive doses of enzyme replacement therapy.

Miscellaneous Problems

Pneumatous Intestinales

Pneumatous intestinales complication has been described in older patients with advanced pulmonary disease (74). Its etiology is uncertain. Air collecting in the colonic wall may track between muscle and mucosa layers, and if severe, can be associated with the formation of submucosal cysts. There rarely are any significant clinical complications of this problem.

Gastrointestinal Malignancy

There have been a number of reports of gastrointestinal malignancy, specifically ileal adenocarcinoma, in older patients with CF (75,76,77). The inflammatory bowel disease survey among U.S. CF clinics identified four further cases and a possible increased risk among the CF population (68). The U.S. Cystic Fibrosis Cancer Study Group has confirmed the increased risk of gastrointestinal malignancy, noting 13 cases in the U.S. cohort and 11 in the European cohort, with all but one case occurring in patients older than 20 years of age (78). Of the 24 cases from the combined cohorts, there were two esophageal cancers, one gastric cancer, three small intestine cancers, nine large intestine cancers, three pancreatic cancers, five biliary cancers, and one retroperitoneal cancer.

The increased risk of digestive cancers compared with other organs in patients with CF

may be related to the level of CFTR expression in the gastrointestinal system. Alternatively, the complications of the disease could predispose to malignancy, such as the occurrence of Barrett's esophagus in those with esophagitis (79), biliary stones, or inflammation predisposing to cholangiocarcinoma and selenium and vitamin E deficiency to ileal adenocarcinoma (80). Further studies no doubt will be forthcoming in this area, but currently the aforementioned studies give a timely warning to those caring for adult patients to be aware of the malignant complications of this disease.

Celiac Disease

There have been anecdotal reports of celiac disease in young children with CF (81,82). Unfortunately, follow-up data on these children have not been provided since the original reports. Primary protein caloric malnutrition per se can be associated with falsely elevated sweat chlorides, which return to within the normal range on nutritional rehabilitation. Moreover, long-standing celiac disease has been associated with the development of secondary pancreatic insufficiency, usually in adults (83). Therefore, in the reported cases, malnutrition associated with celiac disease may have produced a false elevation of the sweat chloride, and the patients may have had secondary pancreatic insufficiency, thus confusing the diagnosis. Nevertheless, celiac disease has been recognized in adult patients with CF in the U.S. survey (68), with a prevalence of 1:1,258 patients. The coexistence of celiac disease and CF needs to be considered in patients whose malabsorption is not controlled by adequate enzyme replacement therapy and the diagnosis confirmed by duodenal biopsy. Patients require a lifelong gluten-free diet, and thus, it is essential that the diagnosis is confirmed histologically.

CLINICAL APPROACH TO ABDOMINAL PAIN

From the aforementioned, a common theme underlying the presentation of gastrointestinal disease in older patients with CF is the presence of abdominal pain with or without the presence of a mass lesion. The causes of abdominal pain and/or approach to their management are outlined in Table 15–3, and all should be considered in the differential diagnosis of this common problem, which may affect more than 25% of older patients. The location of the pain is a helpful discriminating feature—for example, epigastric and chest pain with esophagitis, right upper quadrant pain in patients with biliary tract disease, and gallstones or flank pain in those with renal stones; however, in patients with lower abdominal colicky pain, there are a number of intestinal problems that may be difficult to distinguish on clinical grounds alone. As evident in the previous discussion, right lower quadrant pain with the presence of a palpable mass could be associated with DIOS, intussusception, appendiceal abscess, Crohn's disease, proximal colonic strictures, or cancer. The dilemma for the physician involved is how to most appropriately investigate the patient, to prevent delay in diagnosis of eminently treatable problems, without causing discomfort or inconvenience to a patient who is likely to have moderate to severe pulmonary disease.

In the presence of a nontender palpable mass (in a patient without guarding or rebound tenderness) or evidence of intestinal obstruction (bilious vomiting or overt distension), the simplest investigation is a plain abdominal x-ray to confirm the presence of fecal material in the proximal colon and cecum and determine the presence or absence of intestinal obstruction. A follow-up ultrasound examination will help to define whether there is an intussusception or appendiceal mass.

In the presence of an intraluminal mass without evidence of obstruction, intussusception or appendiceal pathology, intestinal evacuation using oral *Go-lytely* solution is recommended. However, if obstruction is present, a *Go-lytely* enema often is successful in evacuating the fecal mass and relieving the obstruction, thus enabling a washout with oral *Go-lytely*. If the enema fails to relieve the obstruction, a water-soluble contrast enema should be attempted, and

TABLE 15–3. *Approach to abdominal pain in cystic fibrosis*

Upper abdominal pain
  Epigastric
    Esophagitis
    Peptic ulcer disease
      Investigations
        Ba swallow and meal
        Endoscopy
    Pancreatitis (pancreatic sufficient patients)
      Investigations
        Serum amylase
        Serum trypsinogen
        Pancreatography
  Right upper quadrant
    Cholelithiasis
    Biliary tract stones
    Common bile duct stenosis
    Sclerosing cholangitis
      Investigations
        Biliary ultrasound
        Biliary scintigraphy
        Cholangiography
  Loin
    Renal stones
      Investigations
        Urine microscopy
        Ultrasound
        Urological consultation
Lower abdominal pain
  ± Palpable mass
    Consider DIOS
      Investigations
        Plain abdominal radiograph
              ↓
        Conservative management
        Laxatives (mineral/paraffin oil)
          ↓ (no response)
        Intestinal lavage using iso-osmotic electrolyte
        preparation orally *or* via NG tube
          ↓ (no response)
        Contrast enema to assess re-DIOS, Crohn's
          disease, intussusception or stricture
  Guarding + rebound tenderness + ± palpable mass
    Appendiceal disease
      Investigations
        • Ultrasound
        • CT scan
        ↓ If suggestive → surgery
    Crohn's disease
    Fibrosing colonopathy
      Investigations
        • Ba enema
        • Colonoscopy
  Intestinal obstruction + ± palpable mass
    Investigations
      • Plain abdominal radiograph
        Management
          IV fluids
          NG aspiration
      • Contrast enema
      if DIOS
        Colonic lavage, then oral-intestinal lavage
      Intussusception
        Attempt hydrostatic reduction
        ↓ If fails → surgery
      ?Crohn's disease, ?stricture, ?carcinoma
        Colonoscopy, surgery

Ba, barium; CT, computed tomography; DIOS, distal intestinal obstruction syndrome; IV, intravenous; NG, nasogastric.

although usually successful at relieving DIOS, this also will determine whether other problems, for example, intussusception, or strictures, also are present. If symptoms—particularly pain— persist after colonic evacuation, a repeat ultrasound or CT scan is advised to define an appendiceal mass that previously was disguised by the intraluminal fecal mass. In circumstances in which an intramural lesion or stricture are suggested by the aforementioned investigations, colonoscopy should be performed to directly visualize the lesion and perform a biopsy. In determining whether there is acute appendicitis, abscess formation, or perforation, the finding of rebound tenderness and guarding should alert one to this possibility, as should the presence of a limp, which may indicate a local perforation of the appendix into the psoas muscle. Both abdominal ultrasound and CT scan examination may be helpful diagnostically, but ultimately, in the absence of a secure diagnosis of DIOS, intussusception, or Crohn's disease, an exploratory laparotomy will be required.

SUMMARY

Gastrointestinal disease is an evolving area of CF, both in terms of basic research and the emergence of previously unrecognized complications, including fibrosing colonopathy, inflammatory bowel disease, and malignancy. Basic research in human tissue and the recently developed mouse models have begun to unravel the pathophysiology of the intestinal disease by addressing the issues of ion transport abnormalities and the influence of CFTR mutations on intracellular processes, including mucin production and secretion. Ongoing research hopefully will enhance further our understanding of factors involved in the genesis of the gastrointestinal complications of this disease and provide more appropriate therapeutic options to prevent or treat these problems.

The sphere of gastrointestinal complications is vast, and gut disease no longer simply is related to MI or DIOS. It also is evident that many of these complications are complex, requiring considerable experience and a flexible approach. The presentation of DIOS, for example, is common to a variety of complications, including intussusception, Crohn's disease, appendiceal disease, and malignancy; as such, the physician should be aware of these problems, thus enabling appropriate investigation and, by expediting management, preventing excessive morbidity from these complications. Clearly, because the majority of CF populations currently survive into adulthood, there is a need for experienced adult gastroenterologists to be involved continuously in CF care, and not on an *ad hoc* basis, as currently is evident. The emergence of fibrosing colonopathy in children with CF also is a timely warning regarding the inappropriate use of therapy in CF. Although high-dose lipase enzyme replacement promised much in terms of reducing the number of capsules ingested, the excessive use of these preparations in the absence of objective data on fat absorption has led to an unwelcome complication. The future will see an intense research effort to provide a better appreciation of the underlying pathophysiology of gut disease, and this should provide a sound rationale on which to base clinical management of these complex evolving problems.

REFERENCES

1. Durie PR. Cystic fibrosis: gastrointestinal and hepatic complications and their management. *Int Semin Paediatr Gastroenterol Nutr* 1993;2(2):3–9.
2. Orlando RC, Powell DW, Croom RD, et al. Colonic and esophageal transepithelial potential difference in cystic fibrosis. *Gastroenterology* 1989;96(4):1041–1048.
3. Gowen CW Jr, Gowen MA, Knowles MR. Colonic transepithelial potential difference in infants with cystic fibrosis. *J Pediatr* 1991;118(3):412–415.
4. Taylor CJ, Baxter PS, Hardcastle J, et al. Failure to induce secretion in jejunal biopsies from children with cystic fibrosis. *Gut* 1988;29(17):957–962.
5. Berschneider HM, Knowles MR, Azizkhan RG, et al. Altered intestinal chloride transport in cystic fibrosis. *FASEB J* 1988;2(10):2625–2629.
6. Goldstein JL, Shapiro AB, Rao MC, et al. In vivo evidence of altered chloride but not potassium secretion in cystic fibrosis rectal mucosa. *Gastroenterology* 1991;101(4):1012–1019.
7. Veeze HJ, Sinaasappel M, Bijman J, et al. Ion transport abnormalities in rectal suction biopsies from children with cystic fibrosis. *Gastroenterology* 1991;101(2):398–403.

8. O'Loughlin EV, Hunt DM, Gaskin KJ, et al. Abnormal epithelial transport in cystic fibrosis jejunum. *Am J Physiol* 1991;260(5 pt 1):G758–G763.

9. Veeze HJ, Halley DJ, Bijman, et al. Determinants of mild clinical symptoms in cystic fibrosis patients: residual chloride secretion measured in rectal biopsies in relation to genotype. *J Clin Invest* 1994;93(2): 461–466.

10. Marino CR, Gorelick FS. Scientific advances in cystic fibrosis. *Gastroenterology* 1992;103(2):681–693.

11. Crawford I, Maloney PC, Zeitlin PL, et al. Immunocytochemical localization of the cystic fibrosis gene product CFTR. *Proc Natl Acad Sci U S A* 1991;88 (20):9262–9266.

12. O'Loughlin EV, Hunt D, Gaskin K, et al. X-ray microanalysis of cell elements in normal and cystic fibrosis jejunum: evidence for chloride secretion in villi. *Gastroenterology* 1996;110(2):411–418.

13. Ameen NA, Ardito T, Kashgarian M, et al. A unique subset of rat and human intestinal villus cells express the cystic fibrosis transmembrane conductance regulator. *Gastroenterology* 1995;108(4):1016–1023.

14. Hamosh A, Corey M. Correlation between genotype and phenotype in patients with cystic fibrosis: the Cystic Fibrosis Genotype–Phenotype Consortium. *N Engl J Med* 1993;329(18):1308–1313.

15. Kristidis P, Bozon D, Corey M, et al. Genetic determination of exocrine pancreatic function in cystic fibrosis. *Am J Hum Genet* 1992;50(6):1178–1184.

16. Thomaidis TS, Arey JB. The intestinal lesions in cystic fibrosis of the pancreas. *J Pediatr* 1963;63(3): 444–453.

17. Thiru S, Devereux G, King A. Abnormal fucosylation of ileal mucus in cystic fibrosis: I, a histochemical study using peroxidase labelled lectins. *J Clin Pathol* 1990;43(12):1014–1018.

18. King A, McLeish M, Thiru S. Abnormal fucosylation of ileal mucus in cystic fibrosis: II, a histochemical study using monoclonal antibodies to fucosyl oligosaccharides. *J Clin Pathol* 1990;43(12):1019–1022.

19. Al-Awqati Q, Barasch J, Landry D. Chloride channels of intracellular organelles and their potential role in cystic fibrosis. *J Exp Biol* 1992;172:245–266.

20. Barasch J, Kiss B, Prince A, et al. Defective acidification of intracellular organelles in cystic fibrosis. *Nature* 1991;352(6330):70–73.

21. Zhang Y, Doranz B, Yankaskas JR, et al. Genotypic analysis of respiratory mucous sulfation defects in cystic fibrosis. *J Clin Invest* 1995;96(6):2997–3004.

22. Bradbury NA, Dormer RL, McPherson MA. Dissociation between cyclic AMP rise and mucin secretion in response to a beta-adrenergic agonist. *Acta Univ Carol (Med) Praha* 1990;36(1–4):55–57.

23. Forstner JF. Intestinal mucins in health and disease. *Digestion* 1978;17(3):234–263.

24. Gaskin KJ. Hereditary disorders of the pancreas. In: Walker JA, Durie PR, Hamilton JR, Walker-Smith JA, Watkins JB, eds. *Pediatric gastrointestinal disease.* St Louis: Mosby-Year Book, 1996.

25. Snouwaert JN, Brigman KK, Latour AM, et al. An animal model for cystic fibrosis made by gene targeting. *Science* 1992;257(5073):1083–1088.

26. Dorin JR, Dickinson P, Alton EWF, et al. Cystic fibrosis in the mouse by targeted insertional mutagenesis. *Nature* 1992;359(6392):211–215.

27. Gaskin KJ, Durie PR, Lee L, et al. Colipase and lipase secretion in childhood-onset pancreatic insufficiency: delineation of patients with steatorrhea secondary to relative colipase deficiency. *Gastroenterology* 1984; 86(1):1–7.

28. Lapey A, Kattwinkel J, di Sant'Agnese P, et al. Steatorrhoea and azotorrhoea and their relation to growth and nutrition in adolescents and young adults with cystic fibrosis. *J Pediatr* 1974;84(3):328–334.

29. Forstner G, Gall G, Corey M, et al. Digestion and absorption of nutrients in cystic fibrosis. In: Sturgess J, ed. *Perspectives in cystic fibrosis: proceedings of the 8th International Congress on Cystic Fibrosis.* Mississauga: Imperial Press, 1980.

30. Roy CC, Weber AM, Lepage G, et al. Digestive and absorptive phase anomalies associated with the exocrine pancreatic insufficiency of cystic fibrosis. *J Pediatr Gastroenterol Nutr* 1988;7(Suppl 1):S1–S7.

31. Buts JP, Morin CL, Roy CC, et al. One-hour blood xylose test: a reliable index of small bowel function. *J Pediatr* 1978;92(5):729–733.

32. Schaad U, Kraemer R, Gaze H, et al. One-hour blood xylose in cystic fibrosis. *Arch Dis Child* 1978;53(9): 756–757.

33. Frase LL, Strickland AD, Kachel GW, et al. Enhanced glucose absorption in the jejunum of patients with cystic fibrosis. *Gastroenterology* 1985;88(2):478–484.

34. Baxter P, Goldhill J, Hardcastle J, et al. Enhanced intestinal glucose and alanine transport in cystic fibrosis. *Gut* 1990;31(7):817–820.

35. Grubb BR. Ion transport across the jejunum in normal and cystic fibrosis mice. *Am J Physiol* 1995;268(31): G505–G513.

36. Leclercq-Foucart J, Forget PP, Van Cutsem JL. Lactulose rhamnose intestinal permeability in children with cystic fibrosis. *J Pediatr Gastroenterol Nutr* 1987;6 (6):66–70.

37. Escobar H, Perdomo M, Vasconez F, et al. Intestinal permeability to ^{51}Cr-EDTA and orocecal transit time in cystic fibrosis. *J Pediatr Gastroenterol Nutr* 1992;14 (2):204–207.

38. Mack DR, Flick JA, Durie PR, et al. Correlation of intestinal lactulose permeability with exocrine pancreatic dysfunction. *J Pediatr* 1992;120(5):696–701.

39. Murphy MS, Brunetto AL, Pearson AD, et al. Gut hormones and gastrointestinal motility in children with cystic fibrosis. *Dig Dis Sci* 1992;37(2):187–192.

40. Wattchow DA, Furness JB, Gibbins IL, et al. Vasoactive intestinal peptide immunoreactive nerve fibers are deficient in intestinal and nasal mucosa affected by cystic fibrosis. *J Gastroenterol Hepatol* 1988;3(6): 549–555.

41. Barbero GJ, Sibinga MS. Enlargement of the submaxillary salivary glands in cystic fibrosis. *Pediatrics* 1962;29(5):788–793.

42. Leake D, Khaw K-T, Shwachman H. Parotid gland sialograms in cystic fibrosis. *J Pediatr* 1970;76(2):301–304.

43. Blomfield J, Rush AR, Allars HM, et al. Parotid gland function in children with cystic fibrosis and child control subjects. *Pediatr Res* 1976;10(6):574–578.

44. Scott RB, O'Loughlin EV, Gall DG. Gastroesophageal reflux in patients with cystic fibrosis. *J Pediatr* 1985;106(2):223–227.

45. Feigelson J, Girault F, Pecau Y. Gastro-oesophageal reflux and oesophagitis in cystic fibrosis. *Acta Paediatr Scand* 1987;76(6):989–990.

46. Bendig DW, Seilheimer DK, Wagner ML, et al. Complications of gastroesophageal reflux in patients with cystic fibrosis. *J Pediatr* 1982;100(4):536–540.

47. Cucchiara S, Santamaria F, Andreotti MR, et al. Mechanisms of gastro-oesophageal reflux in cystic fibrosis. *Arch Dis Child* 1991;66(5):617–622.

48. Tytgat GNJ, Nicolai JJ, Reman FC. Efficacy of different doses of cimetidine in the treatment of reflux esophagitis: a review of three large, double-blind controlled trials. *Gastroenterology* 1990;99(3):629–634.

49. Koelz HR, Birchler R, Bretholz A, et al. Healing and relapse of reflux esophagitis during treatment with ranitidine. *Gastroenterology* 1986;91(5):1198–1205.

50. Hetzel DJ, Dent J, Reed WD, et al. Healing and relapse of severe peptic esophagitis after treatment with omeprazole. *Gastroenterology* 1988;95(4):903–912.

51. Hakanson R, Sundler F, Carlsson E et al. Proliferation of enterochromaffin-like (ECL) cells in the rat stomach following omeprazole treatment. *Hepatogastroenterology* 1985;32:48–49.

52. Cox KL, Isenberg JN, Ament ME. Gastric acid hypersecretion in cystic fibrosis. *J Pediatr Gastroenterol Nutr* 1982;1(4):559–565.

53. Gaskin KJ, Durie PR, Corey M, et al. Evidence for a primary defect in pancreatic $HCO_3{}^-$ secretion in cystic fibrosis. *Pediatr Res* 1982;16(7):554–557.

54. Graham DY. Treatment of peptic ulcers caused by Helicobacter pylori. *N Engl J Med* 1993;328(5):349–350.

55. Walsh JH, Peterson WL. The treatment of Helicobacter pylori infection in the management of peptic ulcer disease. *N Engl J Med* 1995;333(15):984–991.

56. Shwachman H, Kowalski M, Khaw K-T. Cystic fibrosis: a new outlook. *Medicine* 1977;56(2):129–149.

57. di Sant'Agnese PA, Davis PB. Cystic fibrosis in adults: 75 cases and a review of 232 cases in the literature. *Am J Med* 1979;66(1):121–132.

58. Andersen HO, Hjelt K, Waever E, et al. The age-related incidence of meconium ileus equivalent in a cystic fibrosis population: the impact of high-energy intake. *J Pediatr Gastroenterol Nutr* 1990;11(3):356–360.

59. Cleghorn GJ, Stringer DA, Forstner GG, et al. Treatment of distal intestinal obstruction syndrome in cystic fibrosis with a balanced intestinal lavage solution. *Lancet* 1986;i(8471):8–11.

60. Redel CA, Motil KJ, Bloss RS, et al. Intestinal button implantation for obstipation and fecal impaction in children. *J Pediatr Surg* 1992;27(5):654–656.

61. Coughlin JP, Gauderer W, Stern RC, et al. The spectrum of appendiceal disease in cystic fibrosis. *J Pediatr Surg* 1990;25(8):835–839.

62. Shields MD, Levison H, Reisman JJ, et al. Appendicitis in cystic fibrosis. *Arch Dis Child* 1991;66(3):307–310.

63. Allen ED, Pfaff JK, Taussig LM, et al. The clinical spectrum of chronic appendiceal abscess in cystic fibrosis. *Am J Dis Child* 1992;146(10):1190–1193.

64. McIntosh JC, Mroczek EC, Baldwin C, et al. Intussusception of the appendix in a patient with cystic fibrosis. *J Pediatr Gastroenterol Nutr* 1990;11(4):542–544.

65. Sheehy TW, Holley HP Jr. Giardia-induced malabsorption in pancreatitis. *JAMA* 1975;233(13):1373–1375.

66. Petersen H. Giardiasis (lambliasis). *Scand J Gastroenterol* 1972;7(Suppl 14):1–44.

67. Roberts DM, Craft JC, Mather FJ, et al. Prevalence of giardiasis in patients with cystic fibrosis. *J Pediatr* 1988;112(4):555–559.

68. Lloyd-Still JD. Cystic fibrosis, Crohn's disease, biliary abnormalities, and cancer. *J Pediatr Gastroenterol Nutr* 1990;11(4):434–437.

69. Lloyd-Still JD. Crohn's accounts for increased prevalence of inflammatory bowel disease (IBD) in CF. *Pediatr Pulmonol Suppl* 1992;8:307–308 (abstract).

70. Smyth RL, van Velzen D, Smyth AR, et al. Strictures of ascending colon in cystic fibrosis and high-strength pancreatic enzymes. *Lancet* 1994;343(8889):85–86.

71. Oades PJ, Bush A, Ong PS, et al. High-strength pancreatic enzyme supplements and large-bowel stricture in cystic fibrosis. *Lancet* 1994;343(8889):109 (letter).

72. Borowitz DS, Grand RJ, Durie PR, et al. Use of pancreatic enzyme supplements for patients with cystic fibrosis in the context of fibrosing colonopathy. *J Pediatr* 1995;127(5):681–684.

73. Smyth RL, Ashby D, O'Hea U, et al. Fibrosing colonopathy in cystic fibrosis: results of a case-control study. *Lancet* 1995;346(8985):1247–1251.

74. Hernanz-Schulman M, Kirkpatrick J Jr, Shwachman H, et al. Pneumatosis intestinalis in cystic fibrosis. *Radiology* 1986;160(2):497–499.

75. Davis TH, Sawicka EH. Adenocarcinoma in cystic fibrosis. *Thorax* 1985;40:199–200.

76. Redington AN, Spring R, Batten JC. Adenocarcinoma of the ileum presenting as non-traumatic clostridial myonecrosis in cystic fibrosis. *Br Med J* 1985;290(6485):1871–1872.

77. Siraganian PA, Miller RW, Swender PT. Cystic fibrosis and ileal carcinoma. *Lancet* 1987;2(8568):1158 (letter).

78. Neglia JP, Fitzsimmons SC, Maisonneuve P, et al. The risk of cancer among patients with cystic fibrosis. *N Engl J Med* 1995;332(8):494–499.

79. Hassall E, Israel DM, Davidson AG, Wong LT. Barrett's esophagus in children with cystic fibrosis: not a coincidental association. *Am J Gastroenterol* 1993;88(11):1934–1938.

80. Stead RJ, Hinks LJ, Hodson ME, et al. Selenium deficiency and possible increased risk of carcinoma in adults with cystic fibrosis. *Lancet* 1985;ii(8460):862–863.

81. Goodchild MC, Nelson R, Anderson CM. Cystic fibrosis and coeliac disease: coexistence in two children. *Arch Dis Child* 1973;48(9):684–691.

82. Taylor B, Sokol G. Cystic fibrosis and coeliac disease: report of two cases. *Arch Dis Child* 1973;48(9):692–696.

83. Weizman Z, Hamilton JR, Kopelman HR, Cleghorn G, Durie PR. Treatment failure in celiac disease due to coexistent exocrine pancreatic insufficiency. *Pediatrics* 1987;80(6):924–926.

SECTION IV

Other Systems

Cystic Fibrosis in Adults,
edited by J. R. Yankaskas and M. R. Knowles,
Lippincott–Raven Publishers, Philadelphia, 1999.

16

Pharmacotherapy

Arnold L. Smith, *Morty Cohen, and †Bonnie W. Ramsey

*Department of Molecular Microbiology and Immunology, University of Missouri–Columbia
School of Medicine, Columbia, Missouri; *Children's Hospital and Regional Medical Center;
and †Cystic Fibrosis Research Program, Department of Pediatrics, University of Washington School
of Medicine, Seattle, Washington*

Cystic fibrosis (CF), a disease that affects most epithelial cells in the body, is characterized by multiorgan dysfunction. This disease, caused by one of more than 700 mutations in the cystic fibrosis transmembrane conductance regulator (CFTR) gene, is characterized by loss of cyclic adenosine monophosphate (cAMP)-activated apical and intracellular chloride channels. The most common genotype, ΔF508 homozygosity, also produces an increase in most drug-metabolizing activities; however, detailed studies of other genotypes and drug disposition have not been performed. Studies of many drugs administered to patients with CF have shown that there is a CF-specific increased total body clearance and increased distribution volume. This increased clearance may be the result of increased activity of specific hepatic drug-metabolizing enzymes (such as with acetaminophen or trimethoprim) or increased renal clearance of drugs believed not to be metabolized (such as the aminoglycosides). The increased volume of distribution may be a reflection of an increased proposition of lean body mass (1,2). In addition, multiple metabolic pathways (e.g., oxidation, sulfation, acetylation) appear to be increased, whereas others in the same family (i.e., the cytochrome P450s oxidase) are not affected.

The effect of CF on drug metabolism is of paramount importance because the dose must be tailored—usually increased—specifically for individuals with this disease. In the absence of dosage modification, the administration of conventional doses to patients with CF leads to inadequate serum concentrations and potential loss of efficacy.

Multiple pharmaceutical products are administered to patients with CF for treatment of the primary manifestations of the disease. This includes replacement of pancreatic exocrine deficiency by administration of pancreatic extracts, which provides active proteases and lipases for digestion of foods.

Most commonly, drugs are administered to patients with CF not for the primary chloride secretory lesion but for disease complications. The most prominent of these is chronic endobronchial infection. Intraluminal pulmonary infection is the primary cause of morbidity and mortality in patients with CF. Drugs administered for the chronic pulmonary disease currently consist of antibiotics for the intraluminal infection, bronchodilators, and certain antiinflammatory agents (ibuprofen and glucocorticoids). Drugs to treat this complication are administered systemically or by aerosol (e.g., antibiotics and rhDNase)

For gastrointestinal (GI) disease, patients receive digestive enzymes, fat-soluble vitamins, antacids, and medications to decrease the gastric acidity (see Chapter 15). Because the CF pancreas does not secrete an adequate concentration of bicarbonate into the GI lumen, these patients have abdominal discomfort and pain from unbuffered gastric acid. To treat the symptoms, H_2 blockers or omeprazole, as well as antacids and/or sucralfate, are administered.

PHARMACOKINETICS

Basic Concepts

Patients with CF dispose of most xenobiotics (compounds not normally found within the body but biologically active) differently from patients who do not have CF. Despite widespread GI dysfunction, no intrinsic abnormality in the absorption of hydrophilic polar drugs from the GI tract ever has been demonstrated. The amount of unionized drug present in the GI lumen depends on the pKa of the compound and the intraluminal pH. Although there is decreased pancreatic bicarbonate secretion and duodenal injury due to unbuffered gastric acid, it is unlikely that the pH of jejunal and ileal contents is abnormal. Thus, polar xenobiotic absorption is not different from non-CF subjects. However, the amount of drug reaching the systemic circulation after oral administration can be reduced by presystemic metabolism by the bowel epithelium or the liver. Available data suggest that the epithelium of the small bowel might have increased permeability.

Because of the problems in generating lipid micelles in the GI tract (for lipid absorption), lipid-soluble drugs are absorbed poorly. For example, cyclosporine is a lipid-soluble drug whose absorption is decreased in patients with CF. This occurs because micelles, into which cyclosporine normally partitions, are not formed. Without micelles, there is little cyclosporine absorption. In addition, the cyclosporine can partition into the undigested fats and be eliminated in steatorrhea feces.

As might be predicted, there have been no CF-specific differences in absorption of medication after intramuscular administration. No general statement can be made regarding the differences in drug metabolism seen in patients with CF; that is, not every drug has increased metabolic disposition, and even certain drugs metabolized by different isoforms of the same enzyme complex (e.g., the P450 system) (3)

may not have the CF-specific increased metabolism.

Drug clearance and volume of distribution are independent pharmacokinetic parameters (4). The term "clearance" refers to the rate of loss of a drug from the systemic circulation. Its units are the same as those used to express creatinine clearance, that is, milliliters per minute per kilogram of body weight (or normalized to body surface area), and it is called total clearance (Cl_t). The most common clearance term used is "total body clearance," implying that amount of drug cleared from the blood independent of route of elimination. In reality, it is the sum of hepatic clearance and renal clearance. Total body clearance, as commonly used, refers to drugs that are not cleared by the pulmonary tract (e.g., inhalation anesthetics). The volume of distribution (V_d) of a drug reflects the anatomic space occupied by that drug and the relative degree of protein and tissue binding in the blood and the extravascular space. In reality, it is a proportionality constant relating the plasma concentration of drug to the total amount in the body. The volume of distribution only rarely corresponds to a specific anatomic compartment. For example, if a drug was limited completely to the vascular compartment, then its volume of distribution after intravenous administration would equal the blood volume, that is, 8% of the body weight, or the V_d would be 80 mL/kg. The most useful way to express V_d is the proportionality constant when drug equilibration has been reached after repeated dosing, that is, at steady state (Vd_{ss}).

The drug half-life—or more correctly, the elimination half-life—is a dependent variable related to the volume of distribution and clearance by the following relationship: $t_{1/2} = 0.693 \times Vd_{ss} \div Cl$. Half-life is of benefit to the clinician because it provides a useful index of the amount of drug remaining in the body at a given time after dosing. For example, at the cessation of drug administration, four half-lives must occur before the amount of medication in the body will be less than one tenth of the amount in the original dose. This is important because the half-life of the drug can be related to the duration of the clinical effect and used to adjust the frequency of dosing. For example, antibiotics often are readministered when the serum concentration approximates the minimal inhibitory concentration for the target bacterium: this time can be predicted from knowledge of the serum half-life. Differences in serum half-life do not give any insight into CF-specific differences.

To dissect mechanisms of CF-specific differences in drug metabolism, the contribution of specific renal and nonrenal clearance pathways and the Vd_{ss} must be determined. Calculation of the serum half-life does not provide insight into the mechanisms of CF-specific differences because it is not an independent variable. Systemic clearance and the apparent volume of distribution are independent variables.

The "bioavailability" of a drug is the amount that reaches the systemic circulation after administration. Bioavailability usually is expressed as a percentage of the dose and varies with the route of administration, drug stability (in the GI tract after oral administration), and its physical–chemical characteristics. Oral bioavailability is affected not only by drug stability and absorption rate but also by presystemic (mucosal or hepatic) metabolism. CF-specific decreases in oral bioavailability of hydrophilic drugs appear to be the result of increases in drug clearance, that is, the drug is metabolized by the liver, making a certain fraction of the dose available to the systemic circulation.

Pharmacokinetic Changes Seen in Cystic Fibrosis

Volume of Distribution

In general, in patients with CF, there is a slight increase in the volume of distribution, with this increase more marked in patients with more severe disease. Part of the effect of this phenomenon may be in the normalization of the data, that is, as patients become cachectic, dose based on weight will not reflect accurately all the tissues into which the drug distributes. Patients with CF have a larger extracellular space (as measured by bromide distribution) when normalized to body weight. This difference, however, is lost when body surface area is used as the reference (5). In most studies, the volume of distribution at steady state was normalized to body weight or body surface area. The increased volume of distribution in patients with CF is the result of changes in body composition and is similar to that seen in individuals with other chronic diseases associated with wasting. For example, the Vd_{ss} of gentamicin in patients with CF and those undergoing chemotherapy for leukemia are very similar (6).

Clearance

As noted previously, with most drugs, systemic clearance is the result of a combination of renal clearance and hepatic clearance. Renal clearance involves both secretion and filtration of the parent drug and usually more polar metabolites. In patients with CF, renal plasma flow and glomerular filtration rate are at the high end of normal. The increased total body clearance of cefsulodin is solely the result of the increased glomerular filtration rate (GFR) because cefsulodin has no appreciable tubular secretion (7). Increased renal clearance of other weak organic acids (ß-lactams) has been demonstrated. Ticarcillin is one such antibiotic (8). In a controlled study of ticarcillin pharmacokinetics, Wang et al. (8) found that the saturable rate of ticarcillin secretion by the kidney was significantly lower in patients with CF. The measured affinity for tubular secretion (i.e., the pump; similar to Km) was 33.7 ± 12.2 mg/mL for patients with CF, whereas affinity for controls was 77.6 ± 38.4 mg/mL. The maximum tubular rate of ticarcillin secretion (i.e., the V_{max}) was nearly identical in both groups of patients. With an increased GFR, more ticarcillin is delivered to a more avid pump, resulting in increased renal clearance.

Hepatic clearance is caused by biliary secretion and biotransformation and is dependent on the intrinsic capacity of the liver to carry out these functions, the so-called "intrinsic clearance." Using model drugs as probes of specific elimination pathways, Kearns et al. (9) found that glucuronyltransferase activity was increased as measured by lorazepam clearance, twice the value found in non-CF subjects. In the same study, they found that the biliary secretory capacity, as assessed by measurement of indocyanine green (ICG) clearance, was increased fivefold (8). For drugs that have low intrinsic clearance, their metabolism by liver could be limited by decreased hepatic blood flow. Hepatic blood flow was suspected to be decreased in patients with CF because of the high incidence of subclinical biliary cirrhosis and biliary cholestasis. However, in the studies that have been performed to date, data indicate that hepatic blood flow is normal, if not slightly increased, in individuals with CF (10,11). Hepatic drug metabolism, primarily the intrinsic clearance, is increased with most drugs studied in patients with CF.

Elimination Half-Life (T½)

As a result of the metabolic differences, the elimination half-life of most drugs in patients with CF is shorter. This decrease in half-life is the result of a dramatic increase in total body clearance. In fact, with drugs administered by the oral or intramuscular route with prolonged absorption, the increased total body clearance can "blunt" the serum peak concentration (C_{max}) and drastically shorten the elimination half-life. The decreased C_{max} is of particular importance with antibiotics because efficacy in clinical trials correlates better with that parameter than area under the serum concentration versus time curve (AUC) or the ratio of the AUC to the *in vitro*–determined minimal inhibitory concentration.

Summary

Two major differences in drug disposition by patients with CF affect optimal pharmacotherapy: lower blood concentrations with standard dosing and interpatient differences in drug pharmacokinetics (2). Virtually all drugs are administered safely to patients with CF at doses exceeding those recommended for adults without CF. However, administration of these doses will rarely result in toxic serum concentrations

in the patient with CF. In general, there is no correlation with disease severity and increased total body clearance. Correlations between pharmacokinetic phenotype and a specific CFTR genotype have not been sought. Virtually all studies were done on patients with a clinical diagnosis and abnormal sweat tests. The most prudent course is to monitor serum drug concentrations if it has a low efficacy:toxicity ratio.

SPECIFIC DRUGS

Antibiotics

Antibiotics are, in addition to oral administration of pancreatic extract and vitamins, the most commonly administered drugs to patients with CF. Consequently, they are well studied, with the conclusion that the doses of virtually all antibiotics must exceed those recommended for patients without CF if efficacious but nontoxic serum concentrations are to be achieved.

Orally Administered Antibiotics

Antibiotics, like other drugs, are absorbed passively in their unionized state throughout the small intestine; site-specific absorption has not been demonstrated. Only the uncharged form of the antibiotic is absorbed by diffusion "down" the concentration gradient into the systemic circulation. The amount of an oral dose absorbed into the portal circulation is dependent on the pKa of the antibiotic and the pH of the proximal jejunal contents, with GI transit time minimally affecting absorption because of the large surface area of the small intestinal epithelium available for absorption.

Oral administration of antibiotics usually is used for chronic "suppressive" therapy (Table 16–1). The doses administered usually have been determined empirically, with "clinical improvement" being the commonly sought end point. For orally administered penicillins and cephalosporins, the maximum dose is limited by the GI toxicity. Antibiotics in these classes are weak acids and can cause cramping in the upper GI tract and diarrhea (acid-induced)

TABLE 16–1. *Oral antibiotic administration (suppressive therapy)*

Antibiotic	Dose (mg)	Frequency (hrs)	Comment
Amoxicillin	500	8	Diarrhea at doses > 6 g per day; administered with probenecid
Amoxicillin and clavulanate	875	12	Diarrhea common
Cephalexin	500	6	
Azithromycin[a]	500 then 250	once 24	Aluminum and magnesium antacids decrease absorption not studied in patients with CF
Cefuroxime	500	12	
Cefaclor	500	8	Serum sickness, erythema multiforme occur
Third generation cephalosporin[b]	200	12	Expensive
Ciprofloxacin	750	12[c]	Inhibits theophylline metabolism, analeptic
Chloramphenicol	750	6–8	Hematologic toxicity, monitor blood levels.
Clarithromycin	500	12	Inhibits theophylline metabolism used for atypical mycobacteria
Ofloxacin	400	12	Less studied in CF
Doxycycline	100	12	Can cause hepatotoxicity
Erythromycin	500	8	No *H. influenzae* activity (administer as ethylsuccinate)
TMP/SMX	160/800	12	Can cause erythema multiforme; GI disturbance most common

GI, gastrointestinal; TMP/SMX, trimethoprim/sulfamethoxazole.
[a]Has accumulation kinetics.
[b]Cefpodoxime proxetil is depicted.
[c]Occasionally administered three times a day.

when they reach the colon. For adults without CF, ß-lactams administered at oral doses of 6 to 8 g/day will cause diarrhea.

Other less polar or neutral antibiotics, such as the tetracyclines, fluoroquinolones, sulfonamides, and trimethoprim, are well absorbed. As a result, the maximal oral dose for these drugs is limited by their systemic toxicity.

Penicillinase-Resistant Penicillins/Cephalosporins

All cephalosporins are resistant to degradation by the ß-lactamase produced by *Staphylococcus aureus, Haemophilus influenzae,* and most *Pseudomonas aeruginosa* strains. Certain new cephalosporins (e.g., cefixime) have low intrinsic activity against *P. aeruginosa* independent of the isolate's ability to produce ß-lactamase. Harrison et al. (12) compared dicloxacillin versus cephalexin administered as an oral suspension to children. The total daily dose of each agent was 90 mg/kg, and it was administered with meals. Cephalexin was better tolerated and had fewer GI side effects during the 2-month study. The

mean peak cephalexin concentration at this dose was 27 mg/L, a value expected to be effective against all strains of *Staph. aureus* (except methicillin-resistant strains) and a small percentage of *H. influenzae* strains.

One study (13) reported that there were no CF-specific differences in the pharmacokinetics of cephalexin, cefaclor, and cefadroxil after oral administration. Cefuroxime axetil has modest activity against *Staph. aureus* and *H. influenzae*. It is a second-generation cephalosporin which, via the axetil ester, has increased absorption after oral administration. Cefaclor is minimally better than cephalexin against the same spectrum of bacteria: *Staph. aureus* and *H. influenzae*. With repeated administration of cefaclor, an erythema multiforme–like rash has occurred, and rare patients have developed Stevens-Johnson syndrome.

There are three third-generation cephalosporins that are absorbed modestly after oral administration—ceftibuten, cefpodoxime, and cefixime—and all are available on the market. These antibiotics are active against *Streptococcus pneumoniae, S. pyogenes, H. influenzae,* and

Klebsiella species. They have markedly reduced activity against *Staph. aureus*. Because of their cost and poor activity against *P. aeruginosa*, they have not found wide use in the treatment of pulmonary infections in patients with CF.

Amoxicillin

Amoxicillin is administered to patients with CF, usually those with mild disease, and those culturing *H. influenzae* from their sputum. Amoxicillin is a hydroxylated form of ampicillin, which is better absorbed orally and has an identical antibacterial spectrum.

Peterson et al. (14) administered an average total daily dose of 1.8 g of amoxicillin to patients with CF whose sputum had ampicillin-susceptible *H. influenzae*. This total daily dose was administered in three divided doses and coadministered with probenecid, the latter in doses ranging from 500 to 750 mg per day. The duration of the therapy for patients with pulmonary exacerbation was 2 weeks. In this study, the dose of amoxicillin was compared with pivampicillin. All patients had a detectable response to both therapies between days 3 and 4 of administration, and all had the maximal response by day 10. The magnitude of the improvement in pulmonary function was equivalent with each agent; however, 13% of the patients receiving pivampicillin reported nausea versus only 2% of those receiving amoxicillin. Pivampicillin and bacampicillin are esters of ampicillin that have been designed to increase absorption after oral administration; neither has found widespread commercial acceptance.

Pivampicillin was used as treatment for children with CF with *H. influenzae* bronchitis and compared with amoxicillin. In that study, pivampicillin administration was associated with more treatment failures and more nausea, but there was a lower prevalence of ß-lactamase producing strains at the end of therapy (14).

Augmentin

Amoxicillin formulated in a fixed combination with a ß-lactamase inhibitor (clavulanic acid, Augmentin) commonly is administered to patients whose sputum cultures *H. influenzae*

and *Staph. aureus*, or for *H. influenzae* if they produce ß-lactamase. Virtually all clinical isolates of *Staph. aureus* produce ß-lactamase and approximately one half of the sputum *H. influenzae* produce the enzyme. Currently, there are no reports of the study of the bioavailability or the pharmacokinetics of this drug in patients with CF. Diarrhea is common (approximately 10% of all Augmentin recipients under study conditions) with this agent, a fact that seriously curtails its widespread use in patients with CF.

Penicillins G and V

Penicillins G and V are rarely administered to patients with CF because of the lack of activity against the pathogens commonly infecting these patients. The bioavailability of penicillins G and V is inversely proportional to the gastric emptying time. Although penicillin V is more "acid stable" than penicillin G, the bioavailability of each can be decreased by a slow gastric emptying time, permitting inactivation in the stomach. Factors that slow the gastric emptying time are concomitant administration of fatty meals or the recumbent position. If penicillin G or V is indicated in a patient with CF, remember that intraduodenal administration produces serum concentration almost equivalent to intramuscular administration of the same dose (15). Because many patients with CF have indwelling intraduodenal or intrajejunal tubes for nutritional supplementation, this route can be used, avoiding intravenous or intramuscular administration and achieving high serum concentrations.

Macrolides

Erythromycin has good activity against *Staph. aureus* but poor *in vitro* activity against *H. influenzae*, *P. aeruginosa*, and the other gram-negative bacteria found in the sputum of patients with CF. In Asia, macrolides such as erythromycin have been used with apparent efficacy for bronchitis due to *P. aeruginosa*. However, in the United States, because of macrolides' lack of *in vitro* activity against *P. aeruginosa*, no data on macrolide utility in CF are available. Thus, they have limited usefulness in this patient population. A new antibiotic, clarithromycin, is active against penicillin-susceptible and methicillin-susceptible *Staph. aureus*. It also has some activity against *S. pneumoniae* and *H. influenzae*. Data on its efficacy in patients with CF are not available. Clarithromycin inhibits the metabolism of theophylline; thus, serum levels of this drug need to be monitored while the patient is receiving this antibiotic. Clarithromycin has some effectiveness (in combination with other drugs) in non-CF patients with pulmonary infection due to nontuberculous mycobacteria (NTM). It may find a similar utility in subjects with CF with NTM infections (see Chapter 7).

Azithromycin is a macrolide with an extremely long half-life. It is active against *H. influenzae*, *Staph. aureus*, and *S. pneumoniae*. It may prevent the metabolism of theophylline and triazolam; thus, it needs to be used cautiously in patients receiving these drugs. It has unusual accumulation pharmacokinetics because after a loading dose of 500 mg, 2 to 5 days of 250 mg once daily provides therapeutic tissue concentrations against the aforementioned pathogens for approximately 10 days. Neither clarithromycin nor azithromycin have been studied rigorously in patients with CF.

Fluoroquinolones

All fluoroquinolones have analeptic properties and variably inhibit hepatic P450 activity. Thus, these antibiotics should be used with caution in patients receiving drugs metabolized by that enzyme system; the most common drug interaction in patients with CF is theophylline. Ciprofloxacin is well absorbed orally in subjects with CF and is active against *P. aeruginosa* (16,17). It is the most extensively studied fluoroquinolone in patients with CF, and oral administration is equivalent to intravenous ceftazidime and tobramycin in the treatment of a pulmonary exacerbation (18). It also has been administered as "maintenance therapy."

Ciprofloxacin's action in patients with pulmonary exacerbation appears distinct from other antibiotics in several ways (19). Often, there is no change in the sputum *P. aeruginosa* density, but an improvement in pulmonary function. Another paradoxical effect is the eradication of *P. aeruginosa* from sputum, with organisms undetectable as long as 6 weeks later. However, this was associated with minimal (or no) improvement in pulmonary function (20).

Enthusiasm for the use of fluoroquinolones in patients with CF is dampened by the rapid emergency of resistance (21). However, the mechanism of fluoroquinolone resistance in *P. aeruginosa* (particularly with ciprofloxacin) and its clinical relevance is not clear. Mutants with high-level resistance can be selected in the laboratory in a single step. The DNA gyrase in these mutants no longer is susceptible to inhibition by ciprofloxacin concentrations that are toxic to humans (22). *P. aeruginosa* isolated from patients with CF after ciprofloxacin treatment appear commonly to possess another mechanism. After a course of ciprofloxacin administration, the isolate had decreased susceptibility (defined according to standard laboratory criteria) to that antibiotic. Subsequently, after several months, the same *P. aeruginosa* was scored again as susceptible to ciprofloxacin (23). The mechanism of this transient "adaptive" resistance is not known, but there is an indication that combination therapy (e.g., a fluoroquinolone and a ß-lactam) will mitigate the emergence of this novel resistance.

Ofloxacin and pefloxacin are less well studied in patients with CF but appear to have similar efficacy (24,25). Other fluoroquinolones, such as enoxacin, norfloxacin, and lomefloxacin, are absorbed orally and have activity against *P. aeruginosa* but have not been studied in patients with CF.

Sulfa Antibiotics

Trimethoprim-sulfamethoxazole is used commonly as a suppressive agent in patients independent of the susceptibility of the bacteria isolated from sputum. It is eliminated from the blood of patients with CF at an increased rate (26). As a result, increasing the dose or giving the same dose more often has been suggested (27). It is active against *Staph. aureus* and *H. influenzae*, although all *P. aeruginosa* are scored as intrinsically resistant based on standard clinical bacteriologic criteria. Approximately one half of *Burkholderia cepacia* are susceptible.

Chloramphenicol

Chloramphenicol is active against *H. influenzae* and *Staph. aureus*. A very small fraction of *P. aeruginosa* strains are susceptible to chloramphenicol. Chloramphenicol has wide patient-to-patient differences in metabolism and disposition. As a result, the same dose in patients who are the same age, size, and gender can yield vastly different C_{max} and AUC values. Thus, chloramphenicol serum concentration should be monitored, or the patient should have the hematologic indices regularly monitored for toxicity when this antibiotic is administered. Chloramphenicol appears to be efficacious in patients whose sputum cultures grow primarily *P. aeruginosa* even though they will score as resistant to that antibiotic on *in vitro* testing. The mechanism of this benefit is not clear, but it may be the result of the effects of chloramphenicol on virulence factor production in *P. aeruginosa* or the ability of chloramphenicol to act as an immunosuppressive agent. As noted previously, approximately one half of *B. cepacia* strains are susceptible to chloramphenicol. When given orally, chloramphenicol should be administered in capsule form because the absorption of active drug after the administration of the suspension (which is an inactive palmitate ester) is dependent on pancreatic lipase present in the small bowel lumen (28). Administering pancreatic extract along with chloramphenicol palmitate minimally improves the bioavailability (28).

Chloramphenicol capsules (containing the crystalline antibiotic) are available through the Cystic Fibrosis Foundation pharmacy via a "compassionate-use" protocol.

Parenteral Antibiotics

Antibiotics are administered intravenously to patients with CF primarily for the treatment of a pulmonary exacerbation (Table 16–2). In some centers in Denmark, patients receive a course of intravenous antibiotics at regular fixed intervals as suppressive therapy. The intravenous antibiotics administered for a pulmonary exacerbation usually consist of a ß-lactam and an aminoglycoside. There is wide variation in physician choice of antibiotics for an exacerbation both in the United Kingdom and in the United States. Most commonly, the regimen consists of a ß-lactam active against *P. aeruginosa* (ceftazidime or ticarcillin) plus an aminoglycoside possessing similar activity (such as tobramycin or amikacin).

β-lactams

The ß-lactams used for *P. aeruginosa* infection consist of carbenicillin or ticarcillin, or one of the ureidoacylpenicillins (piperacillin or mezlocillin). There are no data directly comparing the treatment of a pulmonary exacerbation in a patient with CF with one of these ß-lactams versus another. In the laboratory, piperacillin is the most potent ureidoacylpenicillin against *P. aeruginosa* in comparison to the other compounds (29). One factor against routine use of piperacillin is the relatively high incidence of allergic reactions (skin rash or fever) with the drug. In one review, 11 of 31 patients with CF had allergic reactions after piperacillin administration (30). Allergic reactions were least frequent with cephalosporins; 0 of 24 patients treated with cefazolin and 1 of 35 patients treated with ceftazidime (30). Ticarcillin also is available as a fixed combination with clavulanic acid (Timentin, Smith Kline Beecham Pharmaceuticals, Pittsburgh, PA), with the combination having activity against *P. aeruginosa* and *Staph. aureus*. Piperacillin also is available in a fixed combination with tazobactam (a ß-lactamase inhibitor) (available as Zosyn, Lederle Laboratories, Pearl River, NY), which has activity against carbenicillin- and ticarcillin-resistant *P. aeruginosa*. If *Staph. aureus* alone is cultured from sputum, one of the isoxazolyl penicillins commonly is administered (nafcillin, methicillin, or oxacillin). Of these antibiotics, nafcillin is most potent *in vitro* against *Staph. aureus*. This antibiotic must be administered parenterally because the oral bioavailability is low because of first-pass hepatic metabolism. Dilution of the nafcillin in the intravenous in-

TABLE 16–2. *Antibiotic administration for pulmonary exacerbations*

Bacteria in sputum	Antibiotic				
	Drug	Dose (mg)	Route	Frequency (hrs)	Comment
Staph. aureus and	Nafcillin	2000	IV	6	Dilute to < 20 mg/ml for infusion
H. influenzae	Tobramycin	3 mg/kg	IV	8	Has been administered once daily
Staph. aureus	Cefazolin	1000	IV	8	
Staph. aureus (Meth)	Vancomycin	1000	IV	12	Duration of infusion should be > 60 min
Staph. aureus and	Tobramycin	160	IV	8	Do not mix with other drugs
P. aeruginosa	Ceftazidime	2000	IV	8	Infuse over 5 min
or	Ticarcillin-clavulanate	3000	IV	6	Can induce platelet dysfunction
or	Imipenem-cilastatin	500 to 1000	IV	6	Doses > 4 gm associated with nausea and vomiting
or	Piperacillin	4000	IV	6	
or	Aztreonam	2000	IV	8	Major indication is penicillin allergy
P. aeruginosa (alone)	β-lactam listed above and appropriate aminoglycoside				
or	Ciprofloxacin	400	IV	12	Interferes with theophylline metabolism
B. cepacia	TMP/SMX	5 mg/kg[a]	IV	6	Can cause nephrotoxicity
	Chloramphenicol	15 mg/kg	IV	6	Monitor serum levels

IM, intramuscular; IV, intravenous; TMP/SMX, trimethoprim/sulfamethoxazole.
[a]Based on TMP.

fusion solution to less than 20 mg/mL and increasing the duration of infusion to at least 1 hour minimizes drug-associated phlebitis.

Two carbapenems have been used for the treatment of *P. aeruginosa* infection in patients with CF: imipenem and meropenem. Imipenem is metabolized rapidly by renal peptidase, necessitating its coadministration with an inhibitor of that enzyme (cilastatin). In addition, imipenem is very labile, requiring administration shortly after dissolution. In some patients, it causes nausea and vomiting, presumably by an effect on the central nervous system (CNS); some seizures have occurred with high intravenous dosages (31). Additionally, it appears to select for resistant *P. aeruginosa*, particularly when administered at lower doses.

Meropenem has a broader spectrum of activity and is not metabolized by renal dipeptidases. There is only limited experience of the use of meropenem in patients with CF (32,33). Meropenem has the additional advantage in that it has activity against many *B. cepacia* strains and *P. aeruginosa*.

A monobactam (aztreonam) also has been used for the treatment of pulmonary infection due to *P. aeruginosa* in patients with CF (34). The main indication for this antibiotic is administration to those patients who are allergic to cephalosporins or penicillins. There is no cross-allergy between aztreonam and the currently available ß-lactams; clinical efficacy appears equivalent to ticarcillin if both are administered in combination with an aminoglycoside.

Cephalosporins

Antibiotics in this class were not considered initially for patients with CF because of the poor activity of the early drugs against *P. aeruginosa*. Certain derivatives, so-called third-generation cephalosporins have good activity against *P. aeruginosa*; cefoperazone, ceftazidime, and cefsulodin all have more activity against *P. aeruginosa* than ticarcillin. Cefsulodin has potency equivalent to gentamicin against most strains of *P. aeruginosa*, but it is not marketed in the United States. Cefoperazone has been

studied in patients with CF and was found to select for cefoperazone-resistant isolates (35).
This property, along with its propensity to induce hypoprothrombinemic coagulopathy (reversible by vitamin K administration), has discouraged its use in patients with CF.

Ceftazidime has been used extensively in
patients with CF. Patients with CF have "super-
normal" GFRs and because ceftazidime is
cleared almost exclusively by filtration, its total body clearance is increased in CF (7). As a
result, doses at the upper end of those recommended for non-CF patients are used. Ceftazidime is synergistic *in vitro* with tobramycin
and ofloxacin or ciprofloxacin (36,37), an observation also noted in experimental infections.
It is not known whether such synergism will be
observed with combination therapy of pulmonary exacerbations due to *P. aeruginosa* in
patients with CF. Because ceftazidime and
ciprofloxacin often are coadministered, the
physician should be aware that crystallization
of ciprofloxacin in the kidney (due to alkaline
urine) can cause oliguric renal failure. In that
situation, ceftazidime can accumulate and produce seizures. Ceftazidime-associated seizures
have been reported in patients who do not have
CF (38). It is not known whether the analeptic
properties of ciprofloxacin will potentiate ceftazidime neurotoxicity.

Aminoglycosides

Many aminoglycosides have been administered to patients with CF. The dosage requirements are higher for antibiotics of this class because of increased nonrenal elimination (39).
All aminoglycosides have potential renal toxicity, which is reversible as well as irreversible
ototoxicity. The latter, in which there is damage
to the vestibular apparatus or the cochlea, is not
reversible, and its occurrence correlates with cumulative aminoglycoside administration. Auditory acuity at the higher frequencies (> 20,000
Hz; conversation is 6,000 to 10,000 Hz) is affected first, and loss of acuity often is not no-
ticed by the patient (40). Because most patients
with CF are likely to receive multiple courses of
aminoglycoside, tobramycin is preferred for this
patient population because it has slightly less

auditory toxicity in high-risk patients. Gentamicin, amikacin, netilmicin, and sisomicin have
been administered independently to patients
with CF with outcome results not significantly
different those observed with tobramycin. There
have been no parallel comparisons seeking to
determine whether one aminoglycoside has
greater efficacy or less toxicity compared with
another.

During a dosing interval, aminoglycosides
have adverse effects on bacteria after the concentration has decreased below the level at
which antibacterial activity usually is not present. This phenomenon is called the postantibi-
otic effect (PAE) and is seen with most aminoglycosides and gram-negative pathogens (41).
PAE is significant because aminoglycosides
can be administered as a single daily dose because toxicity is dependent on the aminoglycoside being present for an extended period of
time (42). Single daily administration takes advantage of aminoglycoside's PAE while decreasing the likelihood of toxicity because of
the long drug-free interval. Tobramycin was
administered as a single daily dose, at 10 ± 0.4
mg/kg (313 ± 12 mg/M^2), to produce a mean
serum tobramycin concentration of 4 mg/mL
(43). The maximum serum tobramycin concentration was up to 64 mg/L after a 60-minute infusion of the total daily dose in 52 patients with
CF (43). Clinical end points of efficacy were
not different from standard regimens, and there
was no detectable auditory toxicity or nephrotoxicity (43). A recent meta-analysis confirmed
this observation for all aminoglycosides in patients who do not have CF (44)

Cationic Peptide Antibiotics

Colistin and polymyxin have been reserved
almost exclusively for administration via the
aerosol route (see below). However, colistin
has been administered intravenously to older
patients infected with *P. aeruginosa* strains that
were resistant to multiple antibiotics. In these
studies, approximately one third of the patients
have significant neurotoxicity (perioral pares-
thesia or ataxia), with clinical efficacy equivalent to standard regimens for susceptible organisms (45).

Vancomycin

Infection with methicillin-resistant *Staph. aureus* is the primary indication for the administration of vancomycin. This drug has the ability to cause systemic release of histamine, which can result in flushing (the "Red Man" syndrome), nausea, fainting, and itching. These episodes often cause the patient to be erroneously labeled as allergic to vancomycin. Increasing the duration of infusion for more than 60 minutes, premedicating the patient with an antihistamine (such as hydroxyzine pamoate), or both controls this adverse event.

Vancomycin is unique among the antibiotics administered to patients with CF because its disposition is unaltered by the disease. In healthy volunteers, vancomycin is eliminated primarily by glomerular filtration, with the renal clearance being 80% of the creatinine clearance. A recent study of 10 adult patients (46) found that the pharmacokinetics virtually were identical to previously reported healthy volunteers (47). This means that the usual dosage of 15 mg/kg every 8 to 12 hours in patients with normal renal function will produce adequate serum concentrations.

The topic of antibiotic therapy in patients with CF recently has been reviewed (48).

Aerosolized Antibiotics

Direct delivery of aerosol antibiotics to the lower respiratory tract has been used in patients with CF with variable enthusiasm for several years. One reason for the variability was the lack of efficacy in some clinical trials. Efficacy is dependent on delivery of an adequate amount of antibiotic to the medium and small airways. Recognition that generation of a small-particle aerosol is dependent on the nebulizer, the antibiotic being aerosolized (49), and its concentration led to "high-dose" antibiotic aerosol administration (50). In reality, the dose to the lower respiratory tract averages 12 mg, but a large amount of medication (300 to 600 mg) must be placed in the nebulizer because of the inherent inefficiency of such devices. This amount of antibiotic is necessary to overcome sputum binding and antagonism of antibiotic activity. In a taste-masked, placebo-controlled, cross-over study of 71 patients with CF not experiencing an exacerbation, aerosol tobramycin administration improved mean forced expiratory volume in 1 second (FEV_1) and forced vital capacity (FVC) by 9.7% and 6.2%, respectively (50). The rate of emergence of tobramycin resistance in *P. aeruginosa* and the appearance of intrinsically tobramycin-resistant organisms (such as *B. cepacia*) were no different during or after placebo or tobramycin administration. Systemic absorption of aerosolized tobramycin is low, resulting in undetectable auditory toxicity and nephrotoxicity (50). Newer jet nebulizers can generate an aerosol that mimics that produced by older ultrasonic devices (49). Some of these newer devices can produce sputum concentrations (51) predicted to be efficacious from prior studies.

A placebo-controlled parallel study of the efficacy of aerosolized tobramycin was conducted in 520 patients. One half received 300 mg of drug, delivered by a PARI LC+ jet (PARI Respiratory Equipment, Inc., Richmond, VA) with standard PulmoAid (DeVilbiss, Somerset, PA) compressor twice daily, while the other half received a taste-masked placebo. Tobramycin was administered for 28 consecutive days with the succeeding 28 days being "off" drug. Three "on-off" cycles were studied for a total of 24 weeks, when the patients were again evaluated. At the end of treatment, the patients in the tobramycin treatment had a average FEV_1 10% better than baseline, while in the placebo group the average FEV_1 had declined 2% compared to enrollment values. Patients in the tobramycin group were 26% less likely to be hospitalized and 36% less likely to be treated with intravenous antipseu-domonal antibiotics than the placebo group. Voice alteration and tinnitus were more common in the tobramycin group, but there was no detectable systemic aminoglycoside toxicity. The frequency of tobramycin-resistant *P. aeruginosa* increased in the tobramycin group and decreased in the placebo group during the six-month trial. However, there was no relationship between development of tobramycin resistance and response to aerosolized tobramycin. Future trials will clarify the relationship between the degree of susceptibility of the

P. aeruginosa to tobramycin and the response to aerosol administration.

Colistin, a peptide antibiotic in the polymyxin family, has been aerosolized to patients with CF as a means of suppressing *P. aeruginosa* colonization and infection. Current commercially available formulations contain 50% antibiotic and are in the form of an inactive prodrug (methane sulfonate) that must be hydrolyzed to yield active antibiotic. Colistin also is a surface-active agent (49), predisposing it to foaming in the nebulizer. Many *ad hoc* manipulations are used to permit aerosolization. However, several of these manipulations (e.g., heating, adding ethanol) would be expected to inactivate or precipitate the antibiotic. Despite these caveats, aerosol colistin/polymyxin has shown efficacy in several trials. These recently have been summarized (52).

Antibiotic Resistance

Standard laboratory criteria (National Committee for Clinical Laboratory Standards) defining antibiotic susceptibility and resistance are devised for the treatment of non-CF patients with a tissue infection. With *P. aeruginosa*, susceptibility testing is to aid the physician in antibiotic selection, often for seriously ill, immunocompromised individuals with bacteremia. Such *P. aeruginosa* strains often are nosocomial and have markedly different phenotypic properties in comparison with *P. aeruginosa* isolated from patients with CF. Recognizing these facts, it is not surprising that clinicians caring for patients with CF use antibiotic susceptibility testing as a supplement to their clinical judgment: if the patient is improving on a specific antibiotic combination and the laboratory has scored the sputum isolates as susceptible to that combination, then the laboratory results are noted. If, however, the laboratory has scored the same isolates resistant to both antibiotics in the combination, then the results are discounted. Derivation of methods specific for testing of *P. aeruginosa* isolated from CF sputum will place antibiotic selection on a firmer base. In the event that the patient does not respond to the maximum doses of an antibiotic combination and the laboratory has designated the *P. aeruginosa* strain as resistant to all drugs in that class (e.g.,

ticarcillin and tobramycin), then synergy testing with other antibiotics is of value because the resistance to one class may not extend to a closely related class (e.g., aztreonam and meropenem) (53). Testing such isolates against multiple combinations of antibiotics has demonstrated synergy in 30% to 70% of the isolates (54,55). These combinations should include antibiotics not considered normally for therapy for infections due to *P. aeruginosa* (rifampin, for example) (56).

Summary

Antibiotics are the primary drug class administered to patients with CF. In general, more medication is administered at more frequent intervals to mimic the serum concentration versus time curve that is efficacious in non-CF subjects with a variety of infections. A higher dosage used for patients with CF is followed, whether the antibiotics are administered prophylactically or in the treatment of a pulmonary exacerbation. The clinical relevance of antibiotic resistance in *P. aeruginosa* isolated from patients with CF is uncertain. Aerosol antibiotic administration is efficacious because delivery of large amounts of medication exceeds the bacterial resistance threshold and overcomes sputum antagonism.

Bronchodilators

Bronchodilators commonly are administered to patients with CF. It has been estimated that one fourth of all patients with this disease have bronchial reactivity and will have improved lung function after bronchodilator administration. In addition, it has been suggested that bronchodilation will increase the efficacy of chest percussion and postural drainage in patients without reactive airway disease. Data documenting this adjunctive usage are not consistent.

ß-Adrenergic Agonists

The use of ß-adrenergic agonists in CF is controversial because all studies have not shown a consistent benefit. In one study, 127 patients received isoproterenol from a metered-dose inhaler, with the desired dose being 340 μg per inhalation. These patients were followed for 8 years, and a positive response was defined as a 15% change in FEV_1, a 20% change in $FEF_{25\%-75\%}$, or a 20% change in $FEF_{50\%}$. During the study, 40% of the patients were found to have at least one positive response in the 573 pulmonary function tests that were performed (57). In a smaller study, 180 μg of albuterol was administered by a metered-dose inhaler to 11 patients with CF, 11 asthmatic patients, and 11 controls (57). All the patients with CF had a beneficial response based on pulmonary function testing with the magnitude of the bronchodilatation occurring in patients with CF less than that observed in asthmatic patients, but greater than that seen in controls (58).

Theophylline

Administration of theophylline to patients with CF is attractive because it has the ability to increase bronchodilatation and increase mucociliary clearance. It is clear that for theophylline to be used in patients with CF, the serum concentrations must be adjusted. This has not been done in all of the studies of efficacy. For example, in one study in which patients were given 30 mg/kg/day in three divided doses or placebo for a 4-week period, only 1 patient had a consistent improvement and 10 patients had severe adverse effects from the theophylline: headaches, vomiting, nausea. However, the randomly obtained serum theophylline concentrations ranged from 5.6 to 33 mg/L and could not be correlated with any effect or forced expiratory flow rate (58). Workers in Montreal showed that in patients with CF, the total body theophylline clearance was 75 mg/kg per hour in comparison with non-CF controls in which it was 35 mg/kg per hour (59). In addition, the volume of distribution was significantly higher in patients with CF. In controls, it was 444 mL/kg whereas in the patients with CF, it was 590 mL/kg. Most importantly this study demonstrated marked intersubject variability among the patients with CF. Thus, most patients with CF will require larger doses adminis-

tered more often, but serum concentrations must be measured because of the patient-to-patient variability in theophylline disposition.

Antiinflammatory Drugs

Accumulating data suggests that older patients with CF and chronic endobronchial infection have a significant portion of disease dependent on inflammation elicited by the host response to the chronic infection. Recognition of this mechanism in the pathogenesis prompted studies of antiinflammatory drugs in patients with CF.

Glucocorticoids

Glucocorticoids or corticosteroids are very potent antiinflammatory agents. They inhibit the activation and chemotaxis of leukocytes and the synthesis of proinflammatory cytokines. In addition, glucocorticoids decrease mucous secretion and edema of epithelia. In a 4-year, double-blind, placebo-controlled study of patients between 1 and 12 years of age with mild to moderate lung disease, workers in Boston found that patients who received an alternate-date prednisone (at a dose of 2 mg/kg) had better pulmonary function and body weight and fewer hospitalizations (60). No serious side effects were uncovered during this study of 45 patients. Follow-up evaluation of 14 of 17 patients in the original study for an additional 6 years noted growth retardation and glucose intolerance as well as osteoporosis and cataracts. In a large trial sponsored by the Cystic Fibrosis Foundation, 285 patients between 6 and 14 years of age with the disease of the same severity were randomized to placebo, low-dose prednisone (1 mg/kg) or high-dose prednisone (2 mg/kg); all medications were administered on alternate days. Growth retardation, glucose intolerance, and cataracts (a cumulative incidence of 30%) prompted early termination of the high-dose arm. Patients receiving the low-dose prednisone had a better pulmonary function (FEV_1) during the 48 months of study compared with those receiving placebo. However, the beneficial effect was seen within the first 6 months after administration and thereafter reached a plateau. In the same 48-month period, the mean percent predicted FEV_1 in the placebo group decreased from 79% to 74%, a difference that was statistically significant. In the low-dose prednisone group, the FVC on enrollment and the 48 months was not significantly different: 84% versus 83% predicted (62). Also, in the low-dose prednisone group in whom the FVC was better, the beneficial effect was seen only in those culturing *P. aeruginosa* from sputum. Because of the growth retardation in the 1 mg/kg prednisone group, it was concluded that if glucocorticoids are administered to patients with CF, it should be done only for short periods of time (6 months), with reevaluation to determine potential benefit. A study more appropriate to adults was a 12-week comparison of prednisolone at 2 mg/kg every day for 2 weeks, tapered to 1 mg/kg on alternate days for an additional 10 weeks. Compared with the placebo group, the prednisolone-treated group had better pulmonary functions (FVC and FEV_1) (63). Despite these ongoing studies of glucocorticoids in patients with CF, there has been limited study of the pharmacokinetics of these drugs in patients with CF.

When the pharmacokinetics of prednisolone were compared in eight patients with CF versus eight asthmatic controls, it was found that the total body clearance and the V_d both were increased (60% and 46%, respectively) (64). The increased V_d has been suggested to be a reflection of increased tissue binding—a possible explanation for the increased frequency of adverse events seen in the aforementioned trial. Another study in a 16-year-old girl with CF demonstrated normal absorption of methylprednisolone, but a markedly increased metabolic clearance (65). With increased glucocorticoid metabolism, one might suspect that there would be increased metabolic clearance of contraceptive steroids. However, when this was studied in six women with CF, the increased clearance was counterbalanced by increased absorption (66). The net effect was that the AUC was equivalent to that found in non-CF women.

Ibuprofen

Ibuprofen is well absorbed from the GI tract of healthy individuals and eliminated primarily by oxidative metabolism with less than 1% excreted unchanged. Konstan and coworkers (67) examined ibuprofen pharmacokinetics in children with CF and compared it with controls. Their data indicated that the systemic bioavailability was greater than 70% in both patients and controls, consistent with other data on drug absorption. As with other drugs, the total body clearance was increased, as was the apparent volume of distribution. Both of these mechanisms produced a significant decrease in the maximum serum concentration (67). Drug concentration is important in the antiinflammatory effects of ibuprofen. With concentrations less than 35 mg/L, it is markedly antiinflammatory, inhibiting neutrophil migration and degranulation at the infectious focus. In addition, it interferes with the production of neutrophil-derived proinflammatory mediators such as leukotriene B_4 (LTB_4). Concentrations less than 25 mg/L are not only not antiinflammatory, but they may augment the inflammatory process. The Cleveland group then sought to administer ibuprofen to patients with CF to achieve a peak serum concentration between 50 and 100 mg/L. This was achieved with a dose between 20 and 30 mg/kg (68). Using this dose in a 4-year, double-blind, placebo-controlled trial, 85 patients were observed serially. They found that in the youngest age group (5 to 13 years), the rate of loss of pulmonary function (as measured by the FEV_1) was slower for the ibuprofen-treated patients versus controls (68). This beneficial effect also was seen in the percent-predicted FVC but was not as dramatic as the FEV_1.

Acetaminophen

Acetaminophen has antipyretic, analgesic, and weak antiinflammatory properties. It is a weak antiinflammatory agent because it inhibits cyclooxygenase but only at concentrations that are toxic. It commonly is administered to patients with CF for mild analgesia (such as that occurring with chronic sinusitis).

It is well absorbed in patients with CF and eliminated almost exclusively by hepatic metabolism. It is cleared from the body at a 50% greater rate because of the formation of the sulfate metabolite, usually 25% of the dose, and a marked increase in the formation of the acetaminophen glucuronide, usually 50% of the dose (69). Because of the increased disposition, the dose of acetaminophen should be increased in patients with CF to approximately 650 mg every 4 to 6 hours to obtain a therapeutic effect.

Miscellaneous

Cyclosporine

Lung transplantation is being performed increasingly in patients with CF. Immunosuppressant therapy after transplantation often consists of an antiinflammatory glucocorticoid, azathioprine, and cyclosporine. Early studies performed after lung transplant indicated that in comparison with non-CF subjects, the cyclosporine absorption was reduced markedly: a bioavailability of 10% for subjects with CF versus 30% in the non-CF subjects (70,71). Thus, to achieve effective whole-blood concentrations of 300 to 600 ng/mL, the cyclosporine dose had to be increased to as much as 30 mg/kg. Cyclosporine is a hydrophobic antibiotic; it is absorbed by micelles, and, as noted above, micelle absorption is impaired in subjects with CF. A newer formulation in lipid microspheres (Neoral, Sandoz Pharmaceuticals Corp., East Hanover, NJ) markedly increases cyclosporine absorption (72). At a dose of 16 mg/kg, the AUC was increased 2.5-fold and the maximum serum concentration increased 2.7-fold. Thus, the lipid-encapsulated formulation significantly improves the oral bioavailability of cyclosporine in the patients with CF. Because of the increased metabolic transformation of this drug, monitoring of serum concentrations is necessary to ensure a therapeutic effect.

An alternative mean of achieving therapeutic serum concentrations is to inhibit hepatic metabolism by coadministration of ketoconazole. The latter antifungal agent is a potent inhibitor of cytochrome P-450, the major elimination pathway, and often is administered prophylactically to transplant patients to minimize the risk of fungal infection. Standard doses of ketoconazole, 200 mg/day, may permit ready achievement of therapeutic cyclosporine concentrations (73,74). If this approach is to be used, it must be kept in mind that ketoconazole also inhibits the metabolism of calcitriol, bile acids, and steroid hormones (75). Administration of another inhibitor of hepatic drug metabolism, such as a fluoroquinolone antibacterial (e.g., norfloxacin), along with ketoconazole, may produce toxic cyclosporine concentrations (76).

Furosemide

This loop diuretic occasionally is administered to patients with CF to treat their congestive right heart failure because adequate oxygen supplementation usually is sufficient. It is well absorbed from the GI tract but has increased total body clearance in patients with CF. The source of this increased clearance is not apparent because the majority of the increased disposition is caused by nonrenal mechanisms. The data available suggest that increased glucuronidation is partly responsible for the clearance, but partial recruitment of another metabolic disposition pathway or route also may be operative. Paradoxically, despite the increased clearance, the effect of the furosemide was greater (as measured by free-water clearance, or rate of Na^+ clearance) in patients with CF (77).

DRUG INTERACTIONS IN CYSTIC FIBROSIS

Very few drug interactions have been studied specifically in the CF population. The information presented in this chapter concern drugs administered to patients with CF, but the clinical observations have been made in the general population. Drug interactions are categorized as pharmacokinetic or pharmacodynamic based on the type of the interaction.

Pharmacokinetic drug interactions occur because of alterations of absorption, distribution (including protein-binding effects), biotransformation, or clearance of one drug by another. An example of a pharmacokinetic drug interaction is the effect of antacids on ketoconazole. The antacid raises the pH of the stomach and duodenum, causing a decrease in ketoconazole absorption. Pharmacodynamic drug interactions are caused by the additive or synergistic effects of two drugs. An example of a pharmacodynamic interaction is the effect of administration of an aminoglycoside and cyclosporine increasing the likelihood of nephrotoxicity.

The most common types of pharmacokinetic drug interactions are those caused by changes in absorption and biotransformation. Both the rate and extent of absorption of oral medications often are affected by pH, the presence of divalent actions, and the GI transit time. Increasing the pH of the fluid in the lumen of the GI tract (by antacids and/or H_2-blocking agents) ionizes a greater amount of weak acids, decreasing their absorption. Sucralfate's chelation of antibiotics also is an example of a drug interaction that affects absorption. Biotransformation reactions are susceptible to inhibition or induction of the hepatic microsomal enzyme systems, causing a slower or faster rate of drug inactivation. See Table 16–3 for a list of commonly used medications by patients with CF that can inhibit drug metabolism and Table

TABLE 16–4. *Agents that can stimulate metabolism of drugs*

Barbiturates
Phenytoin
Carbamazepine
Rifampin
Rifabutin

16–4 for a list of medications that can stimulate metabolism of medications commonly administered to patients with CF.

The likelihood of whether a particular individual will have a drug interaction if they receive two drugs that interact is dependent on several factors. Genetics, dosage of each potentially interacting agent, age of the patient, and the extent of hepatic dysfunction all play a role in determining the magnitude of a drug interaction. For these reasons, there is a large interpatient variability in the drug interaction.

Most interactions caused by induction or inhibition of drug biotransformation are dependent on the dosage of the agent stimulating or inhibiting the metabolism. The mechanism of inhibition of hepatic metabolism usually is one of competitive inhibition. The substrate and the interacting drug are competing for the same binding sites on the metabolizing enzyme; thus, low doses (below a threshold) cause less inhibition of metabolism of a substrate. The role of genetic make-up in affecting the extent of a drug interaction is less clear: the cytochrome P-450 enzymes are products of a superfamily of genes in which differences in the production of individual isoenzyme will have dramatic effects on drug biotransformation. Fast and slow acetylation of isoniazid is a well-known example of genetic differences in biotransformation.

The elderly also have differences in the extent to which they will have a drug interaction. The elderly are less likely to manifest enzyme induction (78): it is not clear at what age the "elderly" phenotype develops in patients with CF. Age has not been shown to be a factor in the extent to which enzyme inhibition is manifested. Hepatic disease also may suppress biotransformation reactions; however, the effect of chronic low-

TABLE 16–3. *Agents that can inhibit metabolism of drugs*

Chloramphenicol
Ciprofloxacin
Cimetidine
Enoxacin
Erythromycin
Fluconazole
Isoniazid
Itraconazole
Ketoconazole
Metronidazole
Miconazole
Omeprazole
Propoxyphene
Trimethoprim/sulfamethoxazole
Verapamil

grade hepatic disease, such as that seen in patients with CF, does not have a predictable effect on the hepatic drug metabolizing ability.

When prescribing or discontinuing a medication that modifies hepatic microsomal enzyme activity, realize that these effects do not start and stop immediately with the first dose. Inhibition of microsomal enzymes begins within 24 hours of administration of the affecting agent, and the medication that is affected will achieve a new pharmacokinetic steady state in approximately three to four half-lives. The onset of enzyme induction takes approximately 1 week and will maximize after 2 to 3 weeks, resulting in a new steady state serum level of the affected drug at that time.

TABLE 16–5. *Drug interactions with drugs used for cystic fibrosis[a]*

Aminoglycosides	
Amphotericin B	Increased nephrotoxicity
Cyclosporine	Increased nephrotoxicity
Miconazole	Decreased peak blood level of aminoglycoside (altered Vd)
Cephalosporins	
Ranitidine	Decreased absorption of cefpodoxime and cefuroxime after oral administration
Quinolones	
Antacids	Decreased absorption if taken at same time
Sucralfate	Decreased absorption of ciprofloxacin and norfloxacin
NSAID-fenbufen + enoxacin	Case reports of seizures
Imipenem/cilastatin	
Gancyclovir	Increased likelihood of seizures (case reports)
Cyclosporine	Increased CNS toxicity—confusion, agitation and tremor
Theophylline	Increased CNS toxicity
Trimethoprim/sulfamethoxazole	
Gancyclovir	Increased toxicity—skin and bone marrow
Erythromycin	
Astemizole	Increased cardiac arrhythmias
Theophylline	Decreased levels of erythromycin
Corticosteroids	
Amphotericin B	Decreased serum potassium
Erythromycin	Decreased clearance of corticosteroids
Ketoconazole	Decreased clearance of corticosteroids
NSAIDs	Increased GI ulceration
Phenytoin	Decreased corticosteroid effect (due to induction of clearance)
NSAIDs	
Corticosteroids	Increased frequency GI ulcers
Cyclosporin	
Aminoglycosides	Increased nephrotoxicity
Amphotericin B	Increased nephrotoxicity
Cimetidine, ranitidine	Increased cyclosporin levels
Erythromycin	Increased cyclosporine levels
Fluconazole	Increased cyclosporin levels (inhibition of metabolism)
Ganciclovir	Increased toxicity (bone marrow, nephrotoxicity)
Imipenem	Increased cyclosporin levels, CNS toxicity, confusion, agitation, and tremor
Itraconazole	Increased cyclosporin levels
Ketoconazole	Increased cyclosporin levels (inhibition of metabolism)
NSAID	Increased serum creatinine and serum potassium; hypertension
Phenytoin	Decreased serum cyclosporin concentration (enzyme induction)
Theophylline	
Quinolones	
Ciprofloxacin and enoxacin	Increased serum levels of theophylline (enzyme inhibition) (flosequinan, lomefloxacin, rufloxacin, ofloxacin, sparfloxacin, and temafloxacin—minor theophylline effect)
Clarithromycin	Increased theophylline levels (20%) (enzyme inhibition)
Erythromycin	Increased theophylline levels (enzyme inhibition)
Cimetidine	Increased theophylline levels (enzyme inhibition)
Phenytoin	Decreased theophylline levels (enzyme induction)
Imipenam/cilastatin	Increased cyclosporin levels

Table continued on following page

TABLE 16–5. *Continued*

Phenytoin	
Chloramphenicol	Increased phenytoin levels (enzyme inhibition)
Ciprofloxacin	Altered phenytoin levels
Cimetidine	Increased phenytoin levels (enzyme inhibition)
Cotrimoxazole	Increased phenytoin levels (enzyme inhibition)
Fluconazole	Increased phenytoin levels (enzyme inhibition)
Ibuprofen	Increased phenytoin levels
Ranitidine	Increased phenytoin levels in some patients
Amphotericin B	
Ganciclovir	Increased toxicity—bone marrow, skin, GI
Aminoglycosides	Increased nephrotoxicity
Cyclosporine	Increased nephrotoxicity
Flucytosine	
Ganciclovir	Increased toxicity—bone marrow
Amphotericin B	Increased toxicity—bone marrow
Itraconazole	
Antacids, cimetidine, ranitidine, famotidine	Decreased absorption
Cyclosporine	Increased nephrotoxicity
Phenytoin	Decreased effect of itraconazole (due to enzyme induction)
Ketoconazole	
Antacids, cimetidine, ranitidine, famotidine	Decreased absorption
Acyclovir	
Cyclosporine	Increased nephrotoxicity if levels of cyclosporin not watched
Ganciclovir	
Amphotericin B	Increased toxicity—bone marrow, nephrotoxicity
Cyclosporine	Increased nephrotoxicity
Cotrimoxazole	Increased bone marrow, skin
Flucytosine	Increased bone marrow, skin
Imipenam/cilistatin	Increased likelihood of seizures

CNS, central nervous system; GI, gastrointestinal; NSAID, nonsteroidal antiinflammatory drug.
[a]Listing is by the object drug (the drug that is affected).

Many of the interactions discussed in Table 16–5 involve the inhibition of hepatic biotransformation by H_2 blockers. Cimetidine is a predictable inhibitor of a wide variety of biotransformation reactions (with significant interpatient variation), whereas ranitidine and famotidine are less likely to produce enzyme inhibition. Many studies have failed to show any effect of ranitidine and famotidine in hepatic microsomal enzymes activity; however, there are case reports of the inhibition of hepatic drug metabolism by these two H_2 blockers producing significant effects on serum levels.

REFERENCES

1. Kavanaugh RE, Unadkat JD, Smith AL. Drug disposition in cystic fibrosis. In: Davis PB, ed. *Cystic fibrosis.* New York: Marcel-Dekker, 1993:91–130.
2. Kearnes GL. Hepatic drug metabolism in cystic fibrosis: recent developments and future directions, *Ann Pharmacother* 1993;27:74–79.
3. O'Sullivan TA, Wang J-P, Unadkat JD, et al. Disposition of drugs in cystic fibrosis: V, in vivo CYP2C9 activity as probed by (S)-warfarin is not enhanced in cystic fibrosis. *Clin Pharmacol Ther* 1993;54:323–328.
4. Koup GM. Pharmacokinetic concept—drug binding, apparent volume of distribution and clearance. *Eur J Clin Pharmacol* 1981;20:299–305.
5. Miller ME, Kornhauser DM. Bromide pharmacokinetics in cystic fibrosis. *Arch Pediatr Adolesc Med* 1994;148:266–271.
6. Siber GR, Echeverria P, Smith AL, et al. Pharmacokinetics of gentamicin in children and adults. *J Infect Dis* 1975;132:637–651.
7. Hedman A, Alvan G, Strandvik B, et al. Increased renal clearance of cefsulodin due to higher glomerular filtration rate in cystic fibrosis. *Clin Pharmacokinet* 1990;18:168–175.
8. Wang J-P, Unadkat JD, Al-Habet SMH, et al. Disposition of drugs in cystic fibrosis: IV, mechanisms for enhanced renal clearance of ticarcillin. *Clin Pharmacol Ther* 1993;54:293–302.
9. Kearns GL, Mallory GB, Crom WR, et al. Enhanced hepatic drug clearance in patients with cystic fibrosis. *J Pediatr* 1990;117:972–979.
10. O'Sullivan TA, Bauer LA, Horn JR, et al. Disposition of drugs in cystic fibrosis: II, hepatic blood flow. *Clin Pharmacol Ther* 1991;50:450–455.

11. Vergesslich KA, Gotz M, Mostbeck G, et al. Portal venous blood flow in cystic fibrosis: assessment by Duplex Doppler sonography. *Pediatr Radiol* 19:371–374. 1989

12. Harrison CJ, Marks MI, Welch DF, et al. A multicenter comparison of related pharmacologic features of cephalexin and dicloxacillin given for two months to young children with cystic fibrosis. *Pediatr Pharmacol* 1985;5:7–16.

13. Gottschalk B, Forgel F, Wiesemann G, et al. Pharmacokinetics of antibacterials in patients with cystic fibrosis. *Monatsschr Kinderheilkd* 1988;136:475–478.

14. Pedersen M, Stovring S, Morkassel E, et al. A comparative study of amoxycillin and pivampicillin in persistent *Haemophilus influenzae* infection of the lower respiratory tract in children with chronic lung disease. *Scand J Infect Dis* 1986;18:245–254.

15. Smith AL. Oral antibiotic therapy for serious infections. *Ann Rev Med* 1988;39:171–184.

16. Christensson BA, Nilsson-Ehle I, Ljungberg B, et al. Increased oral bioavailability of ciprofloxacin in cystic fibrosis patients. *Antimicrob Agents Chemother* 1992;36:2512–2517.

17. Ansorg R, Muller KD, Wiora J. Comparison of inhibitory and bactericidal activity of antipseudomonal antibiotics against *Pseudomonas aeruginosa* isolates from cystic fibrosis patients. *Chemotherapy* 1990;36: 222–229.

18. Richard DA, Nousia-Arvantitakis S, Sollich V, et al. Oral ciprofloxacin vs. intravenous ceftazidime plus tobramycin in pediatric cystic fibrosis patients: comparison of antipseudomonas efficacy and assessment of safety with ultrasonography and magnetic resonance imaging. *Pediatr Infect Dis J* 1997;16:572–578.

19. Goldfarb J, Stern RC, Reed MD, et al. Ciprofloxacin monotherapy for acute pulmonary exacerbations of cystic fibrosis. *Am J Med* 1987;82:174–179.

20. Shalit I, Stutman HR, Marks MI, et al. Randomized study of two dosage regimens of ciprofloxacin for treating chronic bronchopulmonary infection in patients with cystic fibrosis. *Am J Med* 1987;82: 189–195.

21. Kureishi A, Diver JM, Beckthold B, et al. Cloning and nucleotide sequence of *Pseudomonas aeruginosa* DNA gyrase gyrA gene from strain PA01 and quinolone-resistant clinical isolates. *Antimicrob Agents Chemother* 1994;38:1944–1952.

22. Yonezawa M, Takahata M, Matsubara N, et al. DNA gyrase *gyr*A in quinolone-resistant clinical isolates of *Pseudomonas aeruginosa. Antimicrob Agents Chemother* 1995;39:1970–1972.

23. Diver JM, Schollaardt T, Rabin HR, et al. Persistence mechanisms in Pseudomonas aeruginosa from cystic fibrosis patients undergoing ciprofloxacin therapy. *Antimicrob Agents Chemother* 1991;35:1538–1546.

24. Danisovicova A, Brezina M, Belan S, et al. Magnetic resonance imaging in children receiving quinolones: no evidence of quinolone-induced arthropathy: a multicenter survey. *Chemotherapy* 1994;40:209–214.

25. Kesseler A, Lacassie A, Hugot JP, et al. Arthropathies following the administration of pefloxacin to an adolescent with mucoviscidosis. *Annales de Pediatrie* 1989;36:275–278.

26. Hutabarat RM, Unadkat JD, Sahajwalla C, et al. Disposition of drugs in cystic fibrosis: I, sulfamethoxazole and trimethoprim. *Clin Pharmacol Ther* 1991; 49:402–409.

27. Reed MD, Stern RC, Bertino JS, et al. Dosing implications of rapid elimination of trimethoprim-sulfamethoxazole in patients with cystic fibrosis. *J Pediatr* 1984;104:303–307.

28. Dickinson CJ, Reed MD, Stern RC, et al. The effect of exocrine pancreatic function on chloramphenicol pharmacokinetics in patients with cystic fibrosis. *Pediatr Res* 1988;23:388–392.

29. Fernandes CJ, Stevens DA, Ackerman VP. Comparative antibacterial activities of new ß-lactam antibiotics against Pseudomonas aeruginosa. *Chemotherapy* 1985;31:292–296.

30. Pleasants RA, Walker TR, Samuelson WM. Allergic reactions to parenteral beta-lactam antibiotics in patients with cystic fibrosis. *Chest* 1994;106:1124–1128.

31. Sunagawa M, Matsumura H, Wumita Y, et al. Structural features resulting in convulsive activity of carbapenem compounds: effect of C-2 side chain. *J Antibiotics* 1995;48:408–416.

32. Byrne S, Maddison J, Connor P, et al. Clinical evaluation of meropenem versus ceftazidime for the treatment of *Pseudomonas spp.* infections in cystic fibrosis patients. *J Antimicrob Chemother* 1995;36 (Suppl A):135–143.

33. Webb AK. The treatment of pulmonary infection in cystic fibrosis. *Scand J Infect Dis Suppl* 1995;96: 24–27.

34. Schaad UB, Wedgewood-Krucko J, Guenin K, et al. Antipseudomonal therapy in cystic fibrosis: aztreonam and amikacin versus ceftazidime and amikacin administered intravenously followed by oral ciprofloxacin. *Eur J Clin Microbiol Infect Dis* 1989;8: 858–865.

35. Jewett CV, Ledbetter J, Lyrene RK, et al. Comparison of cefoperazone sodium vs. methicillin, ticarcillin, and tobramycin in treatment of pulmonary exacerbations in patients with cystic fibrosis. *J Pediatr* 1985; 106:669–672.

36. Klepser ME, Patel KB, Nicolau DP, et al. Comparison of the bactericidal activities of ofloxacin and ciprofloxacin alone and in combination with ceftazidime and piperacillin against clinical strains of Pseudomonas aeruginosa. *Antimicrob Agents Chemother* 1995;39:2503–2510.

37. Madaras-Kelly KJ, Moody J, Larsson A, et al. Characterization of synergy between ofloxacin, ceftazidime and tobramycin against *Pseudomonas aeruginosa. Chemotherapy* 1997;43:108–117.

38. Klion AD, Kallsen J, Cowl CT, et al. Ceftazidime-related nonconvulsive status epilepticus. *Arch Int Med* 1994;154:586–589.

39. de Groot R, Smith AL. Antibiotic pharmacokinetics in cystic fibrosis: differences and clinical significance. *Clin Pharmacokinet* 1987;13:228–253.

40. McRorie TI, Bosso J, Randolph L. Aminoglycoside ototoxicity in cystic fibrosis: evaluation by high-frequency audiometry. *Am J Dis Child* 1989;143: 1328–1332.

41. Fobelman B, Craig W. Kinetics of antimicrobial activity. *J Pediatr* 1986;5:835–840.

42. Gilbert DN. Once-daily aminoglycoside therapy. *Antimicrob Agents Chemother* 1991;35:499–305.

43. Powell SH, Thompson WL, Luthe MA, et al. Once-daily vs. continuous aminoglycoside dosing: efficacy and toxicity in animal and clinical studies of gentamicin, netilmicin, and tobramycin. *J Infect Dis* 1983; 147:918–932.

44. Bailey TC, Little JR, Littenberg B, et al. A meta-analysis of extended-interval dosing versus multiple daily dosing of aminoglycosides. *Clin Infect Dis* 1997;24:786–795.

45. Bosso JA, Liptak CA, Seilheimer DK, et al. Toxicity of colistin in cystic fibrosis patients, DICP. *Ann Pharmacother* 1991;25:1168–1170.

46. Pleasants RA, Michalets EL, Williams DM, et al. Pharmacokinetics of vancomycin in adult cystic fibrosis patients. *Antimicrob Agents Chemother* 1996; 40:186–190.

47. Healy DP, Polk RE, Garson ML, et al. Comparison of steady-state pharmacokinetics of two dosage regimens of vancomycin in normal volunteers. *Antimicrob Agents Chemother* 1987;31:393–397.

48. Lindsay CA, Bosso JA. Optimisation of antibiotic therapy in cystic fibrosis patients: pharmacokinetic considerations. *Clin Pharmacokinet* 1993;24:496–506.

49. Weber A, Morlin G, Cohen M, et al. Effect of nebulizer type and antibiotic concentration on device performance. *Pediatr Pulmonol* 1997;23:249–460.

50. Ramsey BW, Dorkin HL, Eisenberg JD, et al. Efficacy of aerosolized tobramycin in patients with cystic fibrosis. *N Engl J Med* 1993;328:2740–2746.

51. Eisenberg J, Pepe M, Williams-Warren J, et al. A comparison of peak sputum tobramycin concentration in patients with cystic fibrosis using jet and ultrasonic nebulizer systems. *Chest* 1997;111:955–962.

52. Smith AL, Ramsey B. Aerosol administration of antibiotics. *Respiration* 1995;62(Suppl 1):19–24.

53. Dib C, Trias J, Jarlier V. Lack of additive effect between mechanisms of resistance to carbapenems and other beta-lactam agents in *Pseudomonas aeruginosa*. *Eur J Clin Microb Infect Dis* 1995;14:979–986.

54. Weiss K, Lapointe JR. Routine susceptibility testing of four antibiotic combinations for improvement of laboratory guide to therapy of cystic fibrosis infections caused by *Pseudomonas aeruginosa*. *Antimicrob Agents Chemother* 1995;39:2411–2414.

55. Saiman L, Mehar F, Niu WW, et al. Antibiotic susceptibility of multiply resistant *Pseudomonas aeruginosa* isolated from patients with cystic fibrosis, including candidates for transplantation. *Clin Infect Dis* 1996;23:532–537.

56. Barclay ML, Begg EJ, Chambers ST, et al. The effect of aminoglycoside-induced adaptive resistance on the antibacterial activity of other antibiotics against *Pseudomonas aeruginosa* in vitro. *J Antimicrob Chemother* 1996;38:853–858.

57. Pattishall EN. Longitudinal response of pulmonary function to bronchodilators in cystic fibrosis. *Pediatr Pulmonol* 1990;9:80–95.

58. Shapiro GG, Bamman J, Kanarek P, et al. The paradoxical effect of adrenergic and methylxanthine drugs in cystic fibrosis. *Pediatrics* 1976;57:740–743.

59. Isles A, Spino M, Tabachnik E, et al. Theophylline disposition in cystic fibrosis. *Am Rev Resp Dis* 124: 417–421. 1983

60. Auerbach HS, Williams M, Kirkpatrick JA, et al. Alternate-day prednisone reduces morbidity and improves pulmonary function in cystic fibrosis. *Lancet* 1985;2:686–688.

61. Rosenstein BJ, Eigen H. Risks of alternate-day prednisone in patients with cystic fibrosis. *Pediatrics* 1991;87:245–246.

62. Eigen H, Rosenstein BJ, FitzSimmons S, et al. A multicenter study of alternate-day prednisone therapy in patients with cystic fibrosis: Cystic Fibrosis Foundation prednisone trial group. *J Pediatr* 1995;126:515–523.

63. Greally P, Hussain MJ, Vergani D, et al. Interleukin-1 alpha, soluble interleukin-2 receptor, and IgG concentrations in cystic fibrosis treated with prednisolone. *Arch Dis Child* 1994;71:35–39.

64. Dove AM, Szefler SJ, Hill MR, et al. Altered prednisolone pharmacokinetics in patients with cystic fibrosis. *J Pediatr* 1992;120:789–794.

65. Green CG, Kraus CK, Lemanske RF, et al. Rapid methylprednisolone clearance in a patient with cystic fibrosis. *Drug Intell Clin Pharm* 1988;22:876–878.

66. Stead R, Grimmer SFM, Rogers SM, et al. Pharmacokinetics of contraceptive steroids in patients with cystic fibrosis. *Thorax* 1987;42:59–64.

67. Konstan MW, Hoppel C, Chai B-L, et al. Ibuprofen in children with cystic fibrosis: pharmacokinetics and adverse effects. *J Pediatr* 1991;118:956–964.

68. Konstan MW, Byard PJ, Hoppel CL, et al. Effect of high-dose ibuprofen in patients with cystic fibrosis. *N Engl J Med* 1995;332:848–854.

69. Hutabarat RM, Unadkat JD, Kushmerick P, et al. Disposition of drugs in cystic fibrosis: III, acetaminophen. *Clin Pharmacol Ther* 1991;50:695–701.

70. Cooney GF, Fiel SB, Shaw LM, et al. Cyclosporine bioavailability in heart–lung transplant candidates with cystic fibrosis. *Transplantation* 1990;42:821–823.

71. Tsang VT, Johnston A, Heritier F, et al. Cyclosporin pharmacokinetics in heart-lung transplant recipients with cystic fibrosis: effects of pancreatic enzymes of ranitidine. *Eur J Clin Pharmacol* 1994;46:261,265.

72. Girault D, Haloun A, Viard L, et al. Sandimmune neoral improves the bioavailability of cyclosporin A and decreases inter-individual variation in patients affected with cystic fibrosis. *Transplantation Proc* 1995;24:2488–2490.

73. Berkovitch M, Bitzan M, Matsui D, et al. Pediatric clinical use of ketoconazole/cyclosporin interaction. *Pediatr Nephrol* 1994;8:492–493.

74. Sorenson AL, Lovdahl M, Hewitt JM, et al. Effects of ketoconazole on cyclosporine metabolism in renal allograft recipients. *Transplantation Proc* 1994;26:2822.

75. Moore LW, Alloway RR, Acchiardo SR, et al. Clinical observations of metabolic changes occurring in renal transplant recipients receiving ketoconazole. *Transplantation* 1996;61:537–541.

76. McLellan RA, Drobitch RK, McLellan H, et al. Norfloxacin interferes with cyclosporine disposition in pediatric patients undergoing renal transplantation. *Clin Pharmacol Ther* 1995;58:322–327.

77. Alvan G, Beermann B, Hjelte L, et al. Increased nonrenal clearance and increased diuretic efficiency of furosemide in cystic fibrosis. *Clin Pharmacol Ther* 1988;44:436–441.

78. Vestal RE, Aging and determinants of hepatic drug clearance. *Hepatology* 1989;9:331–334.

Cystic Fibrosis in Adults,
edited by J. R. Yankaskas and M. R. Knowles,
Lippincott–Raven Publishers, Philadelphia, 1999.

17

Cardiopulmonary and Skeletal Muscle Function and Their Effects on Exercise Limitation

Larry C. Lands and *Allan L. Coates

*Department of Pediatrics and Division of Pediatric Respiratory Medicine, McGill University Health Centre, Montreal Children's Hospital, Montreal, Quebec; and *Department of Pediatrics, University of Toronto Faculty of Medicine, and Division of Pediatric Respiratory Medicine, The Hospital for Sick Children, Toronto, Ontario, Canada*

Advanced cystic fibrosis (CF) and other chronic obstructive lung diseases frequently are accompanied by a progressive inability to perform the physical work of daily living. This exercise ability typically is quantified for clinical assessment by the maximal aerobic capacity achieved during a progressive exercise test. The result of this test primarily is a measure of physical fitness in healthy subjects or in those with mild CF, but in advanced disease, it also predicts the degree of tolerance of daily activities (1). The physical inability to perform normal routine tasks often is cited as a major determinant of the quality of life (2). In addition, recent work suggests that a decreased exercise capacity, independent of lung function or age, is associated with increased mortality in patients with CF (3). Finally, a decreased exercise capacity is associated with lower quality of life scores in patients with CF (4). Therefore, an understanding of the factors that limit exercise ability allows for the implementation of rehabilitation programs appropriate for each patient's requirements. Accordingly, the measurement of exercise ability can be used to assess the effectiveness of rehabilitation. This chapter focuses on the cardiopulmonary and peripheral skeletal muscular responses to exercise in patients with CF and their influence on exercise limitation. Where data for patients with CF are not available, literature pertaining to patients with chronic obstructive pulmonary disease (COPD) will be cited.

EXERCISE LIMITATION AND ITS CAUSES

It has long been recognized that patients with CF are prone to exercise limitation (5–9). Although the most obvious cause for this decrement in exercise ability is the reduction in ventilatory capacity and reserve, other nonventilatory factors, such as peripheral skeletal muscle mass and function and cardiovascular function, may play important roles (Table 17–1).

During exercise, the necessary increase in ventilation is achieved by a progressive increase in respiratory rate and recruitment in tidal volume. In patients with CF, even in those with mild disease, the need to increase the tidal volume is complicated further by an abnormally large dead space (5). This volume recruitment normally is achieved by encroaching on both the inspiratory and expiratory reserve volumes. However, patients with obstructive lung disease may have problems extending their tidal volumes to less than resting functional residual capacity (FRC) because of the combination of gas trapping and expiratory

TABLE 17–1. *Exercise performance in adults with cystic fibrosis*

Pulmonary function may affect exercise performance by:
  · limiting maximal achievable ventilation
  · peripheral skeletal muscle detraining due to inactivity
Nutritional status may affect exercise performance by:
  · loss of muscle mass
  · diminished muscle quality

flow limitation that is accentuated by airway narrowing at lower lung volumes (10). Hence, they increase tidal volume by breathing at lung volumes greater than FRC and thereby achieve higher expiratory flow rates (10,11). Furthermore, the increase in respiratory rate during exercise shortens the absolute inspiratory time and thus requires a marked increase in inspiratory flow if tidal volume is to be increased (10,12). If the subject cannot increase inspiratory flow adequately, inspiration may be prolonged relatively and may encroach into the time available for expiration. This results in the early termination of expiration by the start of the next breath, leading to dynamic hyperinflation and/or carbon dioxide (CO_2) retention (12). Alternatively, a small tidal volume–high

frequency pattern may be adopted to preserve expiratory time and limit the degree of dynamic hyperinflation (10). The higher work of breathing at volumes greater than resting FRC theoretically predisposes to exercising respiratory muscle fatigue. Despite this possibility, progressive, incremental types of exercise testing do not appear to cause such fatigue (13). Furthermore, the increased cost of breathing during exercise testing is small, even in patients with chronic lung disease (14), and may not be measurable during tests with short (1-minute) increments (15).

For the past 15 years, nutritional status, independent of lung function, has been recognized as a cause of exercise limitation in patients with CF (6,8,9). Recent evidence that peripheral skeletal muscle function is a better predictor of exercise capacity than lean body mass in these patients (16) suggests that the exercise limitation caused by malnutrition may be mediated by skeletal muscle loss or dysfunction, or a combination of the two (Figs. 17–1 and 17–2). Patients with CF are prone to decreases in muscle mass because of intestinal malabsorption and mildly increased caloric requirements. These caloric needs increase as lung function deteriorates. In addition to reductions in mass,

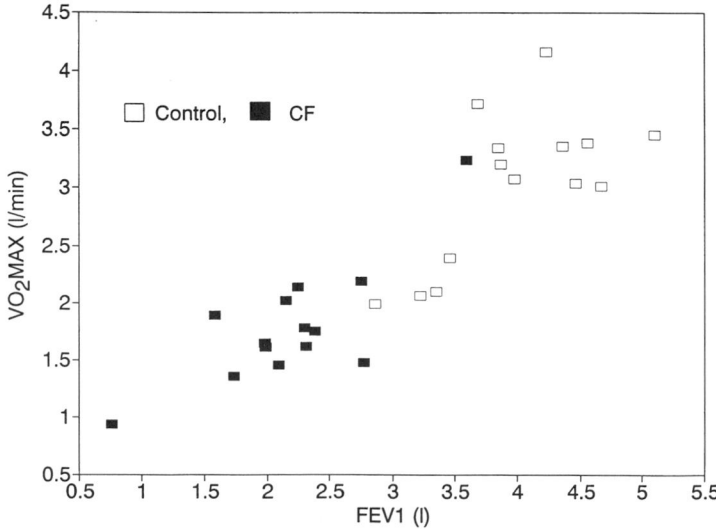

FIG. 17–1. The effect of lung function on exercise ability in healthy adults and those with CF. (Reproduced with permission from reference 16.)

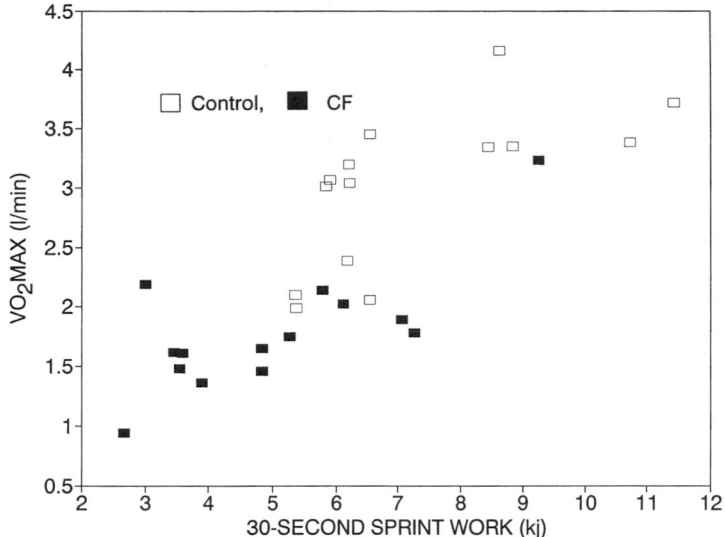

FIG. 17–2. The effect of leg muscle function on exercise ability in healthy adults and those with CF. (Reproduced with permission from reference 16.)

muscle function may be affected adversely by a sedentary lifestyle, an altered electrolyte environment, and oxygen-free radicals (17). All these factors may come into play in patients with CF. Moreover, detraining results in altered muscle metabolism, with a greater reliance on glycolytic products, resulting in higher muscular lactate and CO_2 production, and lower lactate clearance. These alterations in metabolism result in greater ventilatory demands that become more significant for patients with already limited pulmonary reserve.

Oxygen consumption is the difference between oxygen delivery and extraction. Although oxygen delivery depends on cardiac output, it must be recognized that cardiac output responds to metabolic demands, so that up to a certain limit, if oxygen consumption can be increased during exercise, then cardiac output will rise (18). The components of cardiac output—heart rate and stroke volume—both can be affected by lung disease and nutritional status. For most patients with CF, cardiac output is appropriate for the oxygen consumed (8,9,15). However, patients who are malnourished or who have significant airflow limitation may achieve this cardiac output with a reduced stroke volume and an elevated heart rate

response (19). Furthermore, there is some evidence (20) to suggest that severely affected patients may be unable to increase adequately their cardiac output in response to increasing oxygen demands. This may account partially for the improved exercise capacity in response to supplemental oxygen therapy in patients with advanced disease (21).

EXERCISE TESTING

To quantify the degree of functional impairment that accompanies exercise inability, the American Thoracic Society has published guidelines of incapacity based on oxygen consumption (22). Exercise testing is the most efficient way to look at the integration of pulmonary, cardiovascular, and musculoskeletal systems. It also can detect oxyhemoglobin desaturation, although resting lung function, including percent-predicted forced expiratory volume in 1 second (FEV_1) (23), FEV_1/forced vital capacity (FVC) (24), or resting CO diffusing capacity (25), may indicate those patients who are at risk for desaturation. With the addition of some simple auxiliary testing, the factors contributing to exercise limitation can be evaluated. This then can lead to a rational approach to individualizing rehabilitation programs.

There are several excellent texts that discuss many of the practical issues of exercise testing (26,27). There are two issues that need to be highlighted with respect to testing. The first is the method of testing, and the second relates to measuring equipment. Most centers test exercise capacity by a progressive, incremental exercise test, using either a treadmill or cycle ergometer. A cycle ergometer may be preferable for the following reasons. Although it is true that oxygen consumption is higher during a treadmill exercise, a certain amount of balance and coordination is required to do a truly maximal test safely. Furthermore, during exercise on a treadmill, the actual external work performed depends on the settings of the device (speed and elevation) and the weight of the subject, which may vary from test to test. In contrast, cycling allows the subject to be supported by a seat and handlebars, which reduces the risk of falling, and the external work performed depends only on the settings on the device. Furthermore, it is an activity with which most patients are familiar. Thus, if appropriate control populations are used for comparison, it is more likely that useful data can be gleaned from cycle ergometric testing. It also should be stressed that it is preferable for each laboratory to develop its own normative standards, rather than those published by other laboratories. In this regard, using a standard increment, such as 100 kpm/minute (16.35 watts) every minute, allows for direct comparison with control values at the same absolute work loads. However, patients who are more seriously ill may find this increment too large, whereas fit, healthy subjects may find a test using this increment unduly long. This requires adaptation of the test protocol to the population being studied.

In the current era of computerization, it is not unusual to employ a ready-made system for exercise testing with gas exchange. Although the graphics and ease of analysis are impressive, recent experience with some of the difficulties of accurately measuring expired PCO_2 concentrations when subjects are breathing oxygen-enriched gas at a concentration greater than 30% (28) requires verification that the values being reported are the true values. Before purchasing such a system, all the components for gas exchange must be checked—that is, a device to measure minute ventilation, an O_2 analyzer, and a CO_2 analyzer meet the specific requirements for response time and accuracy. It generally is recommended that respiratory equipment employ sampling rates at least five times the natural oscillation of the signal being measured. Another aspect to consider is the size of the mixing chamber on those systems where one is used. Sick patients may have tidal volumes less than 500 mL, whereas healthy athletic adults may exceed 3 L during maximal exercise. If the chamber is overly large, then changes in mixed expired gases will not reflect current changes in gas exchange. Alternatively, a chamber that is too small results in unacceptable variability in the signal. To adapt to the variation in tidal volume associated with both size and severity of disease, it may be useful to have available several mixing chambers of different size or a single mixing chamber whose volume can be varied to roughly match the subject's vital capacity. Many commercially available systems employ a device to measure gas flow and rapidly responsive gas analyzers to measure gas exchange breath by breath. Three signals (flow, O_2, and CO_2) must be analyzed and integrated over time, with the lag time of each of the measuring devices accounted for, to enable the calculation of minute ventilation, O_2 consumption, and CO_2 production. It should be verified that these systems give results comparable to those employing a mixing chamber and that they are suitable for use in the population to be studied.

For the purposes of safety and for investigating oxyhemoglobin desaturation, saturation should be monitored by pulse oximetry. A recent review (29) suggests that there are differences between oximeters, and that for the same equipment, probe placement may affect accuracy. Generally, most devices provide reasonable information for saturations greater than 85%. However, the device's accuracy should be known before purchase. Furthermore, dark skin pigmentation will adversely affect the accuracy of these devices (30).

THE CARDIOVASCULAR SYSTEM

Goldring and colleagues (20) were the first to study cardiac output during exercise in patients with CF. Using right heart catheterizations, they demonstrated that cardiac output increased with oxygen demands in most patients. However, patients with severe obstructive disease had blunted cardiac output responses. Since this initial study, several authors employing CO_2-rebreathing techniques (5,8,9,15) have demonstrated appropriate increases in cardiac output in relation to oxygen consumption. However, malnourished patients and those with advanced lung disease generally achieved this output with a reduced stroke volume and elevated heart rate response.

Several reasons for the reduced stroke volume response in patients with CF are possible. Both nutritional status (8) and cardiopulmonary interaction (19) have been proposed as altering the heart rate response to work. Weight loss often results in reductions in cardiac mass (31), leading to a smaller stroke volume and an increased heart rate response in malnourished patients.

An alternative explanation is that the cardiovascular response is affected by the mass of muscle performing the work. Comparing arm to leg work at equal oxygen consumption, healthy subjects have increased heart rate responses with arm work despite similar cardiac outputs (32). This could result from the inability of the smaller arm muscle mass to cause the same degree of vasodilation as the leg muscles, resulting in smaller stroke volumes and higher heart rates. Smaller muscle masses also may result in greater catecholamine responses, which would elevate the heart rate. Consistent with this effect of muscle mass on heart rate response, Cotes and colleagues (33) found that at a given work load achieved on a cycle ergometer, heart rate related strongly to lean body mass or thigh muscle width. Consistent with these findings, the exaggerated increase in

heart rate (in response to increasing oxygen needs) seen in patients with mild-to-moderate CF could be minimized by controlling for lean body mass (16).

The mechanisms by which lung disease affects stroke volume are multiple (34–36). If hypoxia occurs, then pulmonary vasoconstriction may result. If hypoxia is sustained, then the pulmonary vascular bed can remodel so that pulmonary hypertension becomes fixed (37,38). In addition, the destruction of lung parenchyma in CF reduces the cross-sectional area of the pulmonary vascular bed, further increasing pulmonary vascular resistance (39).

Several studies using radionuclide techniques have demonstrated impaired right and left ventricular responses to supine exercise (40,41). Changes in cardiac filling pressures can be brought on by the exaggerated pleural pressure swings that accompany airflow limitation (42). Recent preliminary data supporting this concept include the finding that, in healthy exercising subjects, decreasing pleural pressure swings with proportional assist ventilation augmented stroke volume and cardiac output (43). Hortop and colleagues (19) noted a strong relation between the stroke volume response and the FEV_1 in patients with CF. Furthermore, the authors suggested that improvement in lung function may result in improved stroke volume responses. The recent work with the aforementioned proportional assist ventilation supports this notion and suggests that such assistance may be of therapeutic benefit.

MEASUREMENT OF CARDIAC OUTPUT

The routine measurement of cardiac output requires the use of noninvasive techniques. Most studies involving patients with CF have employed CO_2-rebreathing methods (5,8,9,15). One recent CF study used pulsed Doppler imaging to measure cardiac output during supine exercise (44). However, the results of this study must be interpreted cautiously because the authors did not find the usual increase in cardiac output when the healthy control subjects were moved from an upright to a supine position. Furthermore, ultrasonic studies can be difficult technically in hyperinflated patients, with inflated lung obscuring the cardiac view. These studies are even more difficult to perform in patients during upright exercise. Because of differences in hemodynamics between supine and upright exercise, results achieved in one position may not be readily applicable to the other position.

In the CO_2-rebreathing techniques, in analogous fashion to the Fick principle, cardiac output is derived by dividing the CO_2 production by the venoarterial CO_2 content difference. Although CO_2 production and arterial PCO_2 can be measured directly, mixed venous PCO_2 is estimated from a rebreathing method. The two rebreathing methods used most frequently are the equilibrium (27,45) and exponential methods (15,46,47). The equilibrium method employs a bag with 10% to 15% CO_2, remainder O_2, whereas the exponential method uses a bag with 4% CO_2, remainder O_2. In both methods, at the end of exhalation, the subject rebreathes from the bag while the end-tidal PCO_2 values are recorded (Fig. 17–3).

Because both methods use relatively high oxygen, the resulting PCO_2 is in blood that is fully saturated. Using the dissociation curves for CO_2 in saturated blood, the venous CO_2 content can be calculated. The arterial CO_2 content can be calculated from the estimate of $PaCO_2$ and the degree of arterial saturation.

The exponential method has several advantages over the equilibrium technique: it technically is simpler to perform, employs a single low (4%), readily tolerable gas concentration, and a bag volume 1.5 to 2 times the tidal volume. The equilibrium technique has been validated in patients with advanced obstructive lung disease (48). The exponential technique has been validated against the equilibrium method in patients with mild-to-moderate CF (15) and, more recently, in patients with severe obstructive lung disease (49).

Although concerns have been expressed about using end-tidal PCO_2 measurements to estimate arterial PCO_2 values in patients with severe airflow limitation (48), Lands and colleagues (50) recently demonstrated that the end-tidal values could be used reasonably to estimate cardiac output in these patients, although estimates of the physiologic dead space/tidal volume ratio were not as accurate.

MUSCLE FUNCTION

Patients with CF are prone to malnutrition and curtailed physical activity because of lung disease. Both of these factors will impact on muscular ability. Although most investigations have concentrated on the ventilatory limitations to exercise in patients with lung disease (51,52), most patients with chronic lung dis-

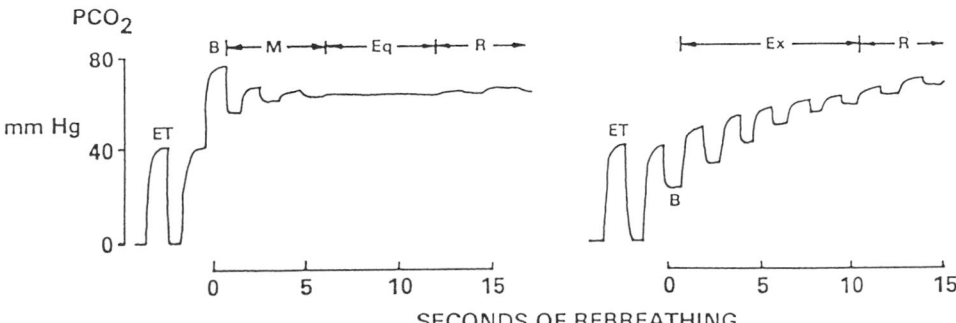

FIG. 17–3. End-tidal PCO_2 tracings for the equilibrium and exponential rebreathing method. Records of PCO_2 during rebreathing in exercise, showing typical records obtained with the equilibrium method (*left*) and the exponential method (*right*). ET, end-tidal PCO_2 before rebreathing; B, initial bag concentration; M, mixing between bag and lungs in equilibrium method; Eq, equilibrium "plateau"; R, recirculation; Ex, "exponential" rise in PCO_2 toward asymptote.

ease will attribute their limitations primarily or partially to sensations of extreme leg exertion (53). Maximal exercise capacity can be characterized further in terms of lung function and peripheral skeletal muscle function (16) (see Figs. 17–1 and 17–2). This appears to be true for both healthy control subjects and patients with CF with mild-to-moderate lung disease, even when controlling for the confounding factors of age, height, and gender. Although lung function is a major factor limiting exercise capacity, muscle function accounts for a significant amount of the residual variability in exercise ability. This recognition of the role of muscle function is important because, unlike respiratory function (54–58), muscular ability is potentially amenable to rehabilitation. Therefore, examination of muscle function in these patients may indicate who is likely to benefit from rehabilitation and the strategies most likely to be beneficial.

PERIPHERAL SKELETAL MUSCLE FUNCTION

Measurement of Peripheral Skeletal Function

Skeletal muscle primarily is composed of two fiber types: type I fibers are slow-twitch, highly oxidative muscles, whereas type II fibers are fast-twitch, primarily glycolytic muscles. Although the force per cross-sectional area is similar for the two fiber types, it is typical that type I fibers are recruited first, whereas type II fibers are recruited for bursts of power and acceleration. Although there is little evidence that fiber type distribution in human muscle can be altered by exercise training, nutritional status, or medications, fibers may undergo changes in cross-sectional area and metabolic capacity.

Muscle strength traditionally has been assessed by manual muscle testing. In this type of examination, a trained examiner assesses the force that the subject can generate against a manual resistance applied by the examiner. Although reasonable reproducibility can be developed by any individual examiner, there is a

fair risk of interobserver differences. In addition, such testing is insensitive to small but significant changes in strength (59).

More recently, quantitative devices have been developed to measure accurately muscle strength and endurance. Although grip strength can be measured readily, this is a measure of small muscle groups that are used frequently, even in bedridden individuals. The measurement of large muscle groups, such as knee extensors, may be more pertinent to muscular ability and exercise capacity. The simplest devices for assessing leg strength will have a strain gauge attached to a limb in a fixed position (60). These allow for the measurement of isometric force at one position, usually chosen as the optimal lever angle for the muscle. In the case of knee extensors, this would be at an angle of 90 degrees.

In addition to these types of devices are those that can measure force during movement. Isokinetic devices (61,62) allow for the measurement of maximal force at all joint angles at a fixed speed of rotation. In contrast to isometric tests, this type of motion is more typical of that employed during daily activities. Because movement is involved, power and work output can be calculated. In addition, force–velocity and power–velocity relations can be examined, giving a broader physiologic study of muscular ability. However, these devices again measure the force across single joints. Other devices, such as the Wingate cycle, will fix the load and measure the speed and thus, the power, which the cyclist can generate over a fixed time period.

Dynamic muscular ability in patients with CF has been assessed by whole-limb isokinetic cycling (16,63,64) and Wingate testing (65,66). An isokinetic cycle fixes the pedalling speed. Strain gauges placed either on the pedal shafts (61) or on the flywheel axle strut (62) measure the force produced by the subject. In addition, whole-leg power and work output can be measured. The measurements made on such a cycle respond to specific types of muscle training in a characteristic manner. Power trainers exhibit high initial forces that rapidly taper off, whereas endurance athletes have lower initial forces that deteriorate slowly. The major advantage of this type of device is that it provides assessment of whole-limb muscle function during the same type of cycling activity employed during exercise testing. Furthermore, when this type of device is used for short-term high-intensity sprints, muscular glycolytic ability can be assessed. During such sprints, there also are dramatic changes in blood chemistries because of rapid fluid and ion shifts and high CO_2 production (64,67). Thus, isokinetic cycling can be a valuable tool for both clinical and more basic types of investigation.

For all these devices, muscular fatigue also can be assessed. For isometric measures, repeated efforts of fixed duration at set time intervals can be done. For isokinetic tests, either the decline in power over set time intervals or the duration at which a set submaximal force can be maintained can be measured. As discussed below, the causes of fatigue are multiple, and more invasive tests are required to ascertain the causes.

Muscle Function in Chronic Lung Disease

Leg strength in patients with chronic lung disease decreases with ventilatory capacity and is a major determinant of exercise ability (68). Furthermore, skeletal muscle weakness contributes to the amount of medical services consumed by patients with chronic lung disease (69). In patients with CF with only mild malnutrition, leg strength is related strongly to lean body mass (63). When expressed per kilogram of lean body mass, leg strength is normal and unaffected by mild malnutrition, suggesting that the quality of the remaining muscle is preserved. Furthermore, patients with CF can improve their skeletal muscle strength with strength training (70).

Strength training in patients with advanced lung disease (mean FEV_1 39% predicted) improves dyspnea and submaximal work endurance times without increasing maximal work capacity (71). The study by Simpson and colleagues (71) demonstrated that patients with advanced disease can tolerate short bursts of high intensity work and that a concentration on improving glycolytic ability and augmenting muscle mass, through strength training, results in improved tolerance of daily activities. The

reason for this is that many daily activities are high-intensity glycolytic events. For instance, climbing a flight of stairs in 5 seconds represents a work load twice the maximal aerobic capacity for a 45-year-old 70-kg man. This is not to imply that significant defects in aerobic capacity are not present in patients with chronic lung disease (72) and that improving maximal exercise capacity would not increase submaximal exercise tolerance. However, dyspnea may preclude patients with chronic lung disease from participating in aerobic training vigorous enough to induce a training response.

Causes of Muscular Weakness

Although the muscular weakness seen in patients with chronic lung disease (53,73) may be attributed to reductions in muscle mass, altered electrolyte distribution (and especially altered transmembrane ion concentration gradients) also may be contributory (74,75). Failure to maintain the same force over time is the hallmark of muscle fatigue. Muscular fatigue generally can be described in terms of central or peripheral fatigue (76). Central fatigue is evidenced by the inability of the subject to voluntarily maintain force generation yet still be able to do so when the muscle is subjected to direct stimulation. This may involve any part of the pathway from the cerebral cortex to the neuromuscular junction. Peripheral fatigue is demonstrated when there is failure of force maintenance, even with direct muscular stimulation. Again, a variety of factors come into play, including failure of propagation of the action potential, excitation–contraction dissociation, diminished contractile ability, and loss of energy supply. As discussed below, electrolyte abnormalities can play an important role in the development of peripheral fatigue. This is further compounded by changes in muscle acid–base status, which fundamentally can affect enzyme regulation and contractile properties.

Electrolyte Disturbances and Muscle Function

Electrolyte disturbances adversely affect muscle function, causing premature loss of force generation (77,78). For instance, decreases in sarcolemmal transmembrane potential, especially when caused by a fall in the transmembrane K$^+$ gradient, may diminish force generation (79,80). Furthermore, exercise training upregulates the expression of muscle Na$^+$-K$^+$-adenosine triphosphatase (Na$^+$-K$^+$-ATPase) pumps, which help to maintain the sarcolemmal transmembrane K$^+$ gradient and potential (81,82), perhaps explaining why there is a correlation between strength and muscle Na$^+$-K$^+$-ATPase pump concentration. Therefore it is conceivable that deconditioning results in downregulation of these pumps or pump activity, with resultant muscular impairment.

In addition, reduced intramuscular Mg^{2+} concentrations in stable patients with chronic lung disease may lower ATP/adenosine diphosphate (ADP) ratios, thus reducing energy availability for muscle contraction and the maintenance of K$^+$ gradients across the sarcolemma (74). This decrease in energy availability may account for the parallel reductions in intramuscular K$^+$ and Mg^{2+} concentrations seen in patients with COPD in acute respiratory failure (75), who cannot maintain ventilatory muscle function.

A more recent cause for electrolyte abnormalities in patients with lung disease is the advent of lung and heart–lung transplantation for end-stage disease. Cyclosporine is a standard part of posttransplantation immunosuppressive therapy. There are a variety of neurological complications secondary to cyclosporine, including hand tremor and, more importantly, encephalopathies, which may result in seizures and even brain

death (83). In addition, hypomagnesemia and hyperkalemia both are frequent occurrences in transplanted patients treated with cyclosporine. As aforementioned, hypomagnesemia may decrease intramuscular energy stores, whereas hyperkalemia may decrease sarcolemmal transmembrane potential, reducing force output. Recently, cyclosporine has been shown to interfere with mitochondrial oxidation in rats (84), which may explain low skeletal muscle ATP production in lung transplant recipients (85). This interference with oxidation could be compensated by an increase in oxygen delivery, although such an increase in cardiac output has been difficult to demonstrate in lung transplant recipients (86,87).

It must be recognized that systemic corticosteroids are another standard therapy in transplant recipients. Corticosteroids may lead to atrophy of fast-twitch (type II) fibers, used for explosive power, and decreases in oxidative enzyme concentrations in slow-twitch (type I) fibers, resulting in alterations in contractile properties of the muscle (88). Functionally, both skeletal and respiratory muscle weakness may develop with steroid use (89). Given the combination of immunosuppressive therapy used in transplantation, it is not surprising that lung transplant recipients have markedly reduced leg muscle function, which limits their exercise ability (87) (Fig. 17–4).

Other medications frequently used in patients with chronic lung disease also can affect muscle function. Those medications that result in potassium depletion, such as diuretics, may

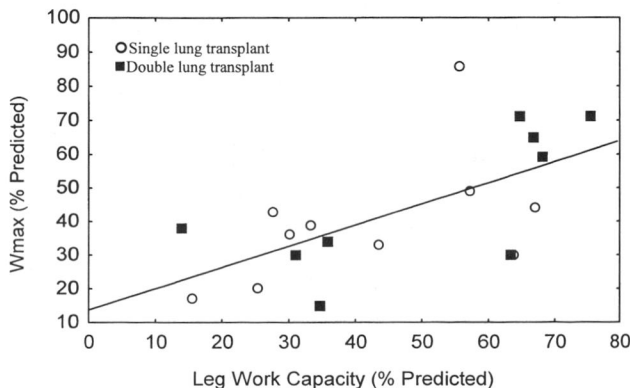

FIG. 17–4. The effect of leg muscle function on exercise ability in lung transplant recipients.

lead to muscular impairment. Alternatively, ß-agonists, by stimulating sarcolemmal Na+-K+-ATPase pumps, may preserve intracellular K+ concentrations and delay the onset of fatigue. There also is evidence to suggest that aminophylline improves muscle contractility in fatigued inspiratory muscles (90).

Oxidant Stress and Muscle Function

Oxidant stress occurs when there is an imbalance between oxidants (oxygen-free radicals and associated substances, such as peroxides) and antioxidant defenses (consisting of vitamins, enzyme systems, and nonenzymatic scavengers). The neutrophilic inflammation seen in the lungs of patients with CF (91) can act as a primary source of oxidants. In addition, patients with CF are predisposed to antioxidant deficiencies. Certain antioxidants, such as vitamin E and beta-carotene, are fat soluble, so their absorption may be impaired in patients with CF (92,93). Additionally, patients with CF are prone to deficiencies in selenium (94), which is required by the antioxidant enzyme, glutathione peroxidase, for activity. Moreover, even when patients with CF have seemingly adequate levels of antioxidants, such as vitamin E, beta-carotene, vitamin C, and uric acid, oxidant stress may occur (95). Thus, this imbalance between oxidants and antioxidants may contribute to the pathogenesis of these patients' lung disease (96–98) and their increased incidence of malignancy (99).

There currently is good evidence that oxidant stress contributes to muscular fatigue (17). Moreover, pretreatment with N-acetylcysteine, a thiol-containing antioxidant that has structural similarities to glutathione, slows the onset of fatigue (100). In addition, Karlsson and colleagues (101) have implicated antioxidant deficiencies in exercise limitation in patients with COPD. Clearly, the role of oxidant stress in both exercise limitation and pulmonary disease needs to be explored further, particularly because there currently are suggestions of possible therapeutic intervention. Accordingly, in addition to supplying adequate

protein and caloric needs for activity and growth, attention also must be paid to micronutrient and vitamin supplementation, which increase the body's defense to oxidant injury. Recent work has suggested that treatment with antioxidants can decrease the amount of oxidant stress that occurs in patients with CF (92,93). In other conditions known to cause oxidative stress, such as exercise (102,103), treatment with antioxidants such as vitamin E (104,105) or a combination of vitamins E and C and beta-carotene (106) also have lessened the degree of lipid peroxidation resulting from oxidant stress. Whether the amelioration of antioxidant defenses will improve or stabilize lung function and exercise performance in patients with CF requires further investigation.

Effects of Training on Muscular Performance and Exercise

Discomfort developed during exercise may lead to curtailment of activity and a sedentary lifestyle. This may lead to reductions in muscle mass, primarily in the type II fiber population, and decreased levels of oxidative enzymes. Most information on the consequences of inactivity has been gained by the exploration of the response to training. Training may be broken down broadly into two categories, namely strength and endurance. Strength training primarily results in muscular hypertrophy of the type II fibers (107). There also is a neural adaptation that affects fiber recruitment and strength development before the onset of hypertrophy (108).

Endurance training results in important metabolic changes that have consequences for the ventilatory demands of exercise (109) (Table 17–2). Although a detailed discussion is beyond the scope of this chapter, there are several adaptations to endurance training that need to be highlighted. With endurance training in healthy populations, at moderate exercise intensities (< 65% maximal) there is a sparing of muscle glycogen achieved primarily by an increased use of fat and, possibly, exogenous glucose as substrates for oxidation (109). In addition, there are

TABLE 17–2. *Effects of endurance training in adults with cystic fibrosis*

More reliance on fat as a fuel
  ·less CO_2 production
  ·glycogen sparing
Increased aerobic capacity
  ·less lactate production
  ·improved lactate clearance

increases in oxidative enzyme capacity favoring fat utilization. Because of stoichiometry, the use of fat as an oxidative substrate produces less CO_2 for the same amount of O_2 consumed. There also is a decrease in the release and an increase in the uptake of lactate (110). These two factors help to limit the amount of acidosis and CO_2 produced during exercise and thus decrease the ventilatory demands. Furthermore, endurance training attenuates the lipid peroxidation caused by oxidant stress during exercise (111).

RESPIRATORY MUSCLE FUNCTION

Muscle strength is determined principally by the muscle mass available to develop tension and the resting length of the muscle. However, with respect to the respiratory muscles, strength, resting length, and mass may be measured only indirectly.

Strength

The simplest measure of respiratory strength is the measurement of mouth pressure during an airway occlusion. For inspiration strength, the pressure generated represents the sum of the tension developed by the diaphragm, the external intercostal muscles, and the accessory muscles, which, in turn, act on the surface area of the lung (which is related to lung volume) to produce a pressure (force/surface area) at the mouth (112). The strategy for pressure development is highly individualized, with some subjects relying mostly on diaphragmatic contraction and others preferring to contract primarily the intercostal muscles (113). Although direct measures of diaphragmatic strength are available, they require the measurement of transdiaphragmatic pressure by esophageal and intragastric balloons during transcutaneous phrenic nerve stimulation (114,115). The relative invasiveness of this type of testing does not lend itself to routine clinical testing; thus, function usually is implied from maximal pressures that can be generated at the mouth.

Muscle Length

When the inspiratory effort occurs at lung volumes greater residual volume (RV), the diaphragm will be shorter than its optimal resting length, and therefore, will not be able to generate its maximum force (116) because of suboptimal actin–myosin cross-bridge linkage (117). Therefore, patients with airflow limitation severe enough to raise the amount of air trapped in the lung at the end of expiration (i.e., those patients who are hyperinflated) will be at a mechanical disadvantage when inspiratory muscle strength is assessed. For this reason, when respiratory muscle function is evaluated using maximal inspiratory pressures generated at the mouth in patients with hyperinflation, the pressures generated should be looked at in relation to the lung volume at which the maximal effort was made (118). This is done easily by expressing the pressure generated as a percent predicted at that lung volume [usually expressed as a percent of total lung capacity (TLC)]. Hence, the inspiratory pressures generated by a patient whose RV is approximately 50% of TLC can be compared with that of a healthy subject whose RV/TLC is 25%.

Hyperinflation also is detrimental because it alters the coupling of the diaphragm to the ribcage. Under normal circumstances, the diaphragm is apposed partially to the ribcage, at the end of expiration. This zone of apposition (119) allows for the contracting diaphragm to descend, while elevating the ribcage, resulting in a decrease in pleural pressure and an increase in thoracic volume. With hyperinflation, the zone of apposition is reduced, diminishing the ability of the diaphragm to generate effective intrapleural pressure, thereby reducing the inspiratory strength (120,121).

A potential adaptive mechanism to chronic hyperinflation is length adaptation. This phenomenon was first demonstrated in a hamster model of emphysema (122), whereby the chronically shortened diaphragm loses sarcomeres. The remaining sarcomeres then stretch out so that actin–myosin cross-bridge linkage is optimized, and the length–tension relationship is returned to normal (123). This last possibility has been difficult to demonstrate in humans. For example, patients with chronic lung disease do not have shortened diaphragms (124), possibly because most of the hyperinflation is assumed by remodelling of the ribcage (125). Furthermore, according to Similowski and colleagues (126), there are no data in the literature concerning sarcomere number in patients with chronic lung disease.

Muscle Mass

Because it is not practical to measure diaphragm weight directly, information, mostly from autopsy series (127), indicates that diaphragm mass increases with body weight. Because muscle mass is related to muscle thickness, a more practical indirect method of assessing diaphragm weight *in vivo* is to use ultrasound to measure diaphragm thickness (128,129). For instance, in their ultrasonic study, Cohn and colleagues (129) demonstrated that inspiratory strength correlated with diaphragm thickness, which, in turn, correlated strongly with body weight.

There currently is no information with respect to diaphragm mass in patients with CF. Furthermore, because the results from patients with COPD (124,130,131) are highly variable (in part, because of variability in methodology and study populations), one cannot make inferences with respect to patients with CF.

Most of the muscle research in CF has concentrated on respiratory muscle function. Despite the presence of low body weights and the mechanical disadvantage of hyperinflation secondary to lung disease, respiratory muscle strength (RMS) usually is preserved in patients with CF (118,132–134). Older patients with CF, however, may not maintain respiratory strength if they are malnourished (134,135). Respiratory muscle endurance appears normal

or increased in patients with CF (63,136). Endurance can be measured by tests of sustained ventilation (137) or repeated measures of static pressures (138).

In patients with CF, although respiratory muscle endurance is normal, it can be enhanced by specific muscle training (118,136), upper limb exercise (136), or a running program (58). However, Asher and colleagues (118) were unable to show any improvement in exercise capacity after this increase in respiratory endurance. In addition, Coates and colleagues (12) showed that CO_2 retention during progressive exercise in patients with CF appeared to be caused by the pattern of ventilation adopted early in the test and not by a progression to a pattern consistent with fatigue. These results suggest that the respiratory impairment in these patients may be acting as a muscle-training stimulus to counteract the effects of malnutrition. If this is true, then inspiratory muscle strength should be relatively maintained with respect to muscle groups not undergoing this stimulus, such as lower limb musculature.

Two studies have compared respiratory and peripheral muscle function in older patients with CF (63,139). Lands and colleagues (63) compared respiratory and peripheral muscle strength in young adults with CF whose nutritional status ranged from well to mildly malnourished (% ideal weight 94.3 ± 9.64). When compared with healthy controls of either gender, the CF group had reductions in lean body mass and leg strength, whereas both their inspiratory and expiratory strengths were within normal limits. In a manner similar to the healthy controls, the male patients with CF demonstrated a correlation between muscular (inspiratory, expiratory, and leg) strength and lean body mass. Inspiratory and expiratory strengths also correlated with leg strength. For the female patients with CF, similar results were found for expiratory and leg strengths, with both correlating with each other and lean body mass. However, inspiratory strength appeared relatively greater, given lean body mass or leg strength. The results for the male patients confirm previous work showing that respiratory muscle strength is related to nutritional status in older males with CF (135). This study also found that the malnourished patients with CF had a shift of the force–frequency curve of the adductor pollicis to the left, a frequent finding in malnourished subjects.

These results suggested that for relatively well-nourished patients with CF, inspiratory strength is better maintained than lean body mass or leg strength. This is supported by the study by Mier and colleagues (139), who found that more patients with CF had normal (i.e., > 75% of predicted) respiratory strength (11 of 25) than had normal leg strength (8 of 25) (63). Furthermore, when Lands and colleagues compared the healthy control male and female patients, the females had reduced lean body mass, respiratory strength, and leg strength. However, when the same analysis was performed on the CF group, the female patients with CF, despite having a lower lean body mass and leg strength, had the same respiratory (both inspiratory and expiratory) strength as the male patients. Because the male and female patients with CF did not differ with respect to relative weight for height, airflow limitation (FEV_1), or the degree of lung hyperinflation (RV/TLC), the inconsistent findings from healthy controls must be attributable to other factors. These factors include a preserved diaphragm mass or improved mechanical coupling of the diaphragm and ribcage, as discussed previously.

REHABILITATION IN CYSTIC FIBROSIS

Although rehabilitation results in little change in pulmonary function, significant training effects can occur, even in patients with moderately severe airflow limitation (140). Thus, improvements in peripheral skeletal muscle function and cardiac function can lead to diminished demands on an already compromised respiratory system. These changes include reduced ventilatory and heart rate response for similar oxygen consumption. However, it is unclear whether these reductions in heart rate and ventilation are associated with any changes in cardiac output.

There are several implications for training that arise from the studies of muscle function cited in the previous section. As strength and endurance are preserved for the inspiratory muscles, respiratory muscle training programs in the CF population need to be tailored to those with demonstrable weakness. Similarly, nutritional supplementation programs may not result in clinically significant increases in respiratory muscle strength in those with normal strength. Keens et al. (136) and Asher et al. (118) demonstrated that the respiratory muscles in CF are trainable, and Charge et al. (141) suggested that respiratory strength can be increased with aggressive nutritional support in severely malnourished patients with CF. However, if the values are normal to begin with, it is difficult to support programs in which exercise compliance frequently is the limiting factor. In support of this, Asher and colleagues (118) found that increased respiratory muscle endurance induced by specific respiratory muscle training did not improve exercise capacity. As aforementioned, CO_2 retention during exercise in patients with CF does not appear to be on the basis of respiratory muscle fatigue. Furthermore, because respiratory muscle training occurs during whole body training (58,136), the more pleasurable activities enjoyed during whole body training may encourage participation and compliance and result in more generalized training benefits. In addition, whole body training can reduce breathlessness in patients with CF (57).

Nutritional support may help peripheral strength if it results in an increase in muscle mass. This may be encouraged by an exercise program stressing strength training rather than aerobic training. This is not to belittle the benefits of endurance training (see Table 17–2), which are an important facet of rehabilitation. As strength increases, the absolute load that may be maintained indefinitely also will increase. Because of the finding of Lands and colleagues (63) that leg strength was decreased but relative endurance was maintained, an exercise program that begins with strength training may be more beneficial than a program consisting solely of endurance activities. It should be recalled that strength training in chronic lung disease improved dyspnea and submaximal exercise endurance times (71). To date, one study has investigated strength training in patients with CF (70). Weight and strength (assessed by manual muscle testing) increased over a 3-month period. Interestingly, there was a decrease in RV and RV/TLC ratio with strength training. This is surprising because although RV typically is achieved by a balance between expiratory muscle strength and chest wall compliance in unobstructed patients, airway closure probably accounts for most of the increase in RV in obstructive lung disease. Thus, these patients with severe airflow limitation (mean FEV_1 42% of predicted) would not have been expected to diminish their RV by increasing expiratory muscle strength.

Exercise training also has been used as a substitute for chest physical therapy (142–144), even during hospitalization (7). However, some of these ambulatory programs require vigorous training and may not effectively remove sputum, especially in adult patients with CF and those with advanced pulmonary disease (145). Currently, although exercise is an excellent adjuvant therapy in patients with CF (146), there is insufficient data to suggest that it may be substituted for the known beneficial effects of conventional chest physical therapy.

During exercise, oxygen supplementation in those patients who desaturate will diminish ventilatory demands and heart rate responses (21,147). This may allow for better tolerance of training sessions.

It also must be recognized that patients with CF will lose excessive amounts of salt through sweating. Although they may be able to acclimatize to heat (148), these patients do so at the cost of salt depletion. Furthermore, they do not voluntarily replenish these losses (149) and thus need to be encouraged to take in both salt and water.

SUMMARY

The inability to perform the physical activity required for daily living can affect adversely the quality of life in patients with advanced CF. Although there is little that can be done to restore pulmonary function in patients with CF, rehabilitation, including physical training and caloric and micronutrient supplementation, can augment muscular function and preserve exercise capacity. In this regard, a recent longitudinal study in adults with CF demonstrated that they were able to increase body mass and maintain maximal exercise capacity, despite losses in lung function (150).

REFERENCES

1. Folgering H, Dekhuijzen R, Cox N, et al. The rationale of pulmonary rehabilitation. *Eur Respir Rev* 1991;1:6:464–471.
2. Guyatt GH, Townsend M, Berman LB, et al. Quality of life in patients with chronic airflow limitation. *Br J Dis Chest* 1987;81:45–54.
3. Nixon PA, Orenstein DM, Kelsey SF, et al. The prognostic value of exercise testing in patients with cystic fibrosis. *N Engl J Med* 1992;327:1785–1788.
4. Orenstein DM, Nixon PA, Ross EA, et al. The quality of well-being in cystic fibrosis. *Chest* 1989;95:344–347.
5. Godfrey S, Mearns M. Pulmonary function and response to exercise in cystic fibrosis. *Arch Dis Child* 1971;46:144–151.
6. Coates AL, Boyce P, Muller D, et al. The role of nutritional status, airway obstruction, hypoxia, and abnormalities in serum lipid composition in limiting exercise tolerance in children with cystic fibrosis. *Acta Paediatr Scand* 1980;69:353–358.
7. Cerny FJ. Relative effects of bronchial drainage and exercise for in-hospital care of patients with cystic fibrosis. *Phys Ther* 1989;69:633–639.
8. Marcotte JE, Canny GJ, Grisdale R, et al. Effects of nutritional status on exercise performance in advanced cystic fibrosis. *Chest* 1986;90:375–379.
9. Marcotte JE, Grisdale R, Levison H, et al. Multiple factors limit exercise capacity in cystic fibrosis. *Pediatr Pulmonol* 1986;2:274–281.
10. Regnis JA, Alison JA, Henke KG, et al. Changes in end-expiratory lung volume during exercise in cystic fibrosis relate to severity of lung disease. *Am Rev Respir Dis* 1991;144:507–512.
11. Stubbing DG, Pengelly LD, Morse JLC, et al. Pulmonary mechanics during exercise in patients with chronic airflow obstruction. *J Appl Physiol* 1980;49:511–515.
12. Coates AL, Canny G, Zinman R, et al. The effects of chronic airflow limitation, increased dead space, and the pattern of ventilation on gas exchange during maximal exercise in advanced cystic fibrosis. *Am Rev Respir Dis* 1988;138:1524–1531.
13. Fitting JW. Respiratory muscle fatigue limiting physical exercise? *Eur Respir J* 1991;4:103–108.
14. Katsardis CV, Desmond KJ, Coates AL. Measuring the oxygen cost breathing in normal adults and pa-

tients with cystic fibrosis. *Respir Physiol* 1986;65: 257–266.

15. Lands LC, Heigenhauser GJF, Jones NL. The determination of cardiac output during progressive exercise in cystic fibrosis. *Chest* 1992;102:1118–1123.

16. Lands LC, Heigenhauser GJF, Jones NL. Analysis of factors limiting maximal exercise performance in cystic fibrosis. *Clin Sci* 1992;83:391–397.

17. Sen CK. Oxidants and antioxidants in exercise. *J Appl Physiol* 1995;79:675–686.

18. Saltin B. Capacity of blood flow delivery to exercising skeletal muscle in humans. *Am J Cardiol* 1988; 62:30E–35E.

19. Hortop J, Desmond KJ, Coates AL. The mechanical effects of expiratory airflow limitation on cardiac performance in cystic fibrosis. *Am Rev Respir Dis* 1988;137:132–137.

20. Goldring RM, Fishman AP, Turino GM, et al. Pulmonary hypertension and cor pulmonale in cystic fibrosis of the pancreas. *J Pediatr* 1964;65:501–524.

21. Marcus CL, Bader D, Stabile MW, et al. Supplemental oxygen and exercise performance in patients with cystic fibrosis with severe pulmonary disease. *Chest* 1992;101:52–57.

22. American Thoracic Society. Evaluation of impairment/disability secondary to respiratory disorders. *Am Rev Respir Dis* 1986;133:1205–1209.

23. Nixon P. Role of exercise in the evaluation and management of pulmonary disease in children and youth. *Med Sci Sports Exerc* 1996;28:414–420.

24. Henke KG and Orenstein DM. Oxygen saturation during exercise in cystic fibrosis. *Am Rev Respir Dis* 1984;129:708–711.

25. Lebecque P, Lapierre J-G, Lamarre A, et al. Diffusing capacity and oxygen desaturation effects on exercise in patients with cystic fibrosis. *Chest* 1987;91:693–697.

26. Wasserman K, Hansen JE, Sue DY, et al. *Principles of exercise testing and interpretation*. Philadelphia: Lea and Febiger, 1987.

27. Jones NL. *Clinical exercise testing*. 4th ed. Toronto: WB Saunders, 1997.

28. Hornby L, Coates AL, Lands LC. Effect of analyzer on the determination of mixed venous PCO_2 and cardiac output during exercise. *J Appl Physiol* 1995;79: 1032–1038.

29. Mengelkoch LJ, Martin D, Lawler J. A review of principles of pulse oximetry and accuracy of pulse oximeter estimates during exercise. *Phys Ther* 1994; 74:40–49.

30. Zeballos RJ, Weisman IM. Reliability of non-invasive oximetry in black subjects during exercise and hypoxia. *Am Rev Respir Dis* 1991;144:1240–1244.

31. Webb JG, Kiess MC, Chan-Yan CC. Malnutrition and the heart. *Can Med Assoc J* 1986;135:753–758.

32. Lewis SF, Taylor WF, Graham RM, et al. Cardiovascular responses to exercise as functions of absolute and relative workload. *J Appl Physiol* 1983;54:1314–1323.

33. Cotes JE, Berry G, Burkinshaw L, et al. Cardiac frequency during submaximal exercise in young adults: relation to lean body mass, total body potassium and amount of leg muscle. *Q J Exp Physiol* 1973;58:239– 250.

34. Moss AJ, Harper WH, Dooley RR, et al. Cor pulmonale in cystic fibrosis of the pancreas. *J Pediatr* 1965;67:797–807.

35. Stern RR, Borkat G, Hirschfeld SS, et al. Heart failure in cystic fibrosis. *Am J Dis Child* 1980;134: 267–272.

36. Moss AJ. The cardiovascular system in cystic fibrosis. *Pediatrics* 1982;70:728–741.

37. Symchych PS. Pulmonary hypertension in cystic fibrosis: a descriptive and morphometric analysis of the pulmonary vasculature. *Arch Pathol* 1971;91: 409–414.

38. Reid L. Structure and function in pulmonary hypertension: new perceptions. *Chest* 1986;89:543–547.

39. Ryland D, Reid L. The pulmonary circulation in cystic fibrosis. *Thorax* 1975;30:285–292.

40. Benson LN, Newth CJL, Desouza M, et al. Radionuclide assessment of right and left ventricular function during bicycle exercise in young patients with cystic fibrosis. *Am Rev Respir Dis* 1984;130:987–992.

41. Geggel RL, Dozer AJ, Flyer DC, et al. Effect of vasodilators at rest and during exercise in young adults with cystic fibrosis and chronic cor pulmonale. *Am Rev Respir Dis* 1985;131:531–536.

42. Culver B, Marini J, Butler J. Lung volume and pleural pressure effects on ventricular function. *J Appl Physiol* 1981;50:630–635.

43. Gallagher CG, Bree T, Zintel TA, Clemens RE, Marciniuk DD, Cujec B. Influence of intrathoracic pressure on cardiac output (CO) during exercise in normal humans. *Am J Respir Crit Care Med* 1996; 153:A648.

44. Perrault H, Coughlan M, Marcotte J-E, et al. Comparison of cardiac output determinants in response to upright and supine exercise in patients with cystic fibrosis. *Chest* 1992;101:42–51.

45. Heigenhauser GJF and Jones NL. Measurement of cardiac output by carbon dioxide rebreathing methods. *Clin Chest Med* 1989;10:255–264.

46. Alves Da Silva G, El-Manshawi A, et al. Measurement of mixed venous carbon dioxide pressure by rebreathing during exercise. *Respir Physiol* 1985;59: 379–392.

47. Jacob S, Hornby L, Lands LC. Measurement of mixed venous PCO_2 for the determination of cardiac output in children during exercise. *Chest* 1997;111:474–480.

48. Mahler DA, Matthay RA, Snyder PE, et al. Determination of cardiac output at rest and during exercise by carbon dioxide rebreathing method in obstructive lung disease. *Am Rev Respir Dis* 1985;131:73–78.

49. Lands LC, Hornby L, Levy RD, et al. Measurement of mixed venous PCO_2 in patients with severe airflow limitation. *Am J Respir Crit Care Med* 1994; 149:A783.

50. Lands LC, Canny G, Xu F, Coates AL. Noninvasive determination of cardiac output in patients with severe airflow limitation. *Am J Respir Crit Care Med* 1996;153:981–984.

51. Cerny FJ, Pullano TP, Cropp GJA. Cardiopulmonary adaptations to exercise in cystic fibrosis. *Am Rev Respir Dis* 1982;126:217–220.

52. Babb TG, Viggiano R, Hurley B, et al. Effect of mild-to-moderate airflow limitation on exercise capacity. *J Appl Physiol* 1991;70:223–230.

53. Killian KJ, Leblanc P, Martin DH, et al. Exercise capacity and ventilatory, circulatory and symptom limitation in patients with chronic airflow limitation. *Am Rev Respir Dis* 1992;146:935–940.

54. Blomquist M, Freyschuss U, Wiman L-G, et al. Physical activity and self treatment in cystic fibrosis. *Arch Dis Child* 1986;61:362–367.

55. Edlund LD, French RW, Herbst JJ, et al. Effects of a swimming program on children with cystic fibrosis. *Am J Dis Child* 1986;140:80–83.

56. Holzer FJ, Schnall R, Landau LI. The effects of a home exercise programme in children with cystic fibrosis and asthma. *Aust Paediatr J* 1984;20:297–302.

57. O'Neill PA, Dodds M, Phillips B, et al. Regular exercise and reduction of breathlessness in patients with cystic fibrosis. *Br J Dis Chest* 1987;81:62–69.

58. Orenstein DM, Frankiln BA, Doershuk CF, et al. Exercise conditioning and cardiopulmonary fitness in cystic fibrosis: the effects of a three-month supervised running program. *Chest* 1981;80:392–398.

59. Aitkens S, Lord J, Bernauer E, Fowler W Jr, et al. Relationship of manual muscle testing to objective strength measurements. *Muscle Nerve* 1989;12:173–177.

60. Hosking GP, Young A, Dubowitz V, et al. Tests of muscle function in children. *Arch Dis Child* 1978;53:224–229.

61. McCartney N, Heigenhauser GJF, Sargeant AJ, et al. A constant-velocity cycle ergometer for the study of dynamic muscle function. *J Appl Physiol* 1983;55:212–217.

62. Lands LC, Hornby L, Desrochers G, et al. A simple isokinetic cycle for the measurement of leg muscle function. *J Appl Physiol* 1994;77:2506–2510.

63. Lands LC, Heigenhauser GJF, Jones NL. Peripheral and respiratory muscle function in adolescents and young adults with CF. *Am Rev Respir Dis* 1993;147:865–869.

64. Lands LC, Heigenhauser GJF, Jones NL. Maximal short-term exercise performance and ion regulation in cystic fibrosis. *Can J Physiol Pharmacol* 1993;71:12–16.

65. Cabrera ME, Lough MD, Doershuk CF, et al. Anaerobic performance assessed by the Wingate test in patients with cystic fibrosis. *Pediatr Exerc Sci* 1993;5:78–87.

66. Boas SR, Joswiak ML, Nixon PA, et al. Factors limiting anaerobic performance in adolescent males with cystic fibrosis. *Med Sci Sports Exerc* 1996;28:291–298.

67. Kowalchuk JM, Heigenhauser GJF, Lindinger MI, et al. Role of lungs and inactive muscle in acid–base control after maximal exercise. *J Appl Physiol* 1988;65:2090–2096.

68. Hamilton AL, Killian KJ, Summers E, Jones NL. Muscle strength, symptom intensity, and exercise capacity in patients with cardiorespiratory disorders. *Am J Respir Crit Care Med* 1995;152:2021–2031.

69. Decramer M, Gosselink H, Verschueren M, Demuynck K, Evers G. Medical consumption is related to muscle weakness in COPD patients. *Am J Respir Crit Care Med* 1994;149:A140.

70. Strauss GD, Osher A, Wang C-I, et al. Variable weight training in cystic fibrosis. *Chest* 1987;92:273–276.

71. Simpson K, Killian K, McCartney N, et al. Randomised controlled trial of weightlifting exercise in patients with chronic airflow limitation. *Thorax* 1992;47:70–75.

72. Belman MJ, Kendregan BA. Exercise training fails to increase skeletal muscle enzymes in patients with chronic obstructive pulmonary disease. *Am Rev Respir Dis* 1981;123:256–261.

73. Rochester DF, Braun NMT. Determinants of maximal inspiratory pressure in chronic obstructive pulmonary disease. *Am Rev Respir Dis* 1985;132:42–47.

74. Moller P, Bergstrom J, Furst P, et al. Energy-rich phosphagens, electrolyte and free amino acids in leg skeletal muscle of patients with chronic obstructive lung disease. *Acta Med Scand* 1982;211:187–193.

75. Fiaccadori E, Del Canale S, Arduini U, et al. Intracellular acid-base and electrolyte metabolism in skeletal muscle of patients with chronic obstructive lung disease and acute respiratory failure. *Clin Sci* 1986;71:703–712.

76. Green HJ. Manifestations and sites of neuromuscular fatigue. In: Taylor AW, Gollnick PD, Green HJ, et al., eds. *Biochemistry of Exercise VII*. Champaign, IL: Human Kinetics Books, 1990:13–35.

77. Russell DM, Prendergast PJ, Darby PL, Garfinkel PE, Whitwell J, Jeejeebhoy KN. A comparison between muscle function and body composition in anorexia nervosa: the effect of refeeding. *Am J Clin Nutr* 1983;38(2):229–237.

78. Lindinger MI, Heigenhauser GJF. Ion fluxes during tetanic stimulation in isolated perfused rat hindlimb. *Am J Physiol* 1988;254:R117–R126.

79. Sjogaard G, Adams RP, Satin B. Water and ion shifts in skeletal muscle of humans with intense dynamic knee extension. *Am J Physiol* 1985;248:R190–R196.

80. Pichard C, Hoshino E, Allard JP, et al. Intracellular potassium and membrane potential in rat muscles during malnutrition and subsequent refeeding. *Am J Clin Nutr* 1991;54:489–498.

81. Klitgaard H, Clausen T. Increased total concentration of Na^+-K^+ pumps in vastus lateralis muscle of old trained human subjects. *J Appl Physiol* 1989;67:2491–2494.

82. McKenna MJ, Schmidt TA, Hargreaves M, et al. Sprint training increases human skeletal muscle Na^+-K^+-ATPase concentration and improves K^+ regulation. *J Appl Physiol* 1993;75:173–180.

83. Maurer JR. Therapeutic challenges following lung transplantation. *Clin Chest Med* 1990;11:279–290.

84. Mercier J, Hokason JF, Brooks GA. Effects of cyclosporin on endurance exercise time and skeletal muscle mitochondrial respiration in rats. *Am J Respir Crit Care Med* 1994;149:A742.

85. Williams TJ, Wang XN, Carey MF, McKenna MJ, Li JL, Fraser SF, Side EA, Snell GI, Walter EH. Low mitochondrial ATP production rate in human skeletal muscle post lung transplant. *Am J Respir Crit Care Med* 1996;153:A828.

86. Mesiano G, Lands LC, Hornby L, Shennib H. Cardiac output following lung transplantation. *Am J Respir Crit Care Med* 1996;153:A826.

87. Lands LC, Smountas AA, Messiano J, et al. Maximal exercise capacity and peripheral skeletal muscle function following lung transplantation. *Am J Resp Crit Care Med* 1998;157(3):A523.

88. Wilcox PG, Hards JM, Bockhold K, et al. Pathological changes and contractile properties of the diaphragm in corticosteroid myopathy in hamsters: comparison to peripheral muscle. *Am J Respir Cell Mol Biol* 1989;1:191–199.

89. Gallagher CG. Respiratory steroid myopathy. *Am J Respir Crit Care Med* 1994;150:4–6.

90. Wanke T, Merkle M, Zifko U, et al. The effects of aminophylline on the force-length characteristics of the diaphragm. *Am J Respir Crit Care Med* 1994; 149:1545–1549.

91. Cantin A. Cystic fibrosis lung inflammation: early, sustained, and severe. *Am J Respir Crit Care Med* 1995;151:939–941.

92. Kneepkens CMF, Lepage G, Roy CC. Role of beta-carotene in cystic fibrosis. *Pediatr Pulmonol* 1993; Suppl 9:169–170.

93. Lepage G, Champagne J, Ronco N, Lamarre A, Osberg I, Sokol RJ. Supplementation with carotenoids corrects increased lipid peroxidation in children with cystic fibrosis. *Am J Clin Nutr* 1996;64:87–93.

94. Dworkin B, Newman LJ, Berezin S, et al. Low blood selenium levels in patients with cystic fibrosis compared to controls and healthy adults. *J Parenter Enteral Nutr* 1987;11:38–41.

95. Langley SC, Brown K, Kelly FJ. Reduced free-radical-trapping capacity and altered plasma antioxidant status in cystic fibrosis. *Pediatr Res* 1993;33:247–250.

96. Ward PA. Neutrophil-mediated oxidant injury to the lung. *Pediatr Pulmonol* 1993;Suppl 9:108–109.

97. Britigan BE. Pseudomonas secretory products, hydroxyl radical production, and lung injury in CF. *Pediatr Pulmonol* 1993;Suppl 9:110–111.

98. Cross CE, Halliwell B. Considerations of free radical injury in CF. *Pediatr Pulmonol* 1993;Suppl 9:112–113.

99. Stead RJ, Redington AN, Hinks LJ, et al. Selenium deficiency and possible increased risk of carcinoma in adults with cystic fibrosis. *Lancet* 1985;8460: 862–863.

100. Reid MB, Stokic DS, Koch SM, et al. N-Acetylcysteine inhibits muscle fatigue in humans. *Am J Resp Crit Care Med* 1994;149:A321.

101. Karlsson J, Diamant B, Folkers K. Exercise-limiting factors in respiratory distress. *Respir* 1992;59(Suppl 2):18–23.

102. Jenkins RR. Free radical chemistry: relationship to exercise. *Sports Med* 1988;5:156–170.

103. Sjödin, Hellsten Westing Y, Apple FS. Biochemical mechanisms for oxygen free radical formation during exercise. *Sports Med* 1990;10:236–254.

104. Sumida S, Tanaka K, Kitao H, et al. Exercise-induced lipid peroxidation and leakage of enzymes before and after vitamin E supplementation. *Int J Biochem* 1989;21:835–838.

105. Goldfarb AH, McIntosh MK, Boyer BT, et al. Vitamin E effects on indexes of lipid peroxidation in muscle from DHEA-treated and exercised rats. *J Appl Physiol* 1994;76:1630–1635.

106. Kanter MM, Nolte LA, Holloszy JO. Effects of antioxidant vitamin mixture on lipid peroxidation at rest and post exercise. *J Appl Physiol* 1993;74: 965–969.

107. Matoba H, Gollnick PD. Response of skeletal muscle to training. *Sports Med* 1984;1:240–251.

108. Narici MV, Roi GS, Landoni L, et al. Changes in force, cross-sectional area and neural activation during strength training and detraining of the human quadriceps. *Eur J Appl Physiol* 1989;59:310–319.

109. Brooks GA, Mercier J. Balance of carbohydrate and lipid utilization during exercise: the "crossover" concept. *J Appl Physiol* 1994;76:2253–2261.

110. MacRae H S-H, Dennis SC, Bosch AN, et al. Effects of training on lactate production and removal during progressive exercise in humans. *J Appl Physiol* 1992;72:1649–1656.

111. Alessio HM, Goldfarb AH. Lipid peroxidation and scavenger enzymes during exercise: adaptive response to training. *J Appl Physiol* 1988;64:1333–1336.

112. Loring SH, De Troyer A. Action of the respiratory muscles. In: Roussos C, Macklem PT, eds. *Lung biology in health and disease: vol 29, the thorax, part a.* New York: Marcel Dekker Inc, 1985:327–349.

113. Laporta D, Grassino A. Assessment of transdiaphragmatic pressure in humans. *J Appl Physiol* 1985;58: 1469–1476.

114. Bellemare F, Bigland-Ritchie B. Assessment of human diaphragm strength and activation using phrenic nerve stimulation. *Respir Physiol* 1984;58:263–277.

115. Similowski T, Gauthier AP, Yan S, et al. Assessment of diaphragm function using mouth pressure twitches in chronic obstructive pulmonary disease patients. *Am Rev Respir Dis* 1993;147:850–856.

116. Smith J, Bellemare F. Effect of lung volume on in vivo contraction characteristics of the human diaphragm. *J Appl Physiol* 1987;62:1893–1900.

117. Dawson MJ. Energetics and mechanics of skeletal muscle. In: Roussos C, Macklem PT, eds. *Lung biology in health and disease: vol 29, the thorax, part a.* New York: Marcel Dekker Inc, 1985:3–43.

118. Asher MI, Pardy RL, Coates AL, et al. The effects of inspiratory muscle training in patients with cystic fibrosis. *Am Rev Respir Dis* 1982;126:855–859.

119. Mead J. Functional significance of the area of apposition of diaphragm to rib cage. *Am Rev Respir Dis* 1979;119(pt 2):31–32.

120. Loring SH, Mead J. Action of the diaphragm on the rib cage inferred from a force-balance analysis. *J Appl Physiol* 1982;53:756–760.

121. Macklem PT, Macklem DM, De Troyer A. A model of inspiratory muscle mechanics. *J Appl Physiol* 1983;55:547–557.

122. Farkas GA, Roussos CH. Adaptability of the hamster diaphragm to exercise and/or emphysema. *J Appl Physiol* 1982;53:1263–1272.

123. Farkas GA, Roussos CH. Diaphragm in emphysematous hamsters: sarcomere adaptability. *J Appl Physiol* 1983;54:1635–1640.

124. Arora NS, Rochester DF. COPD and human diaphragm muscle dimensions. *Chest* 1987;91:719–724.

125. Sharp JT, Beard GA, Sunga M, et al. The rib cage in normal and emphysematous subjects: a roentgenographic approach. *J Appl Physiol* 1986;61:2050–2059.

126. Similowski T, Yan S, Gauthier AP, et al. Contractile properties of the human diaphragm during chronic hyperinflation. *N Engl J Med* 1991;325:917–923.

127. Arora NS, Rochester DF. Effects of body weight and muscularity on human diaphragm muscle mass, thickness and area. *J Appl Physiol* 1982;52:64–70.

128. Wait JL, Nahormek PA, Yost WT, et al. Diaphragmatic thickness-lung volume relationship in vivo. *J Appl Physiol* 1989;67:1560–1568.

129. Cohn DB, Benditt JO, Hoppin Jr FG, et al. Diaphragm thickness: an index of inspiratory muscle strength. *Am Rev Respir Dis* 1993;147:A694.

130. Wilson DO, Rogers RM, Hoffman RM. Nutrition and chronic lung disease. *Am Rev Respir Dis* 1985;132:1347–1365.

131. Thurlbeck WM. Diaphragm and body weight in emphysema. *Thorax* 1978;33:483–487.

132. O'Neill S, Leahy F, Pasterkamp H, Tal A. The effects of chronic hyperinflation, nutritional status, and posture on respiratory muscle strength in cystic fibrosis. *Am Rev Respir Dis* 1983;128:1051–1054.

133. Marks J, Pasterkamp H, Tal A, et al. Relationship between respiratory muscle strength, nutritional status, and lung volume in cystic fibrosis and asthma. *Am Rev Respir Dis* 1986;133:414–417.

134. Lands L, Desmond KJ, Demizio D, et al. The effects of nutritional status and hyperinflation on respiratory muscle strength in children and young adults. *Am Rev Respir Dis* 1990;141:1506–1509.

135. Szeinberg A, England S, Mindorff C, et al. Maximal inspiratory and expiratory pressures are reduced in hyperinflated, malnourished, young adult male patients with cystic fibrosis. *Am Rev Respir Dis* 1985;132:766–769.

136. Keens TG, Krastins IRB, Wannamaker EM, et al. Ventilatory muscle endurance training in normal subjects and patients with cystic fibrosis. *Am Rev Respir Dis* 1977;116:853–860.

137. Nickerson BG, Keens TG. measuring ventilatory muscle endurance in humans as sustainable inspiratory pressure. *J Appl Physiol* 1982;52:768–772.

138. McKenzie DK, Gandevia SC. Strength and endurance of inspiratory, expiratory, and limb muscles in asthma. *Am Rev Respir Dis* 1986;134:999–1004.

139. Mier A, Redington A, Brophy C, et al. Respiratory muscle function in cystic fibrosis. *Thorax* 1990;45:750–752.

140. Casaburi R, Patessio A, Ioli F, et al. Reduction in exercise lactic acidosis and ventilation as a result of exercise training in patients with obstructive lung disease. *Am Rev Respir Dis* 1991;143:9–18.

141. Charge TD, Drury D, Pianosi P, et al. Nutritional rehabilitation and changes in respiratory strength, function, and maximal exercise capacity in cystic fibrosis. *Am Rev Respir Dis* 1991;143:A300.

142. Zach M, Oberwaldner B, Hausler F. Cystic fibrosis physical exercise versus chest physiotherapy. *Arch Dis Child* 1982;57:587–589.

143. Andreasson B, Jonson B, Kornfalt R, et al. Long-term effects of physical exercise on working capacity and pulmonary function in cystic fibrosis. *Acta Paediatr Scand* 1987;76:70–75.

144. Zach MS, Purrer B, Oberwaldner B. Effect of swimming on forced expiration and sputum clearance in cystic fibrosis. *Lancet* 1981;ii:1201–1203.

145. Salh W, Bilton D, Dodd M, et al. effect of exercise and physiotherapy in aiding sputum expectoration in adults with cystic fibrosis. *Thorax* 1989;44:1006–1008.

146. Stanghelle JK. Physical exercise for patients with cystic fibrosis: a review. *Int J Sports Med* 1988;9 (Supplement):6–18.

147. Nixon PA, Orenstein DM, Curtis SE, et al. Oxygen supplementation during exercise in cystic fibrosis. *Am Rev Respir Dis* 1990;142:807–811.

148. Orenstein DM, Henke KG, Green CG. Heat acclimation in cystic fibrosis. *J Appl Physiol* 1984;57:408–412.

149. Bar-Or O, Blimkie CJR, Hay JA, et al. Voluntary dehydration and heat intolerance in cystic fibrosis. *Lancet* 1992;339:696–699.

150. Moorcroft AJ, Dodd ME, Webb AK. Long-term changes in exercise capacity, body mass, and pulmonary function in adults with cystic fibrosis. *Chest* 1997;111:338–343.

Cystic Fibrosis in Adults,
edited by J. R. Yankaskas and M. R. Knowles,
Lippincott–Raven Publishers, Philadelphia, 1999.

18

Endocrine and Renal Disorders in Cystic Fibrosis

Mark K. Robbins and *David A. Ontjes

*Adult Cystic Fibrosis Program, Pulmonary/Critical Care Medicine, University of Virginia Health System, Charlottesville, Virginia; and *Division of Endocrinology, University of North Carolina School of Medicine, Chapel Hill, North Carolina*

Some endocrine organs such as the pancreas may be damaged directly by cystic fibrosis (CF). Dysfunction of several others occurs as a sequel of chronic illness or malnutrition. In this chapter, the pathogenesis of common endocrine and renal disorders in CF is reviewed and guidelines are provided for their clinical management in adults.

GROWTH AND STATURE

Prevalence of Growth Retardation in Cystic Fibrosis

Adolescents and young adults with CF tend to be shorter in stature and lighter in weight than their healthy peers. Growth retardation during childhood and adolescence is common in CF, as it is in other chronic illnesses in children. Figure 18–1 shows the distributions of height and weight of 535 male and female patients with CF followed at the Hospital for Sick Children in Toronto in 1978 (1). The majority of both male and female patients were below the 50th percentile for both height and weight. The height and weight distributions for males are fairly symmetrical, whereas the distributions for females are skewed to the left, suggesting that some girls may be affected disproportionately.

When the patients are further classified into 5-year age groups, it is apparent that weight falls progressively farther below the norm in females as puberty is reached, as shown in Table 18–1. This correlates with a tendency of females with CF to show greater declines than males in both pulmonary function and survival in the teen-age years. The cause of this difference between the genders in the severity of disease after puberty still is unknown.

Pathogenesis of Growth Retardation

Growth retardation can result from undernutrition of any cause. The most important humoral mediator of growth in children is insulin-like growth factor I (IGF-I), which is produced by the liver and other peripheral tissues under the control of pituitary growth hormone. IGF-I, also known as somatomedin C, is a potent mitogen capable of promoting the growth of bone and cartilage as well as soft tissues throughout the body (2). Growth rates in children and adolescents correlate closely with circulating levels of IGF-I under most conditions. In healthy young adults in whom the dietary intake of calories and protein have been restricted experimentally, IGF-I levels are dependent on both total calories and an adequate protein intake (3). Low levels of IGF-I are associated with either a negative energy balance or a negative nitrogen balance. In children with CF, increased resting energy expenditure and poor dietary intake and fat malabsorption often

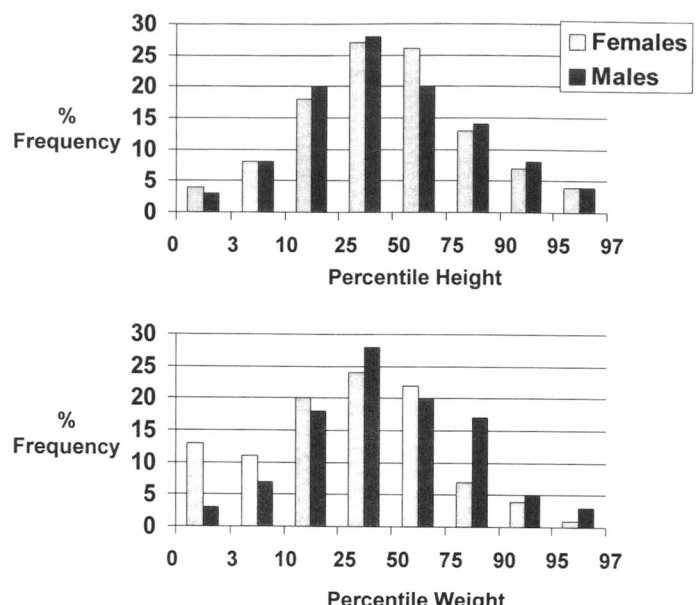

FIG. 18–1. Height and weight distributions by normal percentiles for males and females. Measurements are from 222 female and 293 male patients over 2 years of age attending the Toronto Cystic Fibrosis Clinic in 1978. (Reprinted from reference 1, with permission.)

contribute to a negative energy and nitrogen balance (4).

In patients with CF, levels of IGF-I differ, depending on the assay method. Lee et al. (5) studied six children with CF, all with heights below the third percentile. Using a bioassay of $^{35}SO_4$ incorporation into chick cartilage, they found that somatomedin levels were reduced to approximately 50% of the levels found in healthy children. Both basal and stimulated serum growth hormone levels were normal in the children with CF. In comparison, 11 chil-

TABLE 18–1. *Percentage of patients below the 50th percentile for weight in different age-gender groups*

Age (yrs)	Males	Females
2–4	56	57
5–9	45	48
10–14	58	74
15–19	58	76
20–24	66	81
25–38	64	86

Data from the Hospital for Sick Children in Toronto, 1978 (reference 1).

dren with hypopituitary conditions had abnormally low growth hormone levels and reductions in somatomedin activity of approximately 70% (5). Rosenfeld et al. (6), using a radioreceptor assay for somatomedin C, reported normal levels in 15 children with CF. Their subjects were not as severely retarded in height—only 9 of 15 were below the fifth percentile. In preparing the serum for assay, an initial chromatography step using 0.25 mol/L formic acid was used to separate somatomedin C from serum-binding proteins. The partially purified somatomedin then was measured in a competitive binding assay using placental membranes as the source of receptors. This assay, like the aforementioned bioassay, confirmed low levels of somatomedin in subjects with hypopituitary conditions. The reasons for the discrepancies in the results of these studies in patients with CF are unclear. One possible explanation for the reduced biological activity in the study by Lee et al. (5) could have been the presence of a serum-binding protein acting as an inhibitor of somatomedin activity. Such an inhibitor could have been removed in the preparative chromatography step used by Rosenfeld et al. (6). Further studies in patients with CF-related growth failure using radio-receptor or radioimmunoassay methods are needed.

Reduced production of sex steroids, particularly androgens, also is an important factor in the pathogenesis of growth retardation in adolescents. The usual acceleration of growth occurring at puberty is delayed and blunted in males with CF, as shown in Figure 18–2. Healthy boys reach a peak growth velocity of more than 7 cm per year by 13 years of age at a time when their counterparts with CF are growing at an average of less than 5 cm per year. Boys with CF reach a lower peak at 15 years of age, on the average, but continue to grow for a longer period, often into their early 20s (7). In this respect, their growth patterns resemble males with constitutionally delayed puberty, but the majority of them never reach the 50th percentile for height. Girls with CF show a similar delay and an even greater eventual reduction in stature compared with their healthy counterparts. Both androgens and estrogens increase linear growth in adolescents. These sex steroids also have the effect of causing more rapid skeletal maturation, including closure of the epiphyses of long bones. Once closure has occurred, linear growth can no longer occur. In CF adolescents with delayed puberty, both height and epiphysial closure tend to be retarded proportionately. Thus, growth can continue in response to gradually increasing concentrations of sex steroids over a longer period of time than in healthy adolescents. Unfortunately, malnutrition and other factors relating to the severity of disease often supervene before the full potential for adult stature ever is reached.

Management of Short Stature

Attempts to increase linear growth must be initiated before closure of the epiphyses in late adolescence. Appropriate assessment of the prospects for improving stature should begin with an assessment of nutritional status, the stage of puberty, and bone age, usually by examination of x-ray films of the wrist. The clinician should be most concerned with patients whose stature is more than two standard deviations (SDs) below normal for age and gender and in whom records of height and weight show a subnormal growth rate. A bone age of less than 16 years indicates that the skeleton still is capable of further growth, regardless of the patient's age. Lack of regular menarche in females or a serum testosterone level of less than 100 ng/dL in males indicates that adult sexual development has not yet occurred. Causes of short stature other than malnutrition or delayed sexual development always should be considered. Although their occurrence is relatively uncommon, patients with CF can have defects in growth hormone production, including abnormalities in the gene for growth hormone, leading to deficient growth hormone activity (8). They also may have hypothy-

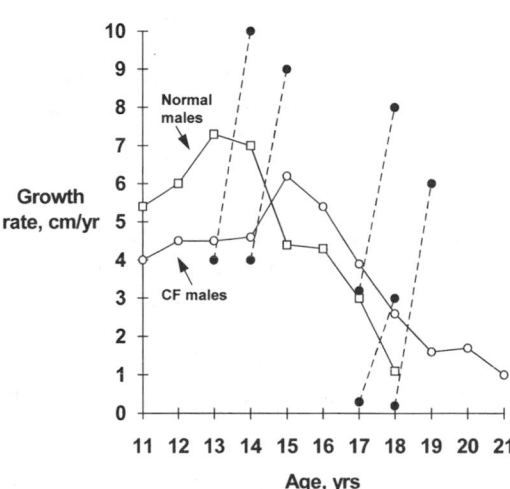

FIG. 18–2. Growth velocity of healthy males and males with cystic fibrosis. □, National Center for Health Statistics–derived 50th percentile growth velocities for healthy subjects; ○, retrospectively obtained, mean growth velocities for 54 male adolescents with cystic fibrosis followed at the Cystic Fibrosis Clinic at Children's Hospital, Stanford, California. ●‑‑‑●, growth velocities of individual subjects with cystic fibrosis in the year before and the year after treatment with testosterone enanthate. (Reprinted from reference 14.)

roidism, another cause of growth failure. Thus, the assessment should include measurement of serum levels of growth hormone after an appropriate stimulant such as L-dopa or clonidine and measurement of serum thyroxine and thyroid-stimulating hormone (TSH; i.e., thyrotropin). In almost all cases, these latter test results will be normal.

In both younger children and adolescents, the first priority should be to improve nutrition. CF genotypes associated with more impaired pancreatic exocrine function and greater malnutrition (homozygous ΔF508 mutation) also are associated with more severe growth retardation (9,10). Pancreatic enzyme supplements can help to improve nutrition and growth in many affected individuals, as described in Chapter 4. Nutritional supplementation of the most malnourished patients can result in significant gains in both weight and height, as described in Chapter 13.

In adolescents with a pubertal delay of 2 years or more, treatment with testosterone or other anabolic steroids can be beneficial. There is enhanced growth in both males and females using anabolic steroids such as norethandrolone or oxandrolone (11–13). These synthetic steroids basically are androgens with the capacity to cause virilization and anabolic effects. Landon and Rosenfeld (14) carefully documented the effects of low-dose testosterone supplements in a controlled trial in male adolescents with CF. Their results in five treated subjects are shown in Figure 18–2. All the subjects had pubertal delay beyond two SDs and serum testosterone levels of less than 100 ng/dL. They also had initial growth velocities far below normal for age. Therapy consisted of 200 mg intramuscular (IM) testosterone enanthate every 3 weeks for a total of four injections. All five subjects responded with marked increases in growth velocity in the subsequent 12 months, from a mean of 2.2 to 7.2 cm per year. Bone age increased in all subjects by a mean of 0.83 years, but not disproportionately to height age. Pulmonary vital capacity and psychological tests of self-image also improved in the treated subjects, but not in untreated controls.

Thus, the efficacy of androgen or anabolic steroid therapy is likely to be greatest in those subjects with the most retarded sexual development and growth. Short-term therapy of up to 6 months in such subjects appears to accelerate growth and improve predicted maximum height because bone age is not advanced disproportionately to height or weight. More prolonged or intensive androgen therapy should be used with caution in adolescents because it may lead to greater acceleration in epiphysial closure and may serve to limit ultimate height. Therapeutic measures that improve growth and stature in adolescents, including improved nutrition and the administration of sex steroids, when appropriate, also may increase the bone mass and strength ultimately achieved in adulthood. This is an important consideration in reducing the risk of osteoporosis later in adult life.

SEXUAL DEVELOPMENT, GONADAL FUNCTION, AND FERTILITY

The average individual with CF in the United States currently lives well beyond puberty and into the reproductive years. Successful pregnancy in women with CF has become relatively common. Virtually all males are infertile, not because they fail to produce sperm, but because they have developmental defects in the ducts that conduct sperm from the testes. Despite the successful sexual development and adaptation of many patients, gonadal function and sex steroid production frequently is diminished. The physician caring for adolescents and adults with CF should be aware of the likelihood that delayed sexual maturation or impaired gonadal function may occur. In many cases, appropriate counseling will be sufficient, but in some cases, sex steroid replacement therapy also may be indicated. The special considerations involved in pregnancy are discussed in Chapter 21.

Sexual Development and Pituitary–Gonadal Function in the Female

Girls with CF undergo menarche approximately 2 years later than their healthy counterparts and are much more likely to have primary amenorrhea beyond the age of 16 years. In a retrospective study from two regional CF centers in the United States, Moshang and Holsclaw (15) found the mean age at menarche to be 14.5 years compared with 12.9 years for all girls in the United States. Neinstein et al. (16) reported a similar mean age of menarche for patients with CF of 14.4 years. In both studies, menarchal delay was related to severity of illness and nutritional status. The best single predictor of menarche is body weight. Of those girls with CF who underwent menarche, 95% had achieved a weight greater than 82 pounds, whereas 75% of those who remained amenorrheic weighed less than 82 pounds (16). Other predictors of menarche included height and the percent of body weight as fat. These predictors of menarche parallel those reported for other chronic diseases, especially diseases involving malnutrition. Patients with the most delayed menarche have been those in whom the diagnosis of CF has been made earliest in life, which undoubtedly correlates with the severity of illness.

Once menarche has occurred, more than 50% of women with CF may have persistent dysfunctional uterine bleeding or oligomenorrhea, probably associated with anovulatory cycles (16). This compares with an estimated prevalence of 20% for dysfunctional bleeding in healthy young women. In those patients in whom normal ovulatory cycles do develop, dysfunctional uterine bleeding or secondary amenorrhea may recur later if their pulmonary disease worsens (17).

The basis of the relationship between body weight, nutritional status, and menarche has been a subject of much interest since the original hypothesis of Frisch and McArthur (18) that the percent body weight as fat was an important determinant of normal menstrual cycles. Most studies of the endocrine mechanisms accounting for suppressed gonadal function in chronic illness or malnutrition point to the hypothalamus as the most critical component. Sexual maturation in both males and females occurs under the control of the central nervous system (19). The primary neurohumoral agent controlling the process is luteinizing-hormone-releasing hormone (LHRH), which is produced by nerve cells in the hypothalamus. LHRH normally is carried via the hypophyseal portal circulation to the anterior pituitary gland, where it stimulates specific epithelial cells to produce and release both luteinizing hormone (LH) and follicle-stimulating hormone (FSH). LH and FSH, in turn, stimulate the gonads to produce germ cells (ova or sperm) and sex steroids (estrogens, progestins, and androgens). For complete sexual maturation to occur in the female, hypothalamic production of LHRH first must increase, the ovaries then must respond with increased production of estrogen, and finally, normal cyclical interactions of gonadotropins and sex steroids resulting in ovulation must be established. Failure of the last step to occur results in irregular, anovulatory menstrual cycles, usually accompanied by a reduced total production of both estrogens and progestins. There is much evidence that in chronic illnesses of many kinds, the normal increases in LHRH secretion occurring at puberty are delayed. In acquired illnesses, or as a result of increasing severity of a congenital illness such as CF, previously acquired adult patterns of LHRH and gonadotropin secretion may be lost, resulting in anovulatory menstrual cycles or secondary amenorrhea.

In pubertal females with CF, the secretion of LH and FSH in response to a test infusion of LHRH was similar to that of pubertal controls (20), although the controls chronologically were younger. This suggests that pituitary function in females with CF inherently is normal. Ovarian production of estradiol in females with CF continues to be less than it is in controls, even after puberty is reached (21). A test dose of LHRH administered to pubertal CF females elicits a normal LH response but a reduced and delayed estradiol response, as shown in Table 18–2. Basal levels of estradiol also tend to be lower.

Other Factors Affecting Female Fertility

Even in those women who have normal ovulatory menstrual cycles, fertility may be reduced. Convincing objective data are difficult

TABLE 18–2. *Effects of a luteinizing hormone-releasing hormone infusion in pubertal cystic fibrosis (CF) and control females*

Subjects	LH (mIU/mL)		FSH (mIU/mL)		Estradiol (pg/mL)		
	Basal	Peak	Basal	Peak	Basal	3 Hr	6 Hr
Control (n = 18)	5.2 ± 1.0	70.4 ± 13.9	4.1 ± 0.4	23.0 ± 3.6	29.7 ± 4.6	46.8 ± 7.1	
CF (n = 23)	11.3 ± 0.7	94.8 ± 16.4	3.5 ± 0.1	14.9 ± 1.5	14.4 ± 2.2	15.7 ± 2.3	25.5 ± 4.3

FSH, follicle-stimulating hormone; LH, luteinizing hormone.
Data from reference 21.

to find, but there is a common impression that pregnancy still is less likely to occur in ovulatory women with CF (22). The female reproductive tract in women with CF is anatomically normal. However, cervical mucus composition is altered, being more viscous and containing less water and electrolytes (23). Whether the abnormally thick mucus actually represents an increased barrier to sperm penetration and fertilization is unknown. Little is known, as well, about possible changes in the intrauterine milieu necessary for implantation and successful nutrition for the fertilized ovum (22). Once pregnancy becomes established, it frequently progresses successfully to term. The issues related to obstetric care for the woman with CF are discussed in Chapter 21.

Sexual Development and Pituitary–Gonadal Function in the Male

Puberty in boys with CF also is delayed. Males typically show a 2- to 4-year lag in the rise of FSH and LH secretion and the increase in testicular size characteristic of puberty. There is a reduced pituitary and gonadal response to a test dose of LHRH in early puberty, as shown in Table 18–3. However, plasma testosterone eventually approaches normal levels in the majority of patients in the late teen-age years (20). Presumably, with continued increases in hypothalamic production of LHRH, the pituitary and testes are capable of developing an adult response pattern.

Male Fertility

Despite the eventual maturation of the pituitary–gonadal axis, virtually all males with CF are infertile because of anatomic abnormalities in the tubules conducting sperm between the testes and the prostate (24). In one series of 25 patients, the vas deferens was absent and epididymal structures were abnormal (25). All patients had infertility and absence of sperm in their semen. Semen volume was reduced, and the content of fructose, normally derived from the seminal vesicles, was diminished. Citric acid and acid phosphatase, normally derived from the prostate, were present in normal or increased concentrations.

Other studies have confirmed the absence of normal wolffian duct–derived structures and have reported normal or moderately decreased

TABLE 18–3. *Effects of a luteinizing hormone-releasing hormone infusion in pubertal cystic fibrosis (CF) and control males*

Subjects	LH (mIU/mL)		FSH (mIU/mL)		Testosterone (ng/dL)		
	Basal	Peak	Basal	Peak	Basal	3 Hr	6 Hr
Control (n = 33)	6.2 ± 1.0	44.4 ± 3.3	3.2 ± 0.4	8.7 ± 1.0	214 ± 48	278 ± 52	
CF (n = 9)	4.0 ± 0.2	35 ± 7.8	2.5 ± 0.1	5.7 ± 1.0	70.7 ± 24.3	90.9 ± 22.2	153 ± 43

FSH, follicle-stimulating hormone; LH, luteinizing hormone.
Data from reference 21.

testicular volumes (22). Leydig cells often appear normal. There usually is active spermatogenesis within the seminiferous tubules, but in some studies, testicular biopsies have shown abnormalities of spermatocytes and spermatids as well as a decreased number of mature sperm. Obstructive azoospermia may be another manifestation of a more generalized abnormality in exocrine ducts, which are a hallmark of CF. Abnormalities of the epididymal ducts and atrophic or absent vas deferens are present even in neonates, suggesting that degenerative changes may begin *in utero*. With puberty, boys with CF begin to demonstrate circulating antibodies against their own spermatozoa (26). Autoimmunity to sperm appears to be secondary to obstruction and not to the underlying genetic abnormality in CF. A similar phenomenon occurs in some healthy men after vasectomy. Whether the fertilizing capacity of CF sperm is impaired by the presence of such antibodies currently is unknown. Theoretically, it may be possible to fertilize a normal ovum with sperm aspirated from the vasa efferentia of the testes, proximal to the site of obstruction. A practical consideration is that a finding of congenital absence of the vas deferens or of azoospermia with antibodies against sperm in a man who has not had a vasectomy strongly suggests CF. Testing frequently has revealed mutations in the cystic fibrosis transmembrane conductance regulator (CFTR) gene in infertile men with these abnormalities, even those not previously known to have CF (27,28).

Management of Impaired Gonadal Function and Reproductive Capacity in the Patient with Cystic Fibrosis

Excessive delay of puberty in boys and girls can have adverse effects on social adaptation as well as general health. Eventual success in marriage and sexual relationships is more likely when there is a reasonably normal rate of sexual development in comparison to peers. Vigorous attempts should be made to optimize nutrition and to control infections because these factors undoubtedly play a role in suppressing the onset of normal puberty. When the onset of puberty is delayed beyond 2 or 3 years in an individual with stable pulmonary disease, the physician also should consider the option of sex steroid administration to enhance secondary sexual development.

Amenorrheic or oligomenorrheic women may be treated with cyclic estrogens and a progestin to promote regular menstrual bleeding. Daily administration of conjugated estrogens in a dose of 0.625 to 1.25 mg, together with cyclic medroxyprogesterone, 5 to 10 mg per day for 10 days each month, will induce regular withdrawal bleeding in a majority of patients. Alternatively, an oral contraceptive containing a combination of a synthetic estrogen such as ethinyl estradiol, 35 to 50 g, and a progestin such as norethindrone, 0.5 to 1 mg, may be given for 21 days each month with the expectation that menstrual bleeding will occur during the week in which the contraceptive is withdrawn. In addition to promoting breast development, estrogens are essential for normal cornification and lubrication of the vaginal mucosa. Estrogens also have beneficial effects on the development of an optimal bone mass in young adult women, thus reducing the likelihood of osteoporotic fractures later in adult life. Some CF centers have been hesitant to prescribe oral contraceptives for fear of certain side effects. In the past, there have been reports of polypoid cervicitis and increased viscosity of bronchial mucus secondary to progesterone use (29). Although such occurrences may be reason for discontinuing estrogen and progestin replacement, the majority of women have no serious side effects (30).

The problem of infertility in the woman with anovulatory cycles and adequate estrogen secretion potentially can be managed by the same methods used in women without CF, provided that the patient's general health and pulmonary function are adequate to support pregnancy. A discussion of the methods for induction of ovulation and *in vitro* fertilization is beyond the scope of this chapter, but further details are presented in Chapter 21.

The male with excessively delayed sexual maturation can be treated with androgens to induce development of facial and body hair, deepening of the voice, enlargement of the penis, and an increase in libido and erections. In addition, androgens and anabolic steroids promote the development of both increased muscle and bone mass. These normal pubertal changes in the male can be essential for the development of a healthy self-image as well as normal sexual potency and relationships.

In the young man with excessive pubertal delay, testosterone may be started at low doses and gradually increased to mimic the process of normal puberty. The preferred drugs for androgen replacement are insoluble esters of testosterone, such as testosterone enanthate and testosterone cypionate. These are given by depot injection, where they are absorbed slowly into the circulation over a prolonged period of time. Typical starting doses for a boy with delayed puberty are 100 to 200 mg intramuscularly every 3 to 4 weeks. After an initial therapeutic trial of 6 to 12 months, further therapy should be suspended to determine whether endogenous testosterone production has become sufficient to sustain pubertal development. Plasma testosterone levels greater than 300 ng/dL usually are sufficient for maintenance of male secondary gender characteristics. For hypogonadal adult males, a typical dose is 300 to 400 mg every 3 to 4 weeks. Testosterone also is available for transdermal administration in the form of medicated patches that are applied to the skin. Although this form of administration is more expensive, it can mimic more closely the normal diurnal rhythm of testosterone secretion and may be more convenient for some patients. Synthetic analogues of testosterone, such as methyltestosterone, have the advantage of being active when taken orally, but are more likely to have undesirable side effects, such as liver toxicity.

In practice, there is little that can be done to promote fertility in the male with azoospermia. Reconstructive surgery to correct the anatomic defect in the spermatic ducts currently is not available. Semen analysis is appropriate in all adult males with CF because patients rarely will have adequate sperm to allow fertility. Further, appropriate counseling is important to enable the patient to adapt to a successful marital relationship. If the likelihood of infertility is disclosed too early, a boy may be unable to clearly differentiate between potency and fertility; if it is disclosed too late, it may create unnecessary marital conflicts (22). Ideally, a young man should understand the problem of infertility sufficiently to discuss it with a potential mate.

It should be emphasized that surveys of married individuals of both genders with CF have shown that sexual problems, although common, are not dramatically more frequent than they are in the general population. In one survey of 30 married patients with CF, 11 marriages were rated by both partners as "aproblematic" and 6 as "good" from the standpoint of sexual relationships (31). In another study of single adult male patients with CF, 63% considered themselves to be "sexually healthy" compared with 72% of age-matched controls (32). As one might expect, sexually healthier male subjects also showed better physical health overall, including more normal physical examination results and vital capacity. Single females with CF as a group had less cognitive desire for sexual contact and greater difficulty in achieving an orgasm. However, 82% reported that they were satisfied, overall, with their sexual lives (32).

THE ENDOCRINE PANCREAS, GLUCOSE HOMEOSTASIS, AND DIABETES

Diabetes is becoming an increasing problem as more individuals with CF survive to adulthood. In 1979, a study from the National Institutes of Health predicted that diabetes would develop in 15% of adult patients with CF (33). In 1991, another survey of patients with CF 25 years of age and older reported that only 35% had normal glucose tolerance, whereas 32% had clinical diabetes and 33% had glucose intolerance (34). The Cystic Fibrosis Registry of 20,096 patients seen in North American clinics in 1995 reported a 5.1% incidence of diabetes mellitus (DM) requiring insulin (35). The incidence in the United States among patients older than 18 years of age was 12.3%. Individual CF centers report a 5% to 15% incidence of clinical diabetes in their patients (36–38). In conclusion, diabetes affects 5% to 15% of patients with CF overall, but as many as 30% of adult patients with CF. The incidence of diabetes in CF increases with age, suggesting that many patients have subclinical disease that will become clinically manifest if they live long enough.

Pathophysiology

All forms of DM are characterized by inability to maintain normal levels of blood glucose and an absolute or relative deficiency of insulin. The most important mechanisms of glucose intolerance, however, vary among different groups of diabetic patients. CF-related diabetes mellitus (CF-DM) resembles classic insulin-dependent diabetes mellitus (IDDM) or juvenile-onset diabetes because both primarily are caused by insulin deficiency, but it differs markedly from noninsulin-dependent diabetes mellitus (NIDDM). Some of the differences between CF-DM, IDDM, and NIDDM are summarized in Table 18–4.

There is little association between the development of diabetes and the severity of pulmonary disease (37), but a strong association exists between pancreatic exocrine insufficiency and impaired pancreatic endocrine function (39). Patients with CF in whom clinical diabetes develops are more likely to have experienced increasing pancreatic insufficiency (PI) in the years before the diagnosis of diabetes (40). Lanng et al. (41) has reported in a Danish population that the common CF genetic defect ΔF508 is associated with PI but not with CF-DM. In contrast to these findings, Hamdi et al. (42) found that in 21 patients older than 18 years of age, CF-DM was more common in ΔF508 homozygotes than in ΔF508 heterozygotes. In a survey of 1,348 European patients

TABLE 18–4. *Comparison between common forms of insulin-dependent diabetes mellitus (IDDM), non-insulin-dependent diabetes mellitus (NIDDM), and cystic fibrosis–related diabetes mellitus (CF-DM)*

	IDDM	NIDDM	CF-DM
Epidemiology			
Incidence in population at risk	1%	10%	8–15%
Presentation	Abrupt	Gradual	Gradual
Peak age of onset (yrs)	10–19	> 40	20–25
Genetic markers			
HLA	HLA types DR3, DR4	No specific HLA types	No specific HLA types (CF genotypes associated with pancreatic exocrine insufficiency)
Immunology			
Antiislet cell antibodies	Present at onset	Absent	May be present secondarily
Hormonal status			
C-peptide levels	Absent or very low	Normal	Decreased
Fasting insulin levels	Absent or very low	Normal or increased	Decreased
Early phase insulin secretion	Absent	Delayed	Reduced and delayed
Overall insulin production	Very low	Normal or increased	Decreased
Glucagon levels	Elevated	Elevated	Normal or low
Clinical features			
Nutritional status	Thin or normal	Obese	Thin
Acute complications	Common (DKA)	Uncommon (hyperosmolar coma)	Uncommon
Long-term complications	Common	Common	Possible
Insulin responsiveness	Normal	Impaired	Normal or increased
Response to sulfonylureas	Unresponsive	Responsive	Variable

HLA, human leukocyte antigen.

with CF, DM was more common in patients homozygous for ΔF508, probably because of the increased frequency of PI (43).

Histopathology

Impaired exocrine function of the pancreas, seen in greater than 90% of adult patients with CF, is associated with ductal blockage, dilation, and fatty replacement. Early reports described "strangulation" of islets by progressive distortion of pancreatic parenchyma (44). Presumably, diabetes was the result of simple physical destruction of islet tissue. More recent studies find a relatively loose correlation between severity of exocrine dysfunction and endocrine dysfunction and suggest that functional changes may occur in the mechanisms controlling insulin secretion (45).

Recent histopathologic studies of islet tissues have advanced our understanding of the pathophysiology of CF-DM. Table 18–5 summarizes the results of several studies of autopsy tissues using cytochemical staining to define changes in distinct islet cell populations. At autopsy, pancreatic tissue from patients with CF, both with and without diabetes, showed an overall loss of islet cells, reduced volume of surviving islets, and alterations of the proportions of cells in remaining islet populations (46–49). Patients with CF-DM have a more severe loss of beta cells, a relative increase in delta cells, and diminished or unchanged alpha cells. Patients with CF without diabetes have changes intermediate between healthy subjects and patients with CF-DM. The loss of beta cells appears to follow a continuum from CF non-DM to CF-DM (Table 18–5). Although the percentage of alpha cells, delta cells, and pancreatic polypeptide (PP) cells in the remaining population actually may increase in CF-DM, the absolute number of these cells in the pancreas may decrease. The overall volume of islet cells is reduced by 42% in patients with CF-DM compared with individuals with CF but not DM (48).

In addition to the loss of beta cells, islet tissue from patients with CF-DM frequently contains amyloid deposits similar to those seen in patients without CF with NIDDM (50). Islet amyloid was detected in 69% of patients with CF with diabetes, 17% of patients with impaired glucose tolerance, and no patients with normal glucose tolerance. The amyloid in both NIDDM and CF-DM is derived from an islet amyloid polypeptide produced within the beta cells and normally secreted together with insulin. Whether such amyloid plays an essential role in the dysfunction or loss of beta cells is unknown, but its presence suggests that the pathogenesis of diabetes in CF may have features in common with the pathogenesis of NIDDM.

Unlike IDDM, there is little evidence that the beta cell destruction in CF-DM is initiated

TABLE 18–5. *Composition of islet cell populations by cell subset in healthy subjects and patients with cystic fibrosis*

Reference	No. of patients	% α	% β	% Δ	% PP cells
Healthy subjects					
Soejima and Landing (48)	Historic controls	18	73–77	4.5	
Abdul-Karim et al. (47)	10	22.3	53.4	15.5	
Lohr et al. (49)	6	23.2	64.4	10.4	2
Cystic fibrosis without DM					
Ianucci et al. (46)	4	26.5	62.5	10.6	0.8
Soejima and Landing (48)	34	43	42.4	11.9	
Abdul-Karim et al. (47)	4	25.4	46.7	26.2	
Cystic fibrosis with DM					
Ianucci et al. (46)	5	33.8	47.4	17.8	1
Soejima and Landing (48)	6	39	30	15	
Abdul-Karim et al. (47)	7	21.9	28.3	29.3	

DM, diabetes mellitus; PP, pancreatic polypeptide.

by an autoimmune process. In one series, anti-islet cell antibodies have been found in 15% of 46 patients with CF compared with 0.5% in control populations. In patients with CF with glucose intolerance, the prevalence of antibodies may increase to as high as 25%. Islet cell antibodies also become more prevalent in patients with CF with increasing age (51). This suggests that the formation of antibodies may occur secondarily with ongoing pancreatic damage. The occurrence of islet cell antibodies in patients with CF is not associated with the HLA histocompatibility antigens DR3 and DR4 that are found in patients with typical autoimmune IDDM.

Alterations in Insulin Secretion

Recent physiologic studies have corroborated histopathologic observations and clarified the nature of the hormonal aberrations accompanying CF diabetes. As suggested by the reduced number of beta cells, patients with CF-DM are insulinopenic. A lesser degree of beta cell dysfunction also occurs in patients with CF but not DM. The insulin response occurring within the first 5 minutes after intravenous (IV) glucose is the most sensitive indicator of beta cell integrity. In patients with CF-DM, the early insulin response to both intravenous and oral glucose always is delayed or blunted. (39,52) A substantial proportion of patients with CF without diabetes also have a reduced early-phase insulin response (40).

Moran et al. (39) reported a continuum of declining early-phase C-peptide responses to IV and oral glucose in the following three subsets of patients with CF: (a) patients with pancreatic sufficiency (PS); (b) patients with PI; and (c) patients with PI with DM (PI-DM). Patients with PS had normal glucose tolerance but a delayed C-peptide response to intravenous glucose. Patients with PI showed a more marked delay in the C-peptide response to oral glucose and a markedly deficient response to intravenous glucose. The PI group also had diminished C-peptide responses to IV arginine. The PI-DM group had severely reduced C-peptide responses to oral glucose and

elevated blood glucose levels. This group also showed the most deficient C-peptide response to IV glucose. In contrast to patients with classic IDDM, none of the patients with CF-DM showed a total loss of C-peptide response. The residual capacity for insulin secretion in most patients with CF-DM probably is sufficient to protect them from development of diabetic ketoacidosis, where circulating insulin levels typically are very low or unmeasurable.

In classic IDDM. 80% to 90% of beta cells must be lost before diabetes ensues, whereas CF-DM can occur with the loss of only 50% of the beta cells (see Table 18–5). Because the loss of insulin secretion may be greater in some patients than can be explained by the loss of beta cells alone, mechanisms involving other islet cell hormones may contribute to the observed abnormalities in glucose regulation.

Somatostatin, a product of delta cells in the pancreatic islets, inhibits the secretion of both insulin and glucagon. It may play a physiologic role as a paracrine regulator of insulin secretion (53). Like insulin and glucagon, somatostatin secretion is stimulated by increased serum levels of certain amino acids, including arginine. There is a relative sparing or an actual increase in delta cells in some forms of experimental diabetes, including diabetes induced by administration of streptozocin to rats (54). Thus, it is of interest that patients with CF-DM exhibit an increased somatostatin release in response to arginine, compared with controls (55). Increased somatostatin could worsen the deficient insulin response in CF-DM by inhibiting beta cell function locally. The inhibition of glucagon by excess somatostatin also might contribute to diminished glucagon secretion under similar conditions. The elevation of somatostatin in patients with CF-DM does not inhibit growth hormone release (56). The changes occurring in islet cell populations and their possible effects on insulin secretion are illustrated in Figure 18–3.

Glucagon, produced by the alpha cells, is an insulin counterregulatory hormone that increases blood glucose. In CF-DM, basal glucagon levels generally are normal but the glucagon response to stimuli may be subnormal (34,39). Patients

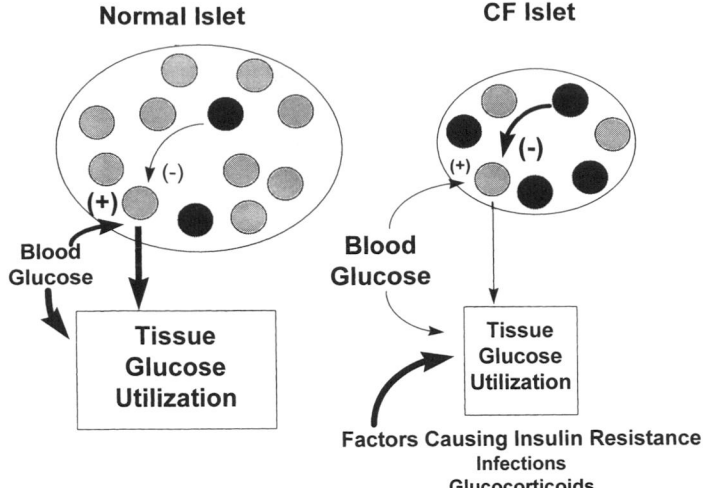

FIG. 18–3. Changes in insulin secretion and glucose homeostasis occurring in cystic fibrosis. Total islet volume and cell number are decreased as pancreatic damage occurs. Within individual islets, there is a disproportionately larger loss of β cells (*light circles*) than of δ cells (*dark circles*). This may lead to an increased inhibitory effect on insulin secretion by somatostatin. The insulin secretory response to hyperglycemia is decreased. Tissue responsiveness to insulin usually remains normal but may be diminished by factors such as infection or glucocorticoid administration. The end result is hyperglycemia and clinical diabetes mellitus.

with CF-DM resemble patients with long-standing IDDM because they have greatly reduced glucagon responses to hypoglycemia. In contrast to patients with IDDM, who generally maintain a glucagon response to arginine, patients with CF-DM show show a greatly reduced glucagon response to this agent (39). This underproduction of glucagon in patients with CF-DM may spare them from the profound hyperglycemia and ketoacidosis seen in patients with type 1 DM. Recovery from insulin-induced hypoglycemia still occurs normally in most patients with CF-DM, probably by other counterregulatory mechanisms (39).

Tissue Responsiveness to Insulin

Glucose intolerance and diabetes can occur as a result of increased resistance to the effects of insulin as well as to insulin deficiency. In typical NIDDM, insulin resistance associated with obesity is a primary cause of defective glucose regulation. In such patients, the principal target tissues, muscle, adipose tissue, and liver, all show diminished responses. Insulin resistance also can result occasionally from increased metabolic clearance or degradation of circulating insulin. In patients with CF, insulin resistance may occur but seldom is a major factor in the pathogenesis of diabetes.

Peripheral use of glucose is modulated in part by alterations in the number and affinity of insulin receptors. In patients with CF, peripheral insulin receptor numbers are increased, possibly in response to the poor nutritional state, but their affinity may be decreased (57). Several investigators have measured tissue responsiveness in CF using the euglycemic clamp technique, giving a constant insulin infusion and maintaining blood glucose at a fixed level by varying the rate of glucose infusion. The metabolic clearance rate for insulin can be estimated using the same technique. Insulin clearance was found to be increased in both CF-DM and patients with CF but not DM, suggesting that insulin may be cleared more rapidly by the CF kidney. (58,59). In those patients who maintain normal glucose tolerance, there may be a compensatory increase in the insulin responsiveness of peripheral tissues to make up for lower prevailing insulin levels. In those patients in whom diabetes develops, peripheral insulin responsiveness may instead be decreased, contributing further to hyperglycemia. The etiology and pathogenic significance of the degree of insulin resistance measured under these experimental conditions still is unclear. Experience with insulin therapy in patients with CF-DM, however, suggests that in the absence of infection or corticosteroid administration, clinical insulin resistance is an uncommon event.

Clinical Manifestations and Diagnosis

Diabetes occurring in patients with CF typically is gradual and insidious in onset. An elevated blood glucose level on routine testing often is the means of diagnosis. Patients may have intermittent periods of hyperglycemia, often precipitated by infections, corticosteroid administration, or increased glucose administration during hyperalimentation, alternating with periods of euglycemia. More patients with CF are undergoing double lung transplantation. At the University of North Carolina (UNC), CF-DM is seen in more than 50% of transplanted patients compared with 20% to 30% before surgery. After transplant, increased food intake, steroid use, and cyclosporine-inhibited insulin release may exacerbate CF-DM. Even when hyperglycemia is established permanently, ketonuria and ketosis are uncommon. Patients with CF-DM often experience symptoms of weight loss and fatigue, but these may be attributed to the underlying long and pancreatic disease. Polyuria and polydipsia also may be overlooked.

Even though it may be easy to control, the development of diabetes has serious implications for the patient with CF. Retrospective analysis of patients enrolled in the Cystic Fibrosis Centre in Copenhagen showed that exocrine pancreatic function, body mass index, and pulmonary function in patients in whom diabetes is destined to develop began to deviate from controls 2 to 4 years before the onset of diabetes (60). A report from the University of Minnesota Cystic Fibrosis Center suggested increased mortality in patients with CF with diabetes (61). These results have been challenged because the overall survival rate of the patients with CF-DM has been similar to the national average for all patients with CF (62). The patients with CF but not DM had a survival of 40 years, exceeding the national expected survival rate.

In patients with classic IDDM, long-term diabetic complications due to microangiopathy are a major cause of death and disability. Microangiopathic complications also are likely to develop in patients with CF-DM if they survive 10 or more years beyond the diagnosis of diabetes. The number of patients in this category has been limited until now, but it is increasing. Sullivan and Denning (63) reported the occurrence of diabetic retinopathy, nephropathy, or neuropathy in 4 of 19 patients with CF-DM under their care.

Diabetes Screening and Diagnosis

The diagnosis of diabetes should be based primarily on blood glucose levels, as summarized in Table 18–6. Because measurements may vary from time to time depending on intercurrent illness, nutrition, and drugs, the diagnosis should be confirmed by two fasting blood glucose tests > 126 mg/dL.

The importance of screening and the value of earlier diagnosis of diabetes in CF has not been evaluated formally in a controlled clinical study. Because effective therapy for diabetes does exist and untreated diabetes may lead to complications, it is reasonable to seek an early diagnosis. A Cystic Fibrosis Consensus Statement on CF-DM (64) recommends screening by a casual blood glucose every year. Hospitalized patients should have a fasting and 2-hour postmeal glucose. If abnormal glucose levels are seen during acute infection, blood glucose should be rechecked when the acute infection is cleared. Glycosylated hemoglobin (HbA1c) is a relatively insensitive screening test for patients and is not recommended for screening.

Diabetes Management in Cystic Fibrosis

There is a growing body of evidence that good control of blood glucose levels reduces

TABLE 18–6. *Criteria for the diagnosis of diabetes in adults*

	Casual glucose (mg/dL)	Fasting glucose (mg/dL)	OGTT 2 hr glucose (mg/dL)
Normal glucose tolerance	<126	<126	<200
CF diabetes mellitus	≥126	≥126	>200
	Requires further testing	Requires further testing	

OGTT, oral glucose tolerance test.

the incidence of long-term complications in IDDM. The Diabetes Control and Complications Trial compared the development of early retinopathy, nephropathy, and neuropathy in a large group of patients with recent-onset IDDM (65). In this 10-year randomized trial, patients were assigned to either a standard treatment group (1 or 2 daily insulin injections) or an intensive treatment group (multiple daily injections or an insulin pump). Average preprandial glucose levels in the intensive treatment group were approximately 150 mg/dL, and glycosylated hemoglobin levels averaged 7% (normal < 6.5%). In the standard treatment group, preprandial glucose levels were approximately 200 to 250 mg/dL, and glycosylated hemoglobin levels averaged 9%. As one might expect, hypoglycemic complications were more common in the intensive treatment group. Intensive treatment also caused a 34% to 76% reduction in the onset and progression of early microangiopathic complications in these young, relatively healthy adults. Intensive therapy of 10 years or more probably would have been required to demonstrate a meaningful difference in clinical morbidity or functional outcomes.

It is unknown whether intensive insulin therapy will prove equally beneficial in patients with CF-DM. No randomized studies in the medical therapy of CF-DM have been done. A retrospective study of 18 patients with CF-DM started on insulin found improvement in pulmonary function and severity of pulmonary infection. These patients with CF-DM had declining lung function and body mass before the diagnosis of DM and initiation of therapy. Insulin therapy correlated with more stable pulmonary

function and increased body mass, suggesting that aggressive insulin treatment was effective because of the deleterious effect of uncontrolled diabetes on pulmonary function (66). Proponents of less aggressive treatment suggest that the reduced life expectancy of patients with CF, their greater susceptibility to hypoglycemia, and the added burdens of caring for a second chronic disease all are factors mitigating against intensive therapy. The Cystic Fibrosis Consensus Conference of 1998 (64) recommended therapy sufficient to achieve optimal metabolic functions and normal growth with minimal hypoglycemia. Ideally, the care giver and patient together should set realistic and achievable goals when initiating or revising diabetic therapy. An initial treatment plan should take into account the factors shown in Figure 18–4. These include the severity of glucose intolerance, as judged by the glycosylated hemoglobin level and the fasting blood glucose; the patient's nutritional status; the existence of any diabetic complications; and the patient's ability to follow a treatment regimen. Any potentially reversible factors contributing to hyperglycemia should be corrected, if possible. Based on the severity of glucose elevation and the tendency of ketosis to develop, it is possible to develop an initial approach for each individual.

Patients having only glucose intolerance, as defined by the criteria in Table 18–6, usually can be managed by dietary modification alone. Patients with mild diabetes with fasting glucose levels in the range of 140 to 200 mg/dL and glycosylated hemoglobin levels of less than 10% may be candidates for a trial of oral hypoglycemic agents. Patients with more severe hyperglycemia and glycosylated hemo-

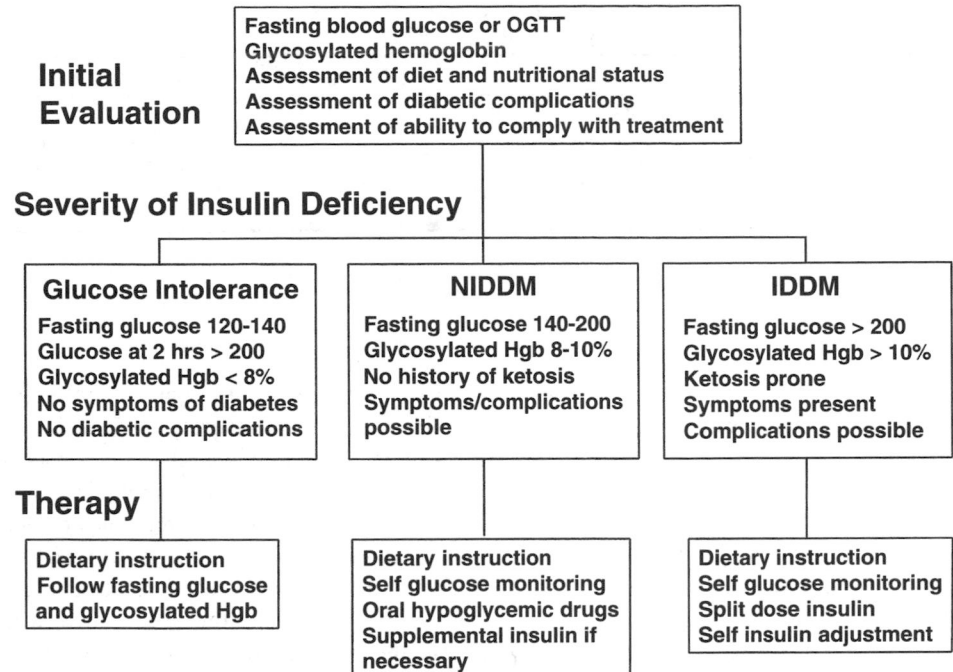

FIG. 18–4. Proposed clinical strategy for management of diabetes in patients with cystic fibrosis based on severity of insulin deficiency. Patients with glucose intolerance but without clinical diabetes usually can be managed with diet and observation. Those with more severe glucose elevations, but with sufficient retention of endogenous insulin secretion to avoid ketosis, often respond adequately to oral hypoglycemic drugs. Insulin supplements may be required during interim infections when insulin resistance increases. Patients without significant endogenous insulin secretion and a tendency toward ketosis require insulin, usually administered at least twice daily. Patients may shift from a milder category to a more severe category because of progressive loss of insulin secretory capacity. For further details, see the text.

globin levels greater than 10% ordinarily should be started on insulin, especially if they have ketonuria or a history of ketoacidosis.

Diet

Dietary management is important in both mild and severe diabetes. The preexisting nutritional problems in CF necessitate a dietary plan that is quite different from the usual recommendation for diabetics, as compared in Table 18–7. Nutritional status often will be impaired more by CF than by diabetes. Assessment may reveal poor weight gain in children or adolescents, weight loss in adults, and decreased somatic energy stores. The combination of increased energy requirements and inadequate calorie intake often demands that a priority be placed on energy supplementation. Thus, the ideal energy intake for a patient with CF-DM may be 100% to 200% of the recommended daily allowance (RDA), whereas for the patient with diabetes alone, it may be 100% or less. Recommended fat intake also is higher for the patient with CF-DM because this affords a way in which total caloric intake may be increased without increasing the bulk amount of food consumed. In addition, the intake of mono- and disaccharides, normally restricted in diabetics, is less restricted in patients with CF-DM to increase overall energy intake. Meals and snacks should be encouraged

TABLE 18–7. *Comparison of dietary recommendations for diabetic patients with and without cystic fibrosis (CF)*

Category	Diabetics without CF	Diabetics with CF
Total energy	100% or less of RDA	100–200% of RDA
Fat content	30% of total calories	30–40% of total calories
Mono-disaccharides	Limited or no intake	Negligible restriction
Salt	Lower than average	Higher than average
No. of meals/snacks	Scheduled and structured	As frequently as possible

Data from reference 64, pp. 3–4.

as frequently as possible and insulin dosage adjusted, as necessary, to meet the intake. As in diabetes without CF, insulin management can be much more successful when snacks are eaten on a predictable regular basis. Pancreatic enzyme replacement must be timed properly to allow assimilation. Enzyme capsules are not needed to cover snacks that contain primarily carbohydrates. Patients treated with insulin must be instructed to have an easily absorbable source of glucose on hand in the event of hypoglycemia. Glucose tablets or gels are available at pharmacies for this purpose.

Oral Hypoglycemics and Insulin

Patients with CF with documented diabetes usually will require hypoglycemic drugs for effective management. Experience with oral hypoglycemic agents is limited in CF, but their greater ease of use warrants a trial in stable patients with milder degrees of glucose intolerance. A recent survey of European CF clinics found 71% of diabetic patients being treated with insulin and 27% being treated with sulfonylureas (38).

The sulfonylureas act primarily by increasing endogenous insulin secretion and secondarily by decreasing peripheral resistance to insulin (67). Zipf et al. (68) have reported a beneficial effect on growth and body composition when sulfonylureas are used in children with CF but only mild glucose intolerance. Because patients with CF-DM rarely have complete insulin deficiency, one would expect most of them to be at least partially responsive

to these agents. Sulfonylureas are unlikely to be effective in more severely underweight patients or in those taking high-dose corticosteroids or those having intercurrent infections. They are contraindicated in pregnancy or in ketosis-prone diabetes. The current sulfonylureas of choice are the so-called second-generation drugs glipizide and glyburide, both of which are metabolized in the liver to inactive derivatives and are active for up to 24 hours. These drugs should be started at a low dose of 2.5 to 5 mg per day and adjusted upward to a maximum dose of 20 mg per day. At daily doses of 10 mg or more, it may be preferable to administer them twice a day. A sustained release form of glipizide currently is available that, when administered once daily at dosages of 5 to 10 mg, provides 24-hour coverage with fewer risks of hypoglycemia.

Insulin should be used initially in patients with more severe diabetes, especially in those who are ketosis prone, severely malnourished, or acutely infected (see Figure 18–4). Insulin also is indicated in those patients who are not adequately controlled with oral agents, as evidenced by glycosylated hemoglobin levels persistently greater than 8% or fasting blood glucose levels averaging more than 150 mg/dL. The insulin dose should be adjusted to maintain glycemic control when the patient is eating a diet adequate for caloric needs. In most patients with CF, twice-daily injections using a mixture of short- and intermediate-acting insulin will provide good control. Typically, the morning dose (administered before breakfast) will be larger than the evening dose (administered before supper) because a larger proportion of calories is consumed during the day. Once-a-day injection regimens tend to be less satisfactory because administration of a large-enough dose in the morning to achieve 24-hour coverage is more likely to cause hypoglycemia during the day. During the initial adjustment period, and whenever there is evidence of unsatisfactory control, glucose monitoring should be done before meals and at bedtime for appropriate adjustments of dosage. Once adjustments have been made successfully and dietary intake is stable, many diabetics can be maintained with glucose monitoring only before breakfast and supper. More intensive insulin regimens with a single dose of ultra-long acting insulin once daily and injections of a short-acting insulin before each meal may be used but are more demanding in terms of monitoring requirements and also more likely to produce hypoglycemia. Minimally, the goals of treatment should be to maintain the patient free of hyperglycemic symptoms and acute diabetic complications, to maintain adequate nutrition and body weight, and to avoid serious hypoglycemic reactions. It usually is possible in compliant patients on a split-dose regimen to maintain fasting glucose levels at less than 150 mg/dL and glycosylated hemoglobin levels at less than 8%. Hayes et al. (69) reported that in 22 patients with insulin-requiring CF-DM treated with two to three injections for 1 year, glycosylated hemoglobin levels were reduced from 11.3% to 7.7% and body weight increased 3.1 kg (69).

Hyperalimentation often will require temporary insulin administration in patients who otherwise have only mild glucose intolerance. One method for providing insulin to patients receiving parenteral hyperalimentation is to add regular insulin to the total parenteral nutrition (TPN) solution at a ratio of one unit of insulin for every 4 to 8 g of carbohydrate. Patients receiving enteral hyperalimentation may require slow infusions of regular insulin or intermittent small subcutaneous injections while the infusion pump is operating. Glucose should be monitored frequently during such infusions to avoid both extreme hyperglycemia and hypoglycemia.

ADRENAL CORTICOSTEROIDS AND ADRENAL CORTICAL FUNCTION IN CYSTIC FIBROSIS

The most important considerations involving adrenal corticosteroids and CF are those related to the use of high-dose glucocorticoids in the therapy of CF lung disease. Spontaneous adrenal cortical insufficiency (Addison's disease) and hyperfunction (Cushing's syndrome) are no more common in individuals with CF than they are in the general population. However, iatrogenic corticosteroid excess is becoming an increasingly common problem in the adult population of patients with CF, many of whom are being treated with high doses of glucocorticoids for varying intervals during their increasing lifetimes. The clinician caring for the patient with CF should understand both the benefits and risks of long-term corticosteroid therapy.

Effects of Corticosteroids on Lung Disease in Cystic Fibrosis

All classes of steroid hormones, including glucocorticoids, act by a similar mechanism. After diffusing into the target cell, the steroid binds to a specific cytoplasmic receptor, causing conformational changes, leading to dimerization and formation of an active steroid-receptor complex. The complex then interacts with specific sequences of DNA on steroid-responsive genes to affect gene expression. The end result of the interaction between the activated glucocorticoid receptor and the genome is the increased (or decreased) accumulation of specific mRNAs within the cell. Changes in the concentration of specific mRNAs ultimately lead to changes in the rate of synthesis of specific proteins that mediate the biological effects of the steroid. Some, but by no means all, of the functional proteins regulated by glucocorticoids are known. Some steroid-dependent proteins are known to be rate-limiting enzymes in important metabolic pathways, such as gluconeogenesis. Others, such as collagen, are essential structural proteins. At higher concentrations, glucocorticoids also affect the synthesis of individual cytokines and key enzymes that mediate immune and inflammatory responses. These latter effects generally are suppressive and are the basis for the use of glucocorticoids as antiinflammatory and immunosuppressant drugs. A detailed discussion of the mechanisms involved is available in several reviews (70,71).

Clinical studies in CF suggest that interleukins (ILs), including IL-1, IL-2, IL-8, and tumor necrosis factor-α (TNF-α) are produced in excess in response to chronic infection (72). These cytokines have chemotactic effects on polymorphonuclear leukocytes and can induce their degranulation, releasing elastase and other proteases. IL-1 and IL-2 also promote proliferation of B lymphocytes and production of immunoglobulins. Increased activity of neutrophil phospholipase A_2 and 5-lipoxygenase leads to increased production of bronchoconstrictive leukotrienes and cyclooxygenase products (thromboxanes and prostaglandins). Colonization of the lung by organisms such as *Aspergillus fumigatus* and mucoid strains of *Pseudomonas aeruginosa* activates immune cells and cytokine production. Although the resulting inflammatory response often is inadequate to eradicate the infection, the damaging effects of inflammation on surrounding lung tissues may be severe and eventually irreversible.

The rationale for the use of glucocorticoids in this setting is to inhibit excessive inflammation, to improve pulmonary function, and to preserve normal pulmonary tissue. Under certain conditions, this ideal may be realized. The most clear-cut benefits from corticosteroid therapy are in allergic bronchopulmonary aspergillosis (73). The benefits of corticosteroids in patients with stable CF lung disease are more uncertain (72). In one clinical trial, longterm administration of prednisolone (2 mg/kg) on alternate days had beneficial effects on pulmonary function, nutritional status, and the need for hospitalization, but the incidence of systemic side effects was unacceptably high (74,75). Preliminary reports indicate that inhaled budesonide in adult patients with CF can bring about reduced bronchial hyperrespon-

siveness to histamine and improved symptom scores, but not improved spirometry results (76).

A more recent use of glucocorticoids is for immunosuppression after lung transplantation in patients with end-stage CF lung disease. In this setting, glucocorticoids are used routinely in very high doses in conjunction with other immunosuppressants for periods of weeks or months after surgery. In successful transplants, it is may be possible to lower the steroid dose gradually to the equivalent of 10 to 20 mg of prednisolone every other day, with the expectation that these doses will be maintained indefinitely.

Complications of Corticosteroid Therapy

Most complications of corticosteroids are predictable from their known pharmacologic effects. The likelihood of a complication usually is proportional to the dose of corticosteroid and the duration of time over which it is given. Untoward effects become increasingly common as the dose exceeds two or three times the daily replacement equivalent. Short-term therapy, even with very high doses, usually can be undertaken with little risk. The longer that high doses are continued, the more inevitable are certain complications, such as osteoporosis. Some complications, including many of the manifestations of Cushing's syndrome, occur in virtually all patients given high doses of glucocorticoids over a prolonged period. Other less predictable effects, such as aseptic necrosis of bone or acute pancreatitis, occur in only a small subset of treated patients and may occur either early or late during the course of therapy. The frequency and time relationships of a number of recognized complications are shown in Table 18–8.

Of the effects listed, glucose intolerance is one of the most critical in the patient with CF. Because of the impairment in ß-cell function already present in many individuals with CF, glucocorticoid therapy is more likely to precipitate clinical diabetes, as it increases peripheral resistance to a limited supply of insulin. Chil-

TABLE 18–8. *Frequency of untoward glucocorticoid effects in relation to duration of therapy*

Common	Sporadic
Early effects (days/wks)	
Weight gain	Anaphylactoid reactions
Mood changes	Hypertriglyceridemia
Glucose intolerance	Peptic ulcers
Transient adrenal	Acute pancreatitis
suppression	
Later effects (mos/yrs)	
Central obesity	Aseptic necrosis of bone
Cutaneous fragility	Cataracts
Myopathy	Glaucoma
Osteoporosis	Hypertension
Prolonged adrenal	Opportunistic infections
suppression	

dren will be prone to the complication of arrested growth and permanently short stature. Older, physically inactive patients will be susceptible to osteoporosis, particularly if they have a reduced capacity to absorb calcium and vitamin D because of PI. Patients who are chronically ill or malnourished may tolerate glucocorticoids poorly because of decreased serum steroid-binding proteins and a proportionate increase in levels of active, unbound drug. One of the most frequently seen sporadic effects in a reported clinical trial of corticosteroids in patients with CF was cataracts (74). Whenever corticosteroid therapy is chosen for an individual patient, the physician must carefully consider the balance of benefits and risks.

High doses of glucocorticoids regularly will suppress secretion of both adrenocorticotrophic hormone (ACTH, i.e., corticotropin) and cortisol in all subjects. The degree and duration of suppression depends on the dose and duration of therapy. Typically, a 3-week course of prednisolone at a dose of 20 mg twice a day will result in a reduction in basal serum levels of both ACTH and cortisol for up to 3 days after the drug is discontinued (77). In contrast, patients receiving continuous high doses of corticoids for 1 year or more may require several months off corticosteroids before basal levels of cortisol and ACTH become normal (78). A defective adrenal response to stress may persist even longer. The concern in managing such patients is that stress may precipitate acute adrenal insufficiency if endogenous secretion of cortisol cannot be raised.

Factors to Consider in Planning a Course of Corticosteroid Therapy

The clinician may choose from a large number of available corticosteroid preparations, the most common of which are compared in Table 18–9. Doses of at least 10 times the daily requirement for replacement commonly are required to achieve acute antiinflammatory or immunosuppressive effects. Once these effects are obtained, it often is possible to reduce the dose and maintain therapeutic benefit. The natural corticosteroids hydrocortisone (cortisol) and cortisone seldom are used as antiinflammatory agents because of their significant mineralocorticoid activity. Synthetic glucocorticoids provide the advantage of having little or no salt-retaining activity, although they retain the capacity to induce all the other complications.

In addition to variations in glucocorticoid and mineralocorticoid potency, the available drugs have widely differing durations of action. This is an important variable in designing a dosage schedule to minimize untoward effects. Short- or intermediate-acting glucocorticoids are preferable to long-acting forms for more chronic maintenance because side effects are decreased when glucocorticoid effects are not continuously present. In terms of side effects, giving 40 mg of prednisone as a single dose once a day is better than giving it in divided doses. Giving 80 mg on an every other day treatment regimen is even better, if adequate control of the disease still can be maintained (79). The complication of osteoporosis may be an exception to the general rule that intermittent therapy is preferable to continuous therapy. In one study of patients with bronchial asthma, treatment for 1 year with 25 mg of prednisone on alternate days still resulted in a 3.5% average reduction in trabecular bone mass (80). Retrospective studies of osteoporotic fractures in steroid-treated patients indicate that bone loss may correlate better with

TABLE 18–9. *Relative potency and duration of action of corticosteroid preparations*

	Relative potency		Replacement dose (mg/day)	Plasma half-life (min)	Biologic half-life (hrs)
Compound	Glucocorticoid	Mineralocorticoid			
Hydrocortisone	1.0	1.0	30	80–120	8–12
Cortisone	0.8	0.8	37	80–120	8–12
Prednisolone	4.0	0.8	7	120–300	12–36
Prednisone	3.5	0.7	7.5	120–300	12–36
Methylprednisolone	5	0.5	6	120–180	12–36
Dexamethasone	30	0	1	150–270	24–72

the cumulative dose rather than the dosing interval (81).

Whenever topical or regional corticosteroid therapy can be used effectively, it is preferable to systemic therapy. Many patients with chronic bronchoconstrictive disease can be managed with aerosolized beclomethasone dipropionate or budesonide at doses up to 400 µg per day, causing relatively few systemic side effects (82,83). More clinical trials are needed to determine the efficacy of inhaled glucocorticoids in patients with CF with inflammatory lung disease.

When glucocorticoids are withdrawn after a long period of therapy, symptoms may be the result of recrudescence of the underlying lung disease, adrenal insufficiency, or both. Often, patients may have subjective withdrawal symptoms, such as nausea, lethargy, weakness, and arthralgia, without objective or laboratory evidence of true adrenal insufficiency. In practice, the greatest difficulties in withdrawal are encountered when the underlying inflammatory or immune disease still is present. Disease activity may increase notably when corticosteroids are reduced to a dose that still is well above that required for physiologic replacement. In that case, the lowering must be done very slowly over a number of weeks or months, and a dose equivalent to physiologic replacement may be difficult to reach. Some patients will remain controlled when the dose is lowered gradually only on alternate days, allowing a transition to an alternate-day treatment regimen. Short- or intermediate-acting steroids always should be used when attempting this transition. Mea-

surement of the endogenous plasma cortisol level in the morning before the daily dose is administered can provide laboratory evidence of endogenous adrenal function if there is doubt. Plasma cortisol levels exceeding 10 µg/dL (275 nmol/L) usually indicate that cortisol production is adequate to meet basal needs, although not necessarily adequate to meet conditions of stress.

CALCIUM BALANCE AND BONE DISORDERS

Adult patients with CF are at increased risk for osteoporosis. Multiple causes may contribute to reduced bone mineral density (BMD). Because of prolonged survival of the CF population, sequelae from decreased bone density, such as pathologic fractures, are becoming more clinically significant. Screening and treatment protocols are in evolution.

Incidence and Etiology of Osteopenia in Cystic Fibrosis

Incidence

Osteoporosis is defined as an abnormal decrease in both bone matrix and mineral content. Decreased bone mass also involves a decrease in strength, which predisposes to increased fractures with minimal or no trauma. The term *osteopenia* is a more general term used to describe reduced bone mass either with or without fractures. BMD measurements are used extensively to assess the degree of osteopenia and to assess the risk of fractures. The correlation between reduced BMD and the likelihood of fractures is well established in populations without CF (84).

The incidence of osteoporosis in the CF population is difficult to define precisely because of variation in the techniques for measuring BMD. Several earlier studies assessed peripheral bone using single-photon absorptiometry (SPA), which can evaluate only the appendicular skeleton, composed mainly of cortical bone. The majority of osteoporotic fractures occur in the axial skeleton, which has a greater component of trabecular bone. Disproportionate bone loss in the axial skeleton may occur in patients with CF and not be assessed adequately by techniques measuring primarily cortical bone. Dual-photon absorptiometry (DPA) and dual x-ray absorptiometry (DEXA) assess axial skeleton sites such as the spine and hip. These are the techniques being used in most current studies. Quantitative computed tomography (QCT) also can measure axial spine density but requires more radiation than DEXA.

Table 18–10 provides a summary of the results of several bone density surveys in adults with CF. In an early study, Hahn et al. (85) compared 21 young adults with CF with age-matched controls and found a 14% decrease in bone mass of the radius by SPA. Gibbens and coworkers (86) used QCT to assess lumbar spine density in 57 adult patients with CF and found an overall 10% reduction in bone density. More recently, Grey et al. (87) evaluated 16 adult patients with CF with DEXA and found significantly reduced bone mass at multiple sites. Grey et al. reported that 69% of patients with CF had reductions greater than one SD at the spine when compared with age-matched controls. Overall, the study group had a mean 12.5% reduction of BMD at the lumbar spine and 11.1% at the femoral neck. Other sites in the proximal femur as well as total body BMD were reduced similarly. There was a positive correlation between total body BMD and body mass index. Bachrach et al. (88) reported even more severe BMD reductions of 25% to 35% in 22 adult patients followed at the Stanford Cystic Fibrosis Center. Fifteen of the 22 had reductions of hip or lumbar spine density of greater than two SDs. At the UNC Cystic Fibrosis Center, the bone density of patients with CF appears to fall progressively below

TABLE 18–10. *Results of bone density measurements in adults with cystic fibrosis*

Study (ref)	Subjects (M/F)	Technique	Site(s) surveyed	Results
Hahn et al. (85)	21 (12/9)	SPA	Distal radius	Mean reduction of 14% in bone mass
Gibbens et al. (86)	57 (29/28)	QCT	Lumbar spine	Mean reduction of 10% in bone mass
Grey et al. (87)	16 (8/8)	DEXA	Lumbar spine, proximal femur, total body	Mean reduction of 12.5% in lumbar spine, 11.1% in femoral neck, 10.5% in total body BMD
Bachrach et al. (88)	22 (8/14)	DEXA	Lumbar spine, femoral neck, total body	Mean reduction of 25% and 35% in lumbar spine for women and men, respectively. Similar reductions in femoral neck.
Aris et al. (91)	20 pretransplant, 20 posttransplant	DEXA	Lumbar spine, femur	Mean reductions of 2 SD below predicted in pretransplant patients and 3 SD below predicted in posttransplant patients

BMD, bone mineral density; DEXA, dual x-ray absorptiometry; QCT, quantitative computed tomography; SD, standard deviation; SPA, single-photon absorptiometry.

non-CF controls with increasing age. In a cross-sectional survey of children ages 5 to 18 years, Henderson and Madsen (89) found that the average BMD of patients with CF declined by approximately one SD every 6 to 8 years in comparison with age-matched controls. In a selected group of CF children in Switzerland, Salamoni et al. (90) found no difference between the whole body bone mineral content of well-nourished CF children and controls matched for gender, age, and height, suggesting that osteopenia is not an inevitable consequence of the disease if good nutrition can be maintained. Patients with more severe manifestations of CF tend to have more severe osteoporosis. In two groups of adult patients with CF before and after lung transplantation, Aris et al. (91) found that 75% of the pretransplant patients and 90% of the posttransplant patients had mean bone densities more than two SDs below age-matched controls. The BMDs in these patients correlated with body mass index and the cumulative dose of glucocorticoids (91). Taken as a group, these studies provide strong evidence that abnormally low BMD is more prevalent in patients with CF than in the normal population.

These bone density surveys all have been performed in younger adults with mean age less than 30 years. They predict that fractures will develop later in life in those patients who survive. In epidemiologic studies of older women who do not have CF, a reduction of BMD by one SD increases the risk of fracture 1.5 to 2.5-fold, whereas a reduction of two SDs increases it fourfold or more (84,92). Data on fracture rates in the CF population are limited. The prevalence of pathologic fractures in some selected populations of adult patients with CF, previously anecdotal, may be as high as 10% to 20%. Three of 22 adult patients with CF studied at the Stanford Cystic Fibrosis Center had experienced atraumatic rib fractures, and 1 had experienced hip fracture (88). Among 45 posttransplant patients with CF at the UNC center, 12 fractures had occurred, corresponding to a rate of 225 fractures per 1,000 person years (91). This rate is comparable to fracture rates reported in postmenopausal women with severe osteoporosis.

Etiology

The cause of osteopenia in CF still is unclear. Most likely, there are multiple factors involved. Some of the factors known to be required for the development and maintenance of an adequate bone mass are illustrated in Figure 18–5. These requirements include the intake and absorption of adequate amounts of calcium and phosphorus from the diet and the formation of adequate new bone by osteoblasts. Excessive resorption of bone by osteoclasts or loss of excessive amounts of calcium in the urine can contribute to bone loss. Thus, the maintenance of a positive calcium balance is a precarious process that can be disrupted easily. Peak bone mass is reached in most healthy individuals at approximately 30 years of age. Beyond that, calcium balance tends to be negative, and gradual bone loss ensues. With aging, as bone mass decreases to a critical level, the risk of fractures increases dramatically. Individuals who fail to accumulate an adequate bone mass when they are younger are at increased risk of developing fractures as they grow older. Some of the factors that may contribute to a negative calcium balance in patients with CF are illustrated in Figure 18–6.

The most commonly proposed cause of osteopenia in CF is malnutrition, resulting from PI, steatorrhea, inadequate nutrient absorption, and increased resting energy expenditure. The mechanism by which malnutrition leads to reduced BMD has not been elucidated fully. Decreased body weight may fail to stress bones to promote growth and remodeling. Specific nutrient or mineral deficiency also may contribute. PI leads to malabsorption of fat and critical fat-soluble vitamins, especially vitamin D, which is essential for normal calcium absorption. Generalized malnutrition and low body weight have been correlated consistently with reduced bone density (86,87,93). Poor nutritional status, as assessed by anthropometric measurements, and disease severity, as measured by Schwachman scores, both are corre-

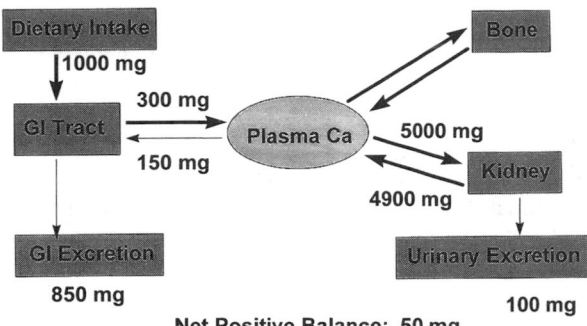

FIG. 18–5. Requirements for a positive calcium balance in the healthy young adult. Dietary calcium intake must be sufficient to allow for a gastrointestinal (GI) absorption of approximately 300 mg per day at a normal absorption efficiency of 30%. There is an obligatory secretion of approximately 150 mg of calcium per day into the gastrointestinal tract. This, plus nonabsorbed dietary calcium, is lost in the stool. Of approximately 5,000 mg per day filtered by the renal glomeruli, 98% or 4,900 mg per day is reabsorbed, causing a net renal loss of 100 mg per day. The net positive body balance of calcium is 50 mg per day, leading to a net gain in skeletal mineral mass.

lated with reduced BMD (86). In a series of 22 adult patients with CF, low body mass index (BMI) and increased disease severity correlated with decreased bone density (87). These patients had normal vitamin D and calcium levels.

Vitamin D deficiency clearly is a factor in some cases of osteomalacia and osteopenia. Vitamin D plays a critical role in gastrointestinal absorption of calcium and is necessary for maintenance of a positive body calcium balance. Serum levels of 25-hydroxyvitamin D (25-OHD) are the best clinical measure of the overall adequacy of vitamin D supply, whereas 1,25-dihydroxyvitamin D (1,25-OH$_2$D) levels reflect the rate at which the biologically active form of the vitamin is being formed within the body. In 21 adolescent patients with CF, low

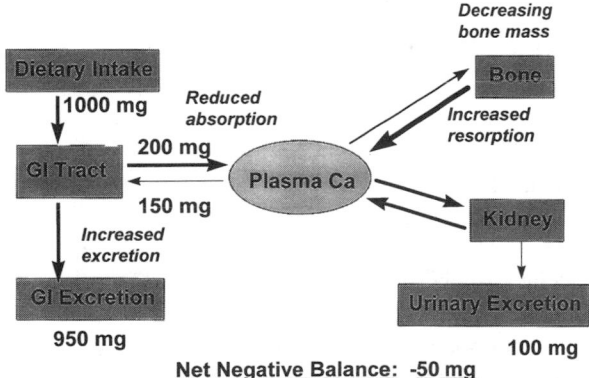

FIG. 18–6. Factors causing a negative calcium balance in the young adult with cystic fibrosis. At the normal dietary intake of 1,000 mg per day, there may be absorption of 200 mg or less because of pancreatic insufficiency and steatorrhea. The obligatory secretion of calcium into the gastrointestinal (GI) tract continues to occur, leading to an excretion of 950 mg per day in the stools. Patients who are physically inactive or who are taking adrenal corticosteroids also will have decreased rates of mineral deposition in bone. The net negative balance is ⁻50 mg per day, leading to a net loss in bone mineral mass.

25-OHD levels correlated with a 14% reduction in BMD (85). In these patients, 25-OHD levels were 36% below normal despite three times the normal intake of vitamin D. In this study, 1,25-$(OH)_2$D was not measured, and only peripheral bone density was assessed. In another early study, 18 patients (ages 6 to 18 years) had low 25-OHD levels but normal bone density as measured by photon beam densitometry of peripheral bone (94). These patients were on a low-fat diet. Most patients with CF no longer receive the low-fat diets prescribed several decades ago. Adequate sunlight is an important factor in the vitamin D supply because it stimulates synthesis of cholecalciferol by the skin. Patients with CF living in northern latitudes in the winter had reduced serum 25-OHD and 1,25 $(OH)_2$ D levels which, however, did not correlate with reduced bone density (95). More recent studies have found normal 25-OHD levels in patients with CF with reduced bone density (86,87). In conclusion, in contrast to earlier studies in which vitamin D replacement might have been inadequate, more recent studies found normal 25-OHD levels, suggesting vitamin D deficiency, per se, is an uncommon or weak correlate of osteopenia. It is possible that gastrointestinal calcium absorption still may be low in some patients with CF despite normal serum levels of vitamin D.

Androgens and estrogens also are important determinants of bone mass. Gender steroid deficiency is associated with increased rates of bone resorption and decreased rates of formation. Inadequate sex steroids during a crucial period of bone development may prevent bone from reaching optimal density and strength, as discussed elsewhere in this chapter. Patients with CF often have a delayed puberty or impaired secretion of sex steroids after puberty (95). Bachrach et al. (88) found low testosterone levels in 7 of 8 adult male patients and amenorrhea in 6 of 14 female patients with CF with osteopenia.

Disease severity has been found to correlate with reduced bone density, but the mechanism remains unknown (86,87). Gibbens et al. (86) found a correlation between low BMD and Shwachman scores. Worse lung function and reduced pulmonary capacity may lead to reduced exercise and inadequate mechanical stress on bone. Cytokines and inflammatory mediators may contribute both to cachexia and bone loss. IL-1 and TNF both promote osteoclastic bone resorption in tissue culture, possibly by stimulating production of IL-6, a direct stimulator of osteoclasts (96). Elevated serum levels of cytokines, such as TNF, in some clinically ill patients with CF may contribute to increased bone-resorbing activity (97,98).

Glucocorticoids, used for treatment of exacerbations of pulmonary disease, have a profound negative effect on BMD. As discussed earlier in this chapter, corticosteroids at high doses reduce calcium absorption, promote calcium excretion, and inhibit osteoblast replication (99). Corticosteroids have a dose-dependent effect on bone density. In a study of patients with asthma, 25 mg of prednisone every other day caused an average reduction in trabecular bone of 3.5% a year. A prednisone dose of 25 mg a day resulted in loss of 17% trabecular bone in 1 year (80). Steroid use also can suppress testosterone and estrogen production. Long-term use of oral steroids in asthma and many other chronic disorders has been associated with osteopenia and fractures.

Clinical Manifestations

Bone loss progresses silently before fractures or bone deformities occur. These fractures typically occur with little or no trauma. The most common osteoporotic fractures in the older non-CF population are those of the vertebral bodies, hip (femoral neck and greater trochanter), and wrist (distal radius). Rib fractures are common in the non-CF population and may be even more common in patients with CF. Fractures of the hip and wrist are clinically obvious because they lead to immediate pain, deformity, and disability. Fractures of the vertebral bodies or ribs also may cause acute pain but sometimes may be overlooked initially because they may be relatively painless.

Healing can occur in osteoporotic bone, but some deformities are irreversible. Compression fractures of the vertebral bodies cause a loss of overall height. Patients with this problem may note shortening of the distance between their shoulders and hips and development of back deformities, including kyphosis and scoliosis. They also may have chronic back pain, especially with prolonged standing.

From the epidemiologic studies already mentioned, one would predict that the adult patient with CF with severe osteoporosis or osteoporotic fractures typically will be one who has more severe pulmonary disease, who is poorly nourished, who has reduced gonadal function, and who has been treated with corticosteroids.

Pathologic fractures occur frequently in the post–lung transplant population. Osteoporotic fractures are likely to become an increasingly common complication after this procedure, especially when there is preexisting bone disease. Lung transplant patients frequently are among the most malnourished and underweight of all patients before surgery. Corticosteroids, given chronically after transplant, often exacerbate previously existing disease (100).

Hypertrophic osteoarthropathy is characterized by swollen painful joints, bone pain, clubbing, and effusions. Joints involved include knees, ankles, wrists, shoulders, and hips. It appears to be correlated with more severe clinical disease. This skeletal complication often presents in young adult patients. A severe form of arthritis in CF had been attributed to circulating immune complexes associated with *Burkholderia cepacia* infection. Treatment of the underlying lung disease may improve symptoms (101). Hypertrophic osteoarthropathy also is associated with other chronic lung infections, tuberculosis, cyanotic heart disease, and biliary cirrhosis.

Clubbing of the distal phalanges occurs in almost all patients with CF. Hyperplasia and hypertrophy in the nail bed result in observable disease. Even very mildly affected patients may demonstrate clubbing. The etiology is unknown. Successful lung transplantation may reverse clubbing.

Evaluation and Management

Bone, once lost, cannot be restored easily, nor can many deformities be reversed. The most effective strategy for management of osteoporosis in patients with CF is prevention. Bone is developed and strengthened during growth in adolescence and childhood. Prevention of osteoporosis in adults with CF begins with proper nutrition and bone development in children. Children with CF should have adequate mineral and vitamin replacement. Proper enzymes are need for fat-soluble vitamin absorption. Gender hormones should be supplemented if there is inadequate maturation. Treatment strategies have been developed for patients diagnosed with osteoporosis. Procedures for evaluation and treatment are outlined in Figure 18–7.

Screening and Risk Assessment

The patient's dietary history, drug history (especially use of corticosteroids), nutritional status, physical activity, and sexual function all are important factors to assess. As recommended in the Cystic Fibrosis Consensus Statement on Nutrition, patients should have weight, height, complete blood counts, albumin, and electrolytes measured yearly. Routine measurements of vitamin D metabolites currently are not recommended.

We recommend that patients with CF with any additional risk factors have baseline measurements of BMD using a technique capable of accurate measurement of axial bone density. Currently, in most medical centers, the preferred technique is DEXA. We have found that DEXA assessment of three sites—spine, proximal femur, and distal radius—is most useful.

In patients with PI and steatorrhea, serum 25-OHD levels will help to ensure that oral intake of vitamin D is adequate. In patients with oligomenorrhea, impaired libido or other evidence of reduced gonadal function, measurements of serum levels of sex steroids (estradiol or testosterone) can help in documenting sex steroid deficiency.

Therapy

The results of BMD measurements, together with the presence of other risk factors, allow a clinical judgment about the degree of risk that

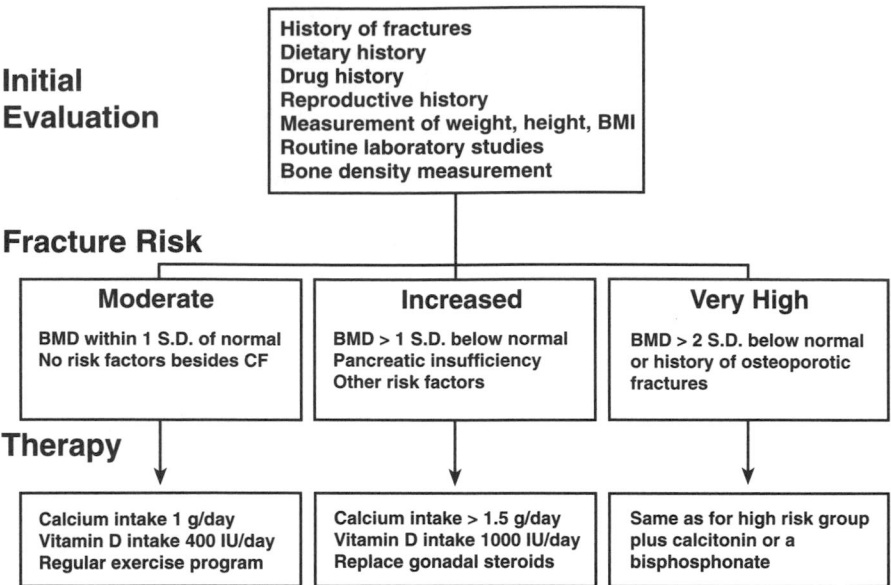

FIG. 18–7. Proposed clinical strategy for evaluation and management of osteopenia in patients with cystic fibrosis based on assessment of fracture risk. The primary method for assessment of fracture risk is measurement of bone mineral density (BMD). Other risk factors, such as pancreatic insufficiency, sex steroid deficiency, and use of adrenal corticosteroids, also are part of the assessment. Existence of either documented osteoporotic fractures or a bone density more than two standard deviations below the mean for an age and gender-matched control population places the individual in the highest risk category. The higher the predicted risk, the more intensive is the recommended therapy. For further details, see the text.

in turn determines the intensity of therapy. The goals of therapy should depend on appropriate endpoints or objectives for the individual patient. Some younger patients may have a normal bone density at the time of assessment but still be at increased risk for the development of osteoporosis because of unavoidable factors, such as the need for corticosteroid therapy. For these individuals, the goals are to prevent bone loss and to maintain existing bone strength. Patients with established osteoporosis already will have a low bone density and may have fractures, deformities, or pain related to their disease. For them, the goals will be to increase bone mass if possible, to prevent further fractures, and to relieve pain.

There have been few therapeutic trials for CF-associated osteoporosis, and the natural history of CF-related bone disease after prolonged survival is unknown. Given these limitations, the therapeutic strategies illustrated in

Figure 18–7 are based largely on clinical experience with osteoporosis in patients who do not have CF, including those with steroid-induced osteoporosis.

Patients with normal bone density and no risk factors other than mild CF should receive at least the RDAs of calcium (1,000 mg per day) and vitamin D (400 international units per day) and engage in regular weight-bearing exercise. Such patients will constitute a minority of the adult CF population.

The majority of individuals are likely to have additional risk factors, such as pancreatic exocrine insufficiency or a BMD more than one SD below normal for their age. These patients should be considered to be in a high-risk category for fractures even though none may have yet developed. For patients in this category, it seems prudent to increase the calcium intake to at least 1,500 mg per day and the vitamin D intake to 1,000 international units per day. Serum 25-OHD levels should be measured during replacement with a target level in the upper range of normal. Regular use of pancreatic enzyme supplements with meals will reduce steatorrhea and improve gastrointestinal efficiency in absorbing the calcium contained in each meal. Women with oligomenorrhea or anovulatory menstrual cycles should be given cyclic estrogen therapy, unless there is a contraindication. Men with low serum testosterone levels should be treated with testosterone replacement.

Patients having a BMD more than two SDs below age-matched normals or a history of prior osteoporotic fractures are in a very high-risk category. In addition to the measures applicable to the aforementioned high-risk group, these patients should be considered candidates for therapy with bone resorption blocking drugs, including calcitonin or bisphosphonates. Short-term clinical trials suggest that these agents can improve bone density in patients with chronic lung diseases and patients on high-dose corticosteroid therapy, although it is unclear yet whether they also can decrease fracture rates.

Bisphosphonates are analogues of pyrophosphate that are incorporated into the hydroxyapatite mineral structure of bone. Once incorporated into the skeleton, these compounds have a very long half-life and can inhibit bone resorption as long as they remain. Several bisphosphonate compounds, including etidronate and alendronate have been shown to be effective both in increasing bone density and decreasing fractures in clinical trials in women with postmenopausal osteoporosis. In a study conducted in the United States by Watts et al. (102), etidronate was administered orally on an intermittent schedule of 400 mg per day for 15 days every 3 months (102). Over the first 2 years of the study, the treated subjects showed a 5% increase in BMD in the lumbar spine and a 50% decrease in vertebral fracture rate compared with controls. With continued treatment, however, the relative advantage shown by the treated group tended to diminish. Etidronate (Didronel) currently is approved in the United States for the treatment of hypercalcemia and

Paget's disease, but not osteoporosis. It is available for both oral (Proctor and Gamble Pharmaceuticals, Cincinnati, OH) and parenteral (MGI Pharma, Inc., Minnetonka, MN) use.

Alendronate (Fosamax, Merck & Co., Inc., West Point, PA) is a more potent second generation bisphosphonate that may provide more sustained benefits when given orally. In a 3-year clinical trial of more than 2,000 postmenopausal women in the United States and Europe, subjects receiving only 10 mg of alendronate per day showed average gains of nearly 10% in spine and 5% in proximal femur BMDs. Spinal fracture rates in the treated subjects were reduced by 48% compared with controls (103). In 1996, alendronate was approved by the U.S. Food and Drug Administration for the treatment of postmenopausal osteoporosis in the United States. It is available for oral administration.

Reid et al. (104) reported a small controlled clinical trial using another bisphosphonate, pamidronate, at a dose of 150 mg per day for 1 year in patients receiving high-dose corticosteroids. The patients receiving pamidronate showed increases in both metacarpal cortical bone area and lumbar spine density, whereas controls, who received only a calcium supplement, showed declines in both of these parameters (104). Pamidronate also has been given by intermittent IV infusion at a dose of 30 mg every 3 months in a pilot study to a group of patients with steroid-dependent asthma or sarcoid lung disease. These patients initially had low BMDs in both the lumbar spine and the proximal femur. After 1 year of therapy, the average BMD had risen significantly by an average of 3.4% in the lumbar spine and had not changed in the femur (105). Presumably, the density would have decreased at both sites without therapy. In the United States, pamidronate (Aredia) is available only for parenteral use and currently is approved for the treatment of hypercalcemia and Paget's disease, but not osteoporosis.

At UNC, an IV pamidronate regimen in several patients with CF with very severe osteoporosis after lung transplantation and steroid administration has improved or stabilized BMD. Our current practice when using bisphosphonates to treat osteoporosis in patients with

CF is to give either pamidronate, 30 mg intravenously every 3 months, or alendronate, 10 mg orally every day, for a period of at least 1 year, with annual measurement of BMD. Future studies should provide more information on the efficacy of the bisphosphonates in CF.

Salmon calcitonin, a peptide hormone, also is effective in reducing rates of bone resorption and is approved by the U.S. Food and Drug Administration for therapy of postmenopausal osteoporosis. Calcitonin is given by subcutaneous injection at doses ranging from 50 to 100 units per day or every other day, or by intranasal administration at a dose of 200 units per day. There are a number of controlled studies documenting improved bone densities in postmenopausal women treated with calcitonin, but few to date demonstrating reduced fracture rates. Calcitonin treatment at a dose of 100 units subcutaneously every other day improved BMD in the radius in a small group of patients with non-CF lung disease receiving corticosteroids (106). In a group of asthma patients, also on corticosteroids, subcutaneous calcitonin at an initial dose of 100 units per day increased BMD in the lumbar spine (107). Calcitonin may have a prolonged benefit after discontinuation of therapy in steroid-dependent asthmatics (108). Intranasal calcitonin at a dose of 200 units per day has been shown to produce significant increases in BMD in postmenopausal women with osteoporosis (109). Side effects of parenteral calcitonin administration, especially nausea, can limit its use in patients already having marginal nutrition. For this reason, intranasal calcitonin, which has fewer side effects, should be a better choice for patients with CF-related osteoporosis. The minimum effective dose of intranasal calcitonin is 200 units per day.

More research is needed to understand the pathophysiology of CF-associated bone disease and its treatment. The clinician who elects to use the more active forms of therapy, such as higher doses of vitamin D, bisphosphonates, or calcitonin, should recognize that the efficacy of such measures still is unproven. Patients treated with these agents should be followed carefully for the occurrence of side effects, and objective methods, such as repeated BMD measurements, should be used to monitor their individual therapeutic responses. As more patients with CF live into adulthood and undergo lung transplantation or even gene therapy, the evaluation and treatment of CF-related osteoporosis should become a routine aspect of care.

DISORDERS OF THYROID HORMONE SECRETION AND METABOLISM

Thyroid disease is relatively common and may occur coincidentally in both children and adults with CF. In addition, changes in thyroid hormone metabolism and secretion may occur secondary to chronic illness due to CF. Thus, the need to evaluate thyroid function and to consider therapy for thyroid disease arises frequently in the patient with established CF. Many of the apparent abnormalities in commonly used thyroid function tests arise not because of intrinsic thyroid disease but because of changes in the extrathyroidal absorption, transport or metabolism of thyroid hormones. Such changes can make it more difficult to recognize and properly treat thyroid disease when it does occur.

Effects of Cystic Fibrosis on Thyroid Function

Intrinsic changes in the structure and function of the thyroid gland can occur in CF, but their significance is uncertain. In some patients with chronic pulmonary infection, secondary amyloidosis affecting the thyroid may develop (110,111). The liver, spleen, adrenal glands, heart, and bowel also may be involved. Patients with amyloidosis involving the thyroid often have goiters, but they rarely have sufficient destruction of thyroid parenchyma to cause hypothyroidism. Developmental disorders of the thyroid also have been described in infants with CF (112), but thyroid dysgenesis probably is no more likely to occur in CF than in the normal population. In general, patients with CF do not appear to have an increased incidence of the more common autoimmune thyroid diseases, such as chronic lymphocytic thyroiditis (Hashimoto's disease) or Graves' disease.

As a chronic illness, CF frequently affects the peripheral transport and metabolism of thyroid hormones. Malnutrition and chronic infection tend to reduce the number of available binding sites for thyroxine (T4) and triiodothyronine (T3) on serum thyroid-binding proteins, especially thyroid-binding globulin and transthyretin (113). The resulting decrease in bound T4 and T3 reduces the circulating concentrations of total T4 and T3. At the same time, 5'-deiodination of T4 to T3 by peripheral tissues, particularly the liver, is reduced in acute and chronic illness. The activity of an alternative deiodination pathway yielding biologically inactive "reverse T3" is enhanced. The result is a profound decrease in the amount of biologically active T3 in the circulation. Systemic inflammation or infection also can suppress TSH secretion, thus leading to a reduced stimulus to the production of both T4 and T3 by the thyroid. These combined changes constitute an adaptation to nonthyroidal illness commonly known as the "sick euthyroid syndrome." The characteristic picture of the patient with the sick euthyroid syndrome is one of low serum T4 levels, even lower serum T3 levels, and a normal or slightly low serum TSH level. Serum levels of reverse T3, if measured, often will be elevated. Recovery of normal thyroid hormone concentration and metabolism occurs when the underlying infection is treated or the nutritional state is improved, suggesting that sick euthyroidism represents a functional adaptation to illness rather than a form of intrinsic thyroid disease. Surveys of patients with CF have shown a high prevalence of reduced circulating T4 and T3 (114). Basal TSH levels commonly are within the normal range, but the increment in T4 and T3 after TRH administration may be reduced.

Some drugs used to treat patients with CF also may induce abnormalities in thyroid function. Iodides, formerly used extensively as expectorants, can suppress thyroid function. In one older prospective study, chronic iodide administration to children with CF resulted in goiter in 50% and caused mild hypothyroidism in some, particularly if they also were treated with sulfonamides (115). High doses of glucocorticoids, sometimes used to treat the inflammatory or allergic components of lung disease, can suppress TSH production and lower circulating thyroid hormone levels.

Finally, the malabsorption resulting from pancreatic exocrine insufficiency can reduce the bioavailability of thyroid hormones given to treat hypothyroidism. The liver excretes thyroxine into the bile as a glucuronide, which then may be reabsorbed after the glucuronide moiety is removed in the gut. The enterohepatic circulation of thyroxine, as well as the absorption of orally administered thyroxine, generally is impaired in diseases causing steatorrhea. Increased fecal losses of thyroxine occur in pancreatic steatorrhea, celiac disease, and inflammatory bowel disease. The subject with normal thyroid function can compensate for these losses by increasing thyroid hormone secretion, but the hypothyroid subject will require larger doses of thyroid hormone replacement. This may be a therapeutic consideration in the hypothyroid patient with CF and PI.

Clinical Manifestations of Thyroid Disease in Cystic Fibrosis

Both hypothyroidism and hyperthyroidism may be overlooked in any patient with another serious chronic illness. Fatigue is a common and nonspecific symptom of both. Weight loss, commonly present in thyrotoxicosis, may be attributed to malabsorption in the patient with CF. Tachycardia may be attributed to pulmonary disease and tremor to side effects from the use of bronchodilators. Pallor, dry skin, and oligomenorrhea, all common in hypothyroidism, also may be seen in any patient with poor nutrition. Goiter in the patient who has not been exposed chronically to iodides should suggest intrinsic thyroid disease.

The key to recognizing thyroid disease is first to suspect it in any patient who demonstrates one or more compatible symptoms and then to perform appropriate laboratory screening tests. For screening purposes, the best test is measurement of the serum TSH using a sensitive radioimmunoassay capable of measuring subnormal as well as high levels. A TSH more than 100% above the upper limit of normal strongly suggests primary hypothyroidism. This diagnosis may be confirmed by measurement of the serum T4, or better, the measurement of the serum-free T4 by a technique such as equilibrium dialysis or ultrafiltration. The latter techniques circumvent many of the problems associated with changes in thyroid hormone-binding proteins in chronically or acutely ill patients. A TSH suppressed to less than 10% of the lower limits of normal almost always indicates clinically significant hyperthyroidism, which may be confirmed by demonstration of an elevated serum-free T4. The rare patient with secondary hypothyroidism due to pituitary disease will have both a low TSH and a low serum-free T4. TSH measurements that are elevated only marginally or are suppressed marginally are more difficult to interpret. Unless the patient has clear-cut signs or symptoms of hypothyroidism or hyperthyroidism, it often is better to repeat the TSH test after a period of observation rather than to treat. Because of the high frequency of low serum levels of T3 in patients with CF, measurement of the serum T3 by radioimmunoassay seldom is a useful test for the diagnosis of intrinsic thyroid disease.

Management of Thyroid Disease in Cystic Fibrosis

Management of thyrotoxicosis usually can be accomplished with either the use of antithyroid drugs (propylthiouracil or methimazole) or thyroid ablation with radioiodine. Complete and lasting remissions with antithyroid drugs alone seldom are obtained. Radioiodine therapy has the disadvantage of producing hypothyroidism in a substantial number of patients but the advantage of providing permanent relief from hyperthyroidism, which may otherwise be difficult to control.

Thyroid hormone replacement for hypothyroidism may present special problems in the patient with pancreatic failure because of poor absorption of oral levothyroxine. This is less likely if steatorrhea is controlled with the use of pancreatic enzymes. By monitoring the serum TSH level, it almost always should be possible to provide an adequate dose of levothyroxine to restore a euthyroid state. The typical replacement dose for adults is 100 to 150 µg per day. A starting dose of 50 to 75 µg usually is appropriate. After beginning replacement therapy and after each new adjustment in dose, a period of 4 to 6 weeks should be allowed before the serum TSH is measured again. The laboratory endpoint in the treatment of both hyperthyroidism and hypothyroidism should be a serum TSH within the normal range.

RENAL FUNCTION AND THE REGULATION OF SALT AND WATER BALANCE

Despite the genetic defect causing ion channel abnormalities in other secretory membranes, primary renal disease is uncommon in CF and is an infrequent cause of death. The CF kidney, however, does have both functional and pathologic abnormalities.

Renal Regulation of Salt and Water Balance

It still is unclear whether the kidney is affected by the electrolyte transport defect that exists in glandular and respiratory epithelial cells elsewhere in the body. Functional alterations of modest proportions have been described in both tubular transport and glomerular filtration. Different investigators have used varying experimental conditions for the measurement of renal function, and the patients studied have had varying severity of illness. This may account for some of the variability in published reports.

Robson et al. (116) studied eight children with moderate to severe pulmonary disease under conditions of both salt restriction and salt loading. The patients had moderate hyponatremia, but they had normal glomerular filtration rates (GFRs) under basal conditions. With salt restriction, glomerular filtration remained normal and urinary sodium excretion decreased, as expected. Water loading was followed by a further decrease in the serum sodium concentration and an increase in the GFR, not seen in healthy subjects. The subnormal free water clearance after water loading was postulated to be caused by an increased reabsorption of both salt and water in the proximal segment of the renal tubule, with delivery of less volume to the distal nephron, where water clearance is regulated. This alteration in renal function would not necessarily indicate an intrinsic defect in tubular transport. Pulmonary disease in CF could lead to a decreased cardiac output and possibly a reduced effective arterial blood volume. These changes could result in turn in an adaptive increase in proximal tubular sodium reabsorption. In the study by Robson et al. (116), the patients with the most severe pulmonary disease tended to be the ones with the most subnormal capacity for free water clearance.

Most other investigators have found normal glomerular filtration and renal plasma flow in children and young adults with CF (117,118). Aladjem et al. (119), while noting a normal basal GFR, reported a subnormal increment in glomerular filtration and a higher fractional excretion of sodium after saline loading. In contrast, Assael et al. (118) found that patients with CF given saline infusions under conditions of maximal water diuresis increased their GFR but not their fractional excretion of sodium. Stenvinkel et al. (120), using lithium clearance to estimate segmental handling of sodium, reported that fractional excretion of sodium was decreased, with increased reabsorption of sodium in both proximal and distal segments of the nephron. These findings, like those of Robson et al. (116), are compatible with the view that overall tubular reabsorption of sodium is increased in many patients with CF.

One clinically important aspect of renal tubular function is the handling of drugs. Patients with CF have lower serum concentrations or increased clearances of a number of antibiotics and other drugs, including dicloxacillin, methicillin, cephalexin, amikacin, gentamicin, tobramycin, and theophylline (117). The reasons for the apparently increased clearance of various drugs are not always well delineated, and in some cases, nonrenal clearance mechanisms

probably are involved. The β-lactam antibiotics may be filtered, secreted, and reabsorbed to variable degrees, depending on the compound. Several of the antibiotics with increased renal clearance, such as dicloxacillin, cefoperazone, and ceftazidime, exist as anions at usual urine pH values. Thus, it is tempting to speculate that tubular reabsorption of certain anions may be impaired in CF (117). Drug metabolism is discussed extensively in Chapter 16.

Actions of Aldosterone

The renin–angiotensin–aldosterone axis is intact in patients with CF. Generally, the responses of mineralocorticoid-regulated transport systems in renal tubules are normal. The effects of aldosterone in the kidney are confined to the distal nephron, where mineralocorticoid receptors are present. These mineralocorticoid effects include increased reabsorption of sodium and increased secretion of potassium and hydrogen ions. The defective transport system responsible for the abnormal chloride permeability and transepithelial potentials in CF airways apparently is not regulated by aldosterone and is not affected by aldosterone antagonists (121).

Aldosterone levels may be elevated in patients with CF exposed to conditions causing increased salt and water losses. In infants and children with CF, chronic salt depletion can lead to secondary hyperaldosteronism with hypokalemia and metabolic alkalosis (122,123). These metabolic abnormalities are corrected readily by replenishment of salt. Clinically significant secondary hyperaldosteronism is not a common problem in adults with CF, but under more stringent salt-losing conditions, a predisposition may become apparent. Although plasma aldosterone was normal at baseline, the levels in athletes with CF were elevated after a marathon race (124). Presumably, aldosterone was elevated secondary to greater salt losses in the sweat. Hypotension and hyponatremia did not occur.

There also are seasonal differences in aldosterone metabolism in patients with CF versus healthy subjects. Aldosterone levels in patients with CF are elevated in summer months when compared with controls. This difference is not seen in the winter. Patients with CF show an increase in the bound fraction of circulating aldosterone and a decrease in metabolic clearance as an adaptation to warm weather (125).

Renal Diseases Complicating Cystic Fibrosis

Patients with CF are exposed chronically to potentially nephrotoxic factors, including bacterial infections, and antibiotics, particularly aminoglycosides. With the higher incidence of DM, liver disease, and cor pulmonale, secondary renal disease also is more likely to occur. Several histopathologic studies of kidneys obtained at autopsy from patients with CF have been reported.

Abramowsky and Swinehart (126) performed morphologic and immunopathologic autopsy studies of the kidneys of 34 patients with CF, ages 4 months to 35 years, 6 of whom had acute renal failure at the time of death. The majority had severe lung disease and cor pulmonale. All 34 patients showed glomerular enlargement, a nonspecific finding in heart failure. Tubulointerstitial histologic lesions also were common, found in 26. Acute tubular injury, including changes of acute tubular necrosis, was frequent. It is likely that a substantial proportion of the tubulointerstitial pathology was related to antibiotic toxicity. Deposits of gentamicin or tobramycin were identified in tubules by immunostaining, using gentamicin and tobramycin antisera. Immunofluorescent staining was positive for immunoglobulins or complement components in 18 of 34 specimens, but specific bacterial antigens were not identified. Elution studies carried out in a few specimens, however, did demonstrate anti-Pseudomonas antibodies. Perhaps surprisingly, none of the specimens showed amyloidosis or specific changes of diabetic glomerulopathy. From these observations, it is clear that CF, like almost any severe chronic illness, frequently leads to renal damage. Heart failure and its associated hemodynamic alterations, immune complexes, or other forms of immune injury and especially drug-related nephrotoxicity all can act in concert to bring about the observed lesions.

Some investigators have postulated that histopathologic changes may result from abnormal renal transport mechanisms that are part of the fundamental lesion in CF. Katz et al. (127) reported microscopic nephrocalcinosis in 35 of 38 autopsy kidneys from patients with CF. The same investigators measured urinary calcium excretion in 14 patients with CF and found hypercalciuria in 5. They postulated a primary abnormality of calcium metabolism in the kidney, possibly mirroring changes in other epithelial tissues.

Other investigators have pointed out that microscopic renal calcium deposits frequently occur in patients with other chronic illnesses. Bentur et al. (128) found microscopic calcium in 5 of 14 CF kidneys at autopsy but also in 6 of 12 kidneys from patients who died of other chronic debilitating diseases, including congenital heart disease and malignancy. These investigators found hypercalciuria in only 4 of 34 patients with CF, and in these, alternative explanations for the hypercalciuria could be identified, including immobilization and corticosteroid administration. Renal ultrasonography in 17 patients failed to demonstrate clinical evidence of nephrocalcinosis. Studies of adult patients with CF have shown an elevated risk of nephrolithiasis (129). Calcium oxalate stones tend to occur in association with malabsorption of any cause. Patients with steatorrhea from chronic inflammatory bowel disease or chronic pancreatitis also have increased oxalate absorption. (130). Hyperoxaluria leads to precipitation of insoluble calcium oxalate in the renal collecting system and may lead to hydronephrosis, infection, or nephrolithiasis.

In summary, there are few, if any, renal histopathologic lesions that are specific for CF. Critically ill patients with CF often have renal failure, but their renal disease usually is a secondary complication of heart failure, infection, drug toxicity, and other associated problems. Further investigation is needed to clarify possible alterations in the tubular handling of electrolytes and drugs.

REFERENCES

1. Gurwitz, D, Corey, M, Francis, PWJ, et al. Perspectives in cystic fibrosis. *Pediatr Clin North Am* 1979; 26:603–615.

2. Underwood LE, Van Wyk JJ. Normal and aberrant growth. In: Wilson JD, Foster DW, eds. *Textbook of endocrinology.* 8th ed. Philadelphia: WB Saunders, 1992:1079–1138.

3. Isley WL, Underwood LE, Clemmons DR. Dietary components that regulate serum somatomedin-C concentrations in humans. *J Clin Invest* 1983;71:175–182.

4. Tomezsko JL, Stallings VA, Kawchak DA, et al. Energy expenditure and genotype of children with cystic fibrosis. *Pediatr Res* 1994;35:451–460.

5. Lee JA, Dickinson LS, Kilgore BS, et al. Somatomedin activity in cystic fibrosis and reserpinized rats: possible explanation for growth retardation. *Ann Clin Lab Sci* 1980;10:227–233.

6. Rosenfeld RG, Landon C, Lewiston N, et al. Demonstration of normal plasma somatomedin concentrations in cystic fibrosis. *J Pediatr* 1981;99:252–254.

7. Landon C, Rosenfeld RG. Short stature and pubertal delay in cystic fibrosis. *Pediatrician* 1987;14:253–260.

8. Mullis PE, Liechti-Gallati S, DiSilvio L, et al. Short stature in a patient with cystic fibrosis caused by a 6.7 kb human growth hormone gene deletion. *Horm Res* 1991;36:4–8.

9. Tummler B, Aschendorff A, Darnedde T, et al. Marker haplotype association with growth in German cystic fibrosis patients. *Hum Genet* 1990;84:267–273.

10. Hamosh A, Corey M. Correlation between genotype and phenotype in patients with cystic fibrosis: the Cystic Fibrosis Genotype–Phenotype Consortium. *N Engl J Med* 1993;329(18):1308–1313.

11. Dennis JL, Panos TC. Growth and bone age retardation in cystic fibrosis. *JAMA* 1965;194:855–858.

12. Dooley RR, Moss AJ, Wright PM, et al. Norethandrolone in cystic fibrosis of the pancreas. *J Pediatr* 1969;74:95–102.

13. Good TA, Bessman SP. Anabolic steroids in cystic fibrosis of the pancreas. *Am J Dis Child* 1976;111:272–277.

14. Landon C, Rosenfeld RG. Short stature and pubertal delay in male adolescents with cystic fibrosis: androgen treatment. *Am J Dis Child* 1984;138:388–391.

15. Moshang T, Holsclaw DS Jr. Menarchal determinants in cystic fibrosis. *Am J Dis Child* 1980;134:1139–1142.

16. Neinstein LS, Stewart D, Wang C-I, Johnson I. Menstrual dysfunction in cystic fibrosis. *J Adolesc Health Care* 1983;4:153–157.

17. Penketh A, Wise A, Mearns MB, et al. Cystic fibrosis in adolescents and adults. *Thorax* 1987;42:526–532.

18. Frisch RE, McArthur JW. Menstrual cycles: fatness as a determinant of minimum weight for height necessary for their maintenance or onset. *Science* 1974;185:949–951.

19. Grumbach M, Styne DM. Puberty: ontogeny, neuroendocrinology, physiology and disorders. In: Wilson JD, Foster DW, eds. *Textbook of endocrinology.*

20. 8th ed. Philadelphia: WB Saunders, 1992:1139–1222.

20. Reiter EO, Stern RC, Root AW. The reproductive endocrine system in cystic fibrosis. *Am J Dis Child* 1981;135:422–426.

21. Reiter EO, Stern RC, Root AW. The reproductive endocrine system in cystic fibrosis: 2, changes in gonadotrophins and sex steroids following LHRH. *Clin Endocrinol* 1982;16:127–137.

22. Stern RC. Cystic fibrosis and the reproductive systems. In: Davis P, ed. *Cystic fibrosis.* New York: Marcel Dekker Inc, 1993:381–399.

23. Kopito LE, Losasky HJ, Shwachman H. Water and electrolytes in cervical mucus from patients with CF. *Fertil Steril* 1973;24:512–516.

24. Seale TW, Flux M, Rennert OM. Reproductive defects in patients of both sexes with cystic fibrosis: a review. *Ann Clin Lab Sci* 1985;15:152–158.

25. Kaplan E, Shwachman H, Perlmutter AD, et al. Reproductive failure in males with cystic fibrosis. *N Engl J Med* 1968;279:65–69.

26. Bronson RA, O'Connor WJ, Wilson TA, et al. Correlation between puberty and the development of autoimmunity to spermatozoa in men with cystic fibrosis. *Fertil Steril* 1992;58:1199–1204.

27. Durieu I, Bey-Omar F, Rollet J, et al. Diagnostic criteria for cystic fibrosis in men with congenital absence of the vas deferens. *Medicine* 1995;74:42–47.

28. Chillon M, Casals T, Mercier B, et al. Mutations in the cystic fibrosis gene in patients with congenital absence of the vas deferens. *N Engl J Med* 1995;332:1475–1480.

29. Dooley RR, Braunstein H, Osher AB. Polypoid cervicitis in cystic fibrosis patients receiving oral contraceptives. *Am J Obstet Gynecol* 1974;118:971–974.

30. Fitzpatrick SB, Stokes DC, Rosenstein BJ, et al. Use of oral contraceptives in women with cystic fibrosis. *Chest* 1984;86:863–867.

31. Levine SB, Stern RC. Sexual function in cystic fibrosis: relationship to overall health status and pulmonary disease severity in 30 married patients. *Chest* 1982;81:422–428.

32. Coffman CB, Levine SB, Althof SE, Stern RC. Sexual adaptation among single young adults with cystic fibrosis. *Chest* 1984;86:412–418.

33. National Institute of Arthritis, Metabolism and Digestive Diseases. Cystic fibrosis: a disease in search of ideas. *Clin Sci* 1979;2:33–418.

34. Lanng S, Thorsteinsson B, Ericksen G, et al. Glucose tolerance in cystic fibrosis. *Arch Dis Child* 1991;66:612–616.

35. Cystic Fibrosis Foundation. *Patient registry, 1995 annual data report.* Bethesda, MD: Cystic Fibrosis Foundation, 1996.

36. Reisman J, Corey M, Canny G, Levison H. Diabetes mellitus in patients with cystic fibrosis: effect on survival. *Pediatrics* 1990;86:374–377.

37. Rodman HM, Doershuk CF, Roland JM. The interaction of two diseases: diabetes mellitus and cystic fibrosis. *Medicine* 1986;65:389–397.

38. Rosenecker J, Eichler I, Baermeier H, Kuehn L. Epidemiology of diabetes mellitus in cystic fibrosis. *Pediatr Pulmonol* 1993;9:277 (abstract).

39. Moran A, Diem P, Klein DJ, et al. Pancreatic endocrine function in cystic fibrosis. *J Pediatr* 1991;118:715–723.

40. De Schepper J, Hachimi-Idrissi S, Smitz J, et al. First phase insulin response in adult cystic fibrosis patients: correlation with clinical and biological parameters. *Horm Res* 1992;38:260–263.

41. Lanng S, Schwartz M, Thorsteinsson B, et al. Endocrine and exocrine pancreatic function and the delta F508 mutation in cystic fibrosis. *Clin Genet* 1991;40:345–348.

42. Hamdi I, Payne SJ, Barton DE, et al. Genotype analysis in cystic fibrosis in relation to the occurence of diabetes mellitus. *Clin Genet* 1993;43:186–189.

43. Rosenecker J, Eichler I, Keuhn L, et al. Genetic determination of diabetes mellitus in patients with cystic fibrosis. *J Pediatr* 1995;127:441–443.

44. Handwerger S, Roth J, Gorden P, et al. Glucose intolerance in cystic fibrosis. *N Engl J Med* 1969;281:451–461.

45. Krueger LT, Lerner A, Katz SM, et al. Cystic fibrosis and diabetes mellitus: interactive or idiopathic? *J Pediatr Gastroenterol Nutr* 1991;13:209–219.

46. Iannucci A, Mukai K, Johnson DB, et al. Endocrine pancreas in cystic fibrosis: an immunohistochemical study. *Hum Pathol* 1984;15:278–284.

47. Abdul-Karim FW, Dahms BB, Velasco ME, et al. Islets of Langerhans in adolescents and adults with cystic fibrosis: a quantitative study. *Arch Pathol Lab Med* 1986;110:602–606.

48. Soejima K, Landing BH. Pancreatic islets in older patients with cystic fibrosis with and without diabetes mellitus: morphometric and immunocytologic studies. *Pediatr Pathol* 1986;6:25–46.

49. Lohr M, Goertchen P, Nizze H, et al. Cystic fibrosis associated islet changes may provide a basis for diabetes: an immunocytochemical and morphometrical study. *Virchows Archiv* 1989;414:179–185.

50. Couce M, O'Brien TD, Moran A, et al. Diabetes mellitus in cystic fibrosis is characterized by islet amyloidosis. *J Clin Endocrinol Metab* 1996;81:1267–1272.

51. Stutchfield PR, O'Halloran SM, Smith CS, et al. HLA type, islet cell antibodies, and glucose intolerance in cystic fibrosis. *Arch Dis Child* 1988;63:1234–1239.

52. Lanng S, Thorsteinsson B, Roder ME, et al. Pancreas and gut hormone responses to oral glucose and intravenous glucagon in cystic fibrosis patients with normal, impaired, and diabetic glucose tolerance. *Acta Endocrinol (Copenh)* 1993;128:207–214.

53. Unger RH, Foster DW. Diabetes mellitus. In: Wilson JW, Foster DW, eds. *Textbook of endocrinology.* 8th ed. Philadelphia: WB Saunders, 1992:1273–1274.

54. Shafrir E. Diabetes in animals. In: Rifkin H, Porte D Jr, eds. *Diabetes mellitus, theory and practice.* 4th ed. New York: Elsevier, 1990:305.

55. Meacham LR, Caplan DB, McKean LP, et al. Preservation of somatostatin secretion in cystic fibrosis patients with diabetes. *Arch Dis Child* 1993;68:123–125.

56. Culler FL, Meacham LR. Effect of hypersomatostatinemia on growth hormone secretion in cystic fibrosis diabetes mellitus. *Neuroendocrinology* 1993;58:473–477.

57. Lippe BM, Kaplan SA, Neufield ND, et al. Insulin receptors in cystic fibrosis: increased receptor number and altered affinity. *Pediatrics* 1980;65:1018–1022.

58. Lanng S, Thorsteinsson B, Roder M, et al. Insulin sensitivity and insulin clearance in cystic fibrosis patients with normal and diabetic glucose tolerance. *Clin Endocrinol* 1994;41:217–223.

59. Moran A, Pyzdrowski K, Weinreb J, et al. Insulin sensitivity in cystic fibrosis. *Diabetes* 1994;43:1020–1026.

60. Lanng S, Thorsteinsson B, Nerup J, Koch C. Influence of the developments of diabetes mellitus on clinical status in patients with cystic fibrosis. *Eur J Pediatr* 1992;151:684–687.

61. Finkelstein SM, Wielinski CL, Elliot GR, et al. Diabetes mellitus associated with cystic fibrosis. *J Pediatr* 1988;112:373–377.

62. Knowles MK, Fernald GW. Diabetes and cystic fibrosis: new questions emerging from increased longevity. *J Pediatr* 1988;112:415–416.

63. Sullivan MM, Denning CR. Diabetic microangiopathy in patients with cystic fibrosis. *Pediatrics* 1989;84:642–647.

64. Consensus Conference on CF-Related Diabetes Mellitus. *Consensus Conferences of the Cystic Fibrosis Foundation,* February 5–6, 1998.

65. The effect of intensive treatment of diabetes on the development and progression of long-term complications in insulin-dependent diabetes mellitus: Diabetes Control and Complications Trial Research Group. *N Engl J Med* 1993;329:977–986.

66. Lanng S, Thorsteinsson B, Nerup J, et al. Diabetes mellitus in cystic fibrosis: effect of insulin therapy on lung function and infections. *Acta Paediatr* 1994;83:849–853.

67. Lebovitz HE. Oral hypoglycemic agents. In: Rifkin H, Porte D Jr, eds. *Diabetes mellitus, theory and practice.* 4th ed. New York: Elsevier, 1990:554–574.

68. Zipf WB, Kien CL, Horswill CA, et al. Effects of tolbutamide on growth and body composition of nondiabetic children with cystic fibrosis. *Pediatr Res* 1991;30:309–314.

69. Hayes DR, Sheehan JP, Ulchaker MM, et al. Management dilemmas in the individual with cystic fibrosis and diabetes. *J Am Diet Assoc* 1994;94:78–80.

70. Munck A, Guyre PM, Holbrook NJ. Physiological functions of glucocorticoids in stress and their relation to pharmacological action. *Endocrine Rev* 1984;5:25–44.

71. Schleimer RP. Effects of glucocorticoids on inflammatory cells relevant to their therapeutic applications to asthma. *Am Rev Respir Dis* 1990;141:S59–S69.

72. Price JF, Greally P. Corticosteroid treatment in cystic fibrosis. *Arch Dis Child* 1993;68:719–721.

73. Mroueh S, Spock A. Allergic bronchopulmonary aspergillosis in patients with cystic fibrosis. *Chest* 1994;105:32–36.

74. Auerbach HS, Williams M, Kirkpatrick JA, et al. Alternate day prednisolone reduces the morbidity and improves pulmonary function in cystic fibrosis. *Lancet* 1985;ii:686–688.

75. Rosenstein BJ, Eigen H. Risks of alternate-day prednisone in patients with cystic fibrosis. *Pediatrics* 1991;87:245–246.

76. van Haren EHJ, Lammers J-WJ, Festen J, et al. The effects of the inhaled corticosteroid budesonide on

lung function and bronchial hyperresponsiveness in adult patients with cystic fibrosis. *Respir Med* 1995; 89:209–214.

77. Webb J, Clark TJH. Recovery of plasma corticotropin and cortisol levels after a three-week course of prednisolone. *Thorax* 1981;36:22–24.

78. Graber AL, Ney RL, Nicholson WE, et al. Natural history of pituitary–adrenal recovery following long-term suppression with corticosteroids. *J Clin Endocrinol Metab* 1965;25:11–16.

79. Fauci AS. Alternate-day corticosteroid therapy. *Am J Med* 1978;64:729–731.

80. Ruegsegger P, Medici TC, Anliker M. Corticosteroid-induced bone loss: a longitudinal study of alternate day therapy in patients with bronchial asthma using quantitative computed tomography. *Eur J Clin Pharmacol* 1983;25:615–620.

81. Dykman TR, Gluck OS, Murphy WA, et al. Valuation of factors associated with glucocorticoid-induced osteopenia in patients with rheumatic diseases. *Arthritis Rheum* 1985;28:361–368.

82. Volovitz B, Amir J, Malik H, et al. Growth and pituitary-adrenal function in children with severe asthma treated with inhaled budesonide. *N Engl J Med* 1993;329:1703–1708.

83. Utiger RD. Differences between inhaled and oral glucocorticoid therapy. *N Engl J Med* 1993;329:1731–1733.

84. Ross PD, Genant HK, Davis JW, et al. Predicting vertebral fracture incidence from prevalent fractures and bone density among non-black, osteoporotic women. *Osteoporos Int* 1993;3:120–126.

85. Hahn TJ, Squires AE, Halstead LR, et al. Reduced serum 25-hydroxyvitamin D concentration and disordered mineral metabolism in patients with cystic fibrosis. *J Pediatr* 1979;94:38–42.

86. Gibbens DT, Gilsanz V, Boechat MI, et al. Osteoporosis in cystic fibrosis. *J Pediatr* 1988;113:295–300.

87. Grey AB, Ames RW, Matthews RD, et al. Bone mineral density and body composition in adult patients with cystic fibrosis. *Thorax* 1993;48:589–593.

88. Bachrach LK, Loutit CW, Moss RB, et al. Osteopenia in adults with cystic fibrosis. *Am J Med* 1994;96: 27–34.

89. Henderson RC, Madsen CD. Bone density in children and adolescents with cystic fibrosis. *J Pediatr* 1996;128:28–34.

90. Salamoni F, Roulet M, Gudinchet F, et al. Bone mineral content in cystic fibrosis patients: correlation with fat-free mass. *Arch Dis Child* 1996;74:314–318.

91. Aris RM, Neuringer IP, Weiner MA, et al. Severe osteoporosis before and after lung transplantation. *Chest* 1996;109:1176–1183.

92. Johnston CC, Slemenda CW, Melton LJ III. Clinical use of bone densitometry. *N Engl J Med* 1991;324: 1105–1109.

93. Mischler EH, Chesney PJ, Chesney RW, et al. Dimineralization in cystic fibrosis detected by direct photon absorptiometry. *Am J Dis Child* 1979;133:632–635.

94. Solomons NW, Wagonfield JB, Rieger C, et al. Some biochemical indices of nutrition in treated cystic fibrosis patients. *Am J Clin Nutr* 1981;34:462–474.

95. Reiter EO, Brugman SM, Pike JW, et al. Vitamin D metabolites in adolescents and young adults with cystic fibrosis: effects of sun and season. *J Pediatr* 1985;106:21–26.

96. Jilka RL, Hangoc G, Girasole G, et al. Increased osteoclast development after estrogen loss: mediation by interleukin-6. *Science* 1992;257:88–91.

97. Levy E, Gurbindo C, Lacaille F, et al. Circulating tumor necrosis factor-alpha levels and lipid abnormalities in patients with cystic fibrosis. *Pediatr Res* 1993;34:162–166.

98. Muchmore JS, Cooper DKC, Ye Y, et al. Prevention of loss of vertebral bone density in heart transplant patients. *J Heart Lung Transplant* 1992;11:959–963.

99. Lukert BP, Raisz LG. Glucocorticoid-induced osteoporosis: pathogenesis and management. *Ann Int Med* 1990;112:352–364.

100. Rich GM, Mudge GH, Laffel GL, et al. Cyclosporine A and prednisone-associated osteoporosis in heart transplant recipients. *J Heart Lung Transplant* 1992; 11:950–958.

101. Dixley J, Reddington AN, Butler RC, et al. The arthropathy of cystic fibrosis. *Ann Rheum Dis* 1988; 47:218–223.

102. Watts NB, Harris ST, Genant HK, et al. Intermittent cyclical etidronate treatment of postmenopausal osteoporosis. *N Engl J Med* 1990;323:73.

103. Liberman UA, Weiss SR, Broll J, et al. Effect of oral alendronate on bone mineral density and the incidence of fractures in postmenopausal osteoporosis. *N Engl J Med* 1995;333:1437–1443.

104. Reid IR, King AR, Alexander CJ, et al. Prevention of steroid-induced osteoporosis with bisphosphonate (APD). *Lancet* 1988;1:143–146.

105. Gallacher SJ, Fenner JAK, Anderson K, et al. Intravenous pamidronate in the treatment of osteoporosis associated with corticosteroid dependent lung disease: an open pilot study. *Thorax* 1992;47:932–936.

106. Ringe JD, Welzel D. Salmon calcitonin in the therapy of corticoid-induced osteoporosis. *Eur J Clin Pharmacol* 1987;33:35–39.

107. Montemurro L, Schiraldi G, Friaoli P, et al. Prevention of corticosteroid-induced osteoporosis with salmon calcitonin in sarcoid patients. *Calcif Tissue Int* 1991; 49:71–76.

108. Luengo M, Picado C, Del Rio L, et al. Treatment of steroid-induced osteopenia with calcitonin in corticosteriod-dependent asthma: a one-year follow-up study. *Am Rev Respir Dis* 1990;142:104–107.

109. Overgaard K, Hansen MA, Jensen SB, et al. Effect of salcatonin given intranasally on bone mass and fracture rates in established osteoporosis: a dose-response study. *BMJ* 1992;305:556–560.

110. Castile R, Shwachman H, Travis W, et al. Amyloidosis as a complication of cystic fibrosis. *Am J Dis Child* 1985;139:728–732.

111. Bontempini L, Ghimenton C, Colombari R, et al. Secondary amyloidosis and cystic fibrosis: a morphological and histochemical study of five cases. *Histol Histopathol* 1987;2:413–416.

112. Depasse C, Chanoine JP, Casimir G, et al. Congenital hypothyroidism and cystic fibrosis. *Acta Paediatr Scand* 1991;80:981–983.

113. Nicoloff JT, LoPresti JS. Nonthyroidal illness. In: Braverman LE, Utiger RD, eds. *The thyroid, a fundamental and clinical text*. 6th ed. New York: JB Lippincott, 1991:357.

114. Knopfle G. The thyroid hormone system in mucoviscidosis. *Klin Padiatr* 1985;197:481–488.
115. Azizi F, Bentley D, Vagenakis A, et al. Abnormal thyroid function and response to iodides in patients with cystic fibrosis. *Trans Assoc Am Physicians* 1974; 87:111–119.
116. Robson AM, Tateishi S, Ingelfinger JR, et al. Renal function in patients with cystic fibrosis. *J Pediatr* 1971;79:42–50.
117. Spino M, Chai RP, Isles AF, et al. Assessment of glomerular filtration rate (GFR) and effective renal plasma flow in cystic fibrosis. *J Pediatr* 1985;107: 64–70.
118. Assael BM, Marra G, Tirelli AS, et al. Renal function in cystic fibrosis. *Int J Pediatr Nephrol* 1986;7:213–216.
119. Aladjem M, Lotan D, Boichis H, et al. Renal function in patients with cystic fibrosis. *Nephron* 1983;34:84–86.
120. Stenvinkel P, Hjelte L, Alvan G, et al. Decreased renal clearance of sodium in cystic fibrosis. *Acta Paedriatr Scand* 1991;80:194–198.
121. Knowles MR, Gatzy JT, Boucher RC. Aldosterone metabolism and transepithelial potential difference in normal and cystic fibrosis subjects. *Pediatr Res* 1985;19:676–679.
122. Kennedy JD, Dinwiddie R, Daman-Willems C, et al. Pseudo-Bartter's syndrome in cystic fibrosis. *Arch Dis Child* 1987;65:786–787.
123. Eigenmann P, Deleze G, Kuchler H. Chronic metabolic alkalosis in an infant with cystic fibrosis. *Eur J Pediatr* 1990;150:669–670.
124. Stanghelle JK, Maehlum S, Skyberg D, et al. Biochemical changes and endocrine responses in cystic fibrosis in relation to a marathon race. *Int J Sports Med* 1988;9 Suppl 1:45–50.
125. Nowaczynski W, Nakielana EM, Murakami T, et al. The relationship of plasma aldosterone-binding globulin to blood pressure regulation in young adults with cystic fibrosis. *Clin Physiol Biochem* 1987;5:276–286.
126. Abramowsky C, Swinehart GL. The nephropathy of cystic fibrosis: a human model of chronic nephrotoxicity. *Hum Pathol* 1982;13:934–939.
127. Katz SM, Krueger LJ, Falkner B, et al. Microscopic nephrocalcinosis in cystic fibrosis. *N Engl J Med* 1988;319:263–266.
128. Bentur L, Kerem, E, Couper R, et al. Renal calcium handling in cystic fibrosis. *J Pediatr* 1990;116:556–560.
129. Strandvik B, Hjetle L. Neprolithiasis in cystic fibrosis. *Acta Paediatr* 1993;82:306–307.
130. Dharmsathaphorn K, Freeman DH, Binder HJ, et al. Increased risk of nephrolithiasis in patients with steatorrhea. *Digest Dis Sci* 1982;27:401–405.

Cystic Fibrosis in Adults,
edited by J. R. Yankaskas and M. R. Knowles,
Lippincott–Raven Publishers, Philadelphia, 1999.

19

The Sweat Gland

Paul M. Quinton

*Department of Biomedical Sciences, University of California at Riverside School of Medicine,
Riverside, California, and Department of Pediatrics, University of California at San Diego
Medical Center, San Diego, California*

The minuscule sweat gland has played a large role in the medical history of cystic fibrosis (CF). It provided the first crude diagnosis of CF several hundred years ago, with an old wives' observation that the child that tastes salty when kissed will soon die, or so it is claimed (1). For 40 years, the sweat gland has been the basis of the most commonly used differential diagnostic test of the disease, the sweat test. The defect in its function provided the first demonstration of Cl⁻ impermeability as a basic cellular defect in CF that is the direct result of mutations in the gene for CF (2–4). It continues to play an important role in descriptions of the functions and regulations of the cystic fibrosis transmembrane conductance regulator (CFTR) (5–10), the protein product of the CF gene. In addition to nasal tissue, it is the only organ that is relatively easily accessible for study both *in vivo* and *in vitro*. It still provides one of the only arenas for investigating actual physiologic function in native human tissue.

In this chapter, a general view of the structure and function of the sweat gland is presented; where and why specific functions fail in CF will be pointed out. We will focus on the role of the CFTR to provide an understanding not only of sweat excretion but also of the principles of fluid and electrolyte transport that are at play in this organ and that create pathophysiology in other epithelia affected in CF. Where appropriate, features that pertain particularly to the adult population will be noted. This information should form the basis for rational inter-pretations of the sweat test, which will be presented and discussed in closing.

DESCRIPTION OF THE SWEAT GLAND

There are no less than two classes of sweat glands. Apocrine sweat glands are associated with pubertal areas, and little is known about their function in CF. It is the eccrine sweat gland that holds our attention in CF. This gland is distributed over the entire body surface except for the ear lobes and the highly vascularized red skin. The number of eccrine sweat glands is fixed at birth and is estimated to be from between 2 to 4 million, or approximately the number of nephrons in the kidneys. Density decreases with greater body surface area so that it is lowest in adults (11). The sweat glands appear at highest density on the forehead (~350 to 400 glands/cm²) and at lowest density on the thigh (~60 glands/cm²) (12,13). The volar surface of the arm, which is the preferred site for sweat testing, is of intermediate density, with 200 to 250 glands/cm². The overall size of the gland also increases with maturation.

Eccrine sweat glands are imbedded in the collagenous matrix of the dermis within 3 to 6 mm of the skin surface. Each gland is a small epithelial structure normally consisting of a single, unbranching tubule approximately 40 μm in diameter and approximately 1 cm in total length. Most of the tubule is coiled randomly on itself into a corpuscle (Figs. 19–1A and 19–1B). The first half of the coil of tubule be-

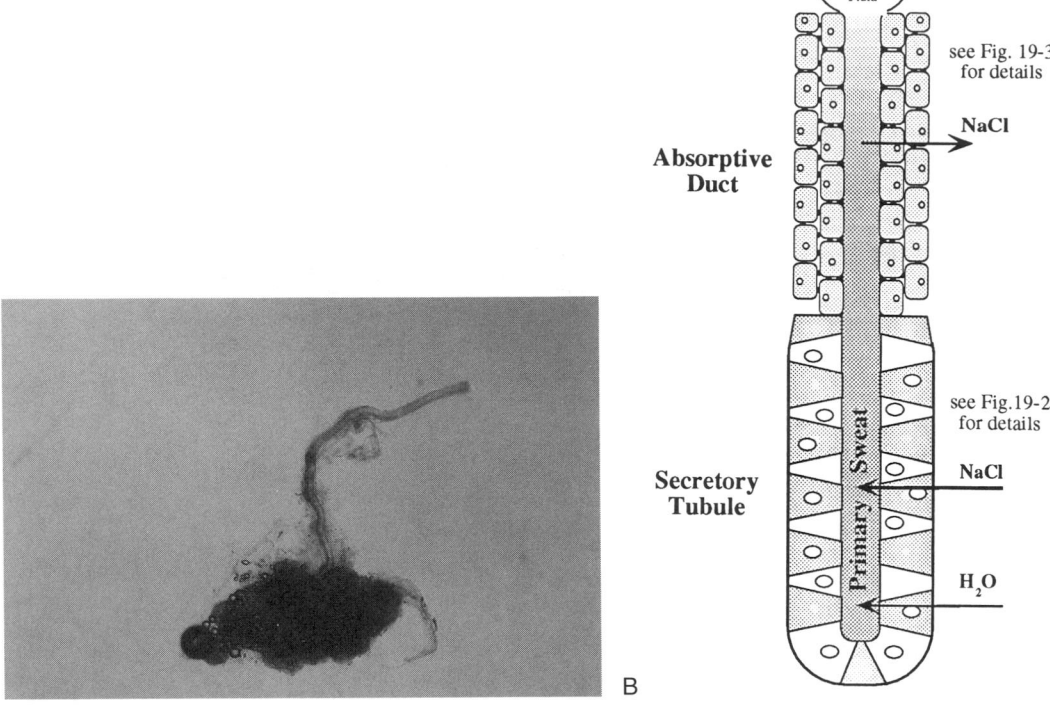

FIG. 19–1. (A) A photomicrograph of a freshly isolated intact human eccrine sweat gland. The straight portion of the reabsorptive duct can be seen extending from the gland corpuscle. Small adipose cells are visible at the periphery of the gland, but the bulk of the gland is composed of the remainder of the sweat duct and the secretory tubule, which are coiled indistinguishably in the corpuscle (150×). **(B)** A schematic model of a single sweat gland depicting the secretory tubule composed of about equal numbers of light and dark cells connected to the reabsorptive duct composed of two concentric layers of cells surrounding a common lumen. NaCl with water is secreted isotonically into the lumen and NaCl (without water) is reabsorbed hypertonically from the lumen by the duct to create hypotonic sweat that is excreted on the skin. See Figures 19–2 and 19–3 for details.

gins with a closed or blind end. It is a purely secretory epithelium referred to as the secretory coil (14,15). Here, the first fluid for sweating, primary sweat, is produced. At the beginning of the second half of the coil, the morphology and function of the tubule change abruptly to that of an absorptive epithelium called the sweat duct. On leaving the corpuscle, the absorptive duct assumes a straight length that leads directly through the dermis to a single sweat pore in the epidermis. The corpuscle of the coil and the straight portion of the duct are well vascularized (16) (see Figs. 19–1A and 19–1B).

The sweat gland is innervated by the autonomic nervous system, but its innervation is an exception to the rule because instead of catecholamines, these autonomic nerve terminals release acetylcholine as the physiologic neurotransmitter to control thermoregulatory sweat secretion. Nonetheless, the gland does respond to adrenergic agonists, although much more weakly (7,17) (see Fig. 19–1B). The purpose of this dual innervation is not known (18).

SWEAT SECRETION

Structure of Secretory Cells

The tubular cells of the secretory coil appear as a pseudostratified epithelium surrounded by an intermittent, noncontinuous network of myoepithelial cells (19). The function of the myoepithelial cells is not well defined, but it generally is believed that they provide structural support for the epithelium, which can be exposed to osmotic pressures apparently capable of generating 500 mm Hg of hydrostatic pressure (20). They also may provide some pulsatile activity for expressing sweat from the gland (21).

The epithelium is composed of two morphologically and physiologically distinct cell types that are dispersed more or less randomly in approximately equal numbers to form the walls of the tubule. These cells are designated light cells and dark cells on the basis of their affinity for basophilic dyes (see Fig. 19–1B). Light cells have very little apical membrane bordering the lumen of the secretory tubule (22). Rather, most of their apical membrane is found along narrow channels formed between two light cells (never with dark cells). These channels are closed near the bases of the two adjoining cells, but open at the opposite end into the lumen. The primary fluid of sweat probably is formed initially in these intercellular canaliculi and then flows into the lumen of the secretory coil (23). These light cells seem to be controlled by both ß-adrenergic [cyclic adenosine monophosphate (cAMP)-mediated] and cholinergic (Ca++-mediated) stimuli. Only the β-adrenergic component of secretion is defective in CF (24–27).

Conversely, the apical membranes of the dark cells constitute most of the luminal membrane of the secretory tubule. Gap junctions appear to closely couple these cells to each other, but not to light cells (22,28). That is, dye or electrical current injected into one cell quickly moves into other adjacent dark cells, but not into light cells. The exact function of these cells is not known, but the presence of numerous vesicles and fluorescent granules has suggested that they are involved with macromolecular secretion (22). These cells seem to be controlled only by cholinergic stimulus, are not sensitive to β-adrenergic agonists, and apparently are not affected in CF (26,27).

Function of Secretory Cells

The coupling between stimulus events, cytoplasmic biochemistry, and electrolyte transport mechanisms have not been worked out nearly as well for Ca++-mediated (cholinergic) as for cAMP-mediated (β-adrenergic) fluid secretion. However, it is the latter that is uniquely defective in CF because of abnormalities in the CF gene product, the CFTR, a Cl⁻ channel (29,30). A brief description of how cAMP-mediated secretion occurs may be instructive in understanding how a defect in the CFTR compromises fluid secretion in CF. But first and perhaps most importantly, it is critical to remember that thermoregulatory Ca++-mediated secretion seems completely normal in CF (7,27,31). Consequently, neither the physiologic response nor the volume of sweat produced by subjects with CF during thermal sweating is abnormal, even though cAMP-mediated secretion is defunct. Patients with CF have no discernible difficulties in thermoregulating; they have difficulties in retaining salt during sweating, which we will consider later in functions of the absorptive duct of the sweat gland.

The components and chemistry of cAMP-mediated (β-adrenergic) secretion might be understood most easily with reference to the model depicted in Figure 19–2A. Following events as we know them, β-adrenergic agonists (norepinephrine) binds to the β-adrenergic receptor and stimulates a G-protein–mediated activation of adenyl cyclase, which increases the intracellular concentration of cAMP. cAMP is removed spontaneously by the action of phosphodiesterase. Increased levels of cAMP bind to and stimulate the catalytic subunits of protein kinase A (PKA). One of the targets of this enzyme is the CFTR, which, when phosphorylated, becomes activated and capable of conducting[a] Cl⁻ ions. In these cells, CFTR is located only in the apical membrane, and when activated and open, it allows Cl⁻ to move out of the cell into the tubule lumen.

For Cl⁻ to move out of the cell, two conditions must be satisfied. First, the electrochemical potential in the cell must be higher than in the lumen. Second, for each Cl⁻ ion that is secreted out of the cell into the lumen, a cation carrying equal charge also must be secreted

---

[a]By *conducting*, we mean passively transporting the ion with electric current.

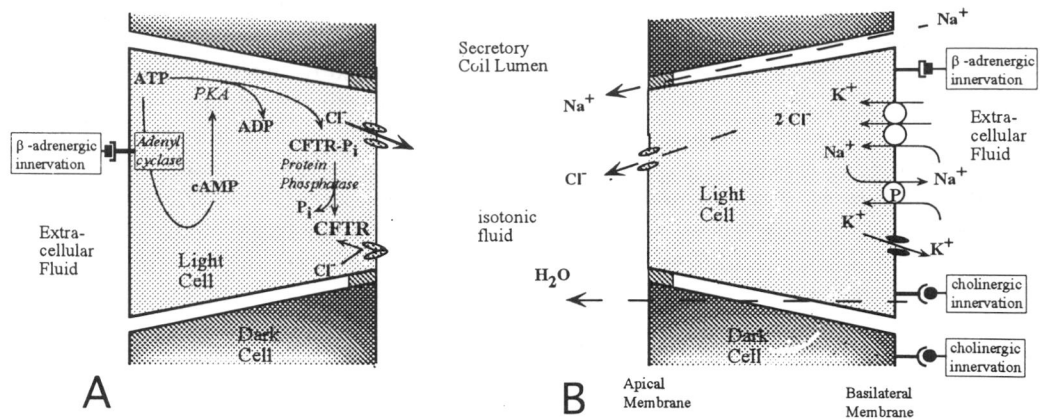

FIG. 19–2. (A) Biochemical events that couple stimulation of the secretory mechanism that is defective in cystic fibrosis (CF). A ß-adrenergic agonist interacts with its receptor to increase intracellular cAMP levels and activate protein kinase A, which in turn activates the CFTR through phosphorylation to initiate secretion. The activated CFTR appears to be deactivated by constitutively active protein phosphatases, which dephosphorylate the CFTR when stimulation terminates. **(B)** Components of secretory mechanism stimulated adrenergically (see Fig. 19–2A) and affected in CF. The Na+/K+-ATPase pump keeps intracellular Na+ low, which maintains a relatively large negative intracellular potential. The negative potential creates an electromotive driving force that drives Cl⁻ out of the cell through the CFTR and keeps intracellular Cl⁻ concentration relatively low. This allows Cl⁻ to enter the cell on the Na/K/2Cl carrier electroneutrally and be secreted across the apical membrane as shown and described. Na+ enters the lumen through the paracellular shunt (tight junction). Light cells are stimulated by both adrenergic and cholinergic receptors, whereas dark cells are sensitive only to cholinergic stimulation. The cholinergic response, which supports normal thermoregulation, is normal in CF.

into the lumen. Otherwise, the requirement for electroneutrality would be violated (which is physiologically impossible).[b]

---

[b]These conditions may seem paradoxical because electrical potentials are the result of separation of charges of opposite sign; one must wonder how an electrical potential is generated if equal numbers of opposite charges must always be transported simultaneously to satisfy electroneutrality. The answer is that although equal numbers of opposite charges must move together, opposite charges may be displaced with respect to each other so that an electrical field is generated. The situation may be visualized simplistically as a group of magnets all moving together and all oriented in the same direction; for each north pole there must always be an equal south pole. The polarity of the field will depend on how the poles are oriented with respect to each other as they move or cross a barrier. In physiology, electroneutrality is never violated. If one species of ion moves in any direction, another ion carrying an equivalent but opposite charge must follow in the same direction, or another ion of the same charge must move in the opposite direction. One can imagine cations displaced and moving slightly ahead of anions to create a positive electric potential or field without separation of charge, or the reverse when anions lead cations.

A couple of important but sometimes neglected biological principals of fluid transport should be observed. First, no animal can secrete[c] hypotonic fluids directly. To do so would constitute active water transport, and there are no water pumps per se in nature. Also, unlike some birds and reptiles, mammals cannot secrete hypertonic fluids (32). Water always moves passively as a function of an osmotic gradient established by the active transport of solutes across a membrane barrier. Water then flows across the barrier according to the difference in osmotic pressures across it. Membranes that are involved in isotonic fluid secretion usually are highly permeable to water so that water moves quickly across them to dissipate

---

[c]The term *excrete* and its derivatives refer to fluid actually leaving the body, whereas the term *secrete* and its derivatives refer to transporting a fluid from the interstitial space into an epithelial compartment still within the body cavity.

or minimize osmotic gradients. These properties permit rapid secretion of large volumes of fluid at low-energy costs.

Second, to form a hypotonic fluid, salts must be extracted from fluid secreted isotonically before the secretion is excreted from the gland. These principals are the basis of the Schwartz-Thaysen two-step model of secretion (33,34), which can be applied to all exocrine glands that secrete a hypotonic fluid. That is, (a) an isotonic primary precursor fluid is elaborated by a secretory epithelium (20,35), and (b) this fluid is modified secondarily by the hypertonic absorption of electrolytes in excess of water across a relatively water-impermeable epithelium. In mammals, hypertonic fluids are formed only by the kidney (32).

Returning to the transport of Cl^- out of the cell, the purpose of the secretory tubule is to secrete isotonic fluid into the lumen. The energy for the process comes from the hydrolysis of adenosine triphosphate (ATP) by the Na^+/K^+-adenosine triphosphatase (ATPase), which is always found in the basolateral membrane (36) and which exchanges three Na^+ ions in the cytoplasm for two K^+ ions in the extracellular fluid (see Fig. 19–2B). In consequence, the cell cytoplasm constantly is low in Na^+ and high in K^+. The Na^+ gradient generated by the Na^+/K^+ pump is directed into the cell and is used as an energy source to accumulate or transport numerous solutes into or out of the cell. One of these substances is Cl^-. Chloride is accumulated in the cell via a coupled carrier, the $Na^+/K^+/2Cl^-$ carrier. As Na^+ moves down its chemical gradient into the cell on the carrier, the movement of 1 K^+ and 2 Cl^- ions are coupled to it (electroneutrality is preserved: 2 + 's and 2 − 's). Under these conditions, when the CFTR opens, Cl^- will spill into the lumen and render the lumen electrically more negative than the interstitial fluid. This electrical gradient in turn drives cations into the lumen through the tight junctions, which form the aforementioned intercellular canaliculi. Electroneutrality is conserved because for each Cl^- ion that moves across the apical membrane, an Na^+ ion moves across the tight junction so that the luminal compartment always will have equal numbers of positive and negative charges. The apical membrane of the secretory cell is of necessity impermeable

to cations (see Fig. 19–2B). If we break this process down into discrete steps beginning with the energy input from ATP hydrolysis by Na^+/K^+-ATPase, we see the following sequence:

- Na^+/K^+-ATPase in the basolateral membrane establishes an Na^+ gradient into cell;
- The $Na^+/K^+/2Cl^-$ carrier uses the Na^+ gradient to accumulate Cl^- in the cell and build an electrochemical gradient for Cl^- to move passively out of the cell;
- The apical membrane CFTR Cl^- channels open by phosphorylation via PKA (β-adrenergic stimulation, followed by increased intracellular cAMP to activate PKA; see Fig. 19–2A);
- Cl^- ions carry negative current out of the cell through the CFTR across the apical membrane into the lumen;
- The resulting electronegative potential in the lumen drives a positive current of Na^+ ions across the tight junctions into the lumen to balance the Cl^- charge, satisfy electroneutrality, and accumulate salt in the lumen;
- The accumulation of Cl^- and Na^+ ions in the lumen increases the luminal osmotic pressure;
- Water moves passively in isotonic proportions from the interstitial compartment to the luminal compartment; and
- Hydrostatic pressure increases in the lumen with the increased fluid volume in the tubule to force luminal fluid into the duct and out of the gland onto the skin as sweat.

Cystic Fibrosis Secretion

In CF, this process either fails or is compromised significantly because the CFTR does not provide a normal Cl^- channel. Most cases of CF in the United States are caused by the ΔF508 mutation, where the CFTR is practically absent from the membrane (5,37,38). Consequently, Cl^- cannot get out of the cell or carry current into the lumen to attract its co-ion, Na^+. Without increased NaCl in the lumen, water cannot move and fluid secretion cannot occur in response to β-adrenergic stimulation. Again, thermoregulatory sweating apparently does not involve CFTR Cl^- channels and is normal in CF.

SALT ABSORPTION

Structure of Absorptive Cells of the Duct

The remaining half of the tubule in the corpuscle of the gland consists of the reabsorptive duct. These epithelial cells are arranged uniquely in a cylindrical bilayer as a functional syncytium. That is, two concentric layers of epithelial cells form the wall of the tubule. Tight junctions appear only between the cells of the inner layer so that only these cells have an apical membrane that forms the barrier to the lumen. All cells of both layers are connected via numerous gap junctions so that the cells of the outer layer can be viewed as an extension of the basolateral membrane of the inner layer cells (see Fig. 19–1B). These intercellular pathways apparently provide free movement of electrolytes and cytoplasmic solutes between all cells in both layers. Tight junctions apparently are tight so that Na^+ and Cl^- both move transcellularly. Innervation of the duct has not been demonstrated.

Function of Duct Cells in Salt Absorption

It is unfortunate that over the past 5 years CF has been characterized repeatedly in the literature and from the podium as a disease of abnormal secretion caused by the lack of the CFTR. Although it is clear that secretion is affected and is abnormal, it is just as clear and, very possibly more important pathologically (39), that salt absorption also is severely defective. The fact that the concentration of salt in CF sweat is abnormally high is one of the most widely known characteristics of the disease (40,41). Other reasons for high sweat NaCl are so rare that this phenomenon almost is pathognomonic for the disease.

So why is sweat so abnormally salty in CF?

Initially, sweat is equally salty in both healthy subjects and those with CF (42); however, normally salt is removed by hypertonic absorption from the primary sweat before it reaches the surface of the skin. In CF, this absorptive process is handicapped severely, and the sweat tends to remain salty. To understand the problem of salt transport in CF glands, it helps to understand the function of salt transport in normal glands.

Mechanisms of Salt Reabsorption

We believe that there are at least two apparently separate mechanisms for the uptake of NaCl from the duct lumen. One mechanism primarily is electroconductive to accommodate rapid uptake of large quantities of salt against relatively smaller Cl^- gradients, and a second mechanism of countertransport exchange[d] is needed to accommodate smaller quantities of salt uptake against relatively larger Cl^- gradients.

Electroconductive Absorption

NaCl absorption via electroconductive absorption is depicted in Fig. 19–3A according to the following sequence:

Na^+/K^+-ATPase, essential to all forms of fluid transport, maintains a low intracellular Na^+ concentration by pumping Na^+ across the basolateral membrane out of the duct cells (see Fig. 19–3A) (23). This action creates an inward gradient for Na^+ movement. The basolateral membrane is relatively impermeable to Na^+, but the apical membrane exhibits a significant Na^+ permeability that can be blocked directly with the diuretic amiloride (3,43).

Na^+ enters the cell from the duct lumen through the Na^+ channel, but because of electroneutrality, Na^+ cannot be transported across the apical cell membrane unless a negative charge accompanies it.

Cl^- carries the negative charge and enters the cell from the lumen only through the CFTR Cl^- channel. We find no evidence for any other Cl^- channels in this membrane. When the Cl^- channel is activated and open, salt absorption proceeds. To our knowledge, the CFTR is the only control point in the absorptive process. We have yet to detect any effect of cAMP on Na^+ conductance (44).

---

[d]An exchanger is a transport mechanism that thermodynamically couples the movement of a species in one direction to the movement of another species in the opposite direction. If the different species carry like charges, the net movement will occur independent of any electrical gradient.

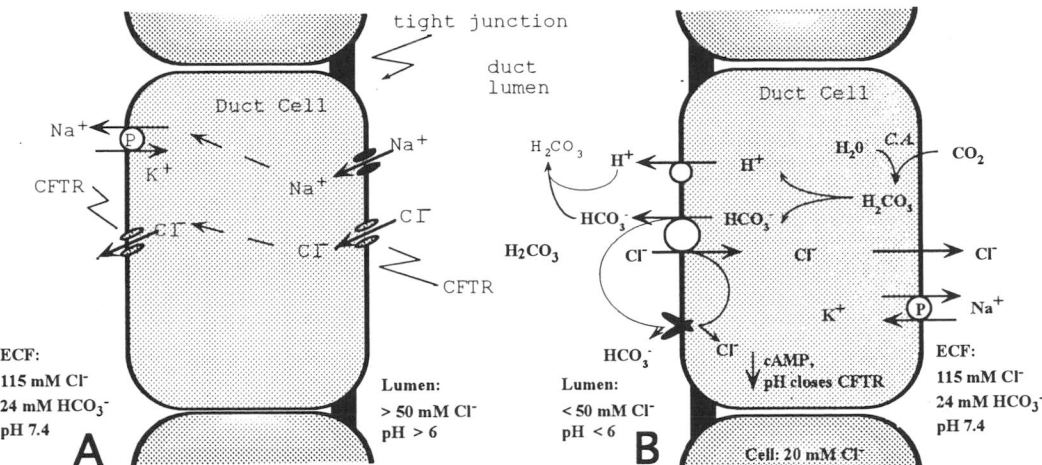

FIG. 19–3. (A) Model of electroconductive mechanism of salt absorption in the sweat duct. Na+ enters the cell across the apical membrane because the intracellular Na+ concentration is kept low by the Na+/K+-ATPase pump, which exports Na+ across the basal membrane to effect transcellular Na+ absorption. These movements of Na establish electrochemical gradients for Cl– to accompany Na+ passively across both membranes. **(B)** Predicted model for electroneutral Cl– absorption in the duct. As the luminal concentration of Cl– decreases to less than approximately 50 mmol/L, the luminal pH also decreases and may move to less than pH 5. The lower luminal pH should bring about a gradient for HCO_3^- movement from the extracellular fluid (ECF) into the cell and from the cell into the lumen. The lower luminal HCO_3^- concentration increases electroneutral uptake of Cl– through the apical Cl–/HCO_3^- exchanger. Low pH and decreased cAMP reduce the activity of PKA, which probably are relevant in closing CFTR so that exchanged Cl– uptake then becomes independent of electrical gradients. The mechanism of Cl– exit through the basal membrane also may be through a Cl–/HCO_3^- exchanger in the basolateral membrane. C.A., carbonic anhydrase.

Once inside the cell, Na+ is extruded by the Na+/K+-ATPase pump in the basolateral membrane.

Cl– again follows passively through the CFTR channel in the basolateral membrane to satisfy electroneutrality.

Even though salt is lost from the luminal fluid and its osmolality is lowered accordingly, water cannot readily accompany the reabsorbed salt because the apical membrane is relatively impermeable to water. Salt therefore is reabsorbed in excess of water so that sweat must become hypotonic as it flows through the duct to the skin surface.

There is little question that most NaCl absorption in the normal duct proceeds via the Cl– electroconductive pathway provided by the CFTR, as described. However, when we as-

sayed to determine the driving forces required for salt absorption to the low levels of 10 to 15 mmol/L Cl– that occur in sweat from healthy subjects, we found that Cl– conductance becomes a liability rather than an asset for Cl– absorption (45). That is, our measurements of intracellular Cl– activity and intracellular potentials showed that when Cl– concentrations in the lumen are less than approximately 40 to 50 mmol/L, the electrochemical gradient favors Cl– secretion back into the lumen rather than Cl– absorption into the cell (45). Clearly, not only must another mechanism for Cl– absorption be present to continue to decrease Cl– concentration to the levels seen in final sweat, but somehow the Cl– conductive pathway of CFTR must be closed. Otherwise, Cl– absorbed by the second mechanism will leak back through the CFTR Cl– conductance into the lumen.

Anion Exchanger Absorption

It has been well established for many years that even though NaCl is higher in final sweat in patients with CF than in healthy subjects (meaning that NaCl absorption is reduced greatly), the final sweat collected from most patients is substantially lower in NaCl than plasma (meaning that substantial salt absorption still occurs). In the past few years, molecular biology has shown us clearly that in most patients with CF, the disease is the result of faulty processing of the CFTR; that is, the protein virtually never reaches its destination in the plasma membrane (5,37,38). We find no evidence of other Cl^- channels in the apical membrane of the duct so we are left with the provocative question of how salt absorption takes place at all in these patients with CF. Two explanations seem most likely. Either small amounts of at least partially functional CFTR Cl^- channels do in fact make it to the membrane so that some reabsorption is supported, or there is more than one mechanism for reabsorption in the sweat duct—one of which is not dependent on CFTR function. Although we cannot exclude the former, we believe that the latter is likely.

The defect in bicarbonate (HCO_3^-) secretion in the CF pancreas (46) is instructive in suggesting a second mechanism for absorption (45) in the duct. In the pancreas, CFTR and Cl^-/HCO_3^- exchange must be coupled functionally because loss of CFTR Cl^- conductance limits pancreatic secretion in CF even though there is no evidence that the exchanger is defective. Anion exchange may be as important for Cl^- absorption in the sweat duct as it is for HCO_3^- secretion in the pancreas. This notion is based on several observations. First, as aforementioned, the electrochemical gradient at low luminal Cl^- concentrations is incompatible with electroconductive Cl^- absorption so that some other means of removing Cl^- from the lumen must present. Second, the pH of sweat at low Cl^- concentrations is very acidic (< 5) (47–49). Third, if Na^+ conductance is blocked with amiloride and Cl^- conductance is blocked by substitution with gluconate (an impermeable

anion), the luminal potential becomes electrically positive. These results strongly suggest active H^+ secretion in the duct. Fourth, cytoimmunologic staining for carbonic anhydrase II (50) is strongly positive in the sweat duct, and this enzyme almost always—if not always—is associated with Cl^-/HCO_3^- exchange. These observations support the idea that a Cl^-/HCO_3^- exchange operates in parallel, with the CFTR Cl^- conductive mechanism for salt absorption. We expect that as long as the Cl^- concentration in the lumen is relatively high, the electroconductive mechanism is the prevalent route of Cl^- absorption. However, when the Cl^- concentration is reduced, Cl^-/HCO_3^- exchange becomes the prevalent, if not exclusive, mode of Cl^- absorption.

Part of a predicted sequence for HCO_3^-/Cl^- exchange absorption of Cl^- is depicted in Figure 19–3B, as follows:

An apical membrane H^+ ion pump actively secretes protons into the lumen, which react with luminal HCO_3^- to form carbonic acid (H_2CO_3). This proton secretion is required to acidify the lumen and remove HCO_3^- from it. Although the anion exchanger continues to add HCO_3^- to the lumen in exchange for Cl^-, the lumen will remain acidic as long as acid secretion exceeds HCO_3^- entry into the lumen.

Carbonic anhydrase catalyzes the carbonic acid to CO_2 plus H_2O, which removes HCO_3^- from the luminal fluid and helps maintain a HCO_3^- gradient from the cell into the lumen. [At physiologic CO_2 levels, the luminal HCO_3^- concentration will approach 0 (< 0.1 mmol/L) as the pH decreases to < 6, but an intracellular pH of 6.8 to 7 is in equilibrium with a HCO_3^- concentration of approximately 6 to 9 mmol/L].

This HCO_3^- gradient out of the cell removes Cl^- from the lumen as HCO_3^- enters the lumen on the exchanger (the apical membrane is impermeable to HCO_3^-).

Intracellular pH decreases with loss of intracellular HCO_3^-.

Lower intracellular pH inhibits PKA activity and supports phosphatase activity, both of which deactivate the CFTR and close CFTR Cl⁻ conductance to block the electroconductive pathway. Because the exchange mechanism is electroneutral and Cl⁻ conductance is blocked, further absorption of Cl⁻ becomes independent of the electrical gradient for Cl⁻ across the apical membrane.[e] Cl⁻ absorption into the cell will continue as long as the chemical gradient for HCO_3^- out of the cell is larger than the chemical gradient for Cl⁻ out of the cell.

In ductal absorptive function, there is a proportional relationship between Cl⁻, HCO_3^-, pH, and sweat rate. When one is high, all tend to be high; when one is low, all tend to be low. The reason for this is that the absorptive capacity of the sweat duct is limited so that at high secretory rates the amount (= volume × concentration) of salt delivered to the duct is large and tends to saturate the absorptive capacity. In this context, HCO_3^- enters the duct lumen from only two sources: (a) in the fluid of the primary sweat secreted from the coil and (b) in exchange for Cl⁻ from the duct. HCO_3^- can leave the duct lumen by only two means: (a) in the fluid of the final sweat and (b) as CO_2 from the product of HCO_3^-, reacting with H⁺ secreted by the duct cells. As long as H⁺ secretion exceeds HCO_3^- delivery, luminal HCO_3^- will be low and the HCO_3^- gradient from cell to lumen will drive Cl⁻ absorption independent of its electrical gradient.

The mechanism of Cl⁻ absorption by anion exchange, or that of any similar mechanism, demands that the state of the CFTR Cl⁻ channel be regulated when electroconductive absorption becomes ineffective. If Cl⁻ transport occurred only through the CFTR and the CFTR never closed, it would be impossible to absorb Cl⁻ beyond the Cl⁻ electrochemical gradient into the cell. Any Cl⁻ absorbed by the exchanger would leak back into the lumen through the open CFTR channel. The fact that CFTR phosphorylation (activation) and dephosphorylation (deactivation) is influenced by intracellular pH provides a mechanism by which the CFTR can be regulated as a function of luminal composition. It is not clear whether regulation is tied to luminal Cl⁻ concentration or whether luminal HCO_3^- simply determines intracellular pH so that at high luminal HCO_3^- (and Cl⁻) concentration, more HCO_3^- accumulates in the cell to increase the cell pH and favor increased net phosphorylation, more open CFTR channels, and electroconductive uptake of Cl⁻ (see Fig. 19–3A). However, at low luminal HCO_3^- (and Cl⁻) concentrations, loss of cell HCO_3^- lowers intracellular pH, favoring dephosphorylation, closed CFTR channels, and uptake via the nonconductive exchanger pathway (see Fig. 19–3B).

Control of Absorption

At this point in our understanding, acute control of salt absorption seems to be exerted only through CFTR. It has long been established that the level of NaCl concentration in the sweat of healthy individuals (51,52)—and to some extent that of CF subjects—(53,54) is a function of circulating aldosterone levels. As in the kidney, this control is exerted over periods of hours or days and occurs via increased expression of amiloride sensitive Na⁺ channels and Na⁺/K⁺-ATPase. Initially, we were not able to detect any acute cAMP-mediated regulation of Na⁺ absorption (ENaC) in the isolated sweat duct (55,56), but recently we have found cAMP-dependent increases in ENaC that appear to depend on activated CFTR. In contrast, CFTR Cl⁻ channels can be turned on or off in a matter of seconds. Acute control of CFTR activation occurs through at least two mechanisms: interaction with ATP and phosphorylation by PKA.

Role of Adenosine Triphosphate

In comparison with findings in other systems where CFTR Cl⁻ channel activity has been studied separately from the cell cyto-

---

[e]In electroneutral exchange mechanisms, each cycle of the exchange transfers an equal number of like charges in opposite directions. Because there is no displacement of net charge, there is no current and the process is independent of electrical gradients. That is, both Cl⁻ and HCO_3^- move on the exchanger only according to their chemical gradients.

plasm, such as with patch clamp (57,58) and planar bilayers (59,60), the concentration of ATP required for CFTR activation in the sweat duct is at least an order of magnitude and perhaps two orders of magnitude higher. We found that Cl⁻ conductance (activation of CFTR Cl⁻ channels) in duct cells is not detectable until the cytoplasmic levels of ATP reach at least 1 mmol/L and does not approach full activation until physiologic levels of 5 mmol/L in the cytoplasmic levels are achieved. Increasing ATP to 10 mmol/L increases Cl⁻ conductance only slightly more (8,61). These levels of ATP reflect those normally found in the cell. There currently is evidence that ATP hydrolysis is required (62–64) to activate and deactivate CFTR channel conductance, but the levels of ATP required for these events also are significantly less than those we require to activate Cl⁻ conductance in the sweat duct.

These requirements and discrepancies suggest that in addition to whatever the need for ATP hydrolysis to change activation states in CFTR (60,63), at least in the sweat duct there seems to be a requirement for nucleotide interaction that is supported only by cytoplasmic levels of ATP concentration. Because one of the most important maintenance functions of any cell is to ensure an adequate energy supply for metabolic processes, we believe that this requirement of the CFTR in the sweat duct for these levels of ATP is integrated with controlling the energy charge of the cell (61). That is, allosteric interaction with ATP as a cofactor is necessary to support Cl⁻ conductance in the duct to the fullest extent needed for physiologic function. This requirement may not involve ATP hydrolysis because, assuming that our protocol truly removes Mg^{++} from the cytoplasm, activation of CFTR is independent of Mg^{++} and to our knowledge all ATP hydrolysis requires Mg^{++}. We anticipate that this control is tied closely to the energy supplies of the cell such that if salt transport activity begins to consume so much ATP that cell reserves become threatened (e.g., cytoplasmic ATP concentrations < 1 to 3 mmol/L), the CFTR begins to shut down, conductance falls, salt transport decreases, ATP consumption declines, and ATP returns to appropriate levels. This feedback mechanism protects vital processes from failing because of energy depletion by auxiliary functions such as transcellular ion transport (65).

Role of Phosphorylation

Although innervation of the sweat duct has not been demonstrated, it is clear that Cl⁻ absorption in the duct is acutely dependent on cAMP. Unlike the secretory tubule, the only apparent route for Cl⁻ transport through duct cells is through the CFTR Cl⁻ channel. Interestingly, not only is the duct apparently insensitive to cholinergic or Ca^{++}-mediated control, but at first impression, it also appeared to be insensitive to β-adrenergic, cAMP-mediated control. This deceit was caused by the fact that, at least under conditions of investigation, when the duct is isolated from the gland, the CFTR channel usually is activated fully and further activation after the application of ß-adrenergic agonists cannot be detected readily (55). However, if small solutes are drained from the cytoplasm by permeabilizing the basolateral cell membrane with a pore-forming agent such as α-toxin, the CFTR Cl⁻ channels deactivate and close within a few minutes. The state of the channels then can be controlled easily by adding back cAMP together with physiologic levels of ATP (8,56). If only cAMP or ATP is added back alone, no activation occurs. This result strongly suggests that the CFTR must be activated both by phosphorylation and by interaction with ATP to support salt transport across the duct cell. It is well established that CFTR Cl⁻ channel activity is controlled by cAMP activation of PKA in numerous other systems (66–69). The simple act of removing and adding back cAMP in the presence of ATP in the sweat duct is strong, although not conclusive, evidence of PKA control. cAMP activation also can be blocked completely by the nonspecific kinase inhibitor staurosporine (56, 67). Other kinases, such as tyrosine kinase (70) and protein kinase G (PKG) (71), have been implicated in controlling CFTR in other systems, but the existence of other kinases in the sweat duct have not been investigated seriously.

Once activated by phosphorylation, CFTR activity is subject to deactivation by endogenous phosphatases. Okadaic acid and calyculin, two inhibitors that are relatively specific for PP1 and PP2 (protein phosphatase 1 and 2, respectively) effectively prevent CFTR Cl$^-$ channels from closing once they have been activated by adding cAMP. If during phosphorylation activation with cAMP, ATP is replaced by an analogue, ATP-γ-S, which can be hydrolyzed by PKA but whose phosphorylation product cannot be hydrolyzed readily by phosphatases (72), the CFTR channels remain open almost indefinitely (9). However, fluoride and vanadate as nonspecific phosphatase inhibitors are considerably less effective blockers of dephosphorylation in the isolated sweat duct (9). Because these nonspecific phosphatase inhibitors are inefficient and because alkaline phosphatase is an ectocytoplasmic enzyme, it is unlikely that alkaline phosphatase has any role in controlling the CFTR in the duct, in contrast to early reports that this enzyme may control the CFTR (69). It seems more likely that PP2 is the endogenous phosphatase that dephosphorylates and deactivates the CFTR in the duct because PP1 neither deactivated nor dephosphorylated the CFTR in transfected cells (67).

Role of pH

If the sweat duct is not innervated but CFTR is under phosphorylation control, we must ask what cytoplasmic factors or conditions control kinase and phosphatase activity. We have observed that cytoplasmic pH may be a determining factor. If the cytoplasmic pH is clamped at 8 or greater by changing the buffered pH of the bathing media of a duct with a permeabilized basolateral membrane after cAMP phosphorylation activation, spontaneous deactivation of the Cl$^-$ channel does not occur. Conversely, if the pH is clamped at pH 6 or less, deactivation is accelerated and, furthermore, CFTR channels cannot be activated by adding back cAMP and ATP at this low pH. If pH is restored to greater than 6, cAMP + ATP will activate the CFTR again, showing that the inhibition is reversible and

not due to nonspecific irreversible effects of low pH, such as denaturation (P. M. Quinton, personal observations, 1996).

Effect of the Defective Cystic Fibrosis Transmembrane Conductance Regulator in Absorption in Cystic Fibrosis Sweat

Electroconductively, the sweat duct is impermeable to Cl$^-$ (2,3). Because cations cannot be transported without an equivalent charge of anions, this defect also renders Na$^+$ effectively impermeable. The CF duct cell has a normal Na$^+$ conductance (permeability) in its membrane (73), but as the cell attempts to absorb it, enormous electrostatic forces are built up that oppose its transport simply because Cl$^-$ with its negative charge cannot follow Na$^+$ with its positive charge. As a consequence, neither Na$^+$ nor Cl$^-$ is absorbed electroconductively in the CF duct, and the sweat that emerges on the skin surface contains an abnormally large amount of NaCl salt.

The electrical nature of the defect produces significant differences in the electrical properties of the CF cell as well. Logically, retention of Cl$^-$ and its negative charge in the lumen causes the lumen to become electrically much more negative relative to the extracellular fluid (blood side of the tissue) than its counterpart in healthy subjects. The luminal potential of the microperfused CF sweat duct is more than six times more negative than that of a normal duct, -85 mV versus -14 mV, respectively (2,3). Viewed another way, because Na$^+$ is permeable in the CF duct, its tendency to move into the cell without Cl$^-$ causes the cell to become positive with respect to the lumen and blocks movement of positively charged Na$^+$ ions into the cell so that neither Cl$^-$ nor Na$^+$ can be transported. This more negative electrical potential is the direct result of decreased Cl$^-$ permeability and is not a result of increased Na$^+$ absorption.

Nonetheless, it is reported (74,75) that Na$^+$ transport is increased in CF airway tissue under conditions in which the effect of the electrical fields generated by Cl$^-$ impermeability are neutralized by external short circuiting; that is, the negative charge normally carried by Cl$^-$ is

TABLE 19–1. *Sweat electrolyte values for healthy subjects and patients with cystic fibrosis (CF)*[a]

Subjects: Gender (age, yrs)	Cl⁻ (range)	Na⁺ (range)	K⁺ (range)
Healthy adults: M (21–>40)	32 (7–87)	40.7 (11–90)	9.6 (6–23)
Healthy adults: F (21–>40)	31 (8–76)	40.4 (10–81)	9.8 (9–25)
Patients with CF: M (21–27)	121 (76–138)	122 (93–138)	16 (11–25)
Patients with CF: F (21–27)	121 (84–141)	123 (87–155)	19 (11–28)

[a]Data from reference 82.

supplied artificially by an external current source to accompany Na^+ when it is transported through the tissue. Na^+ movement then becomes independent of Cl^- movement. We cannot apply this approach to measuring Na^+ movements in the sweat duct because it requires placing an electrode down the center of the lumen of the duct, which seems impossible for a diameter of only 15 μm. Consequently, we do not know whether short-circuited Na^+ transport in the duct would be larger than normal. Calculations from specific resistance and potential measurements in CF and normal ducts indicate that the equivalent short circuits are not different (73). In any case, under physiologic conditions in which short circuiting never is present (open circuit transport), the Na^+ absorption in the CF duct is not increased but is impaired severely (31) (Table 19–1). The effect of a defective CFTR in the CF sweat duct is, as predicted from first principles, to decrease Na^+ transport and to increase the negative electrical potential across the epithelium.

Practical Points of Interest

In addition to esoteric interests in the theory of salt uptake in the human sweat duct, these discussions raise at least two practical points that should be of interest in performing sweat tests. First, in healthy subjects, false-positive results will occur if the absorptive capacity of the duct becomes overloaded by the amount of salt secreted from the secretory coil.[f] When the absorptive machinery is overloaded, salt ab-

sorption is at a maximum, but it is small compared with the total amount of salt being secreted. Consequently, final sweat will be excreted with relatively higher salt concentrations. False-positive results are most likely to occur in adults who have the ability to secrete at very high rates. One should be circumspect about high salt values in sweat secreted at high rates in adults. High rates do not necessarily mean high concentrations, but high concentrations are more likely to occur at high rates, especially if the subject is Na^+ surfeited (low circulating aldosterone), as is the case with many American diets. The sweat glands of children, however, cannot secrete sweat at sufficiently high rates to overload the absorptive capacity of the duct, so this factor is of little consequence for sweat tests in the pediatric group. Teleologically, the reason for the difference between children and adults is that the number of sweat glands is fixed at birth and does not increase with age, stress, or any other factor (13,14). However, in adults, the body surface is larger, so the surface-to-volume ratio is smaller. Thus, the demand on each individual sweat gland for volume in fluid secreted increases with body size (age). However, the increase in the ability to secrete more salt (larger volumes) is not paralleled completely by an increase in the capacity to absorb more salt.

It is clear that virtually all, if not all, CF ducts retain some capacity to absorb salts because Na^+, Cl^-, and HCO_3^- nearly always are found in final CF sweat at concentrations less than those at which they are secreted into the gland lumen as primary sweat (i.e., less than in plasma). This absorption must occur via a non-CFTR mechanism (and probably to some extent via the CFTR if the mutation is expressed and partially functional). In individuals with

---

[f]Recall that amount is volume × concentration or, in this case, rate × concentration; because the concentration is constant (isotonic), the amount secreted into the duct is a strict function of the secretory rate.

CF, this alternate absorptive mechanism may create false-negative (erroneously low) values at low sweat rates when the amount of salt secreted into the lumen is within this limited capacity of the alternative mechanism in the CF duct to absorb salt. It always should be kept in mind that independent of source, CF or normal, values that are reported isotonic, and especially those reported hypertonic to plasma, almost are certainly the result of technical error.

THE SWEAT TEST

The aforementioned discussion provides a theoretical backdrop for understanding factors that affect the production of sweat and its final concentration as it appears on the skin surface. Some of these considerations may have practical importance in performing the sweat test—the test that is almost pathognomonic with CF. The object of the test is to determine quantitatively whether the salt concentration of sweat is abnormally high. There is some problem in establishing what is abnormally high. Unlike plasma, cerebral spinal fluid, glomerular filtrate, or interstitial fluid, the composition of sweat is not constant. We have seen that sweat concentration varies considerably as a function of sweat rate in single glands (31). It is more like urine because its final composition is a function of multiple influences. In addition to rate (76), one of the most important influences is aldosterone levels (77). Like the distal tubule, the sweat duct is an aldosterone target[g]; a low Na^+ diet decreases the sweat salt concentration in patients with CF (53) and in healthy subjects. Conversely, high Na^+ diets increase sweat salt concentration (52,54). Table 19–1 gives a list of a number of electrolytes and compounds and the range of concentrations at which they have been found in normal sweat. After all is said and done, diagnosis from the sweat test is empirical and based on distributions of values between healthy subjects (including heterozygotes) and patients with CF (78,79). The National Cystic Fibrosis Founda-

tion (80) officially recommends considering chloride values that are less than 40 mEq/L as normal, values greater than 60 mEq/L as strongly indicative of the disease, and values between 40 and 60 mEq/L as borderline.

The process of performing a sweat test requires approximately 30 to 40 minutes and includes stimulating a site on the skin with sweating agonists, collecting the resulting sweat, quantitating the volume or weight of sweat collected, and analyzing the sweat for its concentration of Cl^-, Na^+, or both. A brief description of the procedure follows, but the reader is referred to the National Committee for Clinical Laboratory Standards Document C34-A (80) for techniques and details specifically recommended and endorsed by the National Cystic Fibrosis Foundation for its Center Network. Tests should be conducted at accredited centers experienced in the procedure. Experience indicates that tests performed sporadically are much less likely to yield consistently reliable results.

Stimulating the Site

To stimulate sweating, a cholinomimetic drug must be delivered intradermally to the sweat glands. Heating and intradermal injections of drugs are not efficient. After more than 30 years, the most efficient method remains that of Gibson and Cooke (81) who used iontophoresis of pilocarpine, an acetyl cholinesterase-resistant secretagogue. Iontophoresis consists of delivering the drug through the skin by using its ionic form to carry electrical current between two stationary electrodes.

Briefly, areas of approximately 50 cm^2 (7 cm × 7 cm) on the volar and dorsal surfaces of the forearm should be selected and cleaned well. The arm is preferred because it can be manipulated and examined easily, can be stimulated without passing current across any portion of the torso, and has an adequate density of sweat glands. One metal (stainless steel) electrode with a surface area of 25 cm^2 curved to the contour of the arm is strapped firmly to each side of the arm over a slightly larger gauze sponge wetted with 15 mmol/L pilocarpine nitrate so-

---

[g]Unlike the distal nephron, the water permeability is virtually insensitive to antidiuretic hormone (ADH).

lution[h] placed within the selected areas. The objective is to deliver the drug uniformly across an area of skin of approximately 25 cm². Therefore, the density of the electrical current across the area (field) must be even and uniform. If there are spots in the field that are of higher or lower resistance, the current likewise will be uneven. Cleanliness and pressure are the two principal determinants of uniform current. Both the surface of the skin and the surface of the electrode must be free of any oil or grease,[i] which act as insulators, creating high electrical resistance and producing hot spots elsewhere by causing current to flow to areas of lower resistance. Similarly, if the pressure on the electrode is not distributed uniformly, parts of the electrode will be pressed closer to the skin, creating areas of low resistance with increased current, which also will produce hot spots. Hot spots are most likely to occur at edges and corners of unevenly positioned electrodes. Matching the curvature of the arm and the electrode is important in this regard. Not only do hot spots cause poor distribution of the drugs, but also they are very likely to burn the skin. A direct current of approximately 4 milliamperes must be applied for 5 minutes to the 25 cm² electrodes (approximately 0.15 milliamps/cm²), preferably from a battery source (to avoid the possibility of accidental contact with line voltage). The positive electrode (cathode) must be over the site to be stimulated with pilocarpine. Pilocarpine is a cation, positively charged, and will be driven away from this electrode into the skin. The opposite electrode, the anode, is positioned on the contra lateral surface of the same arm over a gauze wetted with saline.

Collecting the Sample

After the glands have been stimulated, the site must be washed rapidly with distilled water and dried with gauze. A precut, preweighed filter paper of low-ash content (e.g., Whatman 40) of approximately 5 cm × 5 cm must be placed over the site and immediately enclosed under a slightly larger piece of clean parafilm or water impermeable plastic and securely taped around the edges to create a hermetic seal.[j] Haste is necessary because the stimulated glands begin to secrete sweat onto the surface, which can evaporate and create erroneously elevated concentrations. For this same reason, the parafilm must be sealed hermetically. Normally, the collection time is approximately 30 minutes. However, if the subject sweats profusely and liquid sweat can be visualized beneath the film, the period can and probably should be shortened. Conversely, if there is doubt about the adequacy of the sample, the period may be extended somewhat. However, it is doubtful that increasing the collection period much longer than 30 minutes will increase significantly the quantity of the sample collected because the highest sweating rates occur initially when the concentration of the agonist still is high in the skin. Not only does the concentration of the drug dissipate within the collection period, but also sweat glands fatigue.

To determine the volume, the preweighed sweat-moistened filter paper (or gauze) must be removed promptly from beneath the film-covered site and hermetically sealed in a preweighed vial. Evaporation from the sample must be avoided at all cost. The sum of the weights (to the nearest mg) of the vial[k] and dry filter paper (before collection) then is subtracted from the total weight of the vial containing the filter paper wetted with the collected sweat. The difference is the net weight of the sample collected. At least 75 µL (10^{-6} L)[l] should be collected. Experienced laborato-

---

[h]The exact concentration is not important but should be between 5 and 20 mmol/L.

[i]Propanol is an excellent solvent for removing oily substances.

[j]Needless to say, cleanliness is essential. Hands should be freshly washed; if gloves are used, they should be powder free, and filter paper should be handled only with clean forceps. If absorbents other than filter paper are used, such as gauze, they should be assayed for the possibility of leaking salts into the sample. That is, they must be salt-free before use.

[k]When weighing the vial, care should be exercised not to contaminate its surface with fingerprints, which erroneously increase its weight.

[l]That is, 75 mg.

ries sometimes can work with less.[m] This volume over a 30-minute period from a 25-cm^2 site equals approximately 0.5 to 1 nL/minute/gland; that is relatively low activity, but recall that this is an average and the initial rates during the collection period certainly will be much higher. In adults, volumes exceeding 200 μL/site/30 minutes are expected.

It is difficult to quantitate a single gland sweat rate because the density of glands varies considerably from individual to individual (11,82). It is not possible to give a reference value for a normal volume of sweat that should be obtained in the aforementioned procedure. Furthermore, a single sweat gland will secrete at maximal rates of between 10 and 20 nL/minute (1 to 2 $\times$ 10^{-8} L/minute) when stimulated initially. This rate would produce a total sweat sample in excess of 1.5 mL per collection period, but as noted, the rate continuously declines after the initial stimulation so that a constant rate during the collection period does not occur and is not to be expected. In adults, samples in excess of 0.5 mL per collection period are not uncommon. Therefore, it is customary and practical to simply ensure that an adequate volume of sweat is obtained for analysis.

Analyzing the Sample

The Cystic Fibrosis Foundation, through its Diagnostic Consensus, recommends that Cl$^-$ be measured for a standard quantitative sweat test. Qualitative tests, for example, sweat conductivity or osmolality assays (83), may be used for screening purposes, but abnormal tests must be confirmed by quantitative assays. Such screening tests are not clinically appropriate for diagnosis of CF in adults. Cl$^-$ and Na$^+$ can be analyzed, but usually the difference between normal and CF

concentrations is somewhat greater for Cl$^-$ than for Na$^+$. This difference is due to the fact that the anion gap or total anions other than Cl$^-$ is smaller in CF sweat than in normal sweat (84, 85). It is recommended that concentrations be determined by coulometric titration with a chloridometer and that Na$^+$ concentration be determined by flame photometry. For a detailed description of these techniques, the reader is referred to the NCCLA document (80).

Interpreting the Result

In the majority of cases, the results clearly should distinguish healthy individuals and individuals with CF. The concentrations of both Na$^+$ and Cl$^-$ in sweat from nonaffected individuals will be less than 40 mmol/L. For example, according to Davis et al. (86), of 166 adults without CF but with other pulmonary disorders, 96% had sweat chloride concentration values of less than 60 mmol/L and 99% had values less than 70 mmol/L. Samples from adult men with values higher than 40 mmol/L should be interpreted cautiously, especially if the volume collected is large (high sweat rate, as noted previously). Before puberty, males and females have approximately equal sweat rates (87). During puberty, the sweat rate for men compared with women approximately doubles. Consequently, men may be more likely to saturate the ductal reabsorptive mechanisms and produce more salt in the sweat.

Some rare inherited metabolic diseases, such as mucopolysaccharidosis type I, can elevate sweat Cl$^-$ in the absence of CF (81). Most such metabolic diseases present in childhood. The most important diseases that present in adulthood and may elevate sweat Cl$^-$ are malnutrition, hypogammaglobulinemia, nephrogenic diabetes insipidus, nephrotic syndrome, pseudohypoaldosteronism, untreated adrenal insufficiency, untreated hypothyroidism, and glucose-6-phosphate dehydrogenase deficiency (88). These diseases generally are diagnosed or excluded by routine clinical evaluations.

---

[m]Some laboratories rely on a commercially available sweat collector, which is a coil of microbore tubing. Theoretically, this device should offer no significant advantage over the classic technique other than convenience. The user should follow the manufacturer recommendations for its application.

Supplementary Assays

Sodium/Chloride Ratios

In some cases, it may be informative to determine the concentrations of both Na^+ and Cl^-. It has been noted rarely, probably because of the lack of precision in most analyses, that in patients with CF the ratio of the Na^+/Cl^- concentrations is less than 1.0 whereas in sweat from healthy subjects, the ratio almost always is greater than 1.0 (31,84,89–91). Thus, if the Cl^- concentration is significantly and consistently less than the Na^+ concentration in the same sample, it is likely that the subject does not have CF.[n]

β-Adrenergic Sweating

It is well established that patients with CF do not respond to β-adrenergic stimulation (7,92–94). Thus, another possibility for interpreting enigmatic results might be to use the iontophoresis procedure to simulate with isoproterenol bitartrate in place of pilocarpine nitrate. The β-adrenergic agonist must be applied with atropine to prevent the adrenergic stimulation from secondarily stimulating release of endogenous acetylcholine, which will stimulate cholinergic sweating. If adequate volumes of sweat are obtained with pilocarpine and virtually no sweat is obtained with isoproterenol, it is likely that the subject has CF. To our knowledge, this test has not been explored using the iontophoresis protocol suggested for pilocarpine. We have used iontophoresis of isoproterenol into a small area of approximately 0.5 cm^2, with clear results in a limited number of patients. Similarly, Sato and Sato first presented the notion of defective β-adrenergically stimulated sweating in CF patients using intradermal injections of isoproterenol plus atropine into small areas of skin (7,92). Caution must be exercised to avoid administering levels

of catecholamines that will induce systemic catecholamine reactions. Acute tachycardia and pupillary dilation may occur in some individuals as a result.

Pitfalls

From the previous discussion, it should be clear that sweat initially is secreted into the secretory tubule in an isotonic fluid with a high NaCl content independent of secretory rate; that is, high means relative to the concentration of sweat secreted from normal glands (20 to 40 mEq/L), but approximately equal to the concentration in interstitial fluid or plasma (140 to 145 mEq/L for Na^+ and 105 to 110 mEq/L for Cl^-). To a very good first approximation, NaCl in CF sweat never can be higher than that of interstitial fluid (there is no hypertonic secretion). The difference of approximately 100 mEq/L between the primary secretion and excreted normal sweat is the result of salt absorption by the duct cells as sweat moves to the skin surface. When Na^+ or Cl^- values higher than those in the plasma are reported, the result most likely is the result of evaporation artifacts or contamination of the collected sample.

SUMMARY

The eccrine sweat gland is the basis for the most common diagnostic test for CF and the basis of much fundamental research on the pathophysiology expressed in CF as well as on fluid transport in human epithelia. The gland clearly demonstrates the function of two types of fluid secretion, cholinergically innervated/Ca^{++}-mediated secretion, which does not depend on the CFTR, and β-adrenergically innervated/cAMP-mediated secretion, which is highly dependent on the CFTR. It also presents two examples of different Cl^- absorption, an electroconductive pathway that is highly dependent on CFTR and a probable nonconductive anion exchange absorption of Cl^-, which probably is not dependent on CFTR. The ability of patients with CF to secrete normal volumes of sweat and thermoregulate properly can be understood in terms of defective CFTR-

---

[n]There have been no clinical studies to our knowledge to firmly establish this phenomenon as a criterion for diagnosis, but in our experience, it holds well and is presented here for the interest of the reader. Clearly, the analysis of both Cl^- and Na^+ must be accomplished with high precision.

dependent and normal non-CFTR–dependent fluid secretory mechanisms. The differing values in concentrations of NaCl appearing in the final sweat of both healthy subjects and those with CF can be understood in terms of decreased hypertonic salt absorption in the CF sweat duct caused by the absence of an electroconductive pathway normally provided by the CFTR. Understanding the impact of the components that contribute to forming final sweat provides a physiologic basis for interpreting the sweat test.

ACKNOWLEDGMENT

This work is supported by the National Cystic Fibrosis Foundation.

REFERENCES

1. Busch R. On the history of cystic fibrosis. *ACTA Universitatis Carolinae Medica* 1990;36:13–15.
2. Quinton PM. Chloride impermeability in cystic fibrosis. *Nature* 1983;301:421–422.
3. Quinton PM, Bijman J. Higher bioelectric potentials due to decreased chloride absorption in the sweat glands of patients with cystic fibrosis. *N Engl J Med* 1983;308:1185–1189.
4. Schulz IJ, Fromter E. *Mikopunktionsuntersuchungen an schweibdrusen von mucoviscidosepatienten und gesunden versuchspersonen.* Mucoviscidose Cystische Fibrose: 2 Deutsche Symposion, Erlangen, April 5, 1968.
5. Kartner N, Augustinas O, Jensen TJ, Naismith AL, Riordan JR. Mislocalization of DF508 CFTR in cystic fibrosis sweat gland. *Nature Genet* 1992;1:321–327.
6. Ram SJ, Weaver ML, Kirk KL. Regulation of Cl⁻ permeability in normal and cystic fibrosis sweat duct cells. *Am J Physiol* 1991;259 (5 pt. 1):C842–C846.
7. Sato K, Sato F. Defective beta adrenergic response of cystic fibrosis sweat glands *in vivo* and *in vitro. J Clin Invest* 1984;73:1763–1771.
8. Quinton PM, Reddy MM. Control of CFTR Cl conductance by ATP levels through non-hydrolytic binding. *Nature* 1993;360:79–81.
9. Reddy MM, Quinton PM. Deactivation of CFTR Cl Conductance by endogenous phosphatases in the native sweat duct. *Am J Physiol Cell Physiol* 1996;270: C474–C480.
10. Riordan J, Burns J, Tsui LC, Reddy MM, Quinton PM, Buchwald M. Utilization of cultured epithelial cells from the sweat gland in studies of the CF defect. *Genetics and Epithelial Cell Dysfunction in Cystic Fibrosis* 1987;254:59–71.
11. Huebner DE, Lobeck CC, McSherry NR. Density and secretory activity of eccrine sweat glands in patients with cystic fibrosis and in healthy controls. *Pediatrics* 1966;38:613–618.
12. Montagna W, Parakal PF. *The structure and function of skin.* New York: Academic Press, 1974.
13. Kuno Y. *Human perspiration.* Springfield, IL: Thomas, 1956.
14. Sato K. The physiology, pharmacology, and biochemistry of the eccrine sweat gland. *Rev Physiol Biochem Pharmacol* 1977;79:51–97.
15. Sato K, Kang WH, Saga K, Sato KT. Biology of sweat glands and their disorders: I, normal sweat gland function. *J Am Acad Dermatol* 1989;20(4):537–565.
16. Quinton PM. Sweating and its disorders. *Annu Rev Med* 1983;34:429–452.
17. Sutcliffe CH, Style PP, Schwarz V. Biochemical studies of sweat secretion in cystic fibrosis. *Proc R Soc Med* 1968;61:297–300.
18. Sato K, Sato F. Pharmacologic responsiveness of isolated single eccrine sweat glands. *Am J Physiol* 1981; 240:R44–R51.
19. Montgomery I, Jenkinson DM, Elder HY, Czarnecki D, Mackie RM. The effects of thermal stimulation on the ultrastructure of the human atrichial sweat gland: I, the fundus. *Br J Dermatol* 1984;110:385–397.
20. Schulz I. Micropuncture studies of the sweat formation in cystic fibrosis patients. *J Clin Invest* 1969; 48(8):1470–1477.
21. Sato K. Pharmacology and function of the myoepithelial cell in the eccrine sweat gland. *Experientia* 1977;33:631–633.
22. Jones CJ, Quinton PM. Dye-coupling compartments in the human eccrine sweat gland. *Am J Physiol* 1989; 256:C478–C485.
23. Quinton PM, Tormey JM. Localization of Na/K-ATPase sites in the secretory and reabsorptive epithelia of perfused eccrine sweat glands: a question to the role of the enzyme in secretion. *J Membr Biol* 1976;29: 383–399.
24. Reddy MM, Quinton PM. Electrophysiologically distinct cell types in human sweat gland secretory coil. *Am J Physiol Cell Physiol* 1992;262(2):C287–C292.
25. Reddy MM, Bell CL, Quinton PM. Evidence of two distinct epithelial cell types in primary cultures from human sweat gland secretory coil. *Am J Physiol* 1992;262:C891–C898.
26. Reddy MM, Bell CL. Distinct cellular mechanisms of cholinergic and ß-adrenergic sweat secretion. *Am J Physiol Cell Physiol* 1996;271:C486–C494.
27. Reddy MM, Bell CL, Quinton PM. Cell specific expression of CF defect among sweat gland secretory cells. *Am J Physiol Cell Physiol* 1997;273:C426–433.
28. Jones CJ, Bell CL, Quinton PM. Different physiological signatures of sweat gland secretory and duct cells in culture. *Am J Physiol* 1988;255:C102–C111.
29. Bear CE, Li C, Kartner N, et al. Purification and functional reconstitution of the cystic fibrosis transmembrane conductance regulator (CFTR). *Cell* 1992;68 (4):809–818.
30. Riordan JR. The cystic fibrosis transmembrane conductance regulator. *Annu Rev Physiol* 1993;55:609–630.
31. Bijman J, Quinton PM. Influence of abnormal Cl⁻ impermeability on sweating in cystic fibrosis. *Am J Physiol* 1984;247:C3–C9.
32. Quinton PM. Water metabolism: protozoa to man. In: Recighl M and Karger S, eds. *Comparative animal nutrition.* Basel, 1979:100–131.

33. Schwartz IL, Thaysen JH, Dole VP. Sodium and potassium excretion in human sweat. *Am J Physiol* 1954; 179:671.

34. Schwartz IL, Thaysen JH. Excretion of sodium and potassium in human sweat. *J Clin Invest* 1956;35: 114–120.

35. Slegers JFG. The mechanism of sweat secretion. *Eur J Physiol* 1964;279:265–273.

36. Ernst SA, Riddle CV, Karnaky KJ. Relationship between localization of Na^+-K^+-ATPase, cellular fine structure, and reabsorptive and secretory electrolyte transport. *Curr Top Membr Transport* 1989;13: 355–384.

37. Cheng SH, Gregory RJ, Marshall J, et al. Defective intracellular transport and processing of CFTR is the molecular basis of most cystic fibrosis. *Cell* 1990;63: 827–834.

38. Ward CL, Omura S, Kopito RR. Degradation of CFTR by the ubiquitin-proteasome pathway. *Cell* 1995;83: 121–127.

39. Smith J, Travis SM, Greenberg EP, Welsh MJ. Cystic fibrosis airway epithelia fail to kill bacteria because of abnormal airway surface fluid. *Cell* 1996;85: 229–236.

40. di Sant'Agnese PA, Darling RC, Perera GA, Shea E. Abnormal electrolyte composition of sweat in cystic fibrosis of the pancreas. *Pediatrics* 1953;12:549–563.

41. Shwachman H, Mahmoodian A, Neff RK. The sweat test: sodium and chloride values. *J Pediatr* 1981;98 (4):576–578.

42. Schulz I, Ullrich KL, Fromter E, et al. Micropuncture experiments on human sweat glands. In: di Sant' Agnese PA, ed. *Research on pathogenesis of cystic fibrosis.* Bethesda: National Institute of Arthritis and Metabolic Diseases, 1964:136–146.

43. Bijman J, Fromter E. Direct demonstration of high transepithelial Cl^- conductance in normal human sweat duct which is absent in cystic fibrosis. *Eur J Physiol* 1986;407(suppl 2):S123–S127.

44. Reddy MM, Quinton PM. Apparent lack of acute regulation of amiloride sensitive Na conductance by PKA in human sweat duct. *Pediatr Pulmonol* 1996; Suppl 13:242.

45. Reddy MM, Quinton PM. Intracellular Cl activity: evidence of dual mechanisms of Cl absorption in sweat duct. *Am J Physiol Cell Physiol* 1994;267:C1136–C1144.

46. Kopelman H, Corey M, Gaskin K, Durie P, Weizman Z, Forstner G. Impaired chloride secretion, as well as bicarbonate secretion, underlies the fluid secretory defect in the cystic fibrosis pancreas. *Gastroenterology* 1988;95:349–355.

47. Hays RM. Antidiuretic hormone and water transfer. *Kidney Int* 1976;9:223–230.

48. Nikolajek WP, Emrich HM. pH of sweat of patients with cystic fibrosis. *Klin Wochenschr* 1976;54:287–288.

49. Bijman J, Quinton PM. Lactate and bicarbonate uptake in the sweat duct of cystic fibrosis and normal subjects. *Pediatr Res* 1987;21:79–82.

50. Briggman JV, Tashian RE, Spicer SS. Immunohistochemical localization of carbonic anhydrase I and II in eccrine sweat glands from control subjects and patients with cystic fibrosis. *Am J Pathol* 1983;112: 250–257.

51. Conn JW. Electrolyte composition of sweat. *Arch Intern Med* 1949;83:416–428.

52. Grand RJ, di Sant'Agnese PA, Talamo RC, Pallavicini JC. The effects of exogenous aldosterone on sweat electrolytes: I, normal subjects. *J Pediatr* 1967;70(3): 346–356.

53. Grand RJ, di Sant'Agnese PA, Talamo RC, Pallavicini JC. The effects of exogenous aldosterone on sweat electrolytes: II, patients with cystic fibrosis of the pancreas. *J Pediatr* 1967;70(3):357–368.

54. di Sant'Agnese PA, Talamo RC, Grand RJ, Pallavicini JC. Effect of aldosterone on normal subjects and patients with cystic fibrosis. In: di Sant'Agnese PA, ed. *Research on pathogenesis of cystic fibrosis.* Bethesda, Maryland: National Institute of Arthritis and Metabolic Diseases, 1964:189–201.

55. Quinton PM, Reddy MM. Regulation of absorption in the human sweat duct. *Adv Exp Med Biol* 1991;290: 159–172.

56. Reddy MM, Quinton PM. cAMP activation of CF-affected Cl^- conductance in both cell membranes of an absorptive epithelium. *J Membr Biol* 1992;130:49–62.

57. Anderson MP, Berger HA, Rich DP, Gregory RJ, Smith AE, Welsh MJ. Nucleoside triphosphates are required to open the CFTR chloride channel. *Cell* 1991;67:775–784.

58. Schultz BD, Venglarik CJ, Bridges RJ, Frizzell RA. Regulation of CFTR Cl^- channel gating by ADP and ATP analogues. *J Gen Physiol* 1995;105(3):329–361.

59. Tilly BC, Winter MC, Ostedgaard LS, O'Riordan C, Smith AE, Welsh MJ. Cyclic AMP-dependent protein kinase activation of cystic fibrosis transmembrane conductance regulator chloride channels in planar lipid bilayers. *J Biol Chem* 1992;267(14):9470–9473.

60. Gunderson KL, Kopito RR. Effects of pyrophosphate and nucleotide analogs suggest a role for ATP hydrolysis in cystic fibrosis transmembrane regulator channel gating. *J Biol Chem* 1995;269(30):19349–19353.

61. Reddy MM, Quinton PM. Hydrolytic and non-hydrolytic interactions in the ATP regulation of CFTR-Cl conductance. *Am J Physiol Cell Physiol* 1996;271: C35–C42.

62. Baukrowitz T, Hwang TC, Nairn AC, Gadsby DC. Coupling of CFTR Cl^- channels gating to an ATP hydrolysis cycle. *Neuron* 1994;12:473–482.

63. Gadsby DC, Nagel G, Hwang TC. The CFTR chloride channel of mammalian heart. *Annu Rev Physiol* 1995;57:387–416.

64. Gunderson KL, Kopito RR. Conformational states of CFTR associated with channel gating: the role of ATP binding and hydrolysis. *Cell* 1995;82(2):231–239.

65. Atkinson DE. *Metabolism and its regulation.* New York: Academic Press, 1977.

66. Hwang TC, Nagel G, Nairn A, Gadsby DC. Regulation of the gating of CFTR Cl channels by phosphorylation and ATP hydrolysis. *Proc Natl Acad Sci U S A* 1994;91(11):4698–4702.

67. Berger HA, Travis SM, Welsh MJ. Regulation of the cystic fibrosis transmembrane conductance regulator Cl^- channel by specific protein kinases and protein phosphatases. *J Biol Chem* 1993;268:2037–2047.

68. Berger HA, Anderson MP, Gregory RJ, et al. Identification and regulation of the cystic fibrosis transmembrane conductance regulator-generated chloride channel. *J Clin Invest* 1991;88:1422–1431.

69. Tabcharani JA, Chang XB, Riordan JR, Hanrahan JW. Phosphorylation-regulated Cl⁻ channel in CHO cells stably expressing the cystic fibrosis gene. *Nature* 1991;352:628–631.

70. Illek B, Fischer H, Santos GF, Widdicombe JH, Machen TE, Reenstra WW. cAMP-independent activation of CFTR Cl channels by the tyrosine kinase inhibitor genistein. *Am J Physiol* 1995;268(4 Pt 1): C886–C893.

71. Tilly BC, Van Gageldonk PGM, Kansen M, VanDenBerghe N, Bijman J, Dejonge HR. Activation of intestinal chloride channels by GTP-binding regulatory proteins. *Biology and Medicine of Signal Transduction* 1990;24:95–100.

72. Yount RG. ATP analogs. *Adv Enzymol* 1975;43:1–56.

73. Bijman J, Quinton PM. Permeability properties of cell membranes and tight junctions of normal and cystic fibrosis sweat ducts. *Eur J Physiol* 1987;408: 505–510.

74. Boucher RC, Stutts MJ, Knowles MR, Cantley L, Gatzy JT. Na⁺ transport in cystic fibrosis respiratory epithelia: abnormal basal rate and response to adenylate cyclase activation. *J Clin Invest* 1986;78:1245–1252.

75. Boucher RC, Chinet T, Willumsen N, Knowles MR, Stutts MJ. Ion transport in normal and CF airway epithelia. *Adv Exp Med Biol* 1991;230:105–118.

76. Hjelm M, Brown P, Briddon A. Sweat sodium related to amount of sweat after sweat test in children with and without cystic fibrosis. *Acta Paediatrica Scandinavica* 1986;75:652–656.

77. Conn JW. Aldosteronism in man: some clinical and climatological aspects: part 1. *JAMA* 1963;183(9): 135–781.

78. di Sant'Agnese PA, Powell GF. The eccrine sweat defect in cystic fibrosis of the pancreas (mucoviscidosis). *Ann N Y Acad Sci* 1962;93:555–599.

79. Shwachman H, Mahmoodian A. Pilocarpine iontophoresis sweat testing results of seven years experience. In: Rossi E, Stoll E, eds. *Modern problems in pediatrics.* Basel/New York: S. Karger AG, 1967:158–182.

80. LeGrys VA, Burritt MF, Gibson LE, Hammond KB, Kraft K, Rosenstein BJ. NCCLS Document C34-A; *Sweat testing: sample collection and quantitative analysis.* Approved guide. In 22nd ed. Villanova, PA: National Committee on Clinical Laboratory Standards, 1994:1–45.

81. Gibson LE, Cooke RE. A test for the concentration of electrolytes in sweat in cystic fibrosis of the pancreas utilizing pilocarpine by iontophoresis. *Pediatrics* 1959;23:545–549.

82. Lobeck CC, McSherry NR. The ionic composition of pilocarpine induced sweat in relation to gland output during aging and cystic fibrosis. In: Rossi E, Stoll E, eds. *Modern problems in pediatrics.* Vol 10. Basel: S Karger AG, 1967:41–53.

83. LeGrys VA. Sweat testing for the diagnosis of cystic fibrosis: Practical considerations. *J Pediatrics* 1996: 129:892–897.

84. Quinton PM. Abnormalities in electrolyte secretion in cystic fibrosis. In: Quinton PM, Martinez RM, Hopfer U, eds. *Fluid and electrolyte abnormalities in cystic fibrosis.* San Francisco: San Francisco Press Inc, 1982:53–76.

85. Quinton PM. Suggestion of an abnormal anion exchange mechanism in sweat glands of cystic fibrosis patients. *Pediatr Res* 1982;16:533–537.

86. Davis PB, DelRio S, Muntz JA, Dieckman L. Sweat chloride concentration in adults with pulmonary diseases. *Am Rev Respir Dis* 1983;128:34–37.

87. Rees J, Shuster S. Pubertal induction of sweat gland activity. *Clin Sci* 1981;60:689–692.

88. Slegers JFG. Patho-physiological studies of the sweat gland. *Eur J Physiol* 1966;290:231–236.

89. Slegers JFG. The secretion and reabsorption of salt and water in the sweat gland: a comparative study between normal subjects and patients suffering from fibrocystic disease. Thesis, University of Nijmegen, Nijmegen, The Netherlands, 1966:1–130.

90. Slegers JFG. A mathematical approach to the two-step reabsorption hypothesis. In: Rossi E, Stoll E, eds. *Modern problems in pediatrics.* Vol 10. Basel: S Karger AG, 1967:74–88.

91. Behm JK, Hagiwara G, Lewiston NL, Quinton PM, Wine JJ. Hyposecretion of beta-adrenergically induced sweating in cystic fibrosis heterozygotes. *Pediatr Res* 1987;22:271–276.

92. Harper S, Quinton PM. Adrenergic and cholinergic stimulation of CF sweat glands. In: Lawson D, ed. *Cystic fibrosis, horizons: Proceedings of the 9th International Cystic Fibrosis Congress.* 9th ed. Brighton, England: John Wiley & Sons, 1984:178.

93. Reddy MM, Bell CL, Quinton PM. Cell specific expression of CF defect in sweat secretory coil. *Pediatr Pulmonol* 1996;Suppl 13:241.

Cystic Fibrosis in Adults,
edited by J. R. Yankaskas and M. R. Knowles,
Lippincott–Raven Publishers, Philadelphia, 1999.

20

Rheumatic Disease in Cystic Fibrosis

Peadar G. Noone and *Barry Bresnihan

*Cystic Fibrosis/Pulmonary Research and Treatment Center, Division of Pulmonary and Critical Care
Medicine, University of North Carolina School of Medicine, Chapel Hill, North Carolina; and
Department of Rheumatology, St. Vincent's Hospital, Dublin, Ireland

Joint disease and cutaneous vasculitis are relatively common in adult patients with cystic fibrosis (CF), with the potential for significant morbidity. Overall, some form of arthropathy occurs in up to 12% of this patient population, with associated vasculitis occurring less commonly (1–8). Although the precise cause of joint disease and vasculitis in CF is unknown, an immunologic basis for at least some of these complications seems likely. Many patients have particularly symptomatic disease requiring drug therapy, with the added potential of problematic side effects.

Patients with CF and chronic lung disease who acquire these additional complications may have further retardation of physical activities, which can impact adversely on their lung disease. A cycle of worsening health status can ensue. A well-defined, structured approach to the diagnosis and management of rheumatic disease is important because physicians who see adult patients with CF will see such complications in their practice. In this chapter an approach to the diagnosis and management of these complications of adult CF is outlined. Although the etiology is uncertain, the current theories regarding the causes of these problems are discussed.

HYPERTROPHIC PULMONARY OSTEOARTHROPATHY

Clinical Features

Hypertrophic pulmonary osteoarthropathy (HPOA) is the association of finger clubbing with chronic proliferative periostitis of long bones and oligosynovitis. HPOA was the first rheumatic disorder reported in patients with CF (9). The median age of onset is approximately 20 years, although occasionally it occurs before the age of 10 years (10–12). Hence, this is a complication that occurs predominantly in younger adults, with few cases described in childhood. In the largest reported series of HPOA in CF where strict diagnostic criteria were applied, a prevalence rate of 8% was reported (12). It may be more common in males, although the number of patients in most series is small. It primarily is manifested by clubbing and chronic symmetrical bone pain or swelling in the regions of the wrist, knee, or ankle. The small joints of the hands and feet rarely are affected. The symptoms usually are symmetric and may be associated with joint effusions, which sometimes are large (6,12). The onset of symptoms usually is insidious, with an increasing level of pain and disability evolving gradually (6). Acute painful exacerbations of HPOA frequently accompany exacerbations of pulmonary infection, unlike other forms of arthropathy encountered in CF (1,4,6). In males, gynecomastia may be present, whereas mastalgia may develop in females (5,11).

Diagnostic Evaluation

Radiographic changes typically are characterized by periosteal new bone formation at the distal ends of the long bones, including the tibia and fibula and the radius and ulna (Fig. 20–1). Occasionally, periosteal changes may involve metacarpal and metatarsal bones. Symptoms may develop without radiographic changes, but conversely, radiographic changes rarely are present in patients without symptoms (13). Technetium-99m (^{99m}Tc) hydroxydiphosphonate bone scanning is a useful diagnostic procedure in early or equivocal cases (4,6). Laboratory investigations may yield an elevated erythrocyte sedimentation rate (ESR), but other investigations are likely to be negative, including rheumatoid factor, antinuclear factor, and tests for circulating immune complexes.

Etiology

The etiology of HPOA is unknown, and unlike the other rheumatic problems associated with CF, it probably does not have an immunologic basis. Several theories have been proposed, including neurogenic and hormonal mechanisms. It seems to occur more frequently in patients with severe lung disease chronically infected with *Pseudomonas aeruginosa* (4). As with other forms of non-CF related HPOA, the syndrome regresses with vagotomy and lung

transplantation, which supports a neural or neuroendocrine role (5,11). However, transplantation also removes a large burden of infection as well as denervating the lung, thus removing a source of bacterial antigens (4). There do not appear to be any specific HLA antigen types involved in the susceptibility of patients with CF to HPOA (14).

Treatment

The treatment of HPOA consists of aggressive treatment for the underlying pulmonary disease (see Chapter 7). Acute symptomatic exacerbations may respond satisfactorily to short courses of antiinflammatory or analgesic medications. However, in some patients, potent analgesia may be required while awaiting resolution of the pulmonary exacerbations. Resolution of the radiographic changes may lag behind remission of the clinical symptoms. The syndrome usually remits after heart–lung or lung transplantation.

EPISODIC ARTHROPATHY

Clinical Features

A characteristic form of intermittent acute arthropathy easily distinguished from HPOA was first described by Newman and Ansell (1). Episodic arthropathy occurs in approximately 2% to 8% of patients with CF. In one study, the mean age at the time of diagnosis of the syndrome was 23 years (4). Others have reported that episodic arthropathy may occur at any age, with a mean age at presentation of 16 years (5,6). Transient self-limiting episodes of acute, often incapacitating, joint pain and swelling involving single or multiple large or small joints are observed. The acute arthropathy usually is asymmetric (Fig. 20–2). Affected joints may be frankly swollen, red, hot, and tender. Sometimes symptoms consist of severe arthralgia without visible joint inflammation. Occasionally, periarticular erythema accompanies arthralgia in the absence of swelling. Fever may be present with exacerbations. Episodes usually resolve within 7 to 10 days but may recur at in-

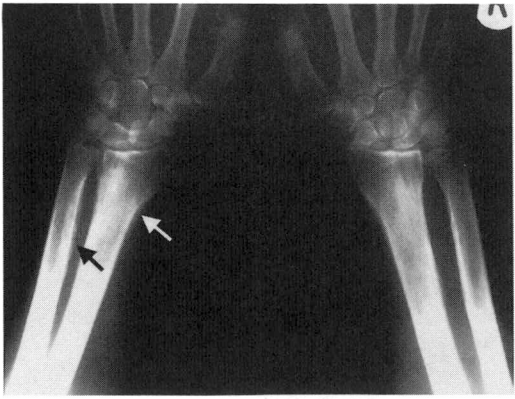

FIG. 20–1. Radiographic features of hypertrophic pulmonary osteoarthropathy (HPOA) in a patient with CF. Periosteal new bone formation is seen along the distal shaft of both radius and ulna (*arrows*).

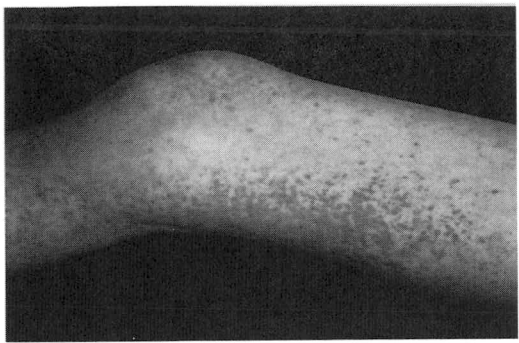

FIG. 20–2. An acute purpuric rash involving the lower limb of an adolescent female patient with CF. The knee joint simultaneously was painful, hot, and swollen.

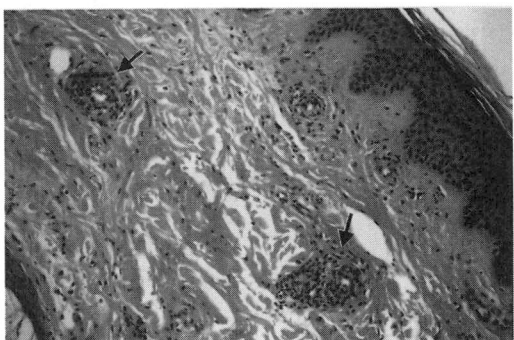

FIG. 20–3. Skin biopsy from a patient with CF during an episode of acute purpura. Several vessels demonstrate features of leukocytoclastic vasculitis, that is, fibrinoid necrosis in the vessel wall with fibrovascular cuffing with neutrophils (*arrows*).

tervals of a few days. Occasionally, episodes last for weeks to years. Episodic arthropathy is almost always nonerosive. The arthropathy is not limited to those patients with severe lung disease and does not necessarily correlate with exacerbations of lung disease. Occasionally, patients may have worsening of lung status in conjunction with joint symptoms, but this may reflect a decrease in physical activity (15).

The joint symptoms may be accompanied by purpuric cutaneous eruptions with histologic features of leukocytoclastic vasculitis (Figs. 20–2 and 20–3) (1,3,5,7,16). The purpuric lesions usually occur discretely on the lower limbs, but they may be seen more diffusely on the upper limbs and trunk. The lesions may be painful, but they rarely are palpable. Others have noted that episodic arthropathy may be accompanied by erythema nodosum (EN) (4,6). Interestingly, in one series, acute EN was accompanied by a high swinging fever in 7 of 12 patients with episodic arthropathy (6).

Diagnostic Evaluation

The diagnosis usually is based on the clinical manifestations. However, it is wise to exclude other forms of joint disease before firmly establishing the diagnosis because other arthopathies may occur in CF. To date, however, there is no specific diagnostic test for episodic arthropathy. Affected patients usually have a high ESR. Rheumatoid factor occasionally is positive (7). Other standard serologic and rheumatology test results usually are negative, including antinuclear antibodies (ANAs). Some patients may have increased levels of circulating immune complexes, low complement levels, and positive anticytoplasmic antibody (ANCA) (8).

Analysis of synovial fluid is useful to address other possible arthopathies but is nonspecific regarding episodic arthropathy, where surprisingly, it usually is quite clear, viscous, and noninflammatory (7). Culture of synovial fluid should be undertaken if infection is being considered. A biopsy of the synovium of an affected joint may reveal inflammation and congestion of the vessel (Fig. 20–4).

Radiologic changes of articular damage usually are absent. However, depending on the time of the radiograph, evidence of soft tissue swelling and effusions may be identified. Periarticular osteopenia is unusual. Rarely, there are features of joint erosion, articular cartilage loss, or more advanced bone damage (4). Periosteal changes have not been described in episodic arthropathy.

Etiology

The etiology of episodic arthropathy is unknown, although there are a number of reasons

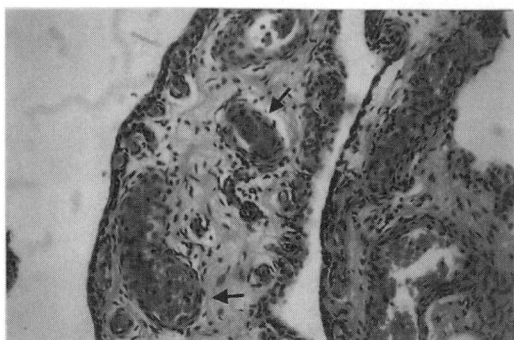

FIG. 20–4. Synovial biopsy from the knee joint of a female patient with CF undergoing an exacerbation of episodic arthropathy. There are two villi of synovium shown, with minimal synovial hypertrophy and inflammatory cell infiltrate. The vessels are congested (*arrows*).

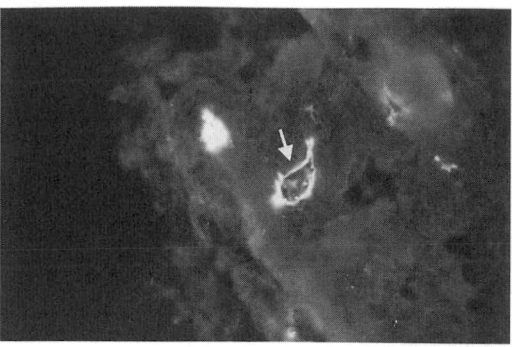

FIG. 20–5. Immunofluorescent staining (*arrow*) of blood vessels in a synovial membrane biopsy obtained from a patient with CF undergoing an acute exacerbation of episodic arthropathy [using an antihuman immunoglobulin (IgG)].

to consider an immunologic mechanism (17). First, circulating immune complexes and lowered serum complement may be identified in some patients undergoing exacerbations. Second, immunoglobulin deposition has been identified in synovial blood vessels in biopsies obtained at the time of acute exacerbations of episodic arthropathy (7) (Fig. 20–5). Finally, during exacerbations of episodic arthropathy, acute cutaneous vasculitis may develop in some patients.

A primary immunologic defect has not been described in CF. The accumulating evidence suggests that the immunologic abnormalities are acquired and the result of chronic bacterial antigenic stimulation (18). The excessive antigen load that results from chronic pulmonary infection produces persistent immune stimulation, polyclonal B-cell activation, hypergammaglobulinemia, and formation of immune complexes (19–21). Circulating immune complexes that contain bacterial antigen have been identified in patients with CF (22–24). Peripheral deposition of immune complexes could account for finding immunoglobulin and complement in involved cutaneous and synovial vessels. In studies using enzyme-linked immunosorbent assay (ELISA) tests for measuring immunoglobulin M (IgM) and IgA rheumatoid factors (RFs), 21% of patients with CF had

elevated serum levels of IgM RF, and 37% had elevated levels of IgA RF (25). RF also may participate in immune complex formation. It has been suggested that RF production in CF was the result of chronic immune stimulation. In a further study, peripheral blood mononuclear cells obtained during acute exacerbations of pulmonary infection in CF were observed to have increased spontaneous *in vitro* synthesis of IgM RF that correlated with the synthesis of immune complexes (26). These observations are of additional interest because there are reports of seropositive rheumatoid arthritis occurring in patients with CF (27,28). A national U.S. study is currently under way, sponsored by the Cystic Fibrosis Foundation, seeking to identify patients with CF and arthritis, to address these issues (29).

Treatment

The treatment of episodic arthropathy usually is symptomatic. Pain usually is a major feature, so adequate analgesia is the first requirement. Nonsteroidal antiinflammatory medication often is very effective, as are short courses of corticosteroids. Because the acute exacerbations usually are of short duration, patients are not likely to require prolonged antiinflammatory drug administration. Long-acting drugs, such as sulfasalazine, hydroxychloroquine, or gold salts, occasionally have been required (4). Symptoms of episodic arthropathy do not necessarily coincide with infective exacerbations of pulmonary disease. Thus, aggressive treatment of underlying lung disease usually does not impact on articular symptoms, although in individual cases it is worth considering.

MISCELLANEOUS ARTHROPATHIES IN CYSTIC FIBROSIS

Rheumatoid Arthritis

Seropositive rheumatoid arthritis has been described in some patients with CF (27,28). The characteristic features of chronic symmetric polyarthritis associated with nodules, joint erosions, and RF are present. It is not known whether the coexistence of rheumatoid arthritis and CF is fortuitous, or whether the two diseases are linked through some immune mechanism. The aforementioned description of increased RF production in some patients with CF raises the intriguing possibility of a causal relationship (17,25,26).

Amyloidosis

Not surprisingly, amyloidosis has been described in a number of adult patients with CF, with involvement of several organ systems, including joints (30–33) (Fig. 20–6). The arthropathy manifests clinically as painless wrist swelling. Renal involvement usually is the dominant feature of amyloidosis in CF, which usually is fatal over a short period of time (30,31). Renal amyloidosis may manifest as proteinuria on routine testing or as overt nephrotic syndrome. Hepatosplenomegaly and goiter resulting from amyloid infiltration also have been described in CF (32,33). Goiter may be accompanied by hypothyroidism and even airway compromise. Patients with amyloidosis always have evidence of widespread involvement of disease, regardless of the presenting organ system (31).

The cause of amyloidosis in CF is unknown. The etiology is likely to be similar to other sit-

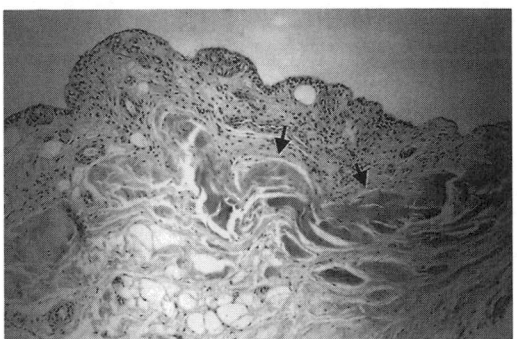

FIG. 20–6. Amyloid deposition in a synovial biopsy of the wrist joint of an adult male patient with CF. The amyloid is the pink amorphous material (*arrows*).

uations in which chronic disease is associated with amyloidosis, for example, other forms of chronic bronchiectasis, or tuberculosis. Abnormal deposition of insoluble fibrillar material, formed from soluble proteins, occurs in the extracellular compartments of major organs. Amyloid P glycoprotein, derived from serum amyloid P, an inhibitor of elastase, also is deposited, which probably contributes to the deposition of amyloid related serum proteins (30). Deposition occurs in most organs but has a special predilection for the kidneys, thyroid gland, and liver and spleen. Interestingly, serum amyloid A (SAA), a low molecular weight protein produced by the liver in response to interleukin 1 (IL-1), IL-6, and tumor necrosis factor (TNF) has been shown to be a good indicator of lung inflammation in patients with CF. Increased levels of SAA also correlate with the presence of pathogens in sputum (34). Whether this has any bearing on the development of amyloid over the long term is unknown. Some authors have speculated that the incidence of amyloid is likely to increase as patients with CF live longer, with more exposure to chronic bacterial infections (31,33). There is no specific treatment for amyloid other than supportive therapy.

Drug-Induced Arthritis

Acute arthritis has been described in patients with CF receiving ciprofloxacin (35). Painful swelling caused by acute synovitis of the knees and wrist is usual. The appearance may resemble an exacerbation of episodic arthropathy. The symptoms resolve rapidly after withdrawal of the drug.

Granulomatous Arthritis

Another chronic arthritis that has been reported in CF is granulomatous arthropathy (36,37); some cases may be sarcoidosis, or others of unknown cause (5) (Fig. 20–7). Erythema nodosum, a frequent manifestation of sarcoidosis also has been reported (4,6). Patients generally are of the younger age group, that is, between 8 and 15 years of age. Other nonpulmonary features of sarcoidosis may be present. Knee arthritis has been prominent, although polyarthritis may be present. The diagnosis of sarcoidosis may be difficult in CF because the characteristic pulmonary features of hilar adenopathy and interstitial markings may be masked by the radiologic changes of CF. As with CF and rheumatoid arthritis, the relationship between CF and sarcoidosis may be coincidental. However, CF and sarcoidosis are characterized by defective cell-mediated immune responses and enhanced B-cell activation (38,39). Hypergammaglobulinemia and immune complex formation are known to cause granulomas in animals, and deposits of immunoglobulin and complement have been demonstrated in sarcoid granulomas (40). Thus, a causal relationship remains a possibility.

Other Arthropathies

Other forms of arthritis may occur in CF and may resemble episodic arthropathy or HPOA. A careful history and examination, together with appropriate investigations, should identify such arthropathies, including septic arthritis, gouty arthritis secondary to hyperuricemia, and arthritis accompanying other systemic complications of CF, such as pancreatitis and small bowel resection. Gout, in particular, has been described in patients with CF as being due to the high content of purines in pancreatic extracts (5). However, this was more a problem with early formulations of pancreatic enzyme extracts and, with the advent of coated tablets, currently is much less common. Overt problematic diabetes mellitus may be complicated by septic arthritis, osteomyelitis, and neuropathic joints, but these complications should be relatively easy to recognize.

VASCULITIS

Clinical Features

Cutaneous vasculitis is a well-recognized complication of CF. It usually occurs in patients older than 20 years of age, although it has been reported in childhood (7,8). In one study, cutaneous vasculitis was recorded in 12 (2.8%) of 430 patients with CF seen over a 22-year period (8). Cutaneous vasculitis usually presents as a painless palpable purpura involving the lower limbs predominantly (see Fig. 20–2), but it may extend to the upper limbs and trunk. The contemporaneous appearance of cutaneous vasculitis and episodic arthropathy has been highlighted in several reports (1,3,5,7,16). In other patients, nonspecific arthralgia or myalgia may be present. No consistent relationship between the onset of cutaneous vasculitis and infective exacerbations of lung disease has been observed. Episodes usually last for several days, often without systemic effects, before resolving spontaneously. Recurrent episodes occur in some patients.

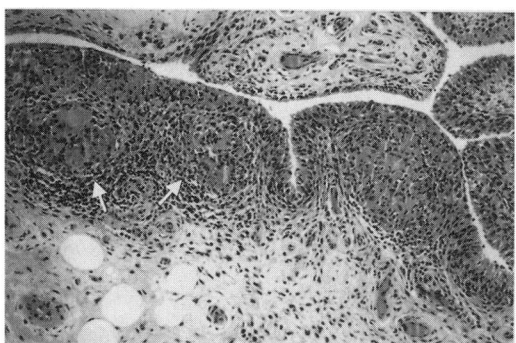

FIG. 20–7. Synovial biopsy from the knee joint of an 8-year-old boy with CF and sarcoidosis. Several noncaseating granulomas, with multinucleated giant cells and a lymphocytic infiltrate, are evident (*arrows*).

Systemic vasculitis involving other organ systems, including the brain, the kidney, and the gastrointestinal tract, is rare, but it may have a fatal outcome (8,41).

Diagnostic Evaluation

Cutaneous vasculitis can be confirmed readily by skin biopsy. Inflammatory cells infiltrating the walls of small vessels and perivascular areas can be demonstrated. The appearances usually are those of leukocytoclastic vasculitis (8) (see Fig. 20–3). Immunofluorescent staining has demonstrated deposits of immunoglobulin and complement in vessel walls. Features of Henoch-Schönlein purpura and Waldenstrom's macroglobulinemia also have been described (8,42).

There is no specific laboratory marker of vasculitis. The ESR usually is elevated. Routine test results for RF and ANAs usually are negative. Increased levels of circulating immune complexes and decreased serum complement have been seen in some patients (7). Positive ANCAs have been observed in 4 of 10 patients with CF and vasculitis and in 0 of 61 control patients with CF (8). However, the specificity of the ANCA pattern has not been characterized, and curiously, patients with CF with systemic vasculitis have been ANCA negative (8,41).

Etiology

There may be several etiologic mechanisms causing vasculitis in CF. There is evidence for an immune-mediated mechanism. Some patients have been shown to have increased levels of circulating immune complexes and decreased serum complement, together with immunoglobulin and complement deposition in vessel walls (7,43). The excessive antigen load associated with chronic bacterial infection will result in sustained immune stimulation. An association between exacerbations of lung disease in CF and increased levels of circulating immune complexes has been shown (26), and bacterial antigen has been demonstrated in circulating immune complexes in CF (22–24).

This phenomenon also has been described in non-CF bronchiectasis associated with severe vasculitis, circulating immune complexes, and local skin immunoglobulin deposition; all of the patients affected were older patients with chronic disease (44). However, attempts to demonstrate bacterial antigen in the vessels in biopsy specimens from patients with CF with vasculitis have not been convincing (8). Further studies employing more sensitive molecular techniques are awaited. The clinical observations that episodes of vasculitis not always are associated with pulmonary exacerbations and, conversely, that exacerbations of lung disease are associated with raised levels of circulating immune complexes that do not invariably result in vasculitis suggest that other mechanisms are involved. The possible role of ANCAs in the pathogenesis of vasculitis in CF also awaits clarification (8,41).

Drug hypersensitivity resulting in vasculitis has been considered a possible mechanism (8). However, no consistent relationship between antibiotic therapy or other therapeutic agents in common usage in CF have been identified, with the exception of ranitidine in a single case (8).

Treatment

Because episodes of cutaneous vasculitis usually resolve spontaneously over several days, no treatment is required in the majority of cases. In patients with persistent vasculitis or with systemic manifestations, treatment with corticosteroids and immunosuppressive therapy has been effective (8,40,41).

SUMMARY

Although a better appreciation of rheumatic disease in CF has emerged over the past decade, further data are needed to elucidate more clearly the etiology of episodic arthropathy and vasculitis. The ongoing U.S. Cystic Fibrosis Foundation–sponsored study may shed more light on pathogenic mechanisms. Pending such data, CF physicians and rheumatologists must remain vigilant to the possibility of these complications in patients who otherwise are relatively healthy. Distinguishing episodic arthropathy and vasculitis from other forms of disease with specific etiologies is of paramount importance and should be done in conjunction with experienced personnel. Amyloid is uncommon, but it may cause considerable morbidity and mortality and always should be considered with unexplained renal or thyroid disease.

REFERENCES

1. Newman AJ, Ansell BM. Episodic arthritis in children with cystic fibrosis. *J Pediatr* 1979;94:594–596.
2. Blau H, Yahav J, Katznelson D. Episodic arthritis in cystic fibrosis. *Prog Rheum* 1984;2:357–360.
3. Schidlow DV, Goldsmith DP, Palmer J, Huang NN. Arthritis in cystic fibrosis. *Arch Dis Child* 1984;59: 377–379.
4. Rush PJ, Shore A, Coblenz C, Wilmot D, Corey M, Levison H. The musculoskeletal manifestations of cystic fibrosis. *Semin Arthritis Rheum* 1986;15:213–225.
5. Phillips BM, David TN, Pathogenesis and management of arthropathy in cystic fibrosis. *J R Soc Med* 1986;79(Suppl 12):44–50.
6. Dixey JJ, Reddington AN, Butter RC et al. The arthropathy of cystic fibrosis. *Br J Rheumatol* 1986;25: 393–395.
7. Bourke S, Rooney M, FitzGerald M, Bresnihan B. Episodic arthropathy in adult cystic fibrosis. *Q J Med* 1987;64:651–659.
8. Finnegan MJ, Hinchcliffe J, Russell-Jones D, et al. Vasculitis complicating cystic fibrosis. *Q J Med* 1989; 72:609–621.
9. Grossman H, Benning CR, Baker DH, Hypertrophic osteoarthropathy in cystic fibrosis. *Am J Dis Child* 1964;107:39–44.
10. Nathansan I, Riddlesberge MM. Pulmonary hypertrophic osteoarthropathy in cystic fibrosis. *Pediatr Radiol* 1980;135:649–651.
11. Braude S, Kennedy H, Hodson M, Batten J. Hypertrophic osteoarthropathy in cystic fibrosis. *Br Med J* 1984;288:822–823.
12. Cohen AM, Yulish BS, Wasser KB, Vignos PN, Jones PY, Sorin SB. Evaluation of pulmonary hypertrophic osteoarthropathy in cystic fibrosis. A comprehensive study. *Am J Dis Chest* 1986;140:74–77.
13. Lipnick RN, Glass RB. Bone changes associated with cystic fibrosis. *Skeletal Radiol* 1992;21:115–116.
14. Rush PJ, Gladman DD, Abraham S, Anhorn KAB. Absence of an association between HLA typing in cystic fibrosis arthritis and hypertrophic osteoarthropathy. *Ann Rheum Dis* 1991;50:763–764.
15. Wulffraat NM, de Graeff Meder ER, Rijkers GT, Van Der Laag H, Kuis W. Prevalence of circulating immune complexes in patients with cystic fibrosis and arthritis. *J Pediatr* 1994;125:374–378.
16. Summers GD, Webley M. Episodic arthritis in cystic fibrosis: a case report. *Br J Rheumatol* 1986;25:393–395.
17. Bresnihan B. Cystic fibrosis, chronic bacterial infection and rheumatic disease. *Br J Rheumatol* 1988;27: 339–341.
18. Thomassen MJ, Demko CA, Doershuk CF. Cystic fibrosis: a review of pulmonary infections and interventions. *Paediatr Pulmonol* 1987;3:334–351.
19. Hoiby N, Schiotz PO. Immune complex mediated damage in the lungs of cystic fibrosis patients with chronic Pseudomonas aeruginosa infection. *Acta Paediatr Scand* 1982;301(Suppl):63–73.
20. Moss RB, Lewiston NJ. Immune complexes and humoral response to Pseudomonas aeruginosa in cystic fibrosis. *Am Rev Respir Dis* 1980;121:23–29.
21. Hassan J, Feighery C, Bresnihan B, Keogan K, FitzGerald MX, Whelan A. Serum IgA and IgG subclasses during treatment for acute respiratory exacerbation in cystic fibrosis: analysis of patients colonised with mucoid or non-mucoid strains of *Pseudomonas aeruginosa. Immunol Invest* 1994;23:1–13.
22. Moss RB, Hsu Y-P. Isolation and characterisation of circulating immune complexes in cystic fibrosis. *Clin Exp Immunol* 1982;47:301–308.
23. Berdischewsky K, Pollack M, Young LS, China D, Oscher AB, Barrett EV. Circulating immune complexes and complement abnormalities in patients with cystic fibrosis. *Pediatr Res* 1980;14:830–833.
24. Wisniesky JJ, Tod EW, Fuller RK, et al. Immune complexes and complement abnormalities in patients with cystic fibrosis. *Am Rev Respir Dis* 1985;132:770–775.
25. Coffey M, Hassan J, Feighery C, FitzGerald MX, Bresnihan B. Rheumatoid factors in cystic fibrosis: associations with disease manifestations and recurrent bacterial infections. *Clin Exp Immunol* 1989;77:52–57.
26. Keogan MT, Callaghan M, Yanni G, et al. Spontaneous in vitro production of rheumatoid factor during infectious exacerbations of cystic fibrosis: correlation with circulating immune complex levels. *Clin Exp Immunol* 1993;91:462–466.
27. Matthieu JP, Stack BHK, Dick WC, Buchanan WW. Pulmonary infection and rheumatoid arthritis. *Br J Chest* 1978;72:57–61.
28. Sagransky DM, Greenwald RA, Gorvoy JD. Sero-positive rheumatoid arthritis in a patient with cystic fibrosis. *Am J Dis Chest* 1980;134:319–320.
29. Fiel SB. Unique challenges and needs of adults with cystic fibrosis. *New insights into cystic fibrosis* 1995; 3:1–6.
30. Castile R, Shwachman H, Travis W, Hadley CA, Warwick W, Missmahl HP. Amyloidosis as a complication of cystic fibrosis. *Am J Dis Child* 1985;139: 728–732.
31. Gaffney K, Gibbons D, Keogh B, FitzGerald MX. Amyloidosis complicating cystic fibrosis. *Thorax* 1993;48:949–950.
32. Sammuels MH, Thompson N, Leichty D, Ridgway EC. Amyloid goiter in cystic fibrosis. *Thyroid* 1995;5: 213–215.
33. Alvarez-Sala R, Prados C, Marcos JS, Carcia Rio F, Vicandi B, Villamore J. Amyloid goiter and hypothyroidism secondary to cystic fibrosis. *Postgrad Med J* 1995;71:307–308.
34. Smith JW, Colombo JL, McDonald TL. Comparison of serum amyloid A and C-reactive protein as indicators of lung inflammation in corticosteroid treated and non-corticosteroid treated cystic fibrosis patients. *J Clin Lab Analysis* 1992;6:219–224.

35. Alfaham M, Holt ME, Goodchild MC. Arthropathy in a patient with cystic fibrosis taking ciprofloxacin. *Br Med J* 1987;259:699.

36. Cooper TJ, Day AJ, Waller PH, Geddes DM. Sarcoidosis in two patients with cystic fibrosis: a fortuitous association? *Thorax* 1987;42:818–820.

37. Soden M, Tempany E, Bresnihan B. Sarcoid arthropathy in cystic fibrosis. *Br J Rheumatol* 1989;28:341–343.

38. Talamo RC, Schwartz RH. Immunologic and allergic manifestations. In: Taussig LM, ed. *Cystic fibrosis.* New York: Thieme-Stratton, 1984:113–131.

39. Daniele RP, Dauber JH, Rossman MD. Immunologic abnormalities in sarcoidosis. *Ann Intern Med* 1980;42:406–416.

40. Ghose T, Landrigan P, Asif A. Localization of immunoglobulin and complement in pulmonary sarcoid granulomas. *Chest* 1974;66:260–268.

41. Parameswaran K, Keaney NP, Veale D. A case of chronic gastrointestinal blood loss in cystic fibrosis. *Respir Med* 1995;89:577–579.

42. Nielsen HE, Lundh S, Jacobsen SV, Hoiby N. Hyper-gamma-globulinaemic purpura in cystic fibrosis. *Acta Paediatr Scan* 1978;67:443–447.

43. Soter NA, Mihm MC, Colten HR. Cutaneous necrotising vasculitis in patients with cystic fibrosis. *J Paediatr* 1979;95:197–201.

44. Hilton AM, Doyle L. Immunological abnormalities in bronchiectasis with chronic bronchial suppuration. *Br J Dis Chest* 1978;72:207–216.

Cystic Fibrosis in Adults,
edited by J. R. Yankaskas and M. R. Knowles,
Lippincott–Raven Publishers, Philadelphia, 1999.

21

Reproductive Issues

Patrick A. Flume and *James R. Yankaskas

*Division of Pulmonary and Critical Care Medicine, Medical University of South Carolina,
Charleston, South Carolina; and *Cystic Fibrosis/Pulmonary Research and Treatment Center,
Division of Pulmonary and Critical Care Medicine, University of North Carolina School of
Medicine, Chapel Hill, North Carolina*

Because patients with cystic fibrosis (CF) are living longer (1), they must deal with issues of normal adulthood, including sexuality and reproduction. In recent decades, patients with CF died before reaching reproductive maturity; currently, however, more patients survive to reproductive age, and they are likely to be of sufficient health to consider parenthood. This fact clearly is borne out by the increasing number of reports of successful pregnancies in women with CF over the last 20 years.

In this chapter, we discuss issues related to reproduction, including sexual development and function in both males and females with CF. We report what is known about pregnancy in women with CF and attempt to provide information that will assist the clinician in guiding the patient and spouse who are considering pregnancy. We also consider other issues, such as contraception, alternatives for the infertile patient, and ethical considerations regarding pregnancy, in this patient population.

REPRODUCTIVE TRACT STRUCTURE AND FUNCTION: MALES

It long has been known that most males with CF are infertile because of obstructive azoospermia (2–5). Infertility is not a universal finding because there are reported cases in which males with CF have a normal semen analysis (6–9) and even have fathered a child (6–8,10,11).

Spermatogenesis occurs in the seminiferous tubules of the testis (Fig. 21–1). The sperm travel through the rete testis and into the head of the epididymis, then into the convoluted tubule of the ductus epididymis, which forms the body and tail of the epididymis before becoming the vas deferens, where the sperm are stored. These ductal structures typically are long with the uncoiled length of the epididymis reaching approximately 4 to 5 m (4). The seminal vesicles join the vas deferens before it becomes the ejaculatory duct, which enters the urethra in the prostate.

In the male with CF, however, the anatomy of the reproductive tract often is grossly abnormal and some portions are difficult to identify. The external genitalia and prostate are normal, but the vas deferens may be absent on physical examination, and rectal ultrasound reveals poorly developed seminal vesicles. Histologic studies have demonstrated absence of the vas deferens and a rudimentary or absent epididymis (3), although the pathology of the male reproductive tract may be quite variable (12). The absence of the vas deferens has been reported in infants as young as 1 month of age (13).

Although the vas deferens and epididymis may be abnormal, analysis of the CF male testicles demonstrates normal spermatozoa with active mitosis (2,3). Careful analysis of semen from the male with CF is consistent with the conclusion that azoospermia is the result of obstruction of the ductal structures (Table 21–1).

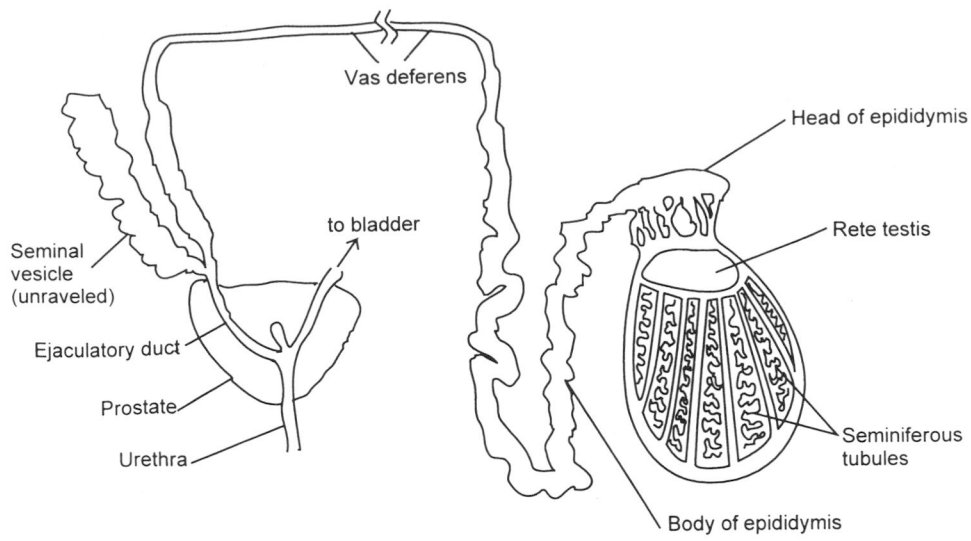

FIG. 21–1. Normal male reproductive tract. This schematic diagram identifies the relationships of the major components.

The volume of ejaculate typically is smaller than normal (2,3). The ejaculate contains elevated citric acid and acid phosphatase levels and diminished fructose concentrations (3,14). These findings may be attributed to the fact that virtually all of the ejaculate is derived from prostatic secretion, which is normal in the male with CF. Citric acid and acid phosphatase in semen is secreted by the prostate (15); fructose in semen is derived primarily from the seminal vesicles (15). Thus, the reduction in fructose is consistent with the absence of secretions from the seminal vesicles (16).

The etiology of the ductal obstruction has been attributed to either a developmental abnormality or atrophy of the ducts due to obstruction by abnormal secretions (4). A developmental anomaly has been proposed because all of the involved structures (i.e., epididymis, vas deferens, seminal vesicles) have a similar origin; that is, all are derived from wolffian duct structures. This has been supported further by the finding that these abnormalities have been seen in infants as young as 1 month of age (13). However, recent findings have demonstrated the presence of the vas deferens in aborted fetuses with CF (12 and 18 weeks postconception) with a normal ductal size compared with non-CF fetuses and without evidence of obstruction (17). These findings lend greater support to an obstruction/atrophy mechanism, as does the finding of portions of normal ducts in some prepubertal males (18,19).

Obstruction of the ducts may be the result of abnormal secretions from the epithelial lining of the male reproductive tract. The epididymis and vas deferens are important not only because they are a conduit for passage of sperm but also because they provide an environment for normal maturation of sperm. The fluid within this conduit may be dependent in part

TABLE 21–1. *Semen analysis*

	CF	Normal
Volume (mL)	1.6	3.5
pH	6.6	8.3
Sperm count (no)	0	$>50 \times 10^6$
Total nitrogen (mg/mL)	5.2	7.0
Citric acid (mg/mL)	23.0	3.4
Acid phosphatase (U/mL)	2.0	0.5
Fructose (mg/mL)	0.1	4.4
Sodium (mEq/L)	162	112
Potassium (mEq/L)	55	24
Calcium (μg/g)	691	181
Zinc (μg/g)	481	90
Magnesium (μg/g)	296	92

Adapted from references 3 and 14.

on local secretion of ions and water, which could be abnormal in the patient with CF; in fact, chloride secretion has been demonstrated in normal (non-CF) epididymal epithelial cells (20,21). Cystic fibrosis transmembrane conductance regulator (CFTR) expression has been demonstrated in the head of the epididymis and vas deferens of tissue from males who do not have CF as well; this expression is noted throughout postnatal life, including newborns and adults (22). It has been suggested that CFTR dysfunction in the epididymis and vas deferens will result in secretory abnormalities throughout life, probably leading to obstructive pathology, as seen in other organs. The finding of abnormalities early in life suggests that the obstruction may occur during gestation. As stated previously, the ductal structures are quite long, that is, there is great opportunity for obstruction to occur in the presence of abnormal secretions. There is little to no expression of the CFTR in the seminal vesicles or prostate. Because the seminal vesicles also are abnormal in CF, it has been proposed that obstructive abnormalities in the epididymis and vas deferens lead to obstruction and atrophy of the seminal vesicles (22).

The finding of azoospermia has been suggested as a clinical criterion for the diagnosis of CF (23). However, as already noted, there are some patients with CF who have a normal ejaculate (6–9), and there are other diseases similar to CF that also include azoospermia. Patients with Young's syndrome have chronic sinopulmonary disease and obstructive azoospermia, yet they have a normal sweat chloride test and pancreatic sufficiency (24). They have a normal vas deferens on physical examination, unlike most patients with CF (24). These patients have been screened for mutations of the CFTR but have been found to have a gene frequency similar to that seen in healthy subjects (25), suggesting the etiology of their azoospermia is the result of something other than a mutation in the CFTR.

Patients with congenital bilateral absence of the vas deferens (CBAVD) have been shown to have a high frequency of CFTR mutations in one or both of their CFTR genes (26–32).

Individuals with CBAVD may have normal, intermediate, or elevated sweat chloride levels, and it has been suggested that CBAVD may be a variant of CF (31). However, a consensus statement by a committee formed by the Cystic Fibrosis Foundation regarding the diagnostic criteria of CF has recommended that patients with CBAVD without overt evidence of chronic pulmonary or pancreatic disease should not be given a diagnosis of CF (27). In addition, Augarten et al. (28) showed that patients with CBAVD and congenital renal malformations (e.g., agenesis of one kidney, ectopic kidney) do not have a mutated CFTR gene, although patients were screened for only nine known mutations. They suggested that some patients with CBAVD may not have CF and reasoned that although both the urinary and reproductive systems are derived from a common origin (i.e., mesodermal tissues), they become separate developmental structures after the seventh week of gestation. They suggested that patients with both CBAVD and renal malformations (i.e., non-CF) have a developmental abnormality that occurs before the seventh week of gestation, whereas those patients without renal malformations (i.e., variant of CF) have an abnormality (e.g., obstruction) that occurs later in pregnancy (28).

The connection between genotype and male genital phenotype has been explored. The most common mutation (ΔF508) seems to be associated with azoospermia because most males with CF are functionally sterile; however, one aborted CF fetus with a normal vas deferens was shown to be homozygous for ΔF508 (17). Heterozygosity for ΔF508 has been shown in a fetus with a normal vas deferens (17) and in a male with a normal semen analysis and who fathered a child (10). Patients with compound heterozygosity (ΔF508/3849 + 10kb C $\rightarrow$ T) also have demonstrated a normal semen analysis (9,11). An individual homozygous for 3849 + 10kb C $\rightarrow$ T also has been shown to have a normal semen analysis and has fathered a child (8).

Mouse models of CF have been developed (33,34); CFTR expression in the mouse epididymis parallels that seen in humans (35).

Despite a severe gene abnormality (i.e., complete absence of the CFTR), the mutant mice have remained fertile (33,34). This finding has been attributed to an alternative Cl⁻ conductance that is activated by luminal adenosine triphosphate (ATP) through P2Y2 nucleotide receptors, which have increased expression in the mouse. The correlation between CFTR expression and effects seen in humans and mice remains to be determined. If they are found to be similar, the variation of pathology seen in the male reproductive tract may be the result of the nature of the intraluminal secretions, which are related to chloride secretion and affected by both CFTR genotype and the presence of alternate channels for chloride conductance.

REPRODUCTIVE TRACT STRUCTURE AND FUNCTION: FEMALES

Unlike the male, the female with CF may be fertile, and pregnancy is not uncommon. Nonetheless, it is widely believed that the female with CF is less fertile than normal (36–38). There are several proposed mechanisms for this belief, but it is clear that circumstances of infertility in the female with CF are different than for the male.

The most notable difference between males and females with CF is that the reproductive anatomy of the female is normal. However, the sexual development of the female with CF is delayed, with menarche occurring at approximately 14.4 years of age, 1.5 years later than normal (39,40). This is associated with a delay in the production of gonadotropins and sex steroids (41), although normal values of gonadotropins and sex steroids will be reached and will be appropriate for the level of sexual maturity (39). The fact that normal levels of gonadotropins and estrogens, as well as the finding of a normal response to gonadotropin-releasing hormone (41), suggests that the etiology of the delay in sexual development cannot be attributed to a primary abnormality in the hypothalamic–pituitary–gonadal axis. A more complete discussion of these findings may be found in Chapter 18.

The delay in sexual maturity has been associated with a reduction in body fat (39,40,42). Females with CF also have a high incidence of menstrual irregularities (40), and it has been suggested that there may be a high prevalence of anovulatory cycles in patients with CF (40). It is not clear whether the menstrual irregularities are a result of weight loss or thinness, but there is a close, complex relationship between undernutrition and poor respiratory function; both have an association with amenorrhea (42). Stead et al. (42) suggested that estimated percent body fat was the best predictor of menstrual function in females with CF. Similarly, a correlation between weight loss and amenorrhea in healthy females has been demonstrated (43).

Although the gross anatomy of the female reproductive tract is normal in CF, there are physiologic abnormalities. Oppenheimer et al. (36) first reported the finding of a thick tenacious mucus plug and a multicystic endocervical polyp obstructing the cervical os of a patient with CF and suggested that these findings might be associated with decreased fertility. A review of histologic sections of the reproductive tract of females with CF revealed an increase in cervical mucus; the hypersecretion of cervical mucus was most prominent in the newborn, and although the frequency of this finding decreased with age, it remained a prominent finding throughout childhood (18).

Kopito et al. (37) studied the characteristics of cervical mucus in three adult women with CF and found that cervical mucus was dehydrated significantly compared with controls; the amount of water was below the minimum level believed to be essential for normal migration of sperm. They also noted abnormally low concentrations of sodium in CF cervical mucus and the absence of ferning (37). These findings led to the common belief that abnormal cervical mucus resulted in plugging of the cervix, serving as a natural barrier to sperm and resulting in infertility.

CFTR expression has been demonstrated in the epithelium and glands of the cervix but not in the ovaries of healthy females (22); it has been suggested that dysfunction of CFTR would result in an abnormal cervical mucus.

CFTR expression has been shown to change during different parts of the estrous cycle of the normal mouse (35), suggesting that the CFTR may participate in regulation of fluids in the normal cycling uterus. The electrolyte pattern measured in cervical mucus of three women with CF was not affected by the menstrual cycle (37); this adds further support to the potential role of the CFTR in contributing to normal cyclical changes in endocervical secretions. Studies in the oviduct of the CF mouse have demonstrated defective cyclic adenosine monophosphate (cAMP)-CFTR–mediated chloride secretion (44), but an alternative Ca^{2+}-mediated pathway maintained normal chloride secretion into the oviduct. It has been suggested that this alternative Cl^- pathway is the reason that fertility in the CF mouse is normal and the reason that there is no obstruction found in the oviducts, whereas obstruction is common in the intestine of the CF mouse where only CFTR-mediated chloride secretion is present (44).

SEXUAL FUNCTION

There is little information available on the effects that chronic disease, especially chronic lung disease, has on sexual function in humans, primarily because these effects are difficult to study because they are not measured easily. In addition, there are conflicting reports on the impact that lung disease has on sexual function. Some data suggest the presence of sexual dysfunction in men with chronic obstructive pulmonary disease (COPD) with a likely correlation between severity of lung disease and degree of sexual dysfunction (45); other studies have attributed the sexual dysfunction found in some patients with COPD to other problems independent of lung disease (46). Although it may be difficult to establish a direct relationship between lung disease and sexual function, it is well accepted that patients perceive that their lung disease has a negative effect on their sex life (47).

There are several ways in which lung disease may adversely affect sexual function. All sexual activities require some increase in ventilation, which may be difficult in patients with se-

vere airways obstruction. The patient may be deconditioned and become fatigued easily. Chronic childhood diseases such as CF place increased stress on the family, which may be associated with problems such as divorce; it is believed that this may lead to future problems with intimacy for the person with CF (48). Chronic pulmonary infection, with cough and sputum production, could lead to a sense of unattractiveness in the individual. The libido may be affected by both the underlying ventilatory impairment and infection as well as the medications used to treat the illness, with a reduced desire for sexual activity.

Despite the aforementioned, studies have demonstrated a remarkably normal sex life for patients with CF. In a study of adolescents with CF (49), a relationship between severity of disease and sexual activity could not be established. Notably, all the patients with CF either already had or intended to have a sexual experience, yet only 75% of their parents believed that their child would ever have a sexual experience. Additionally, only 21% of patients had discussed sexual function with their physician, which may explain why half of the males with CF believed that they could impregnate a girl, a highly unlikely occurrence.

Levine and Stern (50) reported a remarkably normal sexual lifestyle in their review of married persons with CF. Their data indicated that CF was not an independent predictor of impaired sexual function, at least not until the disease became severe enough to interfere with the patient's career. However, when the same authors looked at their unmarried adult patients, they found that persons with CF had more sexual problems when compared with persons without CF (51). The authors could not conclude whether the problems were specific to CF or similar to those found in patients with other chronic diseases.

A common element of the studies of sexual function in patients with lung disease, including CF, is the lack of attention given by the clinician to this subject (49). Patients should be advised that they can expect a reasonably normal sex life, despite any reduction in fertility, and there are techniques that may be used to improve sexual activities for those patients with advanced disease (52). The importance of sexual assessment of patients with lung disease as a part of their complete care cannot be underestimated (47,49,53).

PREGNANCY

The woman with CF who desires children may ask her physician for guidance in her decision to become pregnant. Ethical considerations, such as a shortened life span of the mother-to-be or the potential of having a child with CF, should be discussed early; these issues are dealt with later in this chapter. Of paramount concern to the woman is the effect that pregnancy will have on her health. There is a perceived risk for deterioration in the health of the mother-to-be during pregnancy because it has been associated with an early demise shortly after delivery (54,55). Recent analysis of the effects of pregnancy on the woman with CF has shown that pregnancy is not a significant risk factor for either a decline in pulmonary function or mortality (56). Nonetheless, it is critical for the patient, her spouse, and her physician to make plans early on how the patient will maintain her health, with increased frequency of contact with the physician and more attention to exercise and chest physiotherapy for clearance of airway secretions. A contract should be made between physician and patient that the patient will be treated aggressively, even at the detriment of the fetus, should it become necessary.

It is reasonable to assume that a woman in better health (e.g., better pulmonary function and nutritional status) is likely to have a better outcome than the woman who starts her pregnancy in worse health. Some authors have suggested that certain degrees of pulmonary impairment should be considered contraindications to pregnancy, such as the presence of pulmonary hypertension or a vital capacity less than 1 L or less than 50% predicted (57); these indices can be used only as guidelines because there have been patients who have tolerated pregnancy reasonably well despite more severe pulmonary impairment (58). Some authors

have recommended the use of a scoring system (e.g., Shwachman scores) in advising patients, but such a method has not been shown to be more effective than any other. To develop an understanding of the potential risks of pregnancy in the hopes of providing our patients with sound advice, it is necessary to review the potential complications for the woman with CF and the fetus as well as the outcomes for both that have been reported. In the discussion of potential complications that may occur during pregnancy in the woman with CF, there are three perspectives to consider: (a) the effects of pregnancy on the woman with CF, (b) the effect that CF may have on the pregnant woman, and (c) the effect that CF may have on the fetus.

Effects of Pregnancy on the Woman with Cystic Fibrosis

Virtually the entire respiratory system of the woman is affected during pregnancy, including the airways, thoracic cage, and cardiovascular system; the pertinent effects are listed in Table 21–2. The airway mucosa develops hyperemia and edema that are most pronounced during the third trimester. The enlarging uterus may cause an elevation of the diaphragm of as much as 4 cm; this is offset, however, by a 2-cm increase in the anteroposterior and transverse diameter of the thoracic cage (59,60). There is an increase in cardiac output that reaches 30% to 50% greater than normal near term; this is a result of an increase in heart rate and stroke volume, as well as a decrease in peripheral vascular resistance (59). Total blood volume also increases as much as 35%.

There are additional effects that pregnancy has on the function of the respiratory system.

TABLE 21–2. *Effects of pregnancy on the lung*

Reduced TLC, FRC, and RV
Normal or slightly reduced VC
Reduced airway resistance
Increased minute ventilation ($\uparrow$ Vt, normal RR)
Increased oxygen consumption

FRC, functional residual capacity; RR, respiratory rate; RV, residual volume; TLC, total lung capacity; VC, vital capacity; Vt, tidal volume.

There is a moderate reduction in all lung volumes, including total lung capacity (TLC), functional residual capacity (FRC), and residual volume (RV), that progresses throughout pregnancy (59,60). These changes occur with little to no effect on vital capacity (VC) because there are simultaneous changes in airway resistance. The reduction in airway resistance has been attributed to progesterone-induced relaxation of bronchial smooth muscle (60,61).

Pregnant women experience an increase in breathing, as measured by minute ventilation. This is the result of an increase in tidal volume, with or without an increase in respiratory rate, and results in hypocapnia (61). These effects also have been attributed to an increase in progesterone levels (59). There is an increase in oxygen consumption throughout pregnancy as a result of growing fetal and maternal tissues (59,61).

All women will experience these effects during pregnancy, but some are particularly pertinent to the mother-to-be with CF. The reduction of lung volumes, specifically FRC, may result in problems with clearance of airway secretions. Airway closing volume, the lung volume at which the small airways (< 2-mm diameter) in the dependent portion of the lung begin to close, typically occurs below FRC; however, in the latter part of pregnancy, closing volume may exceed FRC in the pregnant woman (60,61). This could result in impaired clearance of airway secretions for the woman with CF, leading to worsening of pulmonary infection, as well as creating a greater mismatch between ventilation and perfusion with subsequent arterial hypoxemia.

There also is an increase in nutritional requirements because of the growing fetus. The woman with CF already may have difficulty meeting her nutritional requirements because of inadequate caloric intake and impaired absorption. The result may be poor weight gain for the mother-to-be with CF; inadequate maternal weight gain and malnutrition during pregnancy have been associated with poor fetal outcomes (62). Supplemental nutrition may be required to satisfy the needs of the mother-to-be and the fetus; some physicians even have instituted parenteral nutritional support (63). The reader is referred to Chapter 13 for further information on general nutrition issues in CF.

The final important normal change experienced by the pregnant woman that may be pertinent in CF is the increase in plasma volume. This may not be tolerated readily by the woman if there is even mild right heart failure; it has been suggested that this could precipitate cor pulmonale in the patient with severe lung disease (38).

Effects of Cystic Fibrosis on the Pregnant Woman

Usual complications of CF can result in problems during pregnancy; the management of these complications must ensure that treatment is effective for the mother-to-be, yet safe for the fetus. Again, it is imperative that physician and patient plan early for these potential problems so that they may be dealt with promptly and effectively.

The mother-to-be with CF may suffer from chronic sinus and pulmonary infections. Standard chronic therapies, such as inhaled medications and mechanisms of clearance of airway secretions, may be insufficient to control exacerbations of these infections, and treatment may require the use of antibiotics. Hemoptysis often is associated with worsening of pulmonary infection; arterial embolization may be required for massive bleeding (64). Pneumothorax is a common complication of CF; approximately 20% of adults will experience a pneumothorax at some time in their life (64); to our knowledge, there are no reported cases of pneumothorax in the pregnant patient with CF. Because of the potential side effects of medications (e.g., antibiotics) and radiation (i.e., x-rays) on the fetus, the physician may tend to delay institution of therapy or the mother-to-be may be reluctant to seek and accept therapy. It is perilous to both mother-to-be and fetus to delay appropriate therapy; the potential side effects of these therapies are discussed below.

The increase in nutritional requirements during pregnancy have been discussed, and the reader is referred to Chapter 13 for more information regarding general nutritional issues in CF. Most patients with CF have pancreatic insufficiency and may suffer from malabsorption, even with aggressive enzyme replacement. Careful attention must be paid to the pregnant woman's weight gain during pregnancy to ensure that both mother and fetus' nutritional requirements are being met. This will warrant an increase in caloric intake and vitamin supplementation. The physician also must be cognizant of possible glucose intolerance. The incidence of diabetes increases with increasing age. Although the patient with CF may be euglycemic on routine examination, hyperglycemia may be exacerbated during pregnancy. The effects of hyperglycemia are discussed in Chapter 18; the adverse effects of gestational diabetes on the fetus are less clear (65).

Effects of Cystic Fibrosis on the Fetus

Impaired gas exchange may place undue stress on the fetus. Uterine blood flow is impaired by arterial hypoxemia; the fetus is dependent on adequate placental blood flow to meet its metabolic needs. The healthy fetus lives under relatively hypoxic and hypercarbic (fetal $PaCO_2$ is 10 mm Hg > maternal $PaCO_2$) conditions and is dependent on the mother-to-be for delivery of oxygen and removal of carbon dioxide (61). Maternal hypoxia and hypercarbia essentially ensures that the fetus is even more hypoxic and hypercarbic; it is unknown what effects on the fetus may occur under these conditions. The same problems with gas exchange abnormalities can occur with worsening pulmonary infection and hemoptysis; these problems should be dealt with aggressively because as they probably are more likely to have deleterious effects on the fetus than are the treatments for these problems.

Some medications may be harmful to the developing fetus; however, the benefits of treatment with medications often outweigh the risks, and therapy should not be delayed or withheld. The U.S. Food and Drug Administration has classified medications according to their potential risk of complications during pregnancy (Table 21–3). Medications that may

TABLE 21–3. *Classification of medication risks to fetus*

Category	Risk
A	Remote risk
B	Animal studies demonstrate no risk; human studies have not been performed
C	Animal studies demonstrate risk; human studies have not been performed
D	Evidence of risk to human fetus; benefits may outweigh potential risks
X	Evidence of risk to human fetus; risks clearly outweigh any potential benefit

be used to treat pulmonary disease (66) include theophylline (Category C); β-agonists, such as terbutaline (Category B) and albuterol (Category C); and corticosteroids, such as beclomethasone (Category C), triamcinolone (Category D), or flunisolide (Category C). Oral corticosteroids may be used for preterm delivery in the hopes of further maturation of the fetal lungs; short-term use of corticosteroids appears to be safe for the fetus. A greater concern is for the mother-to-be on chronic steroid use who has adrenal suppression and insufficient corticosteroid levels during the increased stress of labor. Inhaled mucolytic agents, such as acetylcysteine (not classified) and Pulmozyme (Category B) (recombinant human DNase, Genentech, Inc., San Francisco), also may be used.

The need for antibiotic therapy during pregnancy is likely to occur in most patients with CF. The pharmacokinetics of certain antibiotics may be altered during pregnancy because of the increased volume of distribution, the decrease in plasma protein concentration, impaired oral absorption (already a problem in CF), and increased renal and hepatic clearance (66). Doses may need to be increased (e.g., cephalosporins) to compensate for these changes (66).

The choices of antibiotics for the mother-to-be with CF is limited by the potential risk to the fetus. Erythromycin (Category B), penicillins (Category B), imipenem-cilastatin (Category B), and cephalosporins (Category B) commonly are used (66). The aminoglycosides (Category C) have only moderate passage across the placenta (20% to 30%) and are used frequently; however, high doses and chronic use of streptomycin has led to ototoxicity (66). Inhaled aminoglycosides result in minimal serum levels and should be tolerated well during pregnancy. The quinolones (Category C) have not demonstrated teratogenic effects, but animal studies have shown deposition in fetal cartilage and irreversible arthropathy; these medications should be avoided during pregnancy until they can be demonstrated to be safe in humans. Trimethoprim (Category C) is contraindicated in the first trimester because it is believed to be teratogenic, like other folate antagonists. Sulfonamides are Category B medications during the first and second trimesters but are Category D medications during the third trimester because they displace bilirubin from albumin, increasing the risk of neonatal kernicterus. The tetracyclines (Category D) inhibit bone growth, discolor teeth, and may be associated with acute fatty liver and renal failure in the pregnant woman. Finally, chloramphenicol (Category C) may cause cardiovascular collapse in the premature newborn ("gray baby syndrome").

There may be hazardous effects of radiation on the fetus, such as growth retardation and increased incidence of childhood leukemia. However, some maternal problems may require extensive use of radiation for diagnostic or therapeutic procedures. An example is the patient with hemoptysis. Arterial embolization may be required for treatment of substantial hemoptysis in the patient with CF (64). There may be reluctance on the part of the physician to expose the fetus to radiation during an embolization procedure, but treatment of hemoptysis should be the same for the pregnant patient as for any other. It has been suggested that a total radiation exposure of less than 5 rads throughout gestation may be safe for the fetus (66,67). The effects of a total exposure of 5 to 10 rads are not clear, but exposures greater than 10 rads are associated with significant fetal effects (66). A typical chest radiograph exposes the fetus to approximately 0.2 rads; a pulmonary angiogram, based on a 40-kg woman with 20 minutes of fluoroscopy time, exposes the fetus to approximately 0.4 rads

(66). Fetal exposure to radiation may be reduced by proper shielding.

Outcome of the Mother

The first reported case of pregnancy in a patient with CF was published in 1960 (68), and there has been an ever-growing number of reported cases since that time (69). Grand et al. (70) reported the first survey of pregnancy in patients with CF, describing 13 pregnancies in 10 patients. There was progressive pulmonary decompensation in five of these patients, which led to death in two patients shortly after delivery. The authors suggested that those patients with a better outcome had better lung function than those whose conditions worsened during pregnancy.

Cohen et al. (54) performed a survey of 119 CF centers in North America and reported 129 pregnancies in 100 patients. Adequate follow-up information was available for 84 patients; 15 patients (18%) died less than 2 years after delivery. This mortality rate was similar to that expected for women with CF of the same age, but it was not controlled for severity of illness (e.g., degree of pulmonary impairment, nutritional status). Nonetheless, the authors suggested that pregnancy should be avoided if the patient's Shwachman (71) or Taussig (72) clinical score is less than 80.

Corkey et al. (73) reported 11 pregnancies in seven patients. Their patients fared better than those previously reported, with only one patient unable to continue the pregnancy to delivery. They found that although there may be a transient reduction in pulmonary function, pregnancy did not appear to affect the general trend of disease.

Palmer et al. (55) reported 11 pregnancies in eight patients; those women who had a successful pregnancy and returned to their pregravid health generally were in good health before pregnancy as opposed to those women whose health deteriorated during pregnancy. The four factors in the study that were associated with a successful outcome included a good Shwachman-Kulczycki clinical score (71), good nutritional status (as measured by weight), nearly normal chest x-ray (CXR), and only mild to moderate airway obstruction, although absolute indices were not defined.

Canny et al. (74) reported the results of 38 pregnancies (34 completed) in 25 women with CF. There was only one death within 2 years after delivery in this group; the improved survival was attributed to the fact that the patients in this survey had less advanced disease (i.e., better lung function and nutritional health) than those in other reports.

There appears to be a general association between pregravid maternal health and the mother's outcome during pregnancy, although there is no clear evidence to support the notion that pregnancy will have an independent negative effect on the mother-to-be. This is borne out in an ongoing review of pregnancy in the Cystic Fibrosis Foundation's Registry Data, perhaps the largest collection of data on pregnancy in CF, which also could not demonstrate a negative effect of pregnancy on the health of the mother-to-be with CF (56). This interpretation of the registry data should be balanced by the knowledge that the pregnancy group is a relatively "select" population; that is, there is an exclusion of patients who chose not to become pregnant or underwent therapeutic abortions on the counsel of their physicians. Although there are no absolute objective measures of impairment that will predict a poor outcome, the physician may use pulmonary function testing and nutritional assessment to advise the patient of potential risks to her health. Some relative contraindications to pregnancy include a rapid decline in pulmonary function in a short period of time (5), frequent exacerbations of infection requiring intravenous antibiotics (5), and malnutrition (e.g., body weight < 70% ideal body weight). The absolute contraindications to pregnancy that most authors would agree on are the presence of cor pulmonale, resting hypoxemia, and hypercarbia.

Outcome of the Infant

Given the potential maternal complications with hypoxemia and malnutrition, as well as the frequent use of medications to treat maternal disease, there is concern for possible fetal complications. Fetal outcomes have been reported, although there is little information to predict outcome. In the survey by Grand et al. (70), 11 of 13 infants were healthy at birth, although 3 were born prematurely; there were two deaths. In the survey by Cohen et al. (54), 97 (75%) of the 129 pregnancies were completed and 31 (25%) were terminated by abortion; the results of 1 pregnancy were not given. Of the abortions, 6 were spontaneous and 25 were therapeutic; the rate of spontaneous abortions in women with CF did not exceed that reported in the general population. Of the completed pregnancies, 86 (89%) resulted in viable infants, a rate significantly lower than that reported for the general population (98%). There also was a considerably higher rate of preterm (< 37 weeks) deliveries (27%) in women with CF compared with the non-CF population (6% to 7%).

Palmer et al. (55) presented infant outcomes with relation to maternal outcomes. They showed that infants of mothers without deterioration during pregnancy all were born at term, whereas the infants of mothers who had worsening of their disease during pregnancy were delivered preterm.

Corkey et al. (73) showed much better results with 10 of 11 pregnancies carried to term; 1 pregnancy was terminated because of worsening maternal disease. In the Canny series (74), 34 of 38 pregnancies were completed, 2 of which were preterm. One infant died of sepsis after birth. Of the four abortions, three were performed therapeutically. It has been suggested that the better infant outcomes reported by Corkey et al. (73) and Canny et al. (74) are due to the milder disease in the mothers in their series compared with other series (69).

BREAST-FEEDING

Breast-feeding previously had been discouraged in mothers with CF; there was concern for the quality of the breast milk and the question of its safety for infants. There also was concern for the safety of the mother because of the increased caloric expenditure associated with breast-feeding. Because breast milk is produced in an exocrine gland, it was presumed that the sodium content in breast milk would be elevated, similar to findings in another exocrine gland, the sweat gland (75). Subsequently, breast milk from a mother with CF was shown to have an elevated sodium concentration (76) with levels that would be unsafe for a child. This finding later was shown to be related to the time at which sodium content was measured in breast milk (77). That is, sodium concentration is increased in colostrum (days 1 to 5 postpartum) then decreases to lower levels in mature milk in women with and without CF (78). Further analysis has shown that breast milk of mothers with CF is physiologically normal, although there may be a reduction in macronutrients during periods of exacerbation of pulmonary disease (78,79).

Sodium concentration is not increased in breast milk, unlike that found in sweat, because of the mechanisms by which sodium is secreted in the mammary and sweat glands. The sweat gland consists of a secretory coil and a reabsorptive duct. Isotonic fluid is secreted into the lumen of the coil, and the sweat is modified in the duct by reabsorption of electrolytes in excess of water, resulting in a hypotonic fluid (80). The sweat of the patient with CF has an increased concentration of sodium because of defective sodium and chloride reabsorption (80). Unlike the sweat gland, the ductal system of the mammary gland does not modify the milk secreted from the acinar cells (81); it has been suggested that this is why exocrine mammary gland function is unaffected in mothers with CF (78).

Of more pressing concern is the nutritional demands that breast-feeding places on the mother with CF. Breast-feeding results in an estimated caloric expenditure of 500 calories/day (82). Although there are mothers with CF whose nutritional status had been affected adversely during breast-feeding (83), this has not been a universal finding (77–79). Recommendations to mothers regarding breast-feeding should be individualized; those mothers who choose to breast-feed should increase their caloric intake to compensate for the increased nutritional demands, and they should be monitored closely to ensure that there is no decline in their health. The physician also must be cognizant of any medications taken by the mother that might be passed to the child through breast-feeding. Some antibiotics reach high levels in breast milk (e.g., erythromycin, trimethoprim, and chloramphenicol), whereas others are excreted poorly (e.g., penicillins, cephalosporins, and sulfonamides) (66). Tetracyclines are excreted in high levels in breast milk but are chelated rapidly with calcium and, therefore, have a low bio-availability to the infant.

FAMILY PLANNING

Planning for Pregnancy

For the patient with CF who desires children, special consideration must be paid to several issues when offering guidance to the couple (52). The impact that pregnancy will have on the health of the woman with CF is of utmost importance, but consideration for how parenthood will affect the mother-to-be with CF cannot be ignored. Caring for an infant can be a physically demanding experience (in addition to the nutritional demands of breast-feeding), and the parent may neglect his or her own health requirements (e.g., not perform adequate chest physiotherapy).

There are ethical considerations as well. The parent with CF, whether male or female, may have a shortened life expectancy. The parent with CF cannot necessarily plan on attending the child's future events (e.g., college graduation), and in some cases, the parent may survive only for the first few years of the child's life. Therefore, the couple should discuss how a shortened life span of one parent will affect their decision to have a child. This should be discussed in context with the growing success of lung transplantation, which may be a therapeutic option for the parent with CF, whose lung function has worsened such that life expectancy is less than 2 years.

Genetic Counseling

It is known that the parent with CF will pass a copy of the abnormal CF gene to the child; thus, the child will be, at least, a known carrier of the CF gene and will require genetic counseling at the appropriate age. It is conceivable that the child could have CF if the other parent is a carrier of an abnormal gene (84). The odds of this occurrence can be estimated after a careful history of the non-CF spouse, with added information from genetic screening. The underlying risk of being a carrier of the CF gene can be predicted if there is a history of CF in a family member or it can be estimated by the frequency occurrence of a mutated CF gene for that person's ethnic background (85–87) (Table 21–4). The risk can be defined further by screening the nonaffected spouse for the presence of a CF mutation. Typical testing used by most commercial laboratories screens for 32 of the most common mutations. This will detect approximately 90% of the mutations in the white population, 97% in the Jewish Ashkenazi population, and 45% in the African American population; some laboratories offer screening of 70 mutations, which increases the detection rate in the white and Ashkenazi populations only slightly but increases the detection rate in the African American population to approximately 60%. Because the tests do not screen for 100% of the CF mutations, the risk of carrying the CF gene never can be zero.

Prenatal diagnosis has become an option for pregnant mothers at risk for carrying a fetus with genetic abnormalities, including CF. This typically is performed by amniocentesis or villous biopsy during the first trimester. It also is possible to test human embryos for CF mutations before implantation (88,89), which is a costly endeavor. The ethical considerations for this technique are beyond the scope of this chapter.

Reproductive Alternatives

Recent medical advances have made the infertility of CF a potentially treatable problem. Because the fertility problem in males with CF is caused by obstruction of the vas deferens, it may be assumed that spermatozoa of the male with CF are viable and could be used for fertilization of ova. Previously, bilateral absence of the vas deferens was considered one of the most difficult cases of infertility to treat (90); however, the introduction of a microsurgical epididymal sperm aspiration technique (91) has provided new hope for couples with this problem. A recent multicenter survey has shown an overall pregnancy rate of 10% with the use of microsurgical epididymal aspiration in males with infertility because of absence of a vas deferens (92). The use of this technique, followed by intracytoplasmic sperm injection into the ova, has resulted in pregnancy rates approaching 50%, with the prediction that greater

TABLE 21–4. *Risk of parent with cystic fibrosis (CF) having a child with cystic fibrosis[a]*

CF mutations detectable (%)	White population		African American population		Ashkenazi population	
	Carrier risk for spouse with negative test	Risk of CF offspring	Carrier risk for spouse with negative test	Risk of CF offspring	Carrier risk for spouse with negative test	Risk of CF offspring
0	1 in 25.5	1 in 51	1 in 63	1 in 126	1 in 29.9	1 in 60
70	1 in 82.7	1 in 165	1 in 208	1 in 416	1 in 97	1 in 194
75	1 in 99	1 in 198	1 in 249	1 in 498	1 in 117	1 in 234
80	1 in 124	1 in 248	1 in 311	1 in 622	1 in 146	1 in 292
85	1 in 164	1 in 328	1 in 414	1 in 828	1 in 194	1 in 388
90	1 in 246	1 in 492	1 in 621	1 in 1,242	1 in 290	1 in 580
95	1 in 491	1 in 982	1 in 1,241	1 in 2,482	1 in 579	1 in 1,158
97	1 in 818	1 in 1,636	1 in 2,068	1 in 4,136	1 in 965	1 in 1,930

[a]Probabilities calculated by Bayesian analysis assuming a population frequency of CF of 1:2500 for the white population (87), 1:17,000 for the African American population (85), and 1:3400 for the Ashkenazi Jewish population (86).

success will be seen as experience grows (90). These techniques offer great promise to the CF male who wishes to father a child.

For women with CF who desire pregnancy but are unsuccessful, intrauterine insemination has been performed successfully in women with CF (93), offering an alternative modality to these patients.

Finally, for the patient with CF who desires children but who cannot conceive for the various aforementioned reasons, adoption remains an option. This is a delicate topic because most adoption agencies will have concern about the predicted survival of the parent with CF.

Birth Control

Some sexually active adults with CF will want to avoid pregnancy. Despite a high likelihood of obstructive azoospermia in the CF male, this cannot be assumed, and semen analysis should be offered. Similarly, although the female with CF may have a reduction in fertility, the potential for fertility is difficult to measure, and contraception is advised.

All conventional methods of contraception have been tried in women with CF, with results similar to those of the general population. Oral contraceptive pills (OCPs) frequently are used. Some authors have recommended against using preparations with very low doses of estrogen because there may be unpredictable absorption from the gut (38). Concern has been raised about the use of OCPs in women with CF because of early reports of polypoid cervicitis and an association between OCPs and a deterioration in pulmonary status (94). A subsequent report noted no deterioration in pulmonary status in 10 women using OCPs (95), and OCPs have been used commonly. In addition, there are theoretical concerns that OCPs may be associated with a higher incidence of cholelithiasis, a problem that already is of higher incidence in CF. It is recommended that women with CF who are started on OCPs be monitored closely.

Surgical sterilization is an excellent option of birth control for the adult with CF or his/her partner. The woman with CF can undergo bilateral tubal ligation, which has a low complication rate and a high success rate. The male partner of the CF woman or the man with a normal semen analysis can consider vasectomy, which has a failure rate of less than 1.2% (96).

Barrier methods, such as a diaphragm or condom, may be used with expectations similar to those of the general population. The patient with CF also should be advised to consider condoms for protection against sexually transmitted diseases. Intrauterine devices have been associated with frequent problems and are not advised.

SUMMARY

Because patients with CF are living into adulthood, there will be an increasing number of patients considering parenthood. Despite a potential reduction in fertility, there are an increasing number of pregnancies reported. For those infertile patients, there are alternatives that will allow them to consider pregnancy. There appears to be an association between maternal health (i.e., pulmonary function and nutritional status) and outcome, both maternal and fetal, during pregnancy. The woman with mild disease is likely to fare well during pregnancy, whereas the woman with severe disease should be advised to avoid or terminate pregnancy. For those patients who desire pregnancy, a careful discussion of the potential complications and their effects on both mother and infant is indicated between the physician and both parents. The pregnant patient with CF requires close monitoring because complications, especially exacerbation of pulmonary infection, are likely, and these problems should be treated aggressively. Genetic counseling is indicated because there is an increased risk of CF in the infant compared with the general population, and the child will be a carrier of a CF gene, at a minimum.

Just as there are many reasons to account for why patients with CF are living longer, so are there many "rewards" that come with this success. One of these rewards is the opportunity to be able to discuss issues of adulthood, such as sex and pregnancy, with our patients. The open discussion of these issues is an important part of a comprehensive program for the care of the patient with CF. Careful preplanning before pregnancy should allow for most situations to be addressed appropriately, leading to a good outcome for all, including patient, spouse, child, and physician.

REFERENCES

1. FitzSimmons SC. The changing epidemiology of cystic fibrosis. *J Pediatr* 1993;122:1.
2. Denning CR, Sommers SC, Quigley HJ. Infertility in male patients with cystic fibrosis. *Pediatrics* 1968;41:7.
3. Kaplan E, Shwachman H, Perlmutter AD, et al. Reproductive failure in males with cystic fibrosis. *N Engl J Med* 1968;279:65.
4. Seale TW, Flux M, Rennert OM. Reproductive defects in patients of both sexes with cystic fibrosis: a review. *Ann Clin Lab Sci* 1985;15:152.
5. Kotloff RM, FitzSimmons SC, Fiel SB. Fertility and pregnancy in patients with cystic fibrosis. *Clin Chest Med* 1992;13:623.
6. Taussig LM, Lobeck CC, Di Sant'Agnese PA, et al. Fertility in males with cystic fibrosis. *N Engl J Med* 1972;287:586.
7. Blanck RR, Mendoza EM. Fertility in a man with cystic fibrosis. *JAMA* 1976;235:1364.
8. Dreyfus DH, Bethel R, Gelfand EW. Cystic fibrosis 3849+10kb C>T mutation associated with severe pulmonary disease and male fertility. *Am J Respir Crit Care Med* 1996;153:858.
9. Stewart B, Zabner J, Shuber AP, et al. Normal sweat chloride values do not exclude the diagnosis of cystic fibrosis. *Am J Respir Crit Care Med* 1995;151:899.
10. Barreto C, Pinto LM, Duarte A, et al. A fertile male with cystic fibrosis: molecular genetic analysis. *J Med Genet* 1991;28:420.
11. Highsmith WE, Burch LH, Zhou Z, et al. A novel mutation in the cystic fibrosis gene in patients with pulmonary disease but normal sweat chloride concentrations. 1994;331:974.
12. Wilschanski M, Corey M, Durie P, et al. Diversity of reproductive tract abnormalities in men with cystic fibrosis. *JAMA* 1996;276:607.
13. Holsclaw D. Cystic fibrosis and fertility. *Br Med J* 1969;1:356.
14. Rule AH, Kopito L, Shwachman H. Chemical analysis of ejaculates from patients with cystic fibrosis. *Fertil Steril* 1970;21:515.
15. Mann TRR. *The biochemistry of semen and of the male reproductive tract*. New York: Wiley, 1964.
16. Gottlieb C, Plöen L, Kvist U, et al. The fertility potential of male cystic fibrosis patients. *Int J Androl* 1991;14:437.
17. Gaillard D, Pigeon F, Delepine B, et al. Vas deferens is normal in fetus with cystic fibrosis. *Pediatr Pulmonol Suppl* 1996;13:246.
18. Oppenheimer EH, Esterly JR. Observations on cystic fibrosis of the pancreas: the uterine cervix. *J Pediatr* 1970;77:991.
19. Valman HB, France NE. The vas deferens in cystic fibrosis. *Lancet* 1969;2:566.
20. Pollard CE, Harris A, Coleman L, et al. Chloride channels on epithelial cells cultured from human fetal epididymis. *J Membr Biol* 1991;124:275.
21. Chan HC, Fu WO, Chung YW, et al. An ATP-activated cation conductance in human epididymal cells. *Biol Reprod* 1995;52:645.
22. Tizzano EF, Silver MM, Chitayat D, et al. Differential cellular expression of cystic fibrosis transmembrane regulator in human reproductive tissues. *Am J Pathol* 1994;144:906.
23. Stern RC, Boat TF, Doershuk CF. Obstructive azoospermia as a diagnostic criterion for the cystic fibrosis syndrome. *Lancet* 1982;1:1401.
24. Handelsman DJ, Conway AJ, Boylan LM, et al. Obstructive azoospermia and chronic sinopulmonary infections. *N Engl J Med* 1984;310:3.
25. Friedman KJ, Teichtahl H, De Kretser DM, et al. Screening Young syndrome patients for CFTR mutations. *Am J Respir Crit Care Med* 1995;152:1353.
26. Anguiano A, Oates RD, Amos JA, et al. Congenital bilateral absence of the vas deferens: a primarily genital form of cystic fibrosis. *JAMA* 1992;267:1794.
27. Rosenstein BJ, Cutting GR. The diagnosis of cystic fibrosis: a consensus statement. *J. Pediatr 1998;* 132: 589–595.
28. Augarten A, Yahav Y, Kerem BS, et al. Congenital bilateral absence of vas deferens in the absence of cystic fibrosis. *Lancet* 1994;344:1473.
29. Culard JF, Desgeorges M, Costa P, et al. Analysis of the whole CFTR coding regions and splice junctions in azoospermic men with congenital bilateral aplasia of epididymis or vas deferens. *Hum Genet* 1994;93: 467.
30. Dumur V, Gervais R, Rigot JM, et al. Abnormal distribution of CF ΔF508 allele in azoospermic men with congenital aplasia of the epidiymis and vas deferens. *Lancet* 1990;336:512.
31. Le Lannou D, Jezequel P, Blayau M, et al. Obstructive azoospermia with agenesis of vas deferens or with bronchiectasis (Young's syndrome): a genetic approach. *Hum Reprod* 1995;10:338.
32. Patrizio P, Ord T, Silber SJ, et al. Cystic fibrosis mutations impair the fertilization rate of epididymal sperm from men with congenital absence of the vas deferens. *Hum Reprod* 1993;8:1259.
33. O'Neal WK, Hasty P, McCray PB, et al. A severe phenotype in mice with a duplication of exon 3 in the cystic fibrosis locus. *Hum Molec Genet* 1993;2:1561.
34. Snouwaert JN, Brigman KK, Latour AM, et al. An animal model for cystic fibrosis made by gene targeting. *Science* 1992;257:1083.
35. Trezise AEO, Linder CC, Grieger D, et al. CFTR expression is regulated during both the cycle of the seminiferous epithelium and oestrous cycle of rodents. *Nature Genet* 1993;3:157.
36. Oppenheimer EA, Case AL, Esterly JR, et al. Cervical mucus in cystic fibrosis: a possible cause of infertility. *Am J Obstet Gynecol* 1970;108:673.
37. Kopito LE, Kosasky HJ, Shwachman H. Water and electrolytes in cervical mucus from patients with cystic fibrosis. *Fertil Steril* 1973;24:512.
38. Geddes DM. Cystic fibrosis and pregnancy. *J R Soc Med* 1992;85:36.
39. Moshang T, Holsclaw DS. Menarchal determinants in cystic fibrosis. *Am J Dis Child* 1980;134:1139.

40. Neinstein LS, Stewart D, Wang C-I, et al. Menstrual dysfunction in cystic fibrosis. *J Adolesc Health Care* 1983;4:153.

41. Reiter EO, Stern RC, Root AW. The reproductive endocrine system in cystic fibrosis: basal gonadotropin and sex steroid levels. *Am J Dis Child* 1981;135: 422.

42. Stead RJ, Hodson ME, Batten JC, et al. Amenorrhea in cystic fibrosis. *Clin Endocrinol* 1987;26:187.

43. Knuth UA, Hull MGR, Jacobs HS. Amenorrhea and loss of weight. *Br J Obstet Gynecol* 1977;84:801.

44. Leung A-YH, Wong PYD, Gabriel SE, et al. cAMP-but not Ca^{2+}-regulated Cl^- conductance in the oviduct is defective in mouse model of cystic fibrosis. *Am J Physiol* 1995;268:C708.

45. Fletcher EC, Martin RJ. Sexual dysfunction and erectile impotence in chronic obstructive pulmonary disease. 1982;81:413.

46. Kass I, Updegraff K, Muffly RB. Sex in chronic obstructive pulmonary disease. *Med Aspects Hum Sexual* 1972;7:33.

47. Hanson EI. Effects of chronic lung disease on life in general and on sexuality: perceptions of adult patients. 1982;11:435.

48. Boyle IR, Di Sant'Agnese PA, Sack S, et al. Emotional adjustment of adolescents and young adults with cystic fibrosis. *J Pediatr* 1976;88:318.

49. Cromer B, Enrile B, McCoy K, et al. Knowledge, attitudes and behavior related to sexuality in adolescents with chronic disability. *Develop Med Child Neurol* 1990;32:602.

50. Levine SB, Stern RC. Sexual function in cystic fibrosis. *Chest* 1982;81:422.

51. Coffman CB, Levine SB, Althof SE, et al. Sexual adaptation among single young adults with cystic fibrosis. *Chest* 1984;86:412–418.

52. Orenstein DM, Knowles MR. Cystic fibrosis and adulthood. In: Orenstein DM, ed. *Cystic fibrosis: a guide for patient and family*, 2nd ed. New York: Lippincott-Raven, 1996:243–260.

53. Vemireddi NK. Sexual counseling for chronically disabled patients. 1978;33:65.

54. Cohen LF, Di Sant'Agnese PA, Friedlander J. Cystic fibrosis and pregnancy: a national survey. *Lancet* 1980;2:842.

55. Palmer J, Dillon-Baker C, Tecklin JS, et al. Pregnancy in patients with cystic fibrosis. *Ann Intern Med* 1983;99:596.

56. FitzSimmons SC, Fitzpatrick S, Thompson B, et al. A longitudinal study of the effects of pregnancy on 325 women with cystic fibrosis. *Pediatr Pulmonol* 1996 (suppl);13:99.

57. Larsen JW. Cystic fibrosis and pregnancy. *Obstet Gynecol* 1972;39:880.

58. Novy MJ, Tyler JM, Shwachman H, et al. Cystic fibrosis and pregnancy: report of a case, with a study of pulmonary function and arterial blood gases. *Obstet Gynecol* 1967;30:530.

59. Elkus R, Popovich J. Respiratory physiology in pregnancy. *Clin Chest Med* 1992;13:555.

60. Weinberger SE, Weiss ST, Cohen WR, et al. Pregnancy and the lung. *Am Rev Respir Dis* 1980;121:559.

61. Noble PW, Lavee AE, Jacobs MM. Respiratory diseases in pregnancy. *Obstet Gynecol Clin North Am* 1988;5:391.

62. Naeye RL. Weight gain and the outcome of pregnancy. *Am J Obstet Gynecol* 1979;135:3.

63. Cole BNL, Seltzer MH, Kassabian J, et al. Parenteral nutrition in a pregnant cystic fibrosis patient. *J Parenter Enteral Nutr* 1987;11:205.

64. Schidlow DV, Taussig LM, Knowles MR. Cystic fibrosis foundation consensus conference report on pulmonary complications of cystic fibrosis. *Pediatr Pulmonol* 1993;15:187.

65. Blank A, Grave GD, Metzger BE. Effects of gestational diabetes on perinatal morbidity reassessed. *Diabetes Care* 1995;18:127.

66. Montella KR. Pulmonary pharmacology in pregnancy. *Clin Chest Med* 1992;13:587.

67. Barron WM. Medical evaluation of the pregnant patient requiring nonobstetric surgery. *Clin Perinatol* 1985;12:481.

68. Siegel B, Siegel S. Pregnancy and delivery in a patient with CF of the pancreas. *Obstet Gynecol* 1960;16:439.

69. Kotloff RM. Reproductive issues in patients with cystic fibrosis. *Semin Respir Crit Care Med* 1994;15:402.

70. Grand RJ, Talano RC, Di Sant'Agnese PA, et al. Pregnancy in cystic fibrosis of the pancreas. *JAMA* 1966; 195:117.

71. Shwachman H, Kulczycki LL. Long-term study of one hundred five patients with cystic fibrosis. *Am J Dis Child* 1958;96:6.

72. Taussig LM, Kattwinkel J, Friedewald WT, et al. A new prognostic score and clinical evaluation system for cystic fibrosis. *J Pediatr* 1973;82:380.

73. Corkey CWB, Newth CJL, Corey M, et al. Pregnancy in cystic fibrosis: a better prognosis in patients with pancreatic function? *Am J Obstet Gynecol* 1981;140:737.

74. Canny GJ, Corey M, Livingstone RA, et al. Pregnancy and cystic fibrosis. *Obstet Gynecol* 1991;77:850.

75. Wood RE, Boat TF, Doershuk CF. State of the art: cystic fibrosis. *Am Rev Respir Dis* 1976;113:833.

76. Whitelaw A, Butterfield A. High breast-milk sodium in cystic fibrosis. *Lancet* 1977;2:1288.

77. Alpert SE, Cormier AD. Normal electrolyte and protein content in milk from mothers with cystic fibrosis: an explanation for the initial report of elevated milk sodium concentration. *J Pediatr* 1983;102:77.

78. Shiffman ML, Seale TW, Flux M, et al. Breast-milk composition in women with cystic fibrosis: report of two cases and a review of the literature. *Am J Clin Nutr* 1989;49:612.

79. Michel S, Mueller DH. Impact of lactation on women with cystic fibrosis and their infants: a review of five cases. *J Am Diet Assoc* 1994;94:159.

80. Quinton PM, Reddy MM. The sweat gland. In: Davis PB, ed. *Cystic fibrosis*. New York: Marcel Dekker Inc, 1993:137–159.

81. Linzell JL, Peaker M. Mechanisms of milk secretion. *Physiol Rev* 1971;51:564.

82. Food and Nutrition Board and National Research Council. Recommended dietary allowances. Washington, DC: National Academy of Sciences, 1974.

83. Welch MJ, Phelps DL, Osher AB. Breast-feeding by a mother with cystic fibrosis. *Pediatrics* 1981;67:664.

84. Herrod HG, Spock A. Mother and daughter with cystic fibrosis. *J Pediatr* 1977;91:276.

85. Kulczycki L, Schauf V. Cystic fibrosis in blacks in Washington, DC: incidence and characteristics. *Am J Dis Child* 1974;127:64.

86. Abelovich D, Lavon I, Lerer I, et al. Screening for five mutations detects 97% of cystic fibrosis (CF) chromo-

somes and predicts a carrier frequency of 1:29 in the Jewish Ashkenazi population. *Am J Hum Genet* 1992; 51:951.

87. Lemna WK, Feldman GL, Kerem B. Mutation analysis for heterozygote detection and the prenatal diagnosis of cystic fibrosis. *N Engl J Med* 1990;322:291.

88. Handyside AH, Lesko JG, Tarin JJ, et al. Birth of a normal girl after in vitro fertilization and preimplantation diagnostic testing for cystic fibrosis. *N Engl J Med* 1992;327:905.

89. Liu J, Lissens W, Silber S, et al. Birth after preimplantation diagnosis of the cystic fibrosis ΔF508 mutation by polymerase chain reaction in human embryos resulting from intracytoplasmic sperm injection with epididymal sperm. *JAMA* 1994;272:1858.

90. Tournaye H, Devroey P, Liu J, et al. Microsurgical epididymal sperm aspiration and intracytoplasmic sperm injection: a new effective approach to infertility as a result of congenital bilateral absence of the vas deferens. *Fertil Steril* 1994;61:1045.

91. Oates RD, Honig S, Berger MJ, et al. Microscopic epididymal sperm aspiration (MESA): a new option for treatment of the obstructive azoospermia associated with cystic fibrosis. *J Assist Reprod Genet* 1992; 9:36.

92. The Sperm Microaspiration Retrieval Techniques Study Group. Results in the United States with sperm microaspiration retrieval techniques and assisted reproductive technologies. *J Urol* 1994;151:1255.

93. Kredentser JV, Pokrant C, McCoshen JA. Intrauterine insemination for infertility due to cystic fibrosis. *Fertil Steril* 1986;45:425.

94. Dooley RR, Braunstein H, Osher AB. Polypoid cervicitis in cystic fibrosis patients receiving oral contraceptives. *Am J Obstet Gynecol* 1974;118:971.

95. Fitzpatrick SB, Stokes DC, Rosenstein BJ, et al. Use of oral contraceptives in women with cystic fibrosis. *Chest* 1984;86:863.

96. Hendry WF. Vasectomy and vasectomy reversal. Brit Med J 1994;73:337–344.

Cystic Fibrosis in Adults,
edited by J. R. Yankaskas and M. R. Knowles,
Lippincott–Raven Publishers, Philadelphia, 1999.

22

Adult Social Issues

James R. Yankaskas and *Gerald W. Fernald

*Cystic Fibrosis/Pulmonary Research and Treatment Center, Division of Pulmonary and Critical Care Medicine, and *Department of Pediatrics, University of North Carolina School of Medicine, Chapel Hill, North Carolina*

Most adults with cystic fibrosis (CF) require regular medical therapy, but they usually are able to pursue the normal activities of society. Despite a chronic illness, most obtain an education, pursue active careers, develop significant personal relationships, and contribute to the community (1,2). However, these achievements are not attained without difficulty. For example, the medical impact of CF may limit some activities and employment options. The presence of a genetic disease may impair the ability to procure medical insurance. Despite their increasing survival rate, medical disabilities develop in most individuals in the course of their lives, and premature death is common. The healthcare needs of adults with CF are met best by a team of professionals who are well trained and experienced in addressing the medical and other problems of CF.

This chapter summarizes the means for dealing with these diverse medical, social, and psychological issues. First, adult CF health systems are described. Various routes to access and use of these resources are identified. Second, the normal adult activities of dating, marriage, education, employment, medical insurance, and disability are addressed. Finally, the psychological stresses associated with CF and the coping mechanisms for dealing with them are addressed. Many adult CF centers have been developed, and the U.S. healthcare system is evolving rapidly in response to economic and political forces. This chapter provides a framework to adapt the available

resources to the best avail. More extensive descriptions of these resources have been published (3).

ADULT CYSTIC FIBROSIS HEALTHCARE

Specialized Cystic Fibrosis Healthcare

Similar to patients with other diseases, adults with CF can expect to achieve the best quality and most cost-efficient medical care from individuals who are trained and experienced in managing this complex disease. As described in Chapter 23, the Cystic Fibrosis Foundation (CFF) approved 114 care, teaching and research centers that provide for the majority of patients with CF throughout the United States. These centers include a program director and a team of nurse coordinators, respiratory and physical therapists, dietitians, social workers, vocational counselors, and others who provide comprehensive care. During the 1980s, centers began to develop adult programs as the number of adults with CF increased. For example, at the University of North Carolina (UNC), adult care developed in parallel with the expanding pediatric CF population (Fig. 22–1). By 1997, more than 35% of patients with CF in the United States were adults, and approximately one third of the CF centers had adult programs. These numbers are expected to continue to increase.

The advantages of care in specialized CF centers include knowledgeable clinicians, their

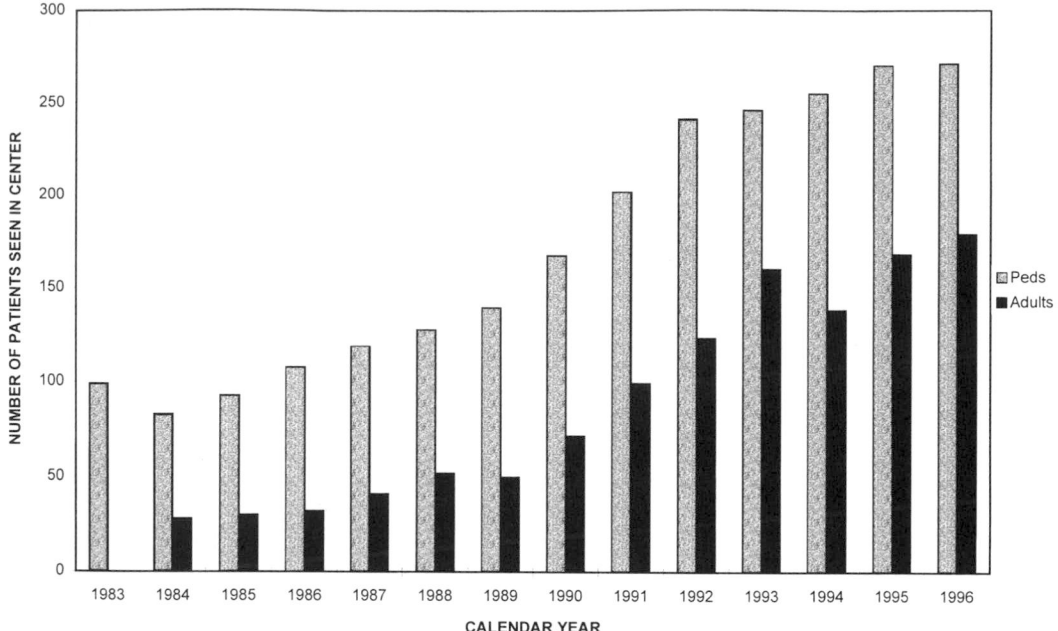

FIG. 22–1. Numbers of pediatric (*shaded bars*) and adult (*solid bars*) patients with CF receiving care at the University of North Carolina Cystic Fibrosis Center.

experience in the recognition and management of CF complications, the prompt dissemination of information about medical advances, and the efficiency of providing specialized services to a group of individuals. The growing number of CFF-sponsored adult care, teaching, and research centers provide such capabilities. They advance the quality and efficiency of CF care through the Cystic Fibrosis Patient Registry and clinical research projects. A number of alternative approaches to providing care for adults with CF are available in areas that have not established an adult CF center.

Although many CF centers have provided care to adult and pediatric patients with common resources, efforts to develop independent adult programs are supported strongly by the CFF. Several organization models provide increasing levels of independent adult care. In Model 1, suitable only for centers caring for fewer than 40 adults, an internist working with pediatric center physicians provides adult care in cohorted outpatient settings, and hospital care in adult units is encouraged. In Model 2,

the adult program director provides routine CF care and hospital care in adult settings, while outpatient care is provided in the pediatric clinic with adults cohorted and team care is provided by the pediatric team. In Model 3, outpatient care is provided in pediatric or adult clinics and team care is provided by pediatric and adult team members. In Model 4, all hospital, outpatient, and team care is provided by independent adult team members.

Whether a full adult program is available, the same advantages that characterize CF care in a comprehensive pediatric center apply to adult CF programs. From the initial diagnosis through the full spectrum of disease progression, involvement of the primary care physician and a close relationship with the CF center must be preserved. The primary care physician can provide routine health supervision and take care of many of the common problems of the patient with CF. The center physician, usually a pulmonologist, provides experience and expertise in managing the details and problems encountered in the course of the disease and has a team of care givers to provide specific advice, guidance, and support. The expectations of the patients toward local medical care and CF center care generally reflect these areas of expertise and focus on the early diagnosis and long-term relationship with the local physician and the expertise and team approach of the CF center.

Developing an Adult Cystic Fibrosis Center

Essential to providing CF care for adult patients are physicians interested in and trained to work with CF and all of its manifestations. Adult pulmonologists are most likely to be trained to meet these expectations if they have been associated with one of the large CF centers. However, general internists or family practitioners can be equally effective if they have the appropriate interest, background, and experience. As demonstrated over the past 3 decades, a team approach to the patients yields the most efficient and effective care for chronically diseased patients.

The selection of a strong clinic coordinator, usually the CF nurse, is the second essential to development of a CF care center. The team then can be expanded by recruiting the participation of social work, nutrition, physical therapy, and/or respiratory therapy specialists. The proportion of time committed to the center will depend on numbers and needs of patients.

Nearly all CF programs currently have a significant number of adult patients; roughly one third of the Cystic Fibrosis Patient Registry is made up of patients older than the age of 18 years (2,4). Many of the larger programs have well-developed adult clinics. Those located within a university hospital or large general hospital benefit from the proximity of internists in the department of medicine. Pediatric centers in free-standing children's hospitals must make arrangements with nearby adult programs. Adolescent clinics may provide a locale for transition but usually are not suited for care of the chronically ill patient.

Recruitment of adult care givers seems to be the first and most difficult step in development of adult CF programs. Only recently has CF been recognized as a rapidly growing compo-

nent of the adult clinic population. Lack of training in this special area and possibly the minimal financial incentives have limited the involvement of internists and family physicians. As adult pulmonary fellowships provide experience with CF, the number of new faculty available to fill these roles is growing. In the interim, a variety of interactions between internists or family practitioners and pediatricians can be developed to provide a suitable clinic setting for care of adults with CF.

One of the most effective beginnings for adult care is to incorporate a physician trained in adult care into an existing pediatric CF center. This will allow the "adult" physician to get to know the older patients and, at the same time, sharpen his/her skills by consulting with the experienced pediatric center physicians. When a critical number of patients is accumulated and separate space and staffing are available, the adult program then can move out of the pediatric clinic.

Variations on this model will extend from those that continue to combine all ages to those that eventually become free-standing adult CF centers. Currently, the CFF recognizes CF adult programs when they serve 40 or more patients and have a designated "adult" physician. The CFF, through its site visit teams, can be an effective means of gaining the support of department chairs and hospital directors, as it has in the past for pediatric centers. Thirty-six CFF accredited adult centers were operating in 1997, and another 31 centers provided care to 40 or more adults with CF. An up-to-date list of centers is maintained by the CFF [1–800–FIGHT CF (1–800–344–4823)].

Entering the Adult Cystic Fibrosis Healthcare System

Developmental Background: Growing Up with Cystic Fibrosis

Early childhood experiences and relationships influence adult behavior. Adults with CF are no exception. In addition to the usual variables of parenting and sibling interactions, the impact of the diagnosis and family reactions to this serious chronic disease create lasting effects on personality development and behavior as the patient with CF matures.

The median age of CF diagnosis is 7 months, but the age at diagnosis ranges from the newborn period into adulthood. As originally described by McCollum and Gibson (5), there is a prediagnostic stage during which parents struggle with possible explanations for their child's failure to thrive, chronic diarrhea, and/or recurrent respiratory problems. Although the diagnosis of CF eventually explains most of these questions, its impact usually is devastating and long-lasting. Immediately after diagnosis, parents struggle with accepting and understanding the disease. A "long-term adaptive" phase then evolves, followed eventually by terminal stages of the disease.

The diagnosis of CF raises problems related to genetics, life expectancy, family planning, and finances. How successfully the family copes with these stresses depends on its strength before diagnosis. It is an enormous challenge for parents to balance prescribed medical care with other family responsibilities, including care of siblings, and yet maintain as normal a lifestyle as possible for the child with CF. Although the literature on the psychology of patients and families with CF tends to emphasize the various maladaptations observed, the few carefully controlled studies suggest that children with CF vary from normal less than children with other chronic conditions (6). They do seem to be less mature, more dependent, worry about their disease, and be less realistic toward career planning.

Observations at UNC suggest a direct correlation between the strength of the family and its ability to understand and cope with the problems of CF. Families able to adapt to the needs of their child with CF seem to maintain the best long-term care. Those who find it difficult to understand and accept the child with CF tend to be either over- or undercompliant. The parental attitudes that bear on such behaviors are present from the start and probably are the most important predictor of the patient's self-concept and behavior toward his/her disease (7).

Review of early childhood circumstances related to the diagnosis and subsequent family interactions often will allow better understanding of the psychosocial status of the adult with CF. Families able to understand the diagnosis in terms of genetic inheritance patterns usually do not continue to blame themselves or their relatives for their child's condition. Those who cannot resolve this conflict will negatively influence the patient with their continued denial, anger, and other maladaptive behavior as parents. When denial translates to hiding the diagnosis from relatives, friends, and even the patient, these conflicts remain unresolved and will need to be dealt with before the patient can achieve a mature adult personality. One of the major challenges of CF center care is to anticipate these problems and provide education and support to families raising a child with CF.

Adolescence: The Second "Disease"

The complexity of adolescent development seems to amplify many of the problems that arise during childhood. Most adolescents are concerned with peer acceptance, appearance, and independence from parents and tend to deny ill health (8,9). Patients with CF also must deal with their disease as they struggle with peer relationships, family, and school. Early teen-agers usually have begun to recognize the significance of their illness and its effect on their future, although outwardly they may deny it. Refusal to allow parents to minister their medications and treatments is common at this age as young adolescents experiment with independence from the family.

In mid adolescence, issues of independence increase and focus on areas of particular teenage interests, including driving cars, dating, sports, and music. Parents who have been overprotective will find it difficult to provide the structured independence necessary for normal resolution of conflicts surrounding these activities. This may result in increased defiance of parental control and even uncontrolled behavior. Such uncontrolled behavior and severe noncompliance may increase the progression of lung disease, risk pregnancy, and produce academic failure. Patients who fail to resolve this stage may continue to rely on parental management of their disease well into adulthood.

With increasing survival expectations and improving health status as a result of modern therapeutic interventions, most adolescents with CF currently progress through puberty at relatively normal rates. Although it is wonderful to see young boys and girls maturing earlier than in the past, this also means that the problems of adolescence arrive at an earlier age, when they may be more difficult to deal with. Families who have struggled from the time of diagnosis will require much counseling and support to allow their adolescent with CF to exercise his or her need for independence. Most CF centers can provide such support and may be able to aid such families.

As adolescence begins to resolve in the late teens and early 20s, most young adults with CF begin to assume a more responsible attitude toward self-care. Hopefully, they have lost little ground during mid adolescence and will be motivated to pursue a more mature lifestyle. The challenges of further education, work, finances, and sexuality become reality once the protective environment of high school is left behind (10). The exact timing of these stages of adolescence varies and greatly influences planning for transfer to an adult medical program.

Achieving Adulthood

As indicated previously, the independence and autonomy most adults eventually attain often are delayed or blocked by childhood and adolescent experiences related to living with this chronic disease. In addition to the psychosocial interaction with parents, family, and friends, real problems of daily self-care face the young adult. If fortunate enough to have the ability and support to continue their education, young adult patients should be urged to prepare for skilled or professional careers. This often means support systems developed in childhood no longer are practicable, and suitable alternatives must be developed. If further education is to be in the community and the student lives at home, a minimum of change may be required. However, many students move to a university setting and will need to develop ways to provide themselves with the necessary medical care, airway clearance techniques, and reasonable nutrition. University campuses associated with CF centers usually have dealt with such challenges and can help students work out appropriate arrangements.

If patients attempt to enter the adult world without further education, they will face even more difficulties in achieving a desired lifestyle. Often, they find themselves financially dependent on their family at a time of life when they need to develop their independence. Family health insurance coverage will be discontinued if they do not maintain student status and the likelihood of finding unskilled employment with a large enough organization to provide comprehensive healthcare is low. As for many adolescents, further education seems an absolute necessity for the future for patients with CF. It prolongs the inevitable challenges of adulthood, and bridges the void of financial earnings and family-based health insurance that face the high school graduate who seeks employment without further education or training.

Many factors will impede the young adult in achieving these necessary goals. Included are mild versus severe disease expression, early or delayed adolescent development, and inappropriate parent–patient interactions. Even when a degree of independence is achieved, severe illness often will dictate a return to a dependent relationship. One of the best examples we have observed that illustrates the importance of these factors is the patient who is diagnosed well beyond adolescence. Having grown up without "having a chronic disease," such patients lack most of the aforementioned attributes. They resemble other adult patients who have acquired a disease after growing up with normal health and psychosocial perceptions. Of course, it is impossible to avoid the effects of the early diagnosis of CF, but such patients illustrate the importance of counseling parents to raise their children with CF "as normally as possible."

Transition to Adult Care

Careful preparation and timing are essential to a smooth transition from pediatric to adult care, whatever the disease (11,12). Most programs use 18 years of age as the average time to make the move. However, this will depend on the maturity of the patient, his/her disease severity, and the attractiveness of the adult clinic. Some adolescents will be ready for the transition earlier than 18 years of age but most will tend to take longer—not uncommonly up to age 21 years. Educational status also may play a role because it may be either ideal or imprudent to combine a new medical system with a move to a college campus. The ideal situation might be when the university campus contains a medical center that provides adult CF care. Given less suitable facilities, it may seem wise to arrange for adult-level care by the age of 21 or 22 years, when most students will have finished their college education.

Preparation of the adolescent for transition to adult care begins by treating him or her as a responsible person. This begins with seeing the patient separately from the parents and encouraging independence in daily medical routines. Because this usually will occur at approximately the time that the patient acquires his or her driver's license, it is an appropriate and significant "rite of passage."

When the adolescent begins to exhibit interest in adult care, he or she can be introduced to the adult clinic team and tour their facilities. This can be a gradual transition of up to 1 year or more while the young adult learns the similarities and differences between the two programs. The process may be more rapid for confident individuals. Often, an admission to the adult medical service will provide the final step. The most successful moves occur at the patient's own pace and should not be forced. However, when the move has been made, there must be no "back-sliding." If the patient is allowed "to come back" to pediatrics, the purpose of the whole transition process and the value of the adult program will be undermined. Most patients will try to maintain contacts in pediatrics, and this should be encouraged as long as it is understood that responsibility for their medical care is in the adult program. No matter how well prepared, most adolescents (and their parents) will find the transition to be stressful; however, few, if any, will not readily adapt to the change.

Perhaps the most influential barrier to a smooth transition is the pediatrician who has cared for the patient and his or her family since early infancy and fails to recognize the need for transition. Although it is difficult to "give up" the patient to adult medicine, the success of adult care easily can be limited by such attitudes. After all, who can best model mature behavior for the patient? Those pediatricians with limited trust in the care delivered by internists should work with the adult care givers to ensure mutual satisfaction. Conversely, demonstration of genuine interest in and knowledge about CF by the internist or pulmonologist will help the pediatrician to "give up" his patients.

Some patients will have medical or psychosocial problems to the extent that clinic attendance and compliance might be lost by forcing the transition on them. They will need to be handled gently and over a period of time. Nevertheless, a new "adult" medical problem, such as diabetes or even pregnancy, eventually will convince both patient and pediatrician that it is time, provided a suitable adult program exists. It also should be remembered that, inevitably, some patients will move to adult care quite willingly but will remain quite immature in their behavior. This behavior will not be unfamiliar to the adult care team, and they should take over where the pediatric team left off.

Referrals to Adult Cystic Fibrosis Centers

Although most of the CF patients acquired by adult programs will come from the transition process, some patients will be referred from outside clinics. Patients 18 years of age or older should be directed to the adult program when they move to an area with an available CF center. Younger adolescents may be welcomed best to the pediatric section and then transitioned, a judgment usually left up to the CF center director, who will receive the referral. Occasionally, adult cases will be suspected or diagnosed with CF and be referred. When this happens, confirmation of the diagnosis, education of patient and appropriate family, or friends, and initial treatment should be offered as it is for new pediatric patients. This may require hospitalization, where all members of the CF team will have access to the patient. Because most CF centers are located in teaching hospitals, this also will make new adult patients with CF available to medical students, residents, nurses, and other support personnel who need to learn to deal with them.

DATING

In the early days of organized CF care, the majority of patients died before reaching sexual maturity. With improved treatment and nutrition, life expectancy is extending into the third and fourth decade of life, and most adolescents develop at normal rates. Thus, adolescents and young adults with CF are physically capable of responding to the opposite sex, although they may be psychologically inhibited. Particularly, those whose self-image has been limited by their own and their parents' perceptions will be shy of seeking companionship or may try to hide their diagnosis for fear of rejection. This is a time when psychosocial counseling may help to resolve childhood problems and allow patients to interact appropriately with their peers. Because there also is a risk that teen-agers will seek sexual gratification for reassurance, peer acceptance, or much needed affection, counseling should include the usual advice about sexually transmitted diseases, contraception, and the risks of pregnancy.

As adolescent patients develop stable dating relationships, they will face difficult decisions depending on how they have handled their disease in the past. Those whose families have encouraged open acceptance of this genetic condition will enter dating with the same open attitude. Those who have been taught to hide their disease from others will face the threat of being found out or eventually having to tell the truth. Experience in counseling adolescents

and adults suggests that most patients find their fear of rejection is out of proportion to reality. They need much supportive counseling to overcome such attitudes, especially those that have persisted since childhood.

Although most adolescents finally make appropriate dating choices, those with low self-esteem seem to take the most risks and make the poorest choices in selecting friends and companions. Whether this behavior is different than that of other adolescents of similar family and socioeconomic background is unknown, but unlikely. Nevertheless, such behavior may result in a few years of social instability, an increased risk of acquiring sexually transmitted diseases, or, for females, pregnancy. Eventually, with support and nonjudgmental counseling, such patients will realize that they are responsible for their own health and begin to act appropriately.

MARRIAGE

As aforementioned, the number of adults with CF reaching marriageable age continues to increase. Although one might assume that few adults with CF would marry, both our own and other published data (1,2) indicate otherwise. Approximately 35% of adults with CF are married, compared with 64% of all adults. If divorced and separated couples are included, the CF marriage rate reaches nearly 45%.

Who do these patients marry? In our experience, they tend to find mates who are accepting of their condition, who are supportive, and who often have professional medical training. This suggests that most of these marriages are carefully worked out between patients and partners who have a mutual understanding of the complex challenges offered by CF.

Dating and marriage raise questions regarding genetic transmission of CF. Every patient needs a careful review of these difficult concepts and any other questions that may be raised. One should be particularly alert for erroneous concepts, ideas, or advice that patients may have received, often from well-meaning but ill-informed "experts." This also is a good time to offer assessment of sperm count to males with CF and to discuss the decreased but still functional fertility in females. If patients are to be referred to urologists or gynecologists for evaluation, one should make sure that these specialists know about CF and how it affects reproductive physiology (see Chapter 21).

Unfortunately, decisions regarding child-bearing by females with CF and their partners often are based on incomplete or misunderstood information. Although clinic personnel should not tell patients what to do, they certainly should provide them with all the basic facts and answer all their questions. If pregnancy occurs, the CF team must work closely with the patient's obstetrician and try to maintain the best possible nutrition and pulmonary status (see Chapter 21). The social worker will be in demand to guide the mother in rearranging her lifestyle, work (or lack of it), finances, insurance, and child care.

EMPLOYMENT

The pursuit of a career is a major component of one's adult life, and the range of possibilities for adults with CF is broad. Of 5,750 adults seen in CF centers in 1995, 58.4% were employed full time or part time and 23.8% were students (2). An individual's aptitude and interests should be considered in selecting the types and level of education and career opportunities. The effects of CF on education and job performance may become considerable. For example, physically strenuous jobs can be productive, enjoyable, and help preserve lung function by encouraging aerobic exercise and airway clearance. However, exposure to occupational hazards, such as inhaled dust or toxins, should be avoided meticulously. In addition, progressive respiratory limitations and the need for treatment of pulmonary exacerbations may significantly limit the ability to perform jobs that require severe physical activity. Consequently, adolescents with CF and young adults should be advised to select educational and training opportunities in occupations that provide the opportunity to continue work performance despite progressive limitations in exercise capability (13). The selection of careers

that provide part-time work and occasional work from home, for example, using computer and Internet technology, may be advisable.

Help with career planning is available from the Division of Vocational Rehabilitation (VR), which has offices in every state. VR offers many services, including modification of existing jobs and vocational testing, that are geared toward developing or maintaining employment. It is useful to consider career planning at high school ages, and referrals at such early ages often are useful. The agency also can assist those who need to change careers or those who need additional education or training to continue working. VR can help frame an educational plan and may provide financial assistance to attend 2- or 4-year college programs, for those who qualify. The CF center can educate the local VR agencies about the current life expectancy and work potential of individuals with CF, and the CF social worker or a high school guidance counselor can assist with referrals.

MEDICAL INSURANCE

Medical insurance is an important issue for all individuals, particularly those with chronic diseases. A recent study of 189 patients with CF seen at one center demonstrated a median survival of 6.1 years for those lacking medical insurance, compared with 20.5 years for those with private insurance or Medicaid (14). Adolescents and young adults may be covered by their parents' medical insurance policy, but these typically exclude children after the age of 19 years unless they retain student status. Some policies provide unlimited coverage, although at an additional expense, to 26 years of age. Medical insurance also can be provided through one's employer, through CHAMPUS, and, for those who qualify, through Children's Special Health Services (formerly, "Crippled Children's" benefits) or Medicaid.

Private employers' health insurance plans often have "preexisting condition" exclusion policies. These typically deny medical expenses associated with preexisting medical conditions for the first 12 months of employment. When taking a new job, one's preexisting medical insurance (whether parental or other) should be continued to cover this exclusionary period. The Federal Comprehensive Omnibus Budget Reconciliation Act (COBRA) requires that employees be offered the opportunity to keep their medical insurance for 18 months after terminating employment (unless fired for gross misconduct). This act provides the opportunity for coverage at the previous level, but the insurance premiums usually are very expensive and must be paid by the individual. In July 1997, the Health Insurance Portability and Accountability Act (HIPAA, also known as the Kassebaum–Kennedy bill) became effective and provides a number of important insurance protections. For example, an employer who provides group health insurance to its employees cannot exclude an individual on the basis of preexisting medical conditions. Insurance coverage based on preexisting medical conditions is limited to a total of 12 months. Insurance portability is required for individuals who change jobs to another employer that provides group health insurance. Other provisions provide for the availability of private insurance for individuals who met previous employment and medical insurance specifications and establish some tax deduction and payment advantages. CF center social workers and insurance experts can provide information and expert advice on these matters.

DISABILITY

Employers may hesitate to hire an individual with CF because of the concern that the disease may limit one's ability to perform adequately. In the United States, capability to meet the job requirements, and not the presence of underlying diseases, is the criterion for determining work disability. The Americans with Disabilities Act (ADA) of 1990 specifically provides legal protection. Per this law, a person with a disability is defined as someone who (a) "has an impairment that substantially limits one or more major life activities"; (b) has a record of such impairment; or (c) is regarded as having such an impairment. Thus, adults with CF may

qualify for protection under this law. Importantly, the disability determination must be made without considering the beneficial effects of treatments. Thus, adults with CF with no significant functional limitations that would affect their work may be protected. The ADA requires that "reasonable accommodation" be made to permit working. Such accommodations may include modifying work hours or providing additional paid or unpaid sick leave.

On applying for a job, honesty about one's physical capabilities and potential limitations is the best policy. Although it is illegal to disqualify an applicant because of an underlying lung disease such as CF, which may not limit one's job performance, it is not mandatory to volunteer this diagnosis during an interview or on a job application. Frankness about the need for intermittent medical leaves to treat obstructive lung disease, however, may be appropriate. Honesty and frankness certainly are the best policies.

Private disability insurance may be hard to procure because of an underlying genetic condition. Some employers, particularly large companies or federal, state, and local governments, offer disability insurance as part of their standard fringe benefits. Disability benefits usually make up a fraction of the prior salary and usually are provided to employees who have worked a specified number of years (often 5 or more).

All individuals employed in the United States contribute to the federal Social Security fund. Individuals who become unable to work because of medical disability may become eligible to receive Social Security disability income (SSDI) (15). Qualification for SSDI is dependent on a favorable determination of disability by the Social Security Administrator, based on specific guidelines. Applications are processed on a state level and typically require 3 to 6 months for approval. Denials are common, and individuals should request reconsideration and may request a hearing before an administrative law judge. Applications that require a hearing may require 12 to 18 months to reach resolution. The benefits of SSDI depend on an individual's duration of work and amount of contributions. Detailed information and assistance is available from the local Social Security Administration.

SSDI does not provide any health insurance coverage for the first 2 years. After 2 continuous years on SSDI, medical insurance through Medicare may become available. Medicare Part A, Hospital Insurance, covers hospital costs and care in skilled nursing facilities. Medicare Part B, Medical Insurance, covers physician costs, diagnostic tests, emergency room visits, outpatient services, durable medical equipment, and some other costs (16). Medicare Part A currently does not require individual payments for most people, but Part B costs approximately $43 per month (deducted from the SSDI payments) for those who choose this benefit. Part B coverage is recommended strongly because much CF care currently is provided in outpatient settings. There may be significant penalties (including delayed eligibility and higher premiums) for not enrolling in Part B when it is offered initially.

Supplemental Security Income (SSI) benefits are paid to individuals with disabilities who have limited financial resources (17). In many states, individuals who receive SSI benefits also qualify for Medicaid. Adult CF center social workers are well versed in the availability of such public and private resources. They can provide valuable guidance in how to select, apply for, and document qualifications for the various programs.

COPING WITH CYSTIC FIBROSIS

Psychological Stresses and Adaptation

Acute and chronic illnesses impose significant emotional stresses on an individual, and CF is no exception. The physical effects of the disease, the time demands of a complicated medical regimen, and uncertainty about the future must be dealt with. These stresses can produce anxiety, depression, interpersonal conflicts, and/or psychosomatic complaints. Fear of death may exacerbate these feelings. There are many different ways to cope with such psychological stresses, including denial, regres-

sion, repression, and confrontation (9,18–20). The benefits of individual coping mechanisms depend on the individual and his or her support systems. In general, better knowledge of the effects of the future and psychological counseling with one's family, friends, or trained professionals often are beneficial in coping with the stress of living with CF (21). Recognizing an individual's coping strategies, his or her limitations, the effects on compliance, healthcare system interactions, and the ability to function can provide important insight into the needs of the individual adult with CF. Psychological counseling by individuals familiar with the stresses of CF in adults can be helpful by providing support, teaching more adaptive coping skills, addressing fears, and teaching anxiety management techniques. Such benefits have been documented for individuals with other diseases and for adults with CF.

Terminal Illness

Progressive respiratory failure ultimately is responsible for death in more than 90% of patients with CF. Early indicators of incipient death from respiratory failure include forced expiratory volume in 1 second (FEV_1) of less than 30% predicted, need for supplemental oxygen, and hypercarbia (see Chapter 8). Late indicators of incipient death include acute exacerbations that do not respond to intensive care, worsening hypercarbia, and refractory hypoxemia (summarized in Chapter 8). A strong relationship between adults with CF and their healthcare providers facilitates adequate education about and planning for medical care during the last stages of life. If lung transplantation is an option, early referral is mandatory (see Chapter 9). The use of supplemental oxygen to treat respiratory failure due to hypoxemia generally is encouraged because it can improve the quality of life and may improve the duration of useful life (see Chapter 8). The use of mechanical ventilation, particularly by nasal or face mask, has been advocated to sustain life while the patient is awaiting lung transplantation. Assisted ventilation also may improve quality of life when nocturnal use improves daytime symptoms. Terminal CF lung disease typically is manifested by progressive obstructive airways disease that becomes refractory to treatment with intensive chest physiotherapy, antibiotics, and bronchodilatory or antiinflammatory drugs. Mechanical ventilation through cuffed endotracheal tubes severely limits mobility, communication, and clearance of secretions. Its use is discouraged by most experienced CF clinicians when no reversible disease or lung transplant option is available.

Most cases of progressive respiratory failure are subacute, developing over several days to weeks. The patient's wishes for intensity and location of care should be determined in advance of irreversible deterioration and should be respected. Hospital, hospice, or home locations may be desirable. Planning for farewells with family members and close friends are delicate issues but are best handled before the severity of respiratory failure severely compromises the patient's ability to communicate. It is appropriate to use anxiety-relieving drugs and narcotics, despite their effects on respiratory drive, to relieve dyspnea and suffering when the chances of recovery are negligible.

SUMMARY

CF presents the adult patient with a large array of challenges in dealing with the normal activities of adulthood. The number of well-trained and experienced adult pulmonologists and subspecialists is increasing steadily. Several healthcare options have been developed in major medical centers and distant locations to meet individual needs. Specialized healthcare teams based in hospitals and clinics include nurses, social workers, occupational and physical therapists, and vocational counselors. They provide the expertise and support necessary to deal with most activities of normal adulthood. Advanced education and employment is possible for most individuals with CF. The medical insurance and disability insurance policies in the United States are in a period of reevaluation and change. Effective lobbying by individuals and representatives of

the CFF should help ensure equitable coverage for individuals with CF. Continuing improvements in clinical care, CF center resources, employee rights, and health and disability insurance are providing opportunities for adults with CF to pursue and enjoy productive and rewarding lives.

REFERENCES

1. Walters S, Britton J, Hodson ME. Demographic and social characteristics of adults with cystic fibrosis in the United Kingdom. *BMJ* 1993;306:549–552.
2. Cystic Fibrosis Foundation. *Patient registry 1995 annual data report.* Bethesda, MD: Cystic Fibrosis Foundation, 1996.
3. Orenstein DM. Cystic fibrosis—a guide for patient and family. 2nd ed. Philadelphia: Lippincott-Raven Publishers, 1997.
4. Fitzsimmons FC. The changing epidemiology of cystic fibrosis. *J Pediatr* 1993;122:1–9.
5. McCollum AT, Gibson LE. Family adaptation to the child with cystic fibrosis. *J Pediatr* 1970;77:571–578.
6. Lloyd-Still DM, Lloyd-Still JD. The patient, the family, and the community. In: Lloyd-Still JD, ed. *The textbook of cystic fibrosis.* Boston: John Wright, PSG Inc, 1983:433–445.
7. Johnson MR, Gershowitz M, Stabler B. Maternal compliance and children's self-concept in cystic fibrosis. *J Dev Behav Pediatr* 1981;2:5–8.
8. DeWet B, Cywes S. The psychosocial impact of cystic fibrosis: a review of research literature. *S Afr Med J* 1984;65:526–530.
9. Cappelli M, McGrath PJ, Heick CE, MacDonald NE, Feldman W, Rowe P. Chronic disease and its impact: the adolescent's perspective. *J Adolesc Health Care* 1989;10:283–288.
10. Mador JA, Smith DH. The psychosocial adaptation of adolescents with cystic fibrosis: a review of the literature. *J Adolesc Health Care* 1988;10:136–142.
11. Schidlow DV, Fiel SB. Life beyond pediatrics: transition of chronically ill adolescents from pediatric to adult health care systems. *Adolesc Med* 1990;74:1113–1120.
12. Landau LI. Cystic fibrosis: transition from paediatric to adult physician's care. *Thorax* 1995;50:1031–1032.
13. Gillen M, Lallas D, Brown C, Yelin E, Blanc P. Work disability in adults with cystic fibrosis. *Am J Respir Crit Care Med* 1995;152:153–156.
14. JR Curtis, Burke W, Kassner AW, Aitken ML. Absence of health insurance is associated with decreased life expectancy in patients with cystic fibrosis. *Am J Respir Crit Care Med* 1997;155:1921–1924.
15. U.S. Department of Health and Human Services. *Disability evaluation under Social Security.* U.S. Department of Health and Human Services, 1995:Social Security Administration Publication No. 64–039, ICN No. 468600 Washington, DC: US Government Printing Office, 1995.
16. U.S. Dept of Health and Human Services. *Your Medicare handbook 1995.* Baltimore, MD: U.S. Depart-

ment of Health and Human Services. Health Care Financing Administration Publication No. HCFA 10050, 21207–5187 Washington, DC: US Government Printing Office, 1995.

17. Social Security Administration. *Social Security: understanding the benefits.* Social Security Administration Publication No. 05–10024, ICN No. 454930. Washington, DC: US Government Printing Office, January 1996.

18. Pinkerton P, Trauer T, Duncan F, Hodson ME, Batten JC. Cystic fibrosis in adult life: a study of coping patterns. *Lancet* 1985;ii:761–763.

19. Moise JR, Drotar D, Doershuk CF, Stern RC. Correlates of psychosocial adjustment among young adults with cystic fibrosis. *J Dev Behav Pediatr* 1987;8: 141–148.

20. Blair C, Cull A, Freeman CP. Psychosocial functioning of young adults with cystic fibrosis and their families. *Thorax* 1994;49:798–802.

21. Hamlett KW, Murphy M, Hayes R, Doershuk CF. Health independence and developmental tasks of adulthood in cystic fibrosis. *Rehabil Psychol* 1996;41: 149–160.

Cystic Fibrosis in Adults,
edited by J. R. Yankaskas and M. R. Knowles,
Lippincott–Raven Publishers, Philadelphia, 1999.

23

The Cystic Fibrosis Foundation

Robert J. Beall

Cystic Fibrosis Foundation, Bethesda, Maryland

In 1955, the Cystic Fibrosis Foundation (CFF) was created by a committed group of parents whose children were threatened by the pathology associated with this disease. These dedicated individuals founded an aggressive organization, targeted to provide unparalleled specialized medical care, to develop breakthrough new treatments, and ultimately, to uncover a cure for cystic fibrosis (CF).

The median life expectancy for individuals with CF reached 31.3 years of age for the first time in 1997. With at least 7,000 patients 18 years of age and older, this improved life expectancy and improved quality of life can be attributed to a number of factors. The CFF and thousands of scientists, medical professionals, and volunteers have played a pivotal role in making these medical achievements possible. This chapter summarizes some of the developments that have led to the improved life expectancy and describes how this unusual organization has helped make these achievements happen.

CYSTIC FIBROSIS FOUNDATION STRUCTURE: FOUNDATION MISSION

The mission of the CFF is to develop treatments and a cure for CF while always working to improve the quality of life for all patients affected by the disease. To meet its goal, the CFF operates as a nonprofit, voluntary health organization to fund CF research, support specialized medical care centers for patients, provide training for medical professionals, and foster public education about the disease. These components substantiate a creative mix of specialized, team-oriented care, applied clinical research, and basic science. The foundation has positioned itself at the forefront of modern medical research by using a business formula that continues to turn financial resources into scientific breakthroughs.

To get the word out about the exciting research, the foundation offers several publication, including *Commitment,* its national newsletter, and a series of CFF fact sheets. The fact sheets also address consumer issues such as financial assistance, treatments, and clinical care. The foundation Web site features CF news and hightlights foundation activities at http://www.cff.org.

A network of 56 chapters across the United States raises dollars to support the programs of the foundation. Hundreds of thousands of volunteers contribute their time, talent, and money at a variety of fundraising events.

FACTORS THAT HAVE CONTRIBUTED TO IMPROVEMENT IN LIFE EXPECTANCY FOR PATIENTS WITH CYSTIC FIBROSIS

There are many medical advances that have contributed to the increasing numbers of individuals surviving into adulthood who are making vital contributions to our society. The CFF activities that have played a central part in these success stories are highlighted in the following sections.

Clinical Research

The foundation has played a pivotal role in the development of new therapies for CF. The fact that Pulmozyme (Genentech Corp., San Francisco), a mucus-thinning drug, went from test tube to U.S. Food and Drug Administration (FDA) approval in less than 5 years demonstrates how CFF programs and resources can push drug development ahead.

This achievement stands out because the average drug development process takes between 12 and 14 years. The foundation decided to mimic the success of Pulmozyme by launching the Therapeutics Development Center (TDC) Program in 1997, the most ambitious program in its history. A special network of CF care centers were selected and trained to form the TDC network, which expedites the early phases of CF clinical trials. At the same time, the foundation offers matching grants to biotechnology and pharmaceutical companies to encourage them to invest in taking an idea for a CF drug through laboratory and preclinical research and into clinical trials.

The CFF's Clinical Research Committee provides guidance both to the foundation and to industry on how to appropriately design clinical studies to maximize patient participation and other resources. The foundation reviews potential trials and sanctions appropriate trials if certain criteria are satisfied, encouraging our centers to participate. Aerosolized tobramycin, which was FDA-approved in 1997, exemplifies a drug development success story "written by" the foundation, industry, CF care centers, and the FDA. Other ongoing CFF-sponsored trials are evaluating CF gene therapy, protein repair therapy, and several mucus-thinning and antibiotic drugs.

Cystic Fibrosis Foundation Care Center Network

The development of the care center network by the CFF occurred in the early 1960s. These centers were established to ensure the rapid translation of new CF therapies and developments directly to the patients. Currently, a network of 114 care centers is recognized as the model program for delivering care to more than 20,000 individuals with this chronic, fatal disease.

In addition to providing care, these centers serve as a focus for CF clinical trials. Using Pulmozyme as an example, more than 900 patients were enrolled in the phase III trial in less than 6 months. Eager patients, coupled with teams of highly qualified researchers and clinicians, worked day and night to test this potential new therapy. The existence of the organized network is a major inducement for drug companies to examine new CF products. Without this comprehensive program, it virtually would be impossible to identify the patients for these trials.

Because of the complexity of CF, researchers must tackle several different clinical challenges at once. They are, therefore, in constant pursuit of new therapies. The foundation's network of care centers has become a growing resource in this type of CF research. Centers collaborate with biotechnology and pharmaceutical companies to perform extensive clinical trials to evaluate new drugs. The TDC network will accelerate the completion of early phases (I and II) of drug development. All accredited centers may be involved in Phase III clinical research.

The care center network initially was started in pediatric pulmonary and gastrointestinal programs. The major challenge in the past decade has been to interest internists to take care of the increasing number of adults with CF. The foundation has initiated unique programs recruiting adult care providers to CF. The CFF currently supports more than 40 adult care satellites in our existing center network. Each of these adult care centers must have an internist as its center director and must follow a minimum of 50 patients. Each of these centers is a part of the existing network to ensure the logical transition of patients from the pediatric setting to the adult care program within the same institution.

Each center is staffed by a team of medical specialists who give state-of-the-art care to patients with CF. Included are pulmonologists, gastroenterologists, nutritionists, pediatricians, physical therapists, nurses, and others.

Manpower Training

The foundation has developed a number of programs to recruit adult care providers into the field of CF. For many years, the foundation supported the subspecialty training of pediatricians to interest them in a career of CF research. More recently, this fellowship training program of the foundation has been extended to internists interested in the field of pulmonology or gastroenterology who are committed to CF care and research. Many of the individuals trained by these mechanisms are assuming leadership roles in the foundation adult care satellites.

National Patient Registry

In addition to providing specialized care, CFF care centers collect medical information on more than 20,000 patients with CF and submit this annually to the CFF's National Patient Registry. From its inception 30 years ago, this centralized data source has become an ideal resource for extensive clinical research on new innovative CF drugs.

Currently, the registry collects data describing demographics, clinical data, and healthcare utilization on all patients cared for in our centers. Information such as pulmonary function, drug usage, and disease complications are a few examples of parameters described.

MECHANISMS TO SUPPORT CYSTIC FIBROSIS RESEARCH

The cornerstone of the progress seen in the improved life expectancy of patients with CF has been the progress in CF research. The foundation has instituted a number of innovative programs directed toward facilitating and pushing CF research ahead. These programs are wide reaching and produce one breakthrough after another.

Cystic Fibrosis Foundation Research Grants

Outstanding researchers are recruited by the foundation and then backed with the resources needed to move the science forward. The foundation strives to keep the momentum in CF research strong by continually building its funding program, always with the idea to develop new ways to manage and control this disease.

Researchers receive support through a variety of funding mechanisms, such as grants to individual investigators and grants to academic institutions. The new investigator and research grants form the backbone of growth in CF science. These grants support both the initial testing of new hypotheses and methods and the application of these methods for the first time to CF. The range of disciplines varies from immunologic studies on *Pseudomonas* infections to molecular investigations of the cystic fibrosis transmembrane conductance regulator (CFTR) protein product of the gene.

Clinical research grants are awarded to support projects directly related to CF treatment and care. Researchers develop diagnostic or therapeutic methods or contribute to understanding the pathophysiology of the disease. Such research must be collaborative between a CFF care center and an academic institution.

The Foundation's Research and Development Program Center Network

The foundation's research grants are centralized through its national office. The CFF brings scientists from different disciplines together to apply their expertise in the fight against CF. By creating a privately funded network of research centers specializing in one disease, the foundation gave birth in the early 1980s to the CFF Research and Development Program (RDP) Center network.

Over the years, these ten foundation-supported centers have turned out one major CF discovery after another. The RDP centers accomplish this by fostering both communication and collaboration, two key ingredients in fast-paced science. Communication is critical because scientific research can become so specialized that even researchers within the same institution become isolated from one another. Ideas that spring from discoveries in CF laboratories are quickly translated into exciting new drug therapies. Increased understanding of the disease at the molecular and cellular levels generates an ever expanding wealth of opportunities to intervene in the disease process.

Request for Applications

Another mechanism that the foundation uses to stimulate innovative research is the request for applications (RFA). Advertisements in scientific journals announce that the foundation has new funding available for various topics in CF. By spreading this wide net, the foundation creates targets of opportunity for enterprising scientists to pursue their research.

These announcements have been particularly successful because the foundation anticipates where the research will be headed and helps steer the advances along. For example, the CFF offered grant money for scientists to develop strategies to deliver CF gene therapy in 1989, before the gene even was identified. Since that time, the foundation has fortified and expanded its gene therapy research support at many top medical institutions.

Over the past few years, RFAs have been issued to foster CF research focusing on topics as diverse as identifying the basic cellular defect, understanding the regulation of ion transport in CF cells, and learning about infection immunity, inflammation, and the role of "antimicrobial peptides" natural antibiotics found on cell surfaces.

Cystic Fibrosis Foundation Support of Unfunded National Institutes of Health Grants

The foundation continues to serve as a launching pad for many outstanding scientists' careers. One way it achieves this is through an innovative program involving CF projects submitted to the National Institutes of Health (NIH) that were rated as excellent but could not be supported. The CFF offers these researchers the opportunity to pursue their research while they prepare to reapply to the NIH at a later date. In this way, the foundation acts as a venture capitalist, investing in the most

novel ideas that often turn into new CF advances.

Cystic Fibrosis-Specific Training and Development Programs

Every year, the foundation hosts the North American Cystic Fibrosis Conference, which brings together more than 2,500 scientists, clinicians, and other care givers with a special interest in CF to exchange information. The conference offers a unique opportunity for participants to stay on top of their fields and to learn about many other diverse aspects of this complex disease. They move the science forward through collaboration, discussing topics ranging from the latest developments in basic science to the clinical "front line" of treating patients. Together, they forge a strong link between state-of-the-art science and specialized patient care. "Adult issues" sessions offer overviews on the special needs of adults with CF. The conference also offers the opportunity for adult clinicians to be exposed to a range of symposia topics and to interact with other CF care givers.

The CFF also hosts consensus conferences in which CF experts in a given area gather to establish guidelines and set standards for patient services. These conferences are held throughout the year and feature topics such as gastrointestinal problems, home therapies, acute pulmonary complications of CF, and lung transplants.

Creative Approach to Cystic Fibrosis Research Process

Peer review committees are in place to ensure that the foundation selects the highest-quality grant proposals to fund. These committees include one for CF research, one for clinical studies, and another for research development and professional training. Similarly, the CFF Center Committee sets standards that must be met by CFF care centers. Members routinely perform site visits to evaluate the centers and review renewal applications for foundation support.

The CFF's Medical Advisory Council (MAC) provides advice and guidance for the entire medical/scientific staff funded by the foundation. Composed of distinguished clinicians and scientists, the MAC develops policies for all CFF medical programs.

VITAL PARTNERSHIPS WITH THE CYSTIC FIBROSIS FOUNDATION

The NIH, the world's leading biomedical research organization, represents a vital force in the effort to advance CF science. By designing specific programs to complement those at the NIH, the foundation often provides initial support that allows researchers to develop and test hypotheses about CF, with the NIH stepping in to provide the long-term support to carry out the ideas.

The foundation has fostered a dynamic relationship with the FDA to facilitate the drug development process. Representatives from the FDA are invited to scientific conferences to offer their input, looking ahead to the drug approval process and what they have learned from experience with other diseases. The foundation and FDA also hold joint meetings such as the landmark forum, to identify ways to better evaluate whether "drugs" such as gene therapy are working.

Another partnership formed by the foundation is with private industry, both biotechnology companies and pharmaceutical companies. These companies take ideas from the laboratory and develop the concepts into new therapies.

The foundation also takes on the role of informing the lay public about CF advances. These advances, seen in turn as visible products, serve to reinforce the commitment of staff and volunteers to achieve even more.

EVOLUTION OF GENE THERAPY FOR CYSTIC FIBROSIS

The foundation has played a critical role in bringing together the investigators, resources, and important scientific information critically essential to developing new technologies and approaches to treatment. The best example has been in the area of gene therapy. In 1988, 1 year before the discovery of the gene, the foundation brought together scientists at the Stone

House Conference on the NIH campus to examine the challenges and opportunities that lie ahead in delivering gene therapy to the airways of patients with CF. It was during this meeting that some of the current leaders in the field first were introduced to CF and to the foundation. The CFF quickly announced an RFA in early 1989 to further stimulate interest in the field. Among the projects supported by this funding mechanism were the first awards in adenovirus and adeno-associated virus gene delivery systems. These first recipients corrected CF cells in the test tube by adding healthy genes just 1 year after the CF gene was discovered. In addition, recipients of these first awards were successful in demonstrating that adenovirus delivery of genes into the airways of animals also was possible.

Based on the success of this RFA, the foundation went to the U.S. Congress in 1992 and presented a unique partnership proposal to key legislators. This resulted in Congress mandating that the NIH establish Gene Therapy Centers for Cystic Fibrosis, to be jointly funded by the NIH and the CFF. Nine Gene Therapy Programs were established, with the NIH supporting the "cores" and shared resources, and the CFF supporting the pilot and feasibility studies. The net effect was an infusion of more than $50 million dollars into this new field of medical pursuit.

In addition to the partnership with the NIH, the CFF has worked closely with the biotechnology industry. In many cases, the CFF has provided the seed money to explore an idea and develop it to the point that industry is ready to take over the next steps. An example of this is the adeno-associated virus research. The CFF initially provided support to investigators at the NIH and a clinical fellow at the Johns Hopkins University to examine the feasibility of using this vector system. Early work led to a partnership with a major biotechnology company and subsequent clinical trials using this gene therapy vector.

The foundation works closely with the FDA to ensure timely review of promising new medications for CF. In 1994, they cosponsored a landmark scientific meeting that brought together the premier researchers in CF gene therapy. Because gene therapy technically is a drug, the FDA has final oversight on studies involving patients who receive this experimental treatment. By sharing information, FDA scientists and CF researchers will be equipped further to move the field forward efficiently and quickly. The efforts by the foundation to collaborate with the FDA have been heralded as highly innovative by the scientific community at large.

PUBLIC POLICY INITIATIVES

The CFF is active on several fronts to secure the highest quality of life for individuals with CF. One way of accomplishing this is to advocate for increased federal investment in biomedical research. Activities include testifying on Capitol Hill for bolstering the NIH budget and orchestrating national letter-writing campaigns to Congress. In turn, the NIH is able to support CF research. Scientists will generate more effective CF treatments that improve the lives of patients, eventually reducing spiraling healthcare costs.

The foundation is concerned equally with the effect of managed care on the way that patients with CF receive medical care. With the tide in healthcare coverage turning away from traditional indemnity insurance plans to health maintenance organizations, the foundation strongly advocates for assured access to specialty care via CF Centers of Excellence for patients with CF. In a managed-care situation, the risk of losing unlimited access to a CF specialty physician is greater because the need to contain costs is paramount. This inability to access the specialty care team within a CF care center can have grievous results in the overall health and well-being of the patient. For this reason, the foundation works hard to ensure the rights of individuals with CF to access specialty care.

On another public policy front, the foundation monitors any new legislation that might stifle the development of new life-saving drugs for CF. Whether under the umbrella of national healthcare reform or other pieces of legislation, special incentives for drug companies to invest in CF drugs always are under fire. As an or-

phan disease affecting less than 200,000 individuals, CF has been a hard disease "to sell." Patients with CF often have had to wait for spillover drugs created for other diseases. The foundation has worked closely with leading biotechnology and pharmaceutical companies to change this. Any added bureaucratic "red tape" in the drug development process could mean a decline in the pipeline of breakthrough drugs for CF.

CYSTIC FIBROSIS
FOUNDATION PHARMACY

With CF research heading in the right direction and fundraising efficiently providing the fuel for that research, the foundation decided in 1988 that it must reduce the burden of rising healthcare costs on people with CF. To accomplish this, the CFF Pharmacy was established to provide prescription drugs at the lowest possible cost to the CF population.

The CFF Pharmacy, a national mail-order pharmacy, helps people with CF afford the medications vital to maintaining their best health. This nonprofit service offers low prices for CF prescriptions, with specially trained pharmacists available to answer patient questions and alleviate concerns. Because of the large volume of medications that are purchased, the CFF Pharmacy saves individuals as much as 50% of the standard drug cost.

Further, customer representatives specially trained in the reimbursement process are available to serve as patient advocates with the insurance companies. Their broad range of experience has enabled them to acquire coverage even when challenged by today's managed care climate.

SUMMARY: WHAT'S AHEAD?

There is no secret to the formula responsible for success in CF research. Outstanding researchers are recruited by the CFF and then supported with the resources needed to push the science forward. The foundation continues to attract the "best in the business." Financial support comes in the form of grants, some to train young clinical and scientific investigators, others to offer research opportunities to veteran scientists at prestigious medical institutions.

The 1990s clearly have become the "Golden Age" of CF science. When researchers discovered the gene in 1989, they had found the blueprint for building a cure. Since then, their Herculean efforts—based on this new tool—have made medical history against the leading fatal, genetic disease in our country. Not only will they cure CF some day, but they will create the stepping stones to cure many other diseases as well. In many ways, the CFF functions as a bridge between the academic research community, industry, care givers, patients, and federal agencies; the more collaboration, the more progress in the laboratory and beyond.

Subject Index

Subject Index

Page numbers followed by t indicate tables; page numbers followed by f indicate figures.